Korean Functional Foods
Composition, Processing and Health Benefits

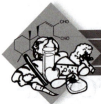

FUNCTIONAL FOODS AND NUTRACEUTICALS SERIES

Series Editor
John Shi, Ph.D.
Guelph Food Research Center, Canada

Korean Functional Foods: Composition, Processing and Health Benefits (2018)
Edited by Kun-Young Park, Dae Young Kwon, Ki Won Lee, and Sunmin Park

Phytochemicals in Citrus: Applications in Functional Foods (2017)
Xingqian Ye

Food as Medicine: Functional Food Plants of Africa (2016)
Maurice M. Iwu

Chinese Dates: A Traditional Functional Food (2016)
Edited by Dongheng Liu, Ph.D., Xingqian Ye, Ph.D., and Yueming Jiang, Ph.D.

Functional Food Ingredients and Nutraceuticals: Processing Technologies, Second Edition (2015)
Edited by John Shi, Ph.D.

Marine Products for Healthcare: Functional and Bioactive Nutraceutical Compounds from the Ocean (2009)
Vazhiyil Venugopal, Ph.D.

Methods of Analysis for Functional Foods and Nutraceuticals, Second Edition (2008)
Edited by W. Jeffrey Hurst, Ph.D.

Handbook of Fermented Functional Foods, Second Edition (2008)
Edited by Edward R. Farnworth, Ph.D.

Functional Food Carbohydrates (2007)
Costas G. Biliaderis, Ph.D. and Marta S. Izydorczyk, Ph.D.

Dictionary of Nutraceuticals and Functional Foods (2006)
N. A. Michael Eskin, Ph.D. and Snait Tamir, Ph.D.

Handbook of Functional Lipids (2006)
Edited by Casimir C. Akoh, Ph.D.

Korean Functional Foods
Composition, Processing and Health Benefits

Edited by
Kun-Young Park
Dae Young Kwon
Ki Won Lee
Sunmin Park

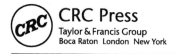

CRC Press
Taylor & Francis Group
Boca Raton London New York

CRC Press is an imprint of the
Taylor & Francis Group, an **informa** business

CRC Press
Taylor & Francis Group
6000 Broken Sound Parkway NW, Suite 300
Boca Raton, FL 33487-2742

© 2018 by Taylor & Francis Group, LLC
CRC Press is an imprint of Taylor & Francis Group, an Informa business

No claim to original U.S. Government works

Printed on acid-free paper

International Standard Book Number-13: 978-1-4987-9965-2 (Hardback)

This book contains information obtained from authentic and highly regarded sources. Reasonable efforts have been made to publish reliable data and information, but the author and publisher cannot assume responsibility for the validity of all materials or the consequences of their use. The authors and publishers have attempted to trace the copyright holders of all material reproduced in this publication and apologize to copyright holders if permission to publish in this form has not been obtained. If any copyright material has not been acknowledged please write and let us know so we may rectify in any future reprint.

Except as permitted under U.S. Copyright Law, no part of this book may be reprinted, reproduced, transmitted, or utilized in any form by any electronic, mechanical, or other means, now known or hereafter invented, including photocopying, microfilming, and recording, or in any information storage or retrieval system, without written permission from the publishers.

For permission to photocopy or use material electronically from this work, please access www.copyright .com (http://www.copyright.com/) or contact the Copyright Clearance Center, Inc. (CCC), 222 Rosewood Drive, Danvers, MA 01923, 978-750-8400. CCC is a not-for-profit organization that provides licenses and registration for a variety of users. For organizations that have been granted a photocopy license by the CCC, a separate system of payment has been arranged.

Trademark Notice: Product or corporate names may be trademarks or registered trademarks, and are used only for identification and explanation without intent to infringe.

Library of Congress Cataloging-in-Publication Data

Names: Pak, Kæon-yæong (Professor of food and nutrition), editor.
Title: Korean functional foods : composition, processing, and health benefits / edited by Kun-Young Park [and three others].
Description: Boca Raton, Florida : CRC Press, 2018. | Includes bibliographical references and index.
Identifiers: LCCN 2017045664| ISBN 9781498799652 (hardback) | ISBN 9781498799669 (e-book)
Subjects: LCSH: Functional foods. | Cooking, Korean. | Diet therapy.
Classification: LCC QP144.F85 K6745 2018 | DDC 613.2--dc23
LC record available at https://lccn.loc.gov/2017045664

Visit the Taylor & Francis Web site at
http://www.taylorandfrancis.com

and the CRC Press Web site at
http://www.crcpress.com

Contents

Series Preface vii

Preface ix

Acknowledgments xi

Editors xiii

Contributors xvii

1. **Korean Foods—History, Culture, and Characteristics** 1
   Cherl-Ho Lee

2. **Korean Diets and Their Tastes** 23
   Dae Young Kwon and Kyung Rhan Chung

3. **Kimchi and Its Health Benefits** 43
   Kun-Young Park and Jaehyun Ju

4. **Lactic Acid Bacteria in Kimchi** 79
   Hak-Jong Choi, Jieun Lee, and Ja-Young Jang

5. **Health Benefits of Doenjang (Soybean Paste) and Kanjang
   (Soybean Sauce)** 101
   Kun-Young Park and Eui-Seong Park

6. **Cheongkukjang** 145
   Sunmin Park and James W. Daily

7. **Biological Functions and Traditional Therapeutic Uses
   of *Kochujang* (Red Pepper Paste)** 165
   Dae Young Kwon and Soon-Hee Kim

8. **Jeotgal (Fermented Fish): Secret of Korean Seasonings** 183
   Ok Kyung Koo and Young Myoung Kim

9. **Sikcho (Korean Vinegar)** 217
   Kwang-Soon Shin and Hoon Kim

10. **Korean Ginseng: Composition, Processing, and Health Benefits** 233
    Boo-Yong Lee

11. **Yangnyeom (Spices) and Health Benefits** 257
    Hye-Kyung Na and Young-Joon Surh

v

12. Seed Oil (Sesame Seed, Perilla Seed) 291
JaeHwan Lee, Mi-Ja Kim, and Mun Yhung Jung

13. Health Benefit Effects of Jukyeom (Bamboo Salt) 319
Hyung-Min Kim, Jaehyun Ju, Phil-Dong Moon, Na-Ra Han, Hyun-Ja Jeong and Kun-Young Park

14. Beneficial Effects of Cheonilyeom (a Mineral-Rich Solar Sea Salt) on Health and Fermentation 341
Jeong-Yong Cho, Lily Jaiswal, and Kyung-Sik Ham

15. Edible Korean Seaweed: A Source of Functional Compounds 359
Sanjeewa K. K. Asanka, Hyun-Soo Kim, and You-Jin Jeon

16. Namul, the Korean Vegetable Dish 385
Young-Eun Lee

17. Bibimbap as a Balanced One-Dish Meal 421
Youn-Soo Cha

18. Korean Alcoholic Beverages: Makgeolli/Yakju 441
Seok-Tae Jeong, Han-Seok Choi, and Ji-Eun Kang

19. Clinical Trials of Some Korean Functional Foods 463
Soo-Wan Chae and Su-Jin Jung

20. Functional Food Industry: Processing and Sanitation 505
Jin-Hee Lee

21. Regulations of Korean Functional Foods 523
Ji Yeon Kim and Yeonkyung Lee

22. Future of Functional Foods in Korea 539
Ki Won Lee, Jong Hun Kim, Sanguine Byun, and Jong-Eun Kim

Index 553

Series Preface

The traditional Eastern terms of therapeutic foods or health foods have been commonly used in Korea for many years. Koreans believe the adage of "food as medicine." Herbs, fruit and vegetable ingredients such as ginger, cinnamon, adlay, mugwort, pomegranate, citron, mushroom, and ginseng, etc., are used in cooking and also used for their therapeutic effects in Korean diet. In the traditional Korean culture, foods are considered to be the fundamental source of life and health, and it is believed that all diseases could be cured by the control of special daily food diets. The Korean food industry has succeeded in producing many special foods of traditional Korean taste. The book *Korean Functional Foods: Composition, Processing and Health Benefits* can provide information related with Korean functional foods and history and culture of Korean foods as well as the comparison of Korean diet tables. Some special foods and diets are explained in the book to describe the relation to their claimed functionality and health benefits. The book covers detailed information of Korean functional foods such as kimchi, soybean products, ginseng, salt, oil seeds, etc. The book also provides information on Korean foods' health benefits, processing technology and methods, and food law and regulations for food manufacture and marketing status. This book is a timely addition to the "Functional Foods and Nutraceuticals Series."

Series Editor
John Shi, Ph.D.
Senior Research Scientist
Guelph Food Research Center
Federal Department of Agriculture and Agri-Food Canada
Canada

Preface

Korea has developed a unique culinary culture, and that story, along with the nutritional and functional benefits that characterize Korean foods, needs to be told. In many ways, the pungent spices that combine with salty fermented fish, soybeans, and cabbage that are consumed with rice, wild vegetables, and seaweed are a reflection of the history of the Korean people.

In this book, we have sought to help people around the world understand both the Korean people and their food and to see how, even though the Korean diet has developed over millennia, it is a diet that stands up to scientific scrutiny for its health benefits in the present. To accomplish this goal, it was necessary to seek out experts who could write authoritatively on different aspects of the history, methods of preparation, and nutritional benefits of individual Korean foods—as well as the Korean diet as a whole. We are proud to have received participation from some of the foremost scientists involved in studying Korean food and nutrition. These people have worked long and hard and sacrificed much of their valuable time and energy to help the editors develop an authoritative treatise on Korean cuisine. A reader who is not familiar with Korean food will be surprised to learn of its delightful uniqueness and how the characteristics that contribute its unique pungent flavors also preserve the food, thereby providing nourishment through the long, bitter Korean winters.

The book begins by explaining the history of Korean food, details the composition of a Korean diet and how the foods are prepared, and then discusses the health benefits of this particular diet. Next, the unique ingredients that go into making Korean foods are explained in detail; most have a chapter devoted to them. Three chapters are devoted to characteristically prepared Korean foods that embody its uniqueness: kimchi, namul (green and yellow vegetables), and bibimbap, which combines all the elements of basic Korean cuisine into one dish. Finally, the book describes modern developments in Korean food manufacturing and dietary habits. Especially important is the modern emphasis on Korean foods as functional foods rather than as simply sustenance foods.

It is our desire that the reader develop an appreciation for the history, culinary art, and nutritional benefits of the Korean diet, which can be recommended as one of the most balanced and healthy diets in the world. The traditional Korean food philosophy, called "yak-sik-dong-won" (medicine and food share the same origin), has accentuated the importance of food. The Korean peninsula has mountainous terrain surrounded by sea; this contributed to the development of a specialized diet composed of steamed rice, seaweed, and herbs as staples. In addition, because of long winter days, fermented foods with solar salt were also developed.

ix

Most Koreans have eaten steamed rice and soup (made of doenjang, vegetables, meats, and/or seaweed) as a staple, as well as other side dishes of kimchi and banchan made with fish, meat, and vegetables. Over the years, the number of side dishes increased from the basic diet ("sam-cheob"—three dishes—and "ban-sang—the dietary table, meaning three more dishes in addition to the basic diet) for people at the lowest social level to seven to nine side dishes for the "nobleman" class. The basic table setting was composed of steamed rice, kimchi, doenjang, and soy sauce; other side dishes were added, based on family wealth and social level.

The fermented foods that are central to the Korean diet are especially timely considering the current interest in beneficial microorganisms as foods. Probiotics themselves and probiotic-fermented foods are subjects of global interest. Healthful ingredients including soybeans, vegetables, and spices are fermented by probiotic bacteria, resulting in high-quality fermented foods with improved taste, health functionalities, storage quality, and even texture. The microbiota residing in our guts are dependent upon what we eat; thus, food has a great impact on overall health.

We, the editors, and the authors are delighted to recommend this journey into the Korean culinary world. It is our desire that this book stimulate interest in learning more about Korean food and, even more importantly, experiencing it.

Acknowledgments

We give special thanks to CRC Press for publishing *Korean Functional Foods: Composition, Processing and Health Benefits,* and to the authors of the chapters of this book. We also appreciate the suggestion of Dr. John Shi—a senior research scientist with the US Federal Department of Agriculture and Agri-Food Canada, as well as an editor for the "Functional Foods and Nutraceuticals" book series for CRC Press—that such a book was needed to bring together the history, art, and science that combine to form the unique dietary creation that has developed along the ocean coasts and in the rugged mountains of the Korean Peninsula.

Editors

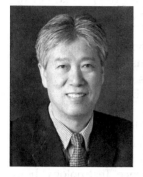

Professor Kun-Young Park has been one of the leading authorities of global fermented functional foods for last 30 years. He got his PhD in food science and technology from the University of Nebraska-Lincoln, in 1982, and did his postdoctoral research work in nutrition at Harvard University, Boston. He has received many national honors and awards from the United States and Korea. He was awarded Phi Tau Sigma by the Honor Society for Food Science in 1982 and the JMF Award for Outstanding Paper in 2010.

He has been president of the Korean Society of Cancer Prevention, president of the Korean Society of Food Science and Nutrition, and president of the Korean Kimchi Association. He was an editor-in chief of the *Journal of Medicinal Food*, as well as senior editor of the *Journal of Carcinogenesis*. Over a period of 20 years, he has edited many academic journals. He is a chair and fellow of the Division of Agricultural and Fishery Sciences in the Korean Academy of Science and Technology. He has published more than 400 research and review papers, and has been invited to or presented more than 800 papers at domestic and international symposia. He has been invited to write many chapters by CRC and Marcel Dekker books.

Prof. Park had been a professor in the Department of Food Science and Nutrition at Pusan National University in Busan, Korea, since 1983, and is working in the Department of Food Science and Biotechnology at Cha University, Pocheon/Seongnam, Gyeonggi-do, South Korea.

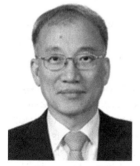

Dae Young Kwon is currently working as a principal research investigator at the Korea Food Research Institute (KFRI) Jeonju, Korea. He has sucessfully served as vice president and president of KFRI. He is a fellow of the Korean Academy of Science and Technology, Seoul, Korea. He obtained his bachelor's degree from the Department of Food Science and Engineering at Seoul National University, Seoul, Korea; he received his MSc, and PhD degrees from the Korea Advanced Institute of Science and Technology (KAIST), Seoul, Korea, in 1986 in the Department of Biological Science and Biotechnology. After completing the PhD, he joined Whitehead Institute, Department of Biology, MIT, Cambridge, Massachusetts, as a postdoctoral fellow until 1989. After finishing his postdoctoral training, he became a research scientist at KFRI, working there in the field of food biological chemistry. He worked as adjunct professor in Sookmyung Women's University from 1997 to 2003. He has been a professor at United University of Science and Technology since 2004. He is president of the Korean Society of Food-Health Communication and the Korean Forum of Fermentation and Food Culture. He has published more than 275 research articles in several renowned Science Citation Index (SCI) international journals in the areas of fermented foods and bioactive food components; those papers have been cited about 6,000 times in SCI journals. He has published five academic books and authored three book chapters. He is also working as editor in chief of the *Journal of Ethnic Foods*, published by Elsevier.

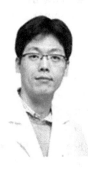

Ki Won Lee is currently working as a professor in the Department of Agricultural Biotechnology, and as a director of the Wellness Emergence Center in the Advanced Institute of Convergence Technology, both in Seoul National University, Seoul, Korea. He obtained his master and PhD degrees from Seoul National University, Republic of Korea. After finishing his postdoctoral career in the Department of Biomedical Informatics and Computational Biology, University of Minnesota (Mayo Clinic and the Hormel Institute), he became a professor in the Department of Bioscience and Biotechnology, Konkuk University, Seoul, Korea, in 2006. His research interests are in identifying molecular targets of various phytochemicals in human disorders, including cancer, cardiovascular disease, obesity, neurodegenerative disease, and photoaging, and in application of these findings to industry. He has published more than 260 papers in SCI/E journals including *Nature Reviews Cancer, Nature Structure, Molecular Biology, Molecular Cell, Lancet, Cancer Research*, and *Journal of the American Chemical Society*. He has also applied for and registered 74 patents and has written seven book chapters.

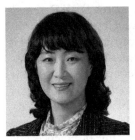

Sunmin Park is a full professor at the Department of Food & Nutrition in Hoseo University, Asan, Korea, a frequently published researcher, and a fellow of the Korean Academy of Science and Technology. Dr. Park earned her undergraduate degree from Ewah Women's University, Seoul, Korea, and a master's degree in biostatistics and a PhD in human nutrition from The Ohio State University, Columbus, Ohio. She worked as a senior scientist at Joslin Diabetes Center in Harvard Medical School, Boston. Her greatest expertise is in the study of diabetes with an emphasis on the etiology of Asian type 2 diabetes. Recently, her research has expanded to include metabolic etiologies of Alzheimer's disease and interactive effects of the gut microbiome on the

Editors

brain and metabolic health. Much of her research has included the effects of traditional Korean fermented foods and their bioactive compounds on metabolic diseases including type 2 diabetes, ischemic stroke, and Alzheimer's disease. Her research has included cellular and animal studies, systematic reviews and meta-analyses, and genome-wide association studies.

Contributors

Sanjeewa K. K. Asanka
Department of Marine Life Science
Jeju National University
Jeju-si, Jeju-do, Republic of Korea

Sanguine Byun
Division of Bioengineering
Incheon National University
Incheon, Republic of Korea

Youn-Soo Cha
Department of Food Science and
    Human Nutrition
Chonbuk National University
Jeonju-si, Jeollabuk-do, Republic
    of Korea

Soo-Wan Chae
Department of Pharmacology
Chonbuk National University
    Medical School
Jeonju-si, Jeollabuk-do, Republic
    of Korea

Jeong-Yong Cho
Department of Food Science and
    Technology
Chonnam National University
Gwangju, Republic of Korea

Hak-Jong Choi
World Institute of Kimchi
Gwangju, Republic of Korea

Han-Seok Choi
National Institute of Agricultural
    Sciences
Wanju-gun, Jeollabuk-do, Republic
    of Korea

Kyung Rhan Chung
The Academy of Korean Sciences
Songnam, Gyonggi-do, Republic
    of Korea

James W. Daily
Daily Manufacturing Inc.
Rockwell, North Carolina, USA

Kyung-Sik Ham
Solar Salt Research Center
Department of Food Science and
    Biotechnology
Mokpo National University
Muan-gun, Jeollanam-do, Republic
    of Korea

Na-Ra Han
Department of Pharmacology
Kyung Hee University
Seoul, Republic of Korea

Lily Jaiswal
Solar Salt Research Center
Department of Food Science and
    Biotechnology
Mokpo National University
Muan-gun, Jeollanam-do, Republic
    of Korea

Ja-Young Jang
World Institute of Kimchi
Gwangju, Republic of Korea

You-Jin Jeon
Department of Marine Life Science
Jeju National University
Jeju-si, Jeju-do, Republic of Korea

xvii

Hyun-Ja Jeong
Department of Food Science and Technology and Research Institute for Basic Science
Hoseo University
Asan-si, Chungcheongnam-do, Republic of Korea

Seok-Tae Jeong
National Institute of Agricultural Sciences
Wanju-gun, Jeollabuk-do, Republic of Korea

Jaehyun Ju
Department of Food Science and Biotechnology
CHA University
Seongnam-si, Gyeonggi-do, Republic of Korea

Mun Yhung Jung
College of Food Science
Woosuk University
Wanju-gun, Jeonbuk, Republic of Korea

Su-Jin Jung
Clinical Trial Center for Functional Foods, Chonbuk National University Hospital
Jeonju-si, Jeonju, Republic of Korea

Ji-Eun Kang
National Institute of Agricultural Sciences
Wanju-gun, Jeollabuk-do, Republic of Korea

Hoon Kim
Skin Biotechnology Center
Kyung Hee University
Suwon-si, Gyeonggi, Republic of Korea

Hyun-Soo Kim
Department of Marine Life Science
Jeju National University
Jeju-si, Jeju-do, Republic of Korea

Hyung-Min Kim
Department of Pharmacology
Kyung Hee University
Seoul, Republic of Korea

Ji Yeon Kim
Department of Food Science and Technology
Seoul National University of Science and Technology
Seoul, Republic of Korea

Jong-Eun Kim
Research Institute of Biotechnology and Medical Converged Science
Dongguk University
Goyang-si, Gyeonggi-do, Republic of Korea

Jong Hun Kim
Department of Agricultural Biotechnology
Sungshin University
Seoul, Republic of Korea

Mi-Ja Kim
Department of Food and Nutrition
Kangwon National University
Samcheok-si, Gangwon-do, Republic of Korea

Soon-Hee Kim
Korea Food Research Institute
Wanju-gun, Jeollabuk-do, Republic of Korea

Young Myoung Kim
Korea Food Research Institute
Wanju-gun, Jeollabuk-do, Republic of Korea

Contributors

Ok Kyung Koo
Department of Food and Nutrition
Gyeongsang National University
Jinju-si, Gyeongsangnam-do,
 Republic of Korea

Dae Young Kwon
Korea Food Research Institute
Wanju-gun, Jeollabuk-do, Republic
 of Korea

Boo-Yong Lee
Department of Food Science and
 Biotechnology
CHA University
Seongnam-si, Kyunggi-do, Republic
 of Korea

Cherl-Ho Lee
Department of Food Science and
 Technology
Korea University
Seoul, Republic of Korea

Jin-Hee Lee
Department of Food Science and
 Biotechnology
CHA University
Seongnam-si, Gyeonggi-do,
 Republic of Korea

JaeHwan Lee
Department of Food Science and
 Biotechnology
Sungkyunkwan University
Suwon-si, Gyeonggi-do, Republic
 of Korea

Jieun Lee
World Institute of Kimchi
Gwangju, Republic of Korea

Ki Won Lee
Department of Agricultural
 Biotechnology
Seoul National University
Seoul, Republic of Korea

Yeonkyung Lee
Amway Korea Ltd.,
Seoul, Republic of Korea

Young-Eun Lee
Department of Food and Nutrition
Wonkwang University
Iksan-si, Jeollabuk-do, Republic
 of Korea

Phil-Dong Moon
Department of Pharmacology
Kyung Hee University
Seoul, Republic of Korea

Hye-Kyung Na
Department of Food Science and
 Biotechnology
Sungshin Women's University
Seoul, Republic of Korea

Eui-Seong Park
Department of Food and Nutrition
Yonsei University
Seoul, Republic of Korea

Kun-Young Park
Department of Food Science and
 Biotechnology
CHA University
Seongnam-si, Gyeonggi-do,
 Republic of Korea

Sunmin Park
Department of Food and Nutrition
Hoseo University
Cheoana-si, Chungcheongnam-do,
 Republic of Korea

Kwang-Soon Shin
Department of Food Science and
Biotechnology
Kyonggi University
Suwon-si, Gyeonggi-do, Republic
of Korea

Young-Joon Surh
College of Pharmacy
Seoul National University
Seoul, Republic of Korea

1

Korean Foods—History, Culture, and Characteristics

Cherl-Ho Lee

CONTENTS

1.1 History of Korean Dietary Culture 1
    1.1.1 Paleolithic Age... 2
    1.1.2 Primitive Pottery Age... 3
    1.1.3 Neolithic Age and the Era of Myth 5
    1.1.4 The Historic Age 8
    1.1.5 Dietary Changes during the Last Century 9
1.2 Health Concept of Korean Functional Food 10
    1.2.1 Taoism.. 10
    1.2.2 Yin and Yang and Five Phases Theory 11
    1.2.3 Traditional Chinese Medicine... 13
    1.2.4 Eastern Medicine and Sasang Typology 14
1.3 Future of Korean Functional Food 16
1.4 Conclusion 19
References... 19

1.1 History of Korean Dietary Culture

The Northeast Asian culture, generally known as a part of Chinese culture to Western society, comprises many segments of ethnic groups, which have each developed their own identity and distinctive culture over time. In the present day, they are referred to in large groups with the names of their countries: China, Mongolia, Korea, Japan, and parts of Russia (Siberia). But until a millennium ago, the ethnic group (or tribe) was more important than the nation in distinguishing the way of life of a people. The early classics of Chinese literature are the products of a long history of the thought, religion, culture, and wisdom of the many tribes in this region. The early historians in China described the existence and the lives of neighboring countries, including the Dong-yi (Eastern Archers). The Eastern Archers have inhabited a wide range of Northeast Asia, from the Shandong Peninsula to the Bohai Corridor, the Manchurian Basin, the Liadong Peninsula, and the Korean

1

Peninsula, which was mostly ruled by Goguryeo until the fifth century AD (Nahm, 1988; Lee and Kim, 2016).

1.1.1 Paleolithic Age

The early existence of human beings in this region is evidenced by early Paleolithic remains (1,800,000–300,000 years ago, BP [before present]) of the early/middle Pleistocene Age in Northern China and the Korean Peninsula. Evidence of the existence of *Homo erectus* (1,800,000–650,000 BP) was found in the Xihoudu, Lantian, and Zhoukoudian sites on the Northern Chinese Mainland, Jinniushan in the Manchurian Basin, and the Sokchangni and Chungbuk Keumkul sites on the Korean Peninsula. Zhoukoudian cave locality I, near Beijing, has yielded the largest number of *Homo erectus* fossils in the world: 40-odd individuals, together with thousands of animal bones, some of which were burnt by roasting (Barnes, 1993). Fossils of early man, *Homo sapiens*, were found in Yokpo Cave (500,000 BP) and Sangwon Cave (400,000 BP) near Pyungyang on the Korean Peninsula (Sohn, 1983).

Recently, several middle Paleolithic (350,000–40,000 BP) remains were found on the Korean Peninsula. The stone tools and animal fauna of the Seungrisan, Jommal Yonggul, Durubong, and Chongongni sites were similar to those of the Dingcun site of China. The fauna and stone tools of the Sokchangni seventh and eighth layers, Chongchongam Cave, Gulpori I, and Sangmu Yongni were comparable to those of the Xujiayao site in Northern China. The earliest Paleolithic remains found in Siberia, at the Irkutsk site near the Angara River and the Ushiki site on the Kamchaka Peninsula, were those of 70,000–130,000 years ago, similar to those found at the Gulpori site (Choi, 1983).

Numerous late Paleolithic (40,000–10,000 BP) sites were found on the Korean Peninsula, in South Manchuria, and on Japanese islands as well as the Chinese mainland. This points to the increase in population and spreading out of people in this region in the late Paleolithic Age (Lee, 1998a). During the glacial periods (Günz, Mindel, Riss, and Würm) of the Pleistocene age, the Yellow and Seto Plains were exposed by lower sea levels, and the East Sea became merely a large lake, which drained through the present Korea Strait. These increased land areas facilitated the movement of humans and animals among and between parts of East Asia (Lee, 1998a). It has also been assumed that the Asian Mongoloids moved to the American continent over the Bering Strait during these periods (Barnes, 1993). However, during the warm interglacial period, the sea levels rose to the present level, and the Korean Peninsula became a land bridge connecting the Japanese islands to Manchuria and the Maritime Province of Siberia. The mobile hunter life of Paleolithic men, who chased after large animals moving periodically with seasonal climate change, continued until the invention of earthenware. Figure 1.1 shows the sites of Paleolithic remains excavated in Northeast Asia, and the migratory route of the mobile hunters from southern Kyushu to northern Manchuria and Siberia through the Korean Peninsula, connected

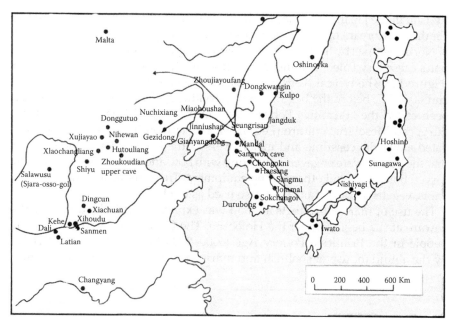

FIGURE 1.1
Paleolithic remains found in Northeast Asia. (From Lee, C. H. 2001. *Fermentation Technology in Korea*. Seoul: Korea University Press.)

by mountain ranges (Lee, 2001). Animal meat, intestines, and blood were the main foodstuffs for these people, and the use of vegetable supplements, such as grass seeds, tree nuts, and wild fruits and roots, increased in the later stages of the Paleolithic era. The people lived in caves in the mountains and gradually moved to the lower plains and river banks in the later part of that era (Lee, 1998a).

The animal meat-eating habit of the early men in Northeast Asia and on the Korean Peninsula gradually appears to have changed to an omnivorous culture by the end of the Paleolithic Age. The utilization of tree nuts and acorns, wild fruits, berries and grapes, grass seeds, roots, and young buds of trees and ferns increased gradually as the inhabitants noticed that abundant plant materials were growing around the previously inhabited caves and dwellings. Traces of pollen of grass, rice (Gramineae), and beans (Leguminosae, Papilionoidiae) have been found to have increased among late Paleolithic remains (Lee, 1998a). With the increase of plant food in the diet, the dwelling sites gradually moved from the mountains to the plains near rivers.

1.1.2 Primitive Pottery Age

Earthenware was likely invented by the people in the coastal area of the Korea Strait comprising the southeast of the Korean Peninsula and the north of

Kyushu in the Japanese Islands during 12,000–8,000 BP (Han, 1983). The use of Chulmun (Korean) or Jomon (Japanese) pottery spread over the whole region of Northeast Asia by the year 6000 BC, and this gradually changed the population's migratory Paleolithic life into a littoral forager life along the coastal line (Figure 1.2). The typical Northeast Asian lifestyle that existed between 10,000 and 4000 BC, before the beginning of Neolithic agricultural settlements, has been called the "Primitive Pottery Age" in order to distinguish it from the European Mesolithic culture (Lee, 1999). The numerous shell mounds excavated along the coastline and major rivers of the Korean Peninsula indicate that the people were engaged in hunting with bow and arrow and fishing with carved bone tools and other fishing equipment. Tree nuts, acorns, wild grains, fruits, vegetables, and roots were also used as foodstuff.

The use of marine products as food was expanded with the use of earthenware at the beginning of the Holocene. The food life of Northeast Asian people in the Primitive Pottery Age (6000–3000 BC) can be characterized by the abundant use of shellfish and marine products together with animal

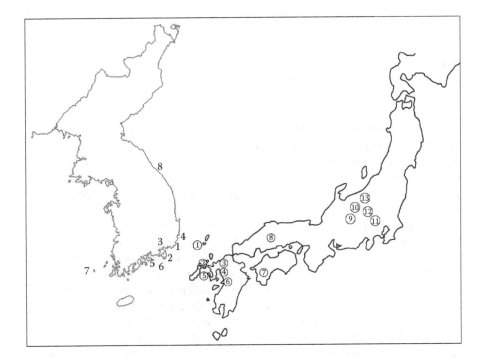

FIGURE 1.2
Primitive Pottery Age remains excavated in the Korea Strait region. (From Han, Y. H. 1983. Regional comparison. In *Korean History 12: Archeology of Korea I*. National History Editorial Committee, 479–521 (in Korean).) Korean Peninsula: 1. Dongsamdong, 2. Dadaepo, 3. Chukgok, 4. Sinamri, 5. Sangnodaedo, 6. Yokjido, 7. Sohuksando, 8. Osanri. Japanese Archipelago: ① Kosijima, ② Fukui, ③ Nisikaratsu, ④ Iwasita, ⑤ Senpukuji, ⑥ Todoroki, ⑦ Kamikuroiwa, ⑧ Mawatari, ⑨ Yangimata, ⑩ Isigoya, ⑪ Hasitate, ⑫ Tazawa, ⑬ Ozawa.

foods from hunting, as evidenced by the numerous shell mounds along the coastline of the Korean Peninsula and Japanese islands. The cooking of fish and vegetables in sea water in earthenware bowls, called chigae today, must have emerged from this period (Lee, 1999). Since the use of earthenware for the storage of cereals, vegetables, meats, and marine products could have naturally resulted in fermentation, fermented foods such as cereal alcoholic beverages, vegetable pickles, and fermented fish and meats were probably developed prior to the beginning of agriculture in this region (Lee and Kim, 2016).

The invention of fermentation technology, which could provide relatively abundant nutrients to the people compared to in previous periods, might have resulted in a sudden increase in population. Human civilization in Northeast Asia actually started at this moment. People lived in caves along the river banks or in semisubterranean pit dwellings as demonstrated by Amsadong remains near Seoul. The long history of fermented food use and chigae culture characterizes the dietary culture of Koreans today.

1.1.3 Neolithic Age and the Era of Myth

The Neolithic Age began with agricultural settlements in Northeast Asia in about 4000 BC. Tribal states, which were based on agricultural and fishery settlements, emerged in this period. The early civilization centers on the Chinese continent were the Bohai Corridor in South Manchuria, represented by Hongshan culture; Cishan in the west of the Central Plain of the Chinese mainland, represented by Yangshao culture; and the Yangzi Delta in the Shanghai area represented by Hemudu culture (Barnes, 1993).

There were three major ethnic groups competing with each other to occupy the Central Plain of China—namely, the eastern tribe, Dong-yi; the western tribe, Hwaxia; and the southern tribe, Miaoman. Figure 1.3 shows the territories of these three tribes in the prehistoric era. The stories of the formation and destiny of these tribes were handed down in the form of myth. Most Chinese and Northeastern mythologies are the stories of thousands of years of struggle between the three tribes, especially between Dong-yi and Hwaxia, to occupy the Central Plain.

According to *Handankogi*, a collection of Korean mythology written between the Silla Era and Chosun Kingdom, the first nation of Dong-yi, Hankuk, was founded near Mount Paektu and the Heilong River in the seventieth century BC by the heavenly god Hannim and was ruled by seven emperors for 3,300 years without any struggle or war (Lim, 1986). In the fortieth century BC, the heavenly God sent one of his sons, Hanung, along with 3,000 followers, including three servants controlling the wind, rain, and clouds, to found a second nation, Baedal, in Shinsi. A bear and a tiger on earth wished to be human beings, so Hanung told them to pray in a dark cave for 100 days and eat only garlic and mugwort in order to become human. The bear followed these instructions successfully and became a woman, Yong-yo, while the tiger could not tolerate the

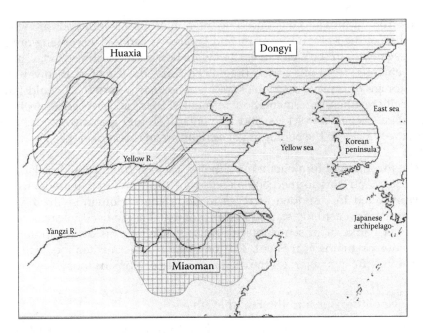

FIGURE 1.3
Prehistoric ethnic grouping in the Central Plain region of China. (From Barnes, G. L. 1993. *China, Korea and Japan: The Rise of Civilization in East Asia*. London: Thames and Hudson.)

suffering. Yong-yo then prayed to have a baby, so Hanung, a son of God, married her and they had a son. This idea of the marriage between a heavenly god and a woman (goddess) of the earth who have children—the people, who are basically the descendants of the heavenly God—is called Samsin (three gods); this concept forms the basis of Asiatic shamanism and folk Taoism, which has been the traditional religion of the Dong-yi. Hanung's kingdom continued with 18 emperors for 1,565 years. The fourteenth emperor, Chiyou (2707 BC), expanded cultivation land and produced copper and iron for the war industry. He appears in the Chinese myth known as the story of "Three Emperors and Five Kings." In 2333 BC, Tangun founded the third nation, Tangun Chosun, the last legendary nation in Korean mythology, which was ended by the forty-seventh emperor, Koyolga, in 295 BC (Lim, 1986). However, historians today consider Tangun Chosun to be the first nation in Korean history (Nahm, 1988).

The legendary nations in Chinese mythology start with Yao followed by Shun, Hsia (2000–1520 BC), and Shang (Yin, 1520–1030 BC). The story of the "Three Emperors and Five Kings" illustrates the formation of the Chinese legendary kingdoms and their struggle with the different tribes. Many of the legendary figures in Korean myths appear in the Chinese myths as a challenging nature or the prime mover of a period. In fact, the Shang period was ruled by the Eastern Archers, the Dong-yi. As with most legendary stories, the Chinese myths were also fabricated intentionally by the powerful elites and kings of the Chinese mainland to justify their legitimacy throughout history. The truths behind the myths are not always possible to prove with evidence, but may be useful in filling the gaps of human history, especially in the case of the lost history of the Dong-yi from 8000 to 2000 BC.

The main early cereal grain cultivated and utilized by the people in Northeast Asia and on the Korean Peninsula appears to be millet, which is the native plant in that region. The oldest rice remains (12,500 BP) were found in Sorori, Korea; these were older than the rice remains found in the Yangzi River region of China (Lee et al., 2015a). Carbonated rice objects have been found in late Neolithic and early Bronze Age remains (2000 BC) in Korea. Rice cultivation was a common practice in the Three Nations Period (third century) of Korea.

When the horse-riding people of the north, the Yemaek tribe of the northeastern Dong-yi, came south to the Korean Peninsula to become agricultural farming settlers, they needed to have a stable protein source to replace their meat from the animal herds. They invented the use of wild soybeans as food by soaking them in water and cooking them properly to eliminate the antinutritional factors in the bean. The Maek tribes are considered to be the first users of soybean as food in history (Lee and Kwon, 2005). Soybeans were cultivated by the nomads who started farming settlements at around Mt. Baekdu, in southern Manchuria, and on the Korean Peninsula at the beginning of the Bronze Age. Among Bronze Age remains in Paldang, near Seoul, a smooth earthen vessel with traces of soybeans on the surface was excavated. Botanists believe that the origin of soybeans is along the line from South Manchuria to the Korean Peninsula, where the most abundant varieties of wild soybeans are found. The first record of soybeans appears in Shyjing, a piece of Chinese literature written in the seventh century BC. The story of soybean introduction into China says that soybeans were brought into China from Sanyung (South Manchuria) in the early seventh century BC by Hwangong of the Chhi dynasty, as he conquered Sanyung during the Chhun Chhiu Period, and it was therefore called Yungsuk (Lee, 1984).

Soybeans played an important role not only in supplying protein but also in providing palatability to the bland diet of cereals and vegetables in the form of fermented soybean products. Weyjyh, Dong-yi joen, and Kokuryo cho of *Sanguojyh*, a history book written in the sixth century in China, describe the people of Kokuryo as good at preparing fermented soybean products. The smell of soy sauce starter, shi, was described in Chinese as gaolixiu, meaning "the smell of the Korean people." Bowuzhi of Jin (AD 265–420) records that Shi originated from a foreign country and the character is part of a dialect. Xintangshu of the Tang period (AD 618–907) names Shi as a special product of Bohai (AD 699–926), a nation founded by refugees from the defeated Koguryo. The production of soy sauce by the Maek tribe, who were originally meat-eating nomads, created a typical Korean dish, bulgoki or Maek-chok— roasted meat marinated with soybean sauce. This dish is considered to be a marriage of meat-eating habits with soy sauce culture, which happened in the crop-farming settlements of the nomads on the Korean Peninsula. In the

Chin dynasty China, marinated roast meat was called Maek-chok, which meant Korean roast meat. The meat diet of the nomads gradually changed because of their changing settlement patterns, as they adapted to the cereal-based food diet of the natives in the southern plains.

1.1.4 The Historic Age

The classics of Korean history, *Samguksaki* (Kim Busik, 1145) and *Samkukyusa* (Ilyon, 1281), describe the founding of Dangun-chosun (2333 BC) and the Three Nations: Silla (57 BC), Koguryo (37 BC), and Paekche (18 BC). The introduction of Buddhism, in AD 372 in Koguryo and in AD 528 in Silla, accelerated the reduction of animal food consumption and encouraged the spread of vegetarian food habits. According to *Samguksaki*, rice, grain-wine, oil, honey, soy sauce, soybean paste, dried meat, and fish sauce were the important food items that were prepared for a wedding in the royal family in Silla in the seventh century. The people of Unified Silla and the succeeding Koryo dynasties were strong Buddhists. During this thousand-year period, nomadic habits centering around animal food mostly disappeared. The extensive use of salted vegetables and soybean products as the major source of protein resulted from this change. The technologies of soy sauce fermentation and rice-wine making were well developed and transferred to neighboring countries. Soybean fermentation technology was transferred from Koguryo to Japan in this period. The document of *Shoso-in* (AD 752) of Japan describes miso, the Japanese name for soybean paste, as a word from a dialect of Koryo (Korea), often called koryojang, which means Korean sauce (Lee, 1984). The ancient Japanese history book *Kojiki* says that a man from Paekche taught them rice-wine making. The memorial tablet of a man called Chin of Silla is kept in a shrine—the Matsuo Taisha in Kyoto—as a god of rice-wine. The rice-wine producers in Japan attend an annual worship ceremony for him, in order to pray for success in their own wine fermenting (Lee, 1995a).

The Chinese Yuan (Mongol) invasion of Koryo in the thirteenth century (1259–1356) brought about the suppression of Buddhism and an increased respect for Confucianism in the Chosun kingdom; it also restored the animal food diet in Korea. Another important thing in the Korean diet is representative fermented foods, such as kimchi and kochujang—typical Korean fermented vegetables and hot soybean paste—which were influenced by red pepper. Recent genetic studies of red peppers showed that the Korean type of red pepper has grown wild for a half a million years in the Korean peninsula (Kwon et al., 2017). The Korean people have known how to make kimchi and kochujang traditionally for more than a thousand years. Kimchi and kochujang can be made only with Korean red pepper—not with central American or tropical Asian red pepper.

During the Chosun kingdom (AD 1382–1910), a well-balanced variety of foods, of both animal and vegetable origins, was utilized. *Imwon Sibyukchi*, an

Korean Foods—History, Culture, and Characteristics

encyclopedia written in 1827 by Seo Yu-Gu, describes the food materials that were used in nineteenth century Korea, including 11 kinds of water, 36 kinds of cereal, 72 kinds of vegetables, 13 kinds of poultry, 34 kinds of fish, and eight kinds of spices. The ideal diet for Koreans was standardized between the fifteenth and nineteenth centuries. *Shieui Jeonseo*, written in the nineteenth century, as well as other books written between the seventeenth and nineteenth centuries, outlines the standard meal of Koreans, consisting more or less of a bowl of cooked rice, a bowl of soup, and a bowl of kimchi as a basic meal. To this basic menu, side dishes are added, forming a three-dish meal (samchop-bansang), five-dish meal (ochop-bansang), seven-dish meal (chilchop-bansang), and so on (Yoon, 1993). A 12-dish meal was served only for the king.

1.1.5 Dietary Changes during the Last Century

Korea opened its gates to western countries in the 1870s, much later than Japan and China. European diplomats, Russians, and missionaries from America introduced cakes and coffee. However, this was soon overshadowed by the Japanese invasion of Korea, and Korea was annexed to Japan for 36 years starting in 1910. One of the statistical records of the colonial regime shows that Japan extorted one-third of the rice produced in Korea every year during this period (Lee, 1995b). The Korean people suffered greatly from the shortage of food, and even defatted soybean flakes were rationed as a rice substitute. Soon after the rehabilitation in 1945, hundreds of thousands of people moved from Communist North Korea to South Korea in order to escape the terror regime of Kim Il-Sung, who was enforcing one-man worship. The total number of refugees from the north to the south during the Korean War (1950–1953) was estimated at two million. The starvation of the people was barely overcome thanks to wheat flour and nonfat dry milk donated by the US aid program. Milk porridges were rationed to the starving people, who had been non-milk-eating people. After experiencing severe lactose intolerance symptoms, people gradually adapted to being able to eat milk porridge. This triggered the explosive consumption of milk products during the economic growth of the 1970s and 1980s, and the rapid Westernization of Korean food habits afterward (Lee, 1995b).

The per-capita GNP of South Korea in the postwar era was 72 USD in 1954 and less than 100 USD until 1962. It increased to 130 USD in 1966 when the first Five-Year Economic Development Plan ended (1962–1966), to 288 USD in 1971 at the conclusion of the second plan, and to 797 USD in 1976 at the close of the third plan. The GDP reached 1,719 USD in 1981, when the fourth plan ended and 2,296 USD in 1986 when the fifth plan concluded. During this period, the proportion of the farming population decreased from 60% of the total population to less than 20%, with a massive inflow into urban centers.

Korea achieved a Green Revolution, producing rice at the level of self-sufficiency in the 1970s, and the term "barley hump," referring to the food shortage, disappeared as the daily rice supply per person exceeded 300 g.

With the rapid development of the food industry after 1980, Korean dietary life changed significantly: The daily intake of animal products per person almost doubled in 5 years, from 98 to 183 g. In particular, there was a significant increase in meat consumption, from 79 to 119 g, and milk consumption rose from 10 to 43 g. Along with such changes in food consumption patterns, degenerative diseases such as diabetes, hypertension, and heart disease started to become important health issues. Therefore, this period has been assessed as one in which South Korea had passed into an era of surplus over the optimal patterns of Korean food consumption. Animal food consumption continued to grow, reaching 230 g in 1995 and 279 g in 2005. The average daily food intake for South Koreans was also on the rise and was estimated to increase 30% in 25 years, from about 1 kg per person in 1980 to 1.3 kg in 2005. The growth in food intake, especially the excessive animal food intake, caused a deterioration of national health, including an increase in obesity and degenerative diseases. The ratio of obesity in Korea in 1995 was 18.8% for men and 22.2% for women, making the average obesity ratio of the population 20.5%. This increased to 26.4% in 1998 and 32.7% in 2000, at which point 38.1% of men and 25.9% of women were obese. The changes in the leading causes of death indicate that the number of people who died of cancer increased by 27% from 1989 to 2009; the number of patients who died of breast cancer doubled, and deaths from colon cancer increased by 3.3 times. During the same period, the number of those who died of diabetes increased by 2.5 times (Lee et al., 2015b).

1.2 Health Concept of Korean Functional Food

The concept of health for Koreans has been formed through history, influenced by the indigenous folk Taoism and the old oriental philosophy of man and the universe, which is represented by the concept of yin/yang and the Five Phases theory. The oldest Chinese medicine book, *The Yellow Emperor's Classic of Medicine*, written in the Chin and Han periods of China (220 BC–AD 220) contains theories of man–universe unity, yin and yang, the Five Phases, the ten calendar signs (the decimal system), earth's twelve branches (the duodecimal system), and other fundamental principles of medical treatment (Ni, 1995). This book was first introduced into Korea in the period of Koguryo King Pyungwon, in year 3 (AD 561). Since then, Chinese medicinal knowledge has greatly influenced the health concepts and food habits of the Korean people.

1.2.1 Taoism

Taoism, the folk religion that originated from the shamanistic beliefs of Northeast Asians, forms the basis of the health concepts found in the

Korean Foods—History, Culture, and Characteristics

traditional diet and medicine of the Korean people (Lee, 1998b). Korean thought about life and health is based on the shamanistic folk philosophy, which sets as the ultimate goal a healthy eternal life. The established Taoism, as developed by early Chinese philosophers, teaches that this goal can be achieved through discipline, mainly with the control of the breath, sex, and food. The principle of this control is the harmony of yin and yang, the negative and positive aspects of the universe. Toward the end of the nineteenth century, tens of thousands of broken tortoise shells and status pieces suggesting longevity were found in the capital city of the Shang (Yin) dynasty on the southern riverbank of Anyang, China. Pictographs on the engraved tortoise shells showed that the basic principles of yin and yang were a part of the Shang dynasty, and that they originated from the legendary saint, Bok-Eui (3000 BC), the god of divination. The Chinese characters, which are used as a writing system today, were developed during the Jou dynasty (1100–220 BC). The theory of interchange developed through the Jou dynasty for 3,000 years, leading to Taoism and Confucianism.

1.2.2 Yin and Yang and Five Phases Theory

The Book of Changes (*Yijing*) is the basis for the yin and yang theory and the principles of the Five Phases; it contains the principles that explain changes in the universe and in nature. Examples of yin/yang that are commonly found in nature include: dark/bright, female/male, inside/outside, center/circumference, weak/strong, empty/full, cold/hot, rise/descend, plants/animals, death/life, moisture/dryness, big/small, sparse/dense, and electron/proton. The important principles applied to the yin/yang relationship are mutual suppression and repulsion, mutual dependence, mutual compensation for equilibrium, and mutual transformation. These principles imply that there is no absolute yin (negative) or yang (positive) in nature, and that everything is relative.

Wood, fire, earth, metal, and water represent the principles of the Five Phases. These imply transition, movement, or passage, rather than the stable, homogeneous chemical constituents such as earth, air, fire, and water, the four eternal elements of ancient Greek science (Magner, 1992). The Five Phases are the principles of changes linked by the relationship between generation and destruction (or suppression), as shown in Figure 1.4 (Magner, 1992; Lee, 1998b).

According to the theories of yin/yang and the Five Phases, all food materials are classified according to their properties and their different tastes. These properties are cool, classified as yin; neutral; or warm, classified as yang. For example, fruits on the tree are considered yang, while roots in the soil are considered yin. The yin property also represents material entities, such as nutrients; the yang property represents functions, like energy. Taste is divided into five groups, representing the Five Phases: sour—wood, bitter—fire, sweet—earth, pungent—metal, and salty—water. As shown in

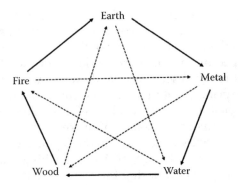

FIGURE 1.4
The five phases. As individual names or labels for the finer ramifications of yin and yang, the five phases represent aspects in the cycle of changes. The five phases are linked by the relationship between generation (—) and destruction (- - -).

Table 1.1, taste can be related to the human body and its organs, senses, and feelings, and even to color, the weather, and the seasons, through classification into the Five Phases. Antagonistic or affinitive relations between tastes and organs/senses are also judged or predicted by the principles of the Five Phases. For example, sour (wood) generates the heart (fire) but suppresses the spleen (earth), and salty (water) is related to the kidney and generates the liver while suppressing the heart. Though simplified unrealistically, Table 1.1 explains the basic notion of the Five Phases applied to food and health practices.

TABLE 1.1

Classification of Materials and Properties according to the Five Phases

Five Phases	Taste	Colors	Weather	Seasons	Bearing
Wood	Sour	Blue	Wind	Spring	East
Fire	Bitter	Red	Hot	Summer	South
Earth	Sweet	Yellow	Wet	Long summer	Center
Metal	Hot	White	Dry	Autumn	West
Water	Salty	Black	Cold	Winter	North

Five Phases	Organs	Intestines	Senses	Tissues	Feeling
Wood	Liver	Gall bladder	Eyes	Tendon	Anger
Fire	Heart	Small intestine	Tongue	Vein	Joy
Earth	Spleen	Stomach	Mouth	Muscle	Love
Metal	Lungs	Large intestine	Nose	Hair	Sorrow
Water	Kidney	Bladder	Ear	Bone	Fear

Korean Foods—History, Culture, and Characteristics

1.2.3 Traditional Chinese Medicine

Traditional societies like China and Korea have a long history of using food as medicine. Traditional Chinese medicine (TCM), for example, in Shennong's *Materia Medica*, divides types of medicine into three categories:

- 120 Upper medicines, which are nontoxic and usable in the long term as food
- 120 Middle medicines, which have a low level of toxicity and are used for chronic diseases
- 125 Lower medicines, which have a high level of toxicity and are used for acute illness

Food is considered the most important medicine to be used for the maintenance of health and prevention of illness, as well as in the first stages of treatment of an illness. The middle or lower medicines are used only when medicinal food (upper medicine) cannot cure a disease. Lists of medicines are found in many traditional Chinese works of literature. They have been developed over thousands of years of experience, mainly through human trials, and have substantiated the effectiveness of the theories of yin/yang and the Five Phases (Lee, 2004).

In TCM, food and medicine commonly have certain health functional properties, such as the four types of chi or ki (energy), the five tastes, descending/ascending, sinking/buoyant, channel tropism, and toxicity. The four types of chi are cold, cool, warm, and hot, which represent the causes of diseases in the body. Cold and cool are considered yin, while warm and hot are yang. Tastes and properties are also classified into yin and yang, as shown in Table 1.2 (Kim et al., 1995). All food materials are classified according to their different tastes and their properties: cool, classified as yin; neutral; or warm, classified as yang.

Healthy food in TCM implies balancing and harmonizing yin and yang and the Five Phases in a diet. A healthy diet must contain an even balance of food materials that have cold/cool (yin) and warm/hot (yang) properties and the five tastes. Therapeutic food (or functional food) means enforcing a certain chi for the imbalanced condition (illness) of a body, and enriching a certain taste to enhance or suppress an organ's function. The effectiveness of functional food has been explained systematically with this principle in TCM (Lee, 1998b).

TABLE 1.2

Classification of Chi, Taste, and Properties into Yin and Yang

	Yin	Yang
Chi	Cold, cool	Warm, hot
Taste	Sour, bitter, salty	Pungent, sweet, umami
Properties	Descending, sinking	Ascending, buoyant

The disease susceptibility and medicine response of individuals are also explained by the differences in chi and personality trait properties. The types of body constitution in TCM are focused on medicinal practice based on the theories of yin/yang and the Five Phases. In contrast, Korean Sasang constitutional typology is based on a combination of neo-Confucianism and the medical tradition of Korea, and describes nature as quaternary (Chae et al., 2003). Traditional Chinese medicine places importance on the harmony between humanity and nature, whereas Sasang typology emphasizes the harmony in social life and developing one's character.

1.2.4 Eastern Medicine and Sasang Typology

Chinese traditional medicine has contributed to the development of Eastern medicine in Korea, in combination with traditional folk medicine, as recorded by Hur Jun in 1610. Eastern medicine was further developed in Korea during the eighteenth and nineteenth centuries, and grew into Sasang medicine (typology): As described by Lee Je-Ma in 1894, Sasang is a unique theory of categorizing people into four body types according to their physical constitutions: taeyang (large yang), taeeum (large yin), soyang (small yang), and soeum (small yin). Figure 1.5 shows a schematic diagram of Sasang types from a biopsychological perspective (Chae et al., 2003). The yang types (taeyang and soyang) are extroverted and the eum (yin) types (taeeum and soeum) are introverted. the taeyang type is very rare in Korea. The body shape of the taeeum type is larger than those of the soeum and soyang types. The personality traits and physical characteristics are symbolically expressed by the organ size: taeyang—large lungs and small liver, soyang—large spleen and small kidney, taeeum—large liver and small lungs, and soeum—large kidney and small spleen (Lee and Choi, 1996). Sasang typology emphasizes

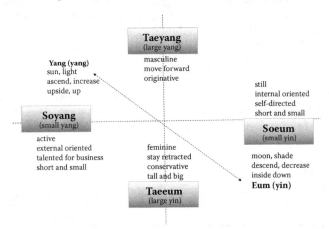

FIGURE 1.5
A schematic diagram of Sasang types from a biopsychological perspective. (From Chae, H. et al. 2003, *Journal of Alternative and Complementary Medicine*, 9(4):519–528.)

Korean Foods—History, Culture, and Characteristics

the importance of individual body types in the diagnosis and treatment of diseases and suggests prescribing different medicinal treatments and food intake for different body constitution types (Lee, 2007).

Many attempts to establish a reproducible and objective method of assessing the Sasang constitution types have been reported after the writing of Lee Je-Ma, but none of the methods has provided reproducible and satisfactory results. A questionnaire developed by KyungHee University (QSCC II) was widely studied for the assessment of Sasang types, and distinctive personality traits associated with Sasang types were demonstrated using psychometric and anthropometric instruments (Chae et al., 2003). Numerous food therapy schemes suggesting beneficial and harmful food items for different Sasang types have been reported and used by TCM doctors and dietitians in Korea (Lee, 2007). Table 1.3 shows an example of a Sasang food list, with foods that are beneficial for different body constitution types (Kim et al., 1995).

Although the assessment of individuals' constitution types is not conclusive, many people in Korea follow Sasang theory in selecting their food and herbal treatments, especially when their health is not satisfactory.

Considering food to be medicine, practitioners of TCM and Eastern medicine have studied each food ingredient for its yin/yang properties and its applicability in diet therapy. Their knowledge has been compiled in numerous classical medicine books in both China and Korea for hundreds of years, and has been practiced in everyday life at the household level as dietary customs. The term *boyak*, which means supplements to replenish weak points in a body, has been used widely in Korea, and the terms *functional food* and *therapeutic food* are, in fact, the scientific terms for *boyak*.

Many reports have suggested that the low-fat intake and high proportion of plant food in the Korean diet might be part of the reason for the lower prevalence of obesity, the lower death rates due to coronary heart disease or high blood pressure, and the lower rates of breast, prostate, and colon cancers than in many other Asian and Western countries (Lee et al., 2002). Koreans believe in the old traditional concept that "food is medicine." Therefore, herbs or fruit ingredients such as ginger, cinnamon, Job's tears, mugwort, pomegranate, citron, mushroom, ginseng, etc., are used in cooking, as well as for therapeutic foods. Food preparation has been likened to prescribing medicine for the individuals in a household. The word *yaknyum*, the general term for seasoning, means "thought of medicine." The enormous size of the health food market in Korea today reflects the country's tradition of food as medicine.

A survey on consumers' attitudes toward health food and their perceptions of health and food habits in Korea revealed that people considered food habits to be the most important factor in the maintenance of health, followed by physical exercise. More than 90% of people believed that food habits were the most important factor determining the health of human beings and that diseases could be cured by adjusting food habits (Lee et al., 1996a). Half of the subjects had made use of health foods (or "functional" foods), and 68% of them believed in their effectiveness (Lee et al., 1996b).

TABLE 1.3

Example of a Sasang Food List

	TaeYang	SoYang	TaeEum	SoEum
Cereals	Buckwheat	Barley, red beans, mung beans, barnyard millet, sesame	Soybeans, Job's tears, sugar, wheat, wheat flour, great millet, perilla, sweet potato, common millet, peanut	Sticky rice, hulled millet, glutinous millet, potato
Fruit	Kiwifruit, grapes, persimmon, cherries, Chinese quince	Watermelon, Korean melon, strawberries, banana, pineapple	Chestnuts, pear, walnuts, gingko nuts, pine nuts, apricot, mum, plum	Apple, mandarin orange, peach, jujube
Vegetables	Water shield, pine needles	Cucumber, Chinese cabbage, pumpkin, lettuce, eggplant, sow thistle, edible burdock bamboo shoot, Asian plantain	Radish, bellflower root, Indian lotus, taro, hemp, bracken, lanceolate root, shiitake mushroom, ear mushroom, matsutake mushroom, *Umbilicariaesculenta*	Water dropwort, Welsh onion, garlic, black pepper, ginger, spinach, carrot, red pepper, crown daisy, onion, mustard
Fishes	Oysters, abalone, conch, shrimp, crucian carp, crab, sea slug, mussels	Flatfish, puffer, turtle, crawfish, carp, snapping, snakehead fish	Freshwater snail, codfish, yellow corvina, small octopus, brown croaker, herring, squid, brown seaweed, laver, kelp	Alaska pollack, loach, eel, snake, catfish
Meats		Pork, eggs, duck	Beef, milk	Chicken, lamb, dog meat, pheasant, goat, sparrow meat

Source: Kim, J. Y. et al. 1995. *Journal of Constitutional Medicine*, 7:263–279.

1.3 Future of Korean Functional Food

Recently, molecular biologists have started to recognize that variations in the genetic makeup of individuals may cause variations in their responses to nutrient intake (Milner, 2004). It is often observed that, even with similar food consumption patterns in a family, one person suffers from obesity while another does not. Food allergies and celiac disease, for example, provide other evidence of genetic variation as it relates to food components (Murray, 2005). With the completion of the Human Genome Project and the powerful tools of molecular biology, it is now possible to elucidate the effects of nutrients or bioactive food ingredients on the regulation of gene expression (i.e., nutrigenomics) or on the impact of variations in gene structure on one's response to food components (i.e., nutrigenetics). Genetic components responsible for differences in dietary response have been proposed for many years by molecular biologists, and research to examine these nutrient–gene interactions has recently begun. Individual genetic variation may possibly be explained by single nucleotide polymorphisms (SNPs).

The health effects of food components are related to specific interactions on a molecular level, SNP in gene regulation, translational control of ribonucleic acid, enzyme regulation (proteomics), and metabolite modulation (metabolomics), which occur as genotypes (Ommen, 2004). On the other hand, in traditional Eastern medicine, numerous phenotypic data on diet response to health have been accumulated and systematically classified by the Sasang body constitution theory. Body constitution is a genomic trait of individuals, which is mainly determined by SNPs. Therefore, it is possible to relate the molecular level genomic studies to the body constitution typology for the scientific substantiation of traditional functional foods (Lee, 2007).

As body constitution types are genomic traits of individuals, it will be possible to determine Sasang types with molecular level genomic studies when sufficient data are accumulated. It is important to identify the genes or SNPs responsible for the phenotypic body constitution types, specifically taeyang, taeeum, soyang, and soeum. Once they have been found, we will be able to classify Sasang constitution types objectively and reliably and be ready to utilize the old wisdom of diet therapy, which has been developed for thousands of years through human trials, as illustrated in Figure 1.6.

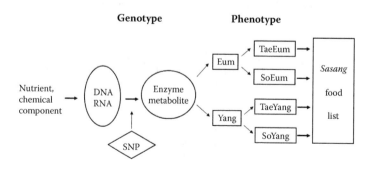

FIGURE 1.6
The relationship between nutrigenetic studies and Sasang body constitution typology. (From Lee, C. H. 2007, *Food Science and Technology Research*, 13(2):89–95.)

An attempt was made to develop marker genes for the classification of Sasang body constitutions (Park, 2006). TCM school students in Korea, who were classified identically by QSCC and by three TCM doctors, were selected; their blood samples were assayed with microarray analysis; and the Sasang-specific genes were identified. About 145 genes were differentially expressed in a microarray, and they were clustered into three groups, respectively: tae-eum, so yang, and so eum. Genes expressed differentially depending on the Sasang constitution types were related to signal transduction, transport, and immune response in their function. Although this study was not conclusive in its classification of the constitution types, it provides the possibility of using microarray analysis and SNP analysis of specific genes for the objective determination of body constitution types (Lee, 2007).

Figure 1.7 illustrates the relationship between nutrigenetic studies and Sasang typology, which have developed toward opposite directions in the East and the West. If we are able to find a channel to relate the Western analytical approach to the Eastern holistic approach, we will achieve great advancement in human nutrition and biomedical research. It will allow us to use all of the data accumulated in Eastern medicine for predicting the health effectiveness of foods. Recent research on nutrigenomic/epigenetic studies may provide a possible way of communicating genomic studies with Sasang typology.

If we are able to identify the genetic markers that are responsible for Sasang typology, we can select food materials useful for an individual with specific markers from the Sasang food list. This will allow Western analytical researchers to communicate with Eastern medical doctors, and to discuss the scientific substantiation of traditional functional foods in the East (Lee and Lee, 2003). It will open a new era of nutrigenomics, and we will be able to

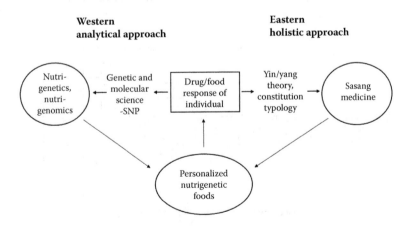

FIGURE 1.7
Collaboration of Western analytical approach and Eastern holistic approach in the field of functional food. (From Lee, C. H. 2007, *Food Science and Technology Research*, 13(2):89–95.)

scientifically substantiate the health benefits of traditional functional foods more easily. It will reduce the variation in experimental results, minimize the cost of finding scientific evidence for functional foods, and consequently prevent the adverse effects of functional food, which often occur in some segments of a population. Personalized or tailor-made functional food that is effective for groups of people with specific body constitutions will be created to enhance their vitality and to treat their health problems.

1.4 Conclusion

Considering food to be medicine, practitioners of traditional medicine in Korea have studied each food ingredient for its properties, taste, and medicinal effects. Their knowledge has been compiled in numerous medicinal books for thousands of years, and has been practiced in everyday life at the household level as part of Korean dietary customs.

Present food law requires scientific substantiation to claim the health effects of a functional food. However, it is not an easy task to verify the physiological and psychological effects of foods made of multiple ingredients. In addition, an individual's response to the intake of a food component varies, as mentioned in the Sasang typology. Consequently, present food regulations restrict the marketing of traditional functional food. There is a strong need to relate the traditional functional food concept to modern scientific methodologies, such as nutrigenomics, in order to be able to use the enormous amount of data compiled in the jewelry box of Eastern medicine, accumulated through a thousand years of human trials.

After the long journey of the food industry through the survival-food age, the convenience-food age, and the functional-food age, we are expecting to usher in a "personalized functional food" era through the collaborative efforts of molecular biologists and Eastern medicine researchers. The new era of personalized functional food will lend great opportunities to future food industries and will contribute greatly to the betterment of the quality of human life.

References

Barnes, G. L. 1993. *China, Korea and Japan: The Rise of Civilization in East Asia.* London: Thames and Hudson.

Chae, H., I. K. Lyoo, S. J. Lee et al. 2003. An alternative way to individualized medicine: Psychological and physical traits of Sasang typology. *Journal of Alternative and Complementary Medicine,* 9(4):519–528.

Choi, B. K. 1983. Comparison of Paleolithic cultures in Northeast Asia. In *Hankuksaron* (Korean History), vol. 12, *Korean Archeology Ia*, 228–306 (in Korean).

Han, Y. H. 1983. Regional comparison. In *Korean History 12: Archeology of Korea I*. National History Editorial Committee, 479–521 (in Korean).

Kim, J. Y., C. W. Kim, B. H. Koh, and I. B. Song. 1995. Justification and usage of food classification according to body constitution. *Journal of Constitutional Medicine*, 7:263–279 (in Korean).

Kwon, D. Y., K. R. Chung, and H. J. Yang. 2017. *The truth of birth and propagation of Korean red pepper (kochu)*. Seoul: Free Academy Press.

Lee, C. H. 1995a. An introduction to Korean food culture. *Korean and Korean American Studies Bulletin*, 6:6–10.

Lee, C. H. 1995b. Changes in the dietary patterns, health, and nutritional status of Koreans during the last century. *Korean and Korean American Studies Bulletin*, 6:32–47.

Lee, C. H. 1998a. The food ways of Paleolithic man in the Northeast Asia and Korean Peninsula. *Korean Culture Research*, 31:415–458 (in Korean).

Lee, C. H. 1998b. Health concepts in the traditional Korean diet: Therapeutic use of foods in East Asia. *Korean and Korean American Studies Bulletin*, 9(1/2):8–18.

Lee, C. H. 1999. The Primitive Pottery Age of Northeast Asia and its importance in Korean food history. *Korean Culture Research*, 32:325–457 (in Korean).

Lee, C. H. 2001. *Fermentation Technology in Korea*. Seoul: Korea University Press.

Lee, C. H. 2004. Functional food of interest to ASEAN: From traditional experience to modern production and trading. *Food Science Biotechnology*, 13(3):390–395.

Lee, C. H. 2007. Harmonization of Eastern and Western health knowledge: Nutrigenetics and Sasang typology. *Food Science and Technology Research*, 13(2):89–95.

Lee, C. H. and M. L. Kim. 2016. History of fermented foods in Northeast Asia. In *Ethnic Fermented Foods and Alcoholic Beverages of Asia* (Ed.: J. P. Tamang). New Delhi: Springer, 1–16.

Lee, C. H., M. R. Kim, and S. J. Rhee. 2015a. *Rice Revolution*. Seoul: Sikanyeon Publishing (in Korean).

Lee, C. H. and T. W. Kwon. 2005. History of soybean utilization. In *Soybean* (Ed.: Soy-world Museum Construction Committee). Seoul: Korea University Press (in Korean).

Lee, C. H. and C. Y. Lee. 2003. Paradigm shift: Harmonization of Eastern and Western food system. In *Bioprocesses and Biotechnology for Functional Foods and Nutraceuticals*. (Eds.: J. R. Neeser and J. B. German). New York: Marcel Dekker, 415–425.

Lee, C. H., H. P. Moon, Y. T. Kim et al. 2015b. *Korea Unification and Food Security*. Seoul: Sikanyeon Publishing.

Lee, C. Y., C. H. Lee, and T. W. Kwon. 2002. Future of foods: Harmonization of Eastern and Western food systems. http://www.worldfoodscience.org/vol3-2/focus-lee.html.

Lee, E. J., S. O. Ro, and C. H. Lee. 1996a. A survey of consumer attitude toward health food in Korea: (1) Consumer perceptions of health and food habits. *Korean Journal of Dietary Culture*, 11:475–485 (in Korean).

Lee, E. J., S. O. Ro, and C. H. Lee. 1996b. A survey of consumer attitude toward health food in Korea: (2) Consumer perceptions of health food. *Korean Journal of Dietary Culture*, 11:487–495 (in Korean).

Lee, J. M. and S. H. Choi. 1996. *Longevity and Life Preservation in Eastern Medicine.* Seoul: KyungHee University Press (in Korean).

Lee, S. W. 1984. *Hankuk Sikpum Sahoesa* (History of Korean Food and Society). Seoul: Kyomunsa, p. 168 (in Korean).

Lim, S. K. 1986. *Handankogi.* Seoul: Jungsinsekeisa (in Korean).

Magner, L. N. 1992. *A History of Medicine.* New York: Marcel Dekker.

Milner, J. A. 2004. Molecular targets for bioactive food components. *Journal of Nutrition,* 9:134.

Murray, J. 2005. Celiac disease: A model of genetically determined food intolerance. In *ILSI Annual Meeting,* Jan. 14–19, New Orleans, LA.

Nahm, A. C. 1988. *Korea, Tradition and Transformation.* Elizabeth, NJ: Holly International Corp.

Ni, Maoshing. 1995. The Yellow Emperor's Classic of Medicine. Boston: Shambhala.

Ommen, B. V. 2004. Nutrigenomics: Exploiting systems biology in the nutrition and health arena. *Nutrition,* 20:4–8.

Park, S. S. 2006. Scientific rationale for Sasang constitution: Development of marker genes for the classification of the constitution. *Proceedings of KCIST-2006 Nutrigenomics: New Perspectives and Applications,* July 20–22, Muju, Korea.

Sohn, P. K. 1983. Human race and residence. In *Hankuksaron* (Korean History), vol. 12, *Korean Archeology Ia,* 187–211 (in Korean).

Yoon, S. S. 1993. *Hankuk Sikpumsa Yongu* (Korean Dietary Culture Studies). Seoul: Shin Kwang Publishing Co (in Korean).

2

Korean Diets and Their Tastes

Dae Young Kwon and Kyung Rhan Chung

CONTENTS

2.1 Korean Diet (K-Diet) 23
2.2 K-Diet as Healthy Diet 25
2.3 Definition 26
2.4 Characteristics 27
2.5 Structure of Bapsang and Representative K-Diet 30
2.6 Siwonhan-Mat: Third Taste of Korean Foods 34
2.7 Understanding Siwonhan-Mat from Linguistic and Literary
  Approaches 36
  2.7.1 Origin of Siwonhada (Infinitive Form of Siwonhan) 36
  2.7.2 Understanding Siwonhan-Mat from a Scientific Approach 37
2.8 Determining Factors of Siwonhan-Mat 39
2.9 Conclusion 39
Acknowledgments 40
References 41

2.1 Korean Diet (K-Diet)

Korea has developed a unique food culture connected to its long agricultural history. Recently, interest in Korean food, especially regarding its health benefits, has greatly increased. However, there are insufficient resources and research available on the characteristics and definitions of Korean cuisine. Although the K-diet has been widely discussed in regard to raw ingredients, traditional cooking methods and technology, fundamental principles, and knowledge, it would be valuable to preserve the traditional methods and knowledge of Korean foods rather than focus on the raw materials themselves. Korean meals have historically been served with bap (cooked rice), kuk (dishes with broth), kimchi, and banchan (side dishes) to be consumed at the same time. As traditional baking or frying were not common methods, Koreans tended to use fermenting, boiling, blanching, seasoning, and pickling. Among these methods, the most characteristic method is fermentation. The process of fermentation enriches food flavors and preserves foods.

Located in Northeast Asia, Korea has an agricultural history that has continued for more than 5,000 years despite its close proximity to China. The Han Chinese, who founded the Three Kingdoms and the Qin, Tang, Song, and Ming dynasties, developed their own language and controlled China until the Qing Dynasty emerged. Korea, from Kochosun and the period of the Three States, including Kokuryo, Baekje, and Silla to Koryo and Chosun, maintained independence from China and developed a unique culture and language. Linguistically, Korean belongs to the Altaic language group along with the Japonic, Mongolic, Tungusic, Hungarian, and Finnish languages. Moreover, the Mongolian spot that is prevalent among Koreans suggests biological differences between Koreans and Chinese. Likewise, Korean food culture has also developed distinctly from Chinese cuisine.

According to Kwon (2015), the development of food technology was prompted by the desire to preserve food resources. For example, in China, frying and pickling were the prevalent methods in reducing water content (a_w) to protect against microbial spoilage of food. In contrast, the limited production of cooking oils in Korea led to the development of the fermentation process for food preservation, which utilizes effective microorganisms against microbial spoilage. While milk was the main ingredient in fermented products such as cheese and yogurt, in countries with strong livestock industries, the main ingredients in Korean fermented foods were grains and vegetables. This was due to their settled lifestyle and focus on agriculture. Korean foods have developed from the necessity of preserving them during hot summers and long, harsh winters on the Korean peninsula characterized by rocky ocean fronts on the east, south, and west, and by rugged mountains on the north. This geographical isolation from neighboring countries and the distinct weather allowed the early Korean people to develop the most enduring cultural legacies of the Korean diet. In this environment, salted beans, fish, and vegetables were preserved by fermentation. Historically, Koreans have made various jang (fermented soy products) (Shin and Jeong, 2015), including kanjang (soy sauce), doenjang (soybean paste), and kochujang (red pepper paste), and diverse types of kimchi (Jang et al., 2015) with vegetables. These unique fermentation techniques are examples of authentic Korean food (Kwon et al., 2014).

Korea has developed unique foods as well as a food culture that is fundamentally distinct from Chinese or Japanese food cultures. Food is one of the key elements of culture and presents possibilities for promulgation of various cultural contents. However, this effect has been diminished by a lack of cohesive definitions and concepts in Korean food culture. Therefore, it is necessary to establish consistent definitions and concepts to be used in relation to the Korean diet.

2.2 K-Diet as Healthy Diet

As leading a healthy lifestyle has become an important global trend, renowned healthy diets, such as the Mediterranean (Willett et al., 1995) and Nordic (Adamsson et al., 2012) diets, have been studied and promoted globally. Moreover, studies on the French diet have reported an interesting epidemiological observation called the French paradox (Ferrieres, 2004), referencing that French people have low incidence of cardiovascular disease (CVD) despite high consumption of saturated fats in their diet. It is presumed that the French lifestyle and consumption of red wine (resveratrol) lower their incidence rates of CVD (Simini, 2000).

Research has suggested that the health benefits of Korean food are due to the diversity of ingredients and cooking methods used in Korean cuisine (*Health Magazine*, 2006). The average life expectancy in Korea is over 80 years despite the popularity of high-salt dishes such as kuk, tang, and kimchi. Excessive salt consumption is a risk factor for CVD. This phenomenon has been referred to as the Korean paradox (Park and Kwock, 2015) and some researchers have claimed that the paradox can be explained by the regular consumption of vegetables and the types of salt used in Korean cuisine. Historically, Koreans have used unrefined, baked, or fermented salts, which may have different health effects compared to refined salt in relation to CVD. Research has shown that consumption of fermented foods like kimchi is not associated with high blood pressure (Song and Lee, 2014). Moreover, high potassium intake assists in discharging salt from the body and, as a result, reduces the risk of CVD (Park and Kwock, 2015).

As problems of overnutrition have become prevalent, the Korean diet (Kwon et al., 2015), characterized by the high consumption of namul (seasoned vegetable dishes) and fermented foods, can bring about positive impacts worldwide. While the health benefits of the Korean diet have been supported by research, resources are needed to further understand the elements of balanced meals in the this diet. Although there are some definitions and characteristics of individual dishes available, there is not a holistic approach to categorizing the data in order to explain the health benefits of Korean food.

The establishment of consistent definitions and concepts in Korean food (K-food) should be based on systematic and scientific research in order to promote its health benefits globally. For that, scholars of the food and nutritional sciences have collaborated and announced the "Seoul Declaration on K-Diet: Korean Heritage and Healthiness." In the postindustrial age, culture is one of the key elements of a country's competitiveness in the global market. Therefore, this chapter will discuss definitions, characteristics, representative K-foods that have been introduced in the Seoul declaration and embody fundamental aspects of a Korean meal (Kwon et al., 2015).

2.3 Definition

K-diet and K-food are two separate concepts. The concept of the K-diet is used to represent traditional Korean food culture, cooking methods, and dietary habits and patterns; K-foods are the food constituents of the K-diet. K-food and K-diet are often described as Korean cuisine, Korean diet, or traditional Korean food. A few elements of defining food culture have been put forward, such as frequently consumed foods, raw ingredients or materials, technology or cooking methods, and the fundamental principles found in the country's dietary patterns. These views put different emphases on food and diet.

The first aspect introduced, which views K-foods as frequently consumed foods, would allow popular foods among youth, such as jajangmyeon (noodles with jang), pizza, or fried chicken, to be considered K-food. The criteria of time period for Korean food would be needed but introduce unneeded complexity. The second idea, which has often been cited by the Korean Ministry of Agriculture, suggests that K-food should be made with ingredients (agricultural products) produced only in Korea (Chung, 2015). According to this view, kimchi made from imported cabbage would not be considered K-food. The third view proposes the use of traditional cooking technology as the key element of K-food in an attempt to overcome this issue. Although it is important to preserve traditional Korean cooking methods, this point of view focuses only on the physical and material aspects of methods. As this view overlooks technological advances, doenjang fermented in jars other than hangari (Korean earthenware crock) would not qualify as K-food.

Therefore, when discussing K-food and K-diet, one should focus on whether certain dishes are made with traditionally used ingredients regardless of the origin of produce, follow traditional cooking methods and principles, and, lastly, preserve the spirit behind traditional Korean food practices. The definition of traditional Korean food by Chung (2009, 2015) reflects these ideas: "Food made with raw materials or ingredients that have been traditionally used in Korea, or with the similar ingredients, use authentic or other similar cooking methods, have historical and cultural characteristics, and have developed and been passed on through people's lives." This meaning contained in Korean food has been interpreted as consistence, patience, consideration, beauty, and appreciation for arts. In the Seoul declaration, the definition of K-diet represents the interpretation as follows:

> K-diet is composed of bab (cooked rice) and kuk, and various banchan with one serving called bapsang. Kimchi is always served at every meal. The principal aspects of K-diet include proportionally high consumption of fresh or cooked vegetables (namul), moderate to high consumption of legumes and fish and low consumption of red meat. Banchan is mostly seasoned with various jang (fermented soy products), medicinal herbs, and sesame or perilla oil.

Korean Diets and Their Tastes

The traditional ingredients of K-food consist of grains and vegetables; however, oceanic regions have used fish and seaweed. Medicinal herbs such as garlic, green onions, and red pepper have also been used to enhance flavor and add to the health benefits of food. Korean fermentation technology has played an important role in preserving these food resources, including legumes, vegetables, and fish. Historically, grains, including rice and barley, were the main source of carbohydrates. Legumes and fish provided protein. Vegetable oils made from sesame or perilla served as a main supply of fat. As metabolic disorders caused by overnutrition have become a serious problem, the Korean diet can be promoted as a healthy alternative. From a sociocultural perspective, the structure of the traditional Korean meal (Kwon et al., 2015), which allows people to share various banchan together, has played an educational role in teaching common etiquette and courtesy to be practiced while eating communal meals (see Figure 1 in Kwon et al., 2015).

2.4 Characteristics

The characteristics of a K-diet include:

1. Various recipes based on rice and grains
2. More fermented foods
3. More vegetables from wild landscapes and the seas
4. More legumes and fish and less red meat
5. More medicinal herbs like garlic, green onion, red pepper, and ginger
6. More sesame and perilla oils
7. Little deep-fat fried cooking
8. More meals based on seasonal produce
9. Various local cuisines
10. More home-cooked meals

These 10 characteristics are explained in more detail next.

Various recipes based on rice and grains: While the main energy source found in Western cuisine is wheat, the predominant Korean dietary energy source is grains such as rice and barley. Bap is served with kuk and banchan (Figure 2.1). Variations of this format, such as kukbap, a dish that combines kuk and bap served in one bowl, and bibimbap (Chung et al., 2015), a dish with mixed bap and banchan, are also popular (Kwon et al., 2015). Sungnyung (Moose, 1911) is the last step of a meal. It is a traditional Korean

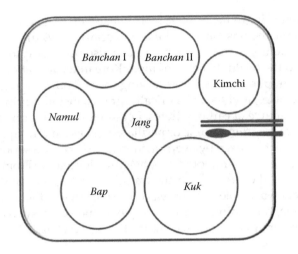

FIGURE 2.1
Diagram of basic bapsang in everyday Korean diet. The structure of the traditional Korean bapsang (see Figure 1 in Kwon et al., 2015). Bap is served alongside kuk, which assists in the swallowing and digestion of the food. In the bapsang, banchan comprises one type of kimchi, one namul, one vegetable dish (banchan I), and one high-protein dish (banchan II), usually made from fish or meat as chim or gui. Jang, or salted dishes such as jangachi and jeotgal, is used to season food and stimulate one's appetite. A variety of bapsang can be constructed using diverse ingredients and cooking methods depending on the season, regions, and one's preference. Overlapping ingredients and methods allow for well-balanced flavors and nutrients.

drink made from the roasted crust of rice that forms on the bottom of a pot after cooking rice.

More fermented foods: Throughout the agricultural history of Korea, fermentation technology has been widely used to enrich the flavors of food by utilizing effective microorganisms against microbial spoilage. Fermented soy products such as kanjang, doenjang, cheongkukjang, (Shin and Jeong, 2015) and kochujang are the fundamental ingredients of various sauces and kuk. Doenjang-kuk, made with vegetables and doenjang, is a traditional iconic kuk. Kimchi is another representative Korean fermented food known for its authenticity and its health benefit of reducing the activity of harmful bacteria. Jeotgal is salted, fermented seafood used to enhance flavor and appetite rather than increase the nutritional value of food. As seen before, traditional fermentation technology has been used to intensify flavors in food beyond its role in food preservation.

More vegetables from wild landscapes and the sea: The Korean diet is characterized by high vegetable intake, which is due to the agricultural environment of the country. Vegetables such as lettuce, peppers, carrots, or cucumbers were often consumed raw with sauces made of kochujang, doenjang, kanjang, or vinegar, and topped with sesame seeds. Cabbage or spinach were often blanched and seasoned with traditional spices. Both raw and dried vegetables were ingredients for kuk, which was flavored with doenjang

(Kang et al., 2016). Kimchi is the most widely enjoyed vegetable dish in Korea. Korean cuisine also includes various types of seaweed dishes made from laver, green algae, kelp, *Hizikia fusiformis*, and *Capsosiphon fulvescens*, all of which are abundant sources of dietary fiber and vitamins.

More legumes and fish and less red meats: Koreans have enjoyed diverse legumes such as soybeans, mung beans, red beans, cowpeas, peanuts, walnuts, and ginkgo nuts. Surrounded on three sides by oceans, Koreans have also consumed fish using various techniques to prepare them, such as grilling, boiling in sauce, and marinating. Because lamb, horse meat, beef, and pork were rare in the agricultural environment, the main source of protein intake was poultry, such as chicken and pheasant.

More medicinal herbs like garlic, green onion, red pepper, and ginger: Compared to the geographically close countries of China and Japan, one of the interesting characteristics of Korean food is the diverse use of yangnyum (a kind of seasoning), created with garlic, green onions, red pepper, and ginger (Surh, 2003). While spices like black pepper have been widely used to hide the unpleasant odors of food in Southeast Asia, medicinal herbs have been used to enhance flavors and increase the food's health benefits (Hu, 1610).

More sesame and perilla oils: Historically, the amount of animal-based and vegetable cooking oils produced in Korea was quite limited. While camellia, castor, sesame, and perilla oils were produced in Korea, mainly sesame and perilla oils were used in cooking. With its distinctive aroma, sesame oil was used in kuk, namul, and bibimbap. Perilla oil was used in pan-frying foods or making yukwa (a puffed rice snack).

Little deep-fat fried cooking: As mentioned before, deep-frying techniques could not have developed in Korea due to the limited production of animal-based and vegetable cooking oils. Instead, cooking methods such as pan-frying or stir-frying, which did not require large amounts of oil, were developed. Jeon, a type of pancake made from flour batter, is the most representative example of this cooking method.

More meals based on seasonal products: Korea has an advanced agricultural industry and four distinctive seasons, which provide an abundance and diversity of ingredients. For this reason, its cuisine has developed recipes that use fresh ingredients available in each season. For example, Koreans make fresh kimchi all year round, utilizing different varieties of seasonal cabbage, except during the winter, as kimchi is stored underground in jars to control temperature for fermentation (Jang et al., 2015).

Various local cuisines: Surrounded by oceans on three sides, Korea lacks extensive plains—mountains cover over 70 percent of its territory. Recipes have been developed based on regional characteristics: grain-based dishes such as bibimbap in the plains (Surh, 2003), seafood dishes in oceanic regions (Kim and Jang, 2015), vegetable dishes such as namul in mountainous regions, and dishes with freshwater fish or clams in regions near rivers. The identification and refinement of these regional recipes and ingredients would be valuable.

More home-cooked meals: The history of agriculture in Korea has shaped a group culture based on family and community. Dedication, communication, and consideration among family members are deeply held values in its culture. As meals are cooked with natural ingredients rather than processed ingredients, usually by mothers, Koreans have believed that food represents a mother's love. This idea has been reflected in the K-diet with jipbap (home-cooked meal) and umma-sonmat (the taste of mother's love).

2.5 Structure of Bapsang and Representative K-Diet

As mentioned in Kwon et al. (2015), it is crucial to analyze the components of a K-diet and identify K-foods representing these characteristics. For easy understanding we adapted our previous paper's report (Kwon et al., 2015) to introduce Korean bapsang as follows (Figure 2.1; also see Figure 1 in Kwon et al., 2015): Korea's traditional meal (bapsang) is generally made up of four constituents:

- Bap (cooked rice) provides calories, the main source of energy.
- Kuk (soup) allows people to chew and swallow rice, in turn supporting the digestive system. Previously, the word kuk was translated into soup; however, kuk is quite different from Western soup (Kwon et al., 2015; Kang et al., 2016).
- Banchan (side dishes) make up the third element and make the food taste better to support digestion while replenishing the body with nutrition. Usually, namul, legumes, and fish comprise banchan.
- Jang (sauce, yangnyum) which stimulates people's appetites (Hwang et al., 2005; Shin and Jeong, 2015). Yangnyum includes herbs like garlic, green onions, red pepper, and onions. Unlike spices that are often used to cover or remove unpleasant smells of food, Korean yangnyum is used to enhance flavors and increase the health benefits of the foods it is combined with (Surh, 2003).

The kinds of bap (cooked rice) that are used in main dishes include steamed rice, boiled barley, and multigrain rice. As for kuk, doenjang kuk, miyok (sea mustard) kuk, and beef kuk are commonly eaten. Kimchi is always there as part of banchan, as are others, including roasted meat, vegetables, and salad dressed with garlic and chili powder; vegetables served as cooked or fresh namul; cooked namul seasoned with sesame seed/oil or perilla seed/oil, and fresh vegetables seasoned with vinegar—also served as side dishes. The most basic seasoning used to make the food savory is kanjang (fermented soy sauce; jang in Korean means fermented soy sauce or paste), doenjang

Korean Diets and Their Tastes 31

(fermented soybean paste), vinegar, kochujang, and jeotkal (fermented fish sauce from anchovies, shrimp, etc.) (Shin and Jeong, 2015). Jeotkal can be eaten as a side dish itself and more often is used as seasoning (Hwang et al., 2005). In Korea, people drink sungnyung (like tea made from leftover scorched rice) to finish off a meal (Moose, 1911). By using these four fundamental foods, Korean people have been developing their own unique meals (bapsang) by choosing one or more elements in each category.

Key elements of the Korean meal structure have been established and the 100 most representative K-foods have been selected according to these elements (see Table 2.1). Most Korean meals are composed of banchan served with bap, but they are often misunderstood as main dishes by Westerners. Although some modern Korean restaurants offer food served in courses, the traditional Korean meal is served all at once on the table. One-bowl dishes are not included in the bap category in Table 2.1 as one-bowl dishes and rice cakes are consumed during busy farming seasons or on special occasions, such as weddings, sixtieth birthdays, and ancestral rites (Kwon et al., 2015). Examples of one-bowl meals include kuksu (a noodle dish), kukbap made from kuk and bap, bibimbap (Chung et al., 2015) made from bap and banchan mixed with jang, and theokkuk made from rice cake and consumed on New Year's Day. The kuk category includes kuk and kuk-based one-bowl dishes (Kwon et al., 2015), such as chigae, jeonkol, and tang. The banchan category consists of kimchi, namul, and banchan made from protein sources such as meat and fish. The jang category comprises jang, which is used for seasoning and stimulating one's appetite. This includes salted banchan, such as jangachi, jeotgal, and other types of yangnyum. Drinks, such as sungnyung, theok, and hankwa are included in the dessert category. Although this classification is disparate from the traditional Korean meal structure (Yoon, 1999), it is helpful for sharing with those who are familiar with the theories and concepts of modern food science. More discourse will be needed to refine this table to effectively bridge this approach between traditional understanding and modern food science.

While cuisine from the Korean royal court has been widely studied and is currently served in restaurants, this chapter focuses on food traditionally consumed by the common people. The traditional Korean meal table, or bapsang, is categorized by the purpose of the meal. It differs depending on whom the meal is for and the occasion for the meal. For example, a meal for guests would be different compared to a meal for elders of a family. Food consumed during celebrations such as birthdays and weddings would not be the same as food for funerals and ancestral rites. Each Korean holiday, including *Seollal* (New Year's Day), *Boreum* (day of the full moon), *Chuseok* (Korean Thanksgiving Day at full moon in mid-autumn), *Dano* (the fifth day of the fifth month of the year according to the lunar calendar), *Chilseok* (July 7 in the lunar calendar), and *Dongji* (winter solstice), is celebrated with unique and seasonal dishes such as spring bapsang, summer bapsang, autumn bapsang and winter bapsang).

TABLE 2.1

Categories of Korean Bapsang (Figure 2.1) and Representative Korean Foods

Category	Subcategory		Representative Korean Foods (K-Food)
Bap			Ssalbap (white rice, brown rice, black rice), boribap, kongbap, okokbap, nurungji (sungnyung)
Kuk	Kuk		Doenjangkuk, bukeokuk, kongnamulkuk, miyok-kuk, soegogimukuk, torankuk
	Chigae		Kimchichigae, doenjangchigae, cheongkukjangchigae, sundubuchigae, oigamjeong
Banchan	Kimchi		Baechukimchi (bossamkimchi), kkakdugi, oisobagi, chonggakkimchi, mulkimchi (dongchimi, nabakkimchi), yeolmukimchi, gatkimchi
	Namul	Saengchae	Saengchae (radish, cucumber), juksunkyeojachae, buchumuchim, dalraemuchim, miyokmuchim, paraemuchim
		Sukchae	Kongnamul, sikeumchinamul, dorajinamul, kosarinamul, beoseotnamul, aehobaknamul, gajinamul, chwinamul, naenginamul, gondrenamul, meowideulkkaejeuptang, japchae, tangpyeongchae (mukmuchim), gujeolpan
	Banchan	Chim	Kalbichim, suyuk, saengseonchim, sundae, kaetnipchim
		Gui	Kimgui, saengseongui, bulgoki, teok-kalbi, bukeogui, deodeokgui, borigulbi
		Jorim	Saengseonjorim, soegokijangjorim, kongjaban, yeongeunjorim, dubujorim
		Bokeum	Myeolchibokeum, ojingobokeum, jeyukbokeum, teokboki, dakbokeum, oibokeum (oibaetduri)
		Jeon	Saengseonjeon, chaesojeon (squash, eggplant, burdock, shiitake), hwauangjeok (pasanjeok), nokdubindaeteok, haemulpajeon, buchujeon, dubumuchim, yukjeon
		Hoe	Saengseonhoe, hongeohoe, kanghoe (green onions, water parsley), dureupsukhoe
		Dried banchan	Bukak, ssam (loose leaf lettuce, perilla leaf, crown daisy)
Jang	Jang		Jang (doenjang, cheongkukjang, kochujang, kanjang)
	Jeolim		Jangachi
	Jeotgal		Jeotgal (sikhae)
Miscellaneous	One-bowl food		Bibimbap, theokmandutkuk (theok-kuk, mandutkuk), kuksu (naengmyeon, kalkuksu, kongkuksu, kuksujangkuk)
	Teok, hankwa		Shaped teok (songpyeon), pounded teok (injeolmi), steamed teok (baekseolki, ssukseolki, siruteok, jeungpyeon, yaksik), pan-fried teok (hwajeon), boiled teok (gyeongdan), yakkwa, yugwa, dasik
	Beverage		Sikhye, sujeongkwa, omija-cha, hwachae

Korean Diets and Their Tastes 33

As seen previously, the Korean bapsang varies according to the purpose of the meal. This section introduces jeongwol daeboreumsang (a kind of bapsang at first full moon of the year) as an example of a holiday meal, and kaeul bapsang (bapsang for autumn) as an example of a seasonal bapsang (a kind of bapsang served at autumn).

Jeongwol daeboreum bapsang: Koreans traditionally used the lunar calendar, so a full moon was considered to have special importance, and it was believed that days with a full moon were filled with yin/yang (see Chung et al., 2015). The celebration of the first full moon, which falls on the 15th day of the lunar calendar, is the biggest holiday along with the eighth full moon, chusoek. During the celebration people wish for good health and fortune in the upcoming year by playing traditional games and sharing meals (Figure 2.2). In the morning of jeongwol daeboreum, people make okokbap with five grains (glutinous rice, red beans, beans, sorghum, millet) and dried namul (bracken, mushroom, eggplant, squash, cucumber, dried radish greens, aster), which is preserved from

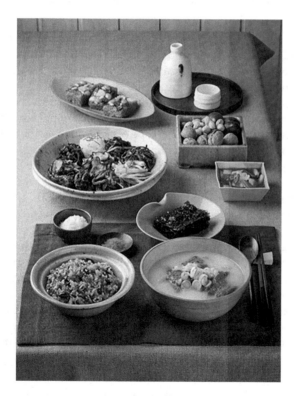

FIGURE 2.2
Jeongwol daeboreum-sang. This bapsang is served on jeongwol daeboreum-sang, the 15th day of the lunar calendar. It consists of okokbap, gomkuk, namul from the past year (eggplant, bracken, squash, dried radish greens, aster, pepper, cucumber, mushroom), kimgui, nabakkimchi, yaksik, and bureom. People share gwibalgisul with the meal and wish for good health and fortune in the upcoming year. Gwibalgi means "ear-quickening."

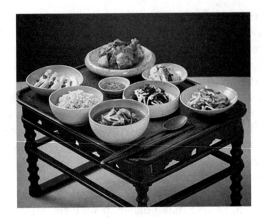

FIGURE 2.3
Kaeul bapsang, an example of a simple seasonal bapsang. New-harvest rice, aukdoenjangkuk, dakdoritang, dububuchim, beoseotnamul, paraemuchim, and chongkak kimchi are served with kanjang.

the past year to be consumed in the winter. These dried namul are first soaked in water, blanched, then seasoned or stir-fried. Dried namul is a great source of nutrients, dietary fiber, minerals, and vitamin D, which is difficult to source during the winter season. Cracking bureom and nuts, such as walnuts and ginkgo nuts, is another popular tradition believed to prevent skin problems through the consumption of unsaturated fatty acid. People also enjoy the custom of kwibalkisul, which is sharing a type of rice wine together while wishing good fortune for the year ahead. Kwibalki means "ear quickening."

Kaeul bapsang: Bapsang served in the fall follows the basic structure of the K-diet described in Figure 2.3. This structure of bapsang was established in the Chosun Dynasty. It consisted of bap made with new-harvest rice and other grains, kuk, kimchi, and various banchan. Depending on the available ingredients, mothers would make banchan using an appropriate cooking method, such as the ones suggested in Table 2.1, and then they would season with jang, garlic, green onions, ginger, red pepper powder, and sesame or perilla oil. In this sense, banchan can be considered a bricolage food. Banchan typically consists of 80 percent namul dishes and 20 percent high-protein dishes that are made with meat, fish, eggs, or tofu. The varieties of banchan offer a healthy, balanced diet that is rich in nutrients and phytochemicals. All dishes are served on a table at once so people can consume them based on their need and preference.

2.6 Siwonhan-Mat: Third Taste of Korean Foods

While there are several ways to describe the characteristics of food, such as smell, taste, color, and nutrient content and composition, the most frequently used is taste (mat; 맛). Taste is the sensory impression of food in the mouth reacting with taste buds along with smell and trigeminal nerve stimulation. Taste can be defined in both a narrow physiological way and in a broad general sense (Ryu, 2015). According to the physiological definition, taste is the chemical sensation produced when a substance reacts with taste receptor cells in the taste buds, which is then transferred through chemical reaction to the central nervous system by way of gustatory nerves. Research has revealed that there are five basic tastes: sweet, sour, salty, bitter, and umami (spicy), which was found in the twentieth century by Japanese scientists (Bear et al., 2006; Ryu, 2015).

However, in some cases, this physiological approach is inadequate to fully explain the characteristics of tastes found in food. Alternatively, taste in a broader sense includes the sense of pain that stimulates somatosensory nerves such as the spiciness of peppers and astringency of persimmons. Experiential characteristics of tastes such as siwonhan-mat (Lee et al., 2013; Kang et al., 2015), kipeun-mat and eolkeunhan-mat (taste, a little spicy and hot) (Ryu, 2015) are also included in taste in this broader sense. In addition, the sense of temperature, such as cool and hot, plays an important role in enjoying food (Choi, 2009).

As we have seen, taste is crucial in assessing the quality of food and initiating preference. Generally, the flavor and quality of processed foods are determined solely by taste sensed through receptors on the tongue. However, there is a unique taste, beyond the chemical or physiological definition of taste, found in traditional foods of various countries. This unique taste, the third taste, is not experienced through gustatory cells. The diverse sensations of food touching soft tissues in the mouth, swallowing food in the throat, digestion in the stomach, and appreciating the color of foods are examples of the third taste (Li et al., 2002). Therefore, in order to understand the ethnic food of a country, one is required to understand cultural expressions and the components of food found in that country.

In this sense, studying traditional Korean food, or K-diet, entails a thorough understanding of the unique tastes of Korean food. Despite the importance of food culture currently, there is a lack of funding for research on the tastes of Korean food beyond the five basic tastes. A scientific and systematic evaluation of the tastes found in Korean food is needed in order to develop and improve the exposure of Korean traditional food in the global market.

A substantial number of expressions in the Korean language describe the third taste or compounded taste (Kim, 2008; Lee et al., 2013; Yang et al., 2015). Lee et al. (2013) have listed the third tastes of Korean food:

- Mat-itneun: delicious
- Mat-upneun: unsavory
- Siwonhan: fresh, pleasureful and feel good digestibility
- Kipeun, kkalkkeumhan: clean

- Keoljukhan: thick or juicy
- Jeongkalhan: neat or nicely presented
- Kosohan: delicate or aromatic
- Hyangkeuthan: fragrant or fresh
- Tateuthan: warm or heated
- Sangkeumhan: fresh or refreshing
- Chagaun: cool or cold
- Neukkihan: repellent or oily

Generally, compounded taste refers to taste created through combinations of the five basic tastes (saltiness, sourness, sweetness, bitterness, and spiciness/umami). However, compounded tastes in Korean food indicate combined tastes acquired from the tongue and other organs in the body. For example, jeongkalhan-mat and kalkkeumhan-mat are compounded tastes using taste buds and vision. Kosohan-mat, hyangkeuthan-mat and sangkeumhan-mat are tastes using taste buds and smell. The combinations of pain, taste, and temperature are also found in expressions related to Korean food. Of all the compounded tastes found in Korean food, siwonhan-mat (Bear et al., 2006; Ryu, 2015) is considered the most important one and is often referred to as the third taste. Siwonhan-mat is a refreshing and pleasurable compounded taste experienced through taste buds and body organs, and it includes the sensation of food touching soft tissues in the mouth, swallowing food in the throat, and digestion in the stomach (Kang et al., 2015).

2.7 Understanding Siwonhan-Mat from Linguistic and Literary Approaches

2.7.1 Origin of Siwonhada (Infinitive Form of Siwonhan)

According to the *National Korean Language Dictionary* (Hangeulhakhoe, 1991), the usage of "siwonhada" includes: "The weather is refreshing," "The broth of this kuk (soup) is cool," "I am relieved of my worries," and "He is merry and cheerful, affable and amiable, and clean and neat." This demonstrates siwonhada's wide use of describing combinations of mind and work, words and behavior, and words related to the body, food, and space (Song, 2011). The diverse usage of siwonhada suggests that it conveys more than just a mere description of temperature. For example, when someone says the kukmul (broth) is siwonhada, it describes the experience of having hot broth calming the stomach. It does not describe the surface temperature of the broth, but the sensation resulting from consuming the food. Kuk with fermented kimchi or

Korean Diets and Their Tastes 37

dried pollack with kan are also dishes described with siwonhada. Kan means balancing the salt concentration to enhance the flavor of food (Song, 2009). The most common seasoning in Korean cuisine is soy sauce. Salt and soybean paste are also widely used. In this case, siwonhada is used to represent the refreshing sensation experienced during digestion as well. When explaining low temperatures with food, "chagapda" (cool) is used instead of siwonhada.

Starting in the fifteenth century, siwonhada began being used in diverse contexts to describe a refreshing and pleasurable sensation (Song, 2009). Starting in the late nineteenth century, siwonhada started being used in association with food when quenching thirst with liquids such as water or broth (Song, 2011), and when describing low-temperature food. Moreover, cathartic emotions from stories, novels, or movies are often described as siwonhada as well. These references suggest that the linguistic origin of siwonhada is "being relieved of worries" (Hangeulhakhoe, 1991). Also, siwonhada means that it is pleasant and vital when cool and refreshing air is inhaled and a hot bath makes the body reboost energy (qi). Therefore, siwonhan-mat refers to the refreshing and soothing tastes of food regardless of its temperature.

People who are not familiar with the origin of siwonhada and non-Korean speakers often perceive the meaning of the word as "cool" and raise questions about the usage of siwonhada when eating hot soup. When entering a bath, Koreans (generally, adults) often describe the feeling as siwonhada. It is a hard concept to grasp for children, who often perceive siwonhada as cool or cold. As a result, siwonhada is frequently perceived as cool, or another antonym of hot. Some scholars have tried to explain this misunderstanding through the concept of polysemy (Lee, 2011), viewing siwonhada only as a temperature-related word.

However, Song's conclusion (2009, 2011) is solely based on the perception of siwonhada as a temperature-related word (Agenda Research Group, 2005) without considering that the meaning of siwonhada is also associated with the combination of mind and work, words and behavior, and words related to the body, food, and space. In other words, the original meaning of siwonhada was distorted when it started being used to describe food. Various usages of siwonhada indicate that the antonym of the word is "pressured" or "greasy/oily" rather than "warm" or "hot."

In addition, the incorrect translation of Korean words also contributes to the misunderstanding of the words' meanings. For example, "maepda" (spicy) and siwonhada are often translated into hot and cool—temperature-related words. The erroneous meaning of siwonhada would be spread this way due to mistranslation. Therefore, it would be desirable to retain the original concept of siwonhada rather than translating the word as "cool."

2.7.2 Understanding Siwonhan-Mat from a Scientific Approach

According to the evolutionary point of view, the development of the sense of taste is closely related with human survival instincts (Ryu, 2015; Lee et al.,

2013). For example, the sense of taste would have been an important determining factor when consuming new food substances in a primitive age. In modern society, however, the sense of taste serves the function of fulfilling one's desire through the consumption of food (Agenda Research Group, 2005; Ko et al., 2014; Ryu, 2015). For this reason, the sense of taste is often regarded as the most enjoyable sense.

According to the physiological definition of taste as a chemical reaction experienced through taste buds, taste can be split into five basic categories: sweetness, sourness, saltiness, bitterness, and umami (Bear et al., 2006; Ryu, 2015). More recently, research has revealed the existence of thermoreceptors: sensory receptors responsible for the sense of pain and temperature. Thermoreceptors react with various temperature levels. However, extremely high or low temperatures activate not only thermoreceptors but also pain receptors, which results in a simultaneous sensation of temperature and pain (Bear et al., 2006). TRPV1, also known as the capsaicin receptor, is the first isolated thermoreceptor and is activated by temperatures greater than 42°C and the chemical compound found in hot chili peppers, capsaicin. TRPM8 is activated by temperatures lower than 25°C (McKemy, 2011). Examples of tastes sensed through thermoreceptors are spiciness, astringency, and temperature-related tastes such as hot and cool.

Historically, Koreans have tried to describe the characteristics of food through a health lens (Anonymous, 200 BC; Kim et al., 2012) with four attributes (Anonymous, 500 BC; Kim et al., 2012) and five tastes (Anonymous, 500 BC; Ko et al., 2014). In Korea and China, medicinal and food ingredients are categorized by the four attributes or natures. The four medicinal natures are cold, hot, warm, and cool. As for food, it can be divided into three categories: neutral, warm/hot, and cool/cold. Warming ingredients decrease oxygen consumption and slow metabolic activity in the body. In addition, they hinder fluid intake and suppress the central nervous system. Warming ingredients also have anti-inflammatory properties and have the effect of raising yang (qi) and warming the body by improving circulation and dispelling cold. On the other hand, cooling ingredients increase oxygen consumption and metabolism. They also promote fluid intake and stimulate the central nervous system. In addition, cooling ingredients have nourishing and detoxifying effects on the blood (Anonymous, 500 BC; Kim et al., 2012). Despite a long agricultural history in Korea, the main purpose of farming was to survive, so it would have been difficult to develop an appreciation of the smells, colors, or tastes of food. In other words, Korean food and its food culture are deeply related to survival and can be conceptualized by the idea of yaksikdongwon (medicine and food arise from the same source). About 2,500 years ago, Hippocrates recognized that food was as important as medicine in humans by saying, "Let food be thy medicine and medicine be thy food." Similarly, in Asia the importance of food in life is acknowledged with the expression "Medicine and food come from the same source" a long time ago (Chung et al., 2016). The similarity between the five traditional tastes of Korean food (sweet, sour, salty, bitter, spicy) and the modern five basic tastes suggests a scientific value of food analysis in Korea. Although much research on the characteristics of food related to the four attributes has been conducted, more work is needed to discuss the key elements of the four attributes in order to support the idea with scientific evidence.

The meaning of siwonhan-mat can be properly understood in the context of health and survival, rather than the mere appreciation of smell, color, and taste. Siwonhan-mat characterizes Korean food and is a vital concept to understand in Korean food culture.

2.8 Determining Factors of Siwonhan-Mat

As mentioned previously, siwonhan-mat is a refreshing taste that is associated with the sensation of food touching soft tissues in the mouth, swallowing food in the throat, and digestion in the stomach. An antonym of siwonhan-mat is not thateuthan-mat, but rather neukihan-mat, which describes an unpleasant indigestive feeling.

It is presumed that siwonhan-mat is composed of several elements other than the five basic tastes, such as salinity, acidity, spiciness, and a feeling of refreshment. For example, siwonhan-mat is often experienced through kuk or tang (Kwon et al., 2015), types of Korean dishes with broth, and in this case, siwonhan-mat is associated with the proper kan (Song, 2009) of the dish. More research on determining the exact elements of siwonhan-mat should be conducted to allow further understanding of this taste. Kuk is often mistranslated as "soup." Korean kuk is not the same as Western soup, which is served before the main dish rather than with the main dish like kuk. Kuk helps with digestion when rice is served; they go together like coke and hamburgers.

2.9 Conclusion

When defining the K-diet, various components are considered, such as raw materials or ingredients, traditional cooking methods, technology, and fundamental principles and knowledge. However, it would be preferable to establish the definition of Korean food by focusing on the preservation of traditional methods and core principles. The Korean meal table is characterized by servings of bap, kuk, and banchan on one table. While various cooking methods are used in Korean cuisine, the most representative method is fermentation, which enhances both the flavor and preservation of the food.

The K-diet is composed of bap (cooked rice) and kuk, and various banchan with one serving called babsang. Kimchi is always served at every meal. The principal aspects of the K-diet include proportionally high consumption of vegetables, moderate to high consumption of legumes and fish, and low consumption of red meat. Banchan is mostly seasoned with various jang (fermented soy products), medicinal herbs, and sesame or perilla oil. This chapter has provided the features of the K-diet, as well as an introduction to K-food and the traditions and health value of the K-diet and K-food. Moreover, this is vital to promote the cultural values of Korea (K-value) by bringing together traditional principles and scientific evidence.

Siwonhan-mat is a refreshing and pleasurable taste experienced through the body rather than by a sense of smell or taste. It is frequently misunderstood as chagapda, or cool, and this misunderstanding began with the mistranslation of siwonhada, using words to describe temperature, such as cool. This has resulted in confusion over the original meaning of siwonhada. Koreans experience siwonhan-mat the most when having kuk or tang with proper kan, which balances the salt concentration of the food and gives rise to a seasoning that is closely associated with siwonhan-mat. Further research on this subject should be conducted to understand the exact determining factors of siwonhan-mat. In Korean cuisine, soy sauce, salt, and soybean paste are commonly used seasonings. Koreans enjoy the distinctive taste of fermented foods, such as soy sauce and soybean paste. Haejang-kuk and kongnamul-haejang-kuk are iconic dishes with siwonhan-mat. Understanding siwonhan-mat is necessary for understanding Korean food and Korean food culture. This chapter plays an important role in making this connection for those learning about Korean food. Siwonhan-mat is a unique, exclusive sensation experienced by Koreans and some from other countries who have had the pleasure of eating the dishes described in the chapter.

Acknowledgments

This work was done with support from the project of nutritional epigenomics study on a Korean healthy diet (E0150302-01,02), in part from the Korea Food Research Institute. I would like to thank the following scholars for their contributions to establishing the definitions and characteristics of Korean food: Soon Hee Kim, Myung Sunny Kim, Hye Jeong Yang, Min Jung Kim, Dae Ja Jang from the Korea Food Research Institute, Myoung Sook Lee from SungShin Women's University, Yong Soon Park from Hanyang University, Hae Jeong Lee from Gachon University, Songnam, Soon-A Kang from Hoseo University, Hyun Sook Lee from Dongseo University, Kyung-Eun Lee from Seoul Women's University, and Young-Eun Lee from Wonkwang University.

References

Adamsson, V., A. Reumark, T. Cederholm, B. Vessby, U. Riserus, and G. Johansson. 2012. What is a healthy Nordic diet? Foods and nutrients in the nordiet study. *Food Nutrit. Res.* 56.

Agenda Research Group. 2005. Globalization of Korean food and related culture. Seoul, Korea.

Anonymous B.C. 200. New-nongbonchokyung. China.

Anonymous B.C. 500. Hwangje-naekyung. China.

Bear, M. F., B. W. Connors, and M. A. Paradiso. 2006. *Neuroscience: Exploring the Brain,* Philadelphia, PA, Lippincott Williams and Wilkins.

Choi, H. S. 2009. *All Human Senses,* Seoul, Korea.

Chung, H. K. 2009. Cultural properties and aesthetics of Korean foods, Seoul, *Proceedings of Conferences for World Society of Comparative Literatures.*

Chung, H. K. 2015. The meaning and symbolism of Korean food culture. *Asia Rev.,* 5:97–121.

Chung, H. K., K. R. Chung, and H. J. Kim. 2016. Understanding Korean food culture from paintings, *J. Ethn Foods,* 3:42–50

Chung, K. R., H. J. Yang, D. J. Jang, and D. Y. Kwon. 2015. Historical and biological aspects of bibimbap, a Korean ethnic food. *J. Ethn. Foods,* 2:74–83.

Ferrieres, J. 2004. The French paradox: Lessons for other countries. *Heart,* 90:107–111.

Hangeulhakhoe. 1991. *Grand Dictionary of Hangeul,* Seoul, Korea.

Health Magazine. 2006. World's five healthiest foods.

Hu, J. 1610. *Donguibogam.* Korea.

Hwang, H. S., B. R. Han, and B. J. Han. 2005. *Korean Traditional Foods,* Seoul, Korea, Kyomunsa.

Jang, D. J., K. R. Chung, H. J. Yang, K. S. Kim, and D. Y. Kwon. 2015. Discussion on the origin of kimchi, representative of Korean unique fermented vegetables. *J. Ethn. Foods,* 2:126–136.

Kang, S. A., H. J. Oh, D. J. Jang, M. J. Kim, and D. Y. Kwon. 2016. Siwonhan-mat: The third taste of Korean foods. *J. Ethn. Foods,* 3:61–68.

Kim, C. G. 2008. A study on meaning of the taste adjective. *Eomunhak,* 100:1–30.

Kim, K., S. Park, S., M. Yang, and Y. Choi. 2012. *Siklyobonchohak,* Korea, Esongdang.

Kim, S. H. and D. J. Jang. 2015. *Fabulous Korean Ethnic Foods, Namdo,* Seoul, Korea, Elsevier Korea.

Ko, B. S., S. Park, and K. J. Chung. 2014. *Korean Traditional Medicine and Nutrition,* Daejeon, Korea, Korea Institute of Oriental Medicine.

Kwon, D. 2015. Why ethnic foods? *J. Ethn. Foods,* 2:91.

Kwon, D. Y., K. R. Chung, H. J. Yang, and D. J. Jang. 2015. Gochujang (Korean red pepper paste): A Korean ethnic sauce, its role and history. *J. Ethn. Foods,* 2:29–35.

Kwon, D. Y., D. J. Jang, H. J. Yang, and K. R. Chung. 2014. History of Korean gochu, gochujang, and kimchi. *J. Ethn. Foods,* 1:3–7.

Lee, J., S. Jeong, J. O. Rho, and K. Park. 2013. A study of adjectives for sensory evaluation of taste in Korea Language. *Sci. Emot. Sensibility,* 16.

Lee, S. Y. 2011. A study on contronymy in Korean. *J Korean Linguistics,* 61:265–289.

Li, X., L. Staszewski, H. Xu, K. Durick, M. Zoller, and E. Adler. 2002. Human receptors for sweet and umami taste. *Proc. Natl. Acad. Sci. USA,* 99:4692–4696.

Mckemy, D. D. 2011. A spicy family tree: TRPV1 and its thermoceptive and nociceptive lineage. *EMBO J*, 30:453–455.

Moose, J. R. 1911. *Village Life in Korea*, Nashville, TN, House of ME Church.

Park, J. and C. K. Kwock. 2015. Sodium intake and prevalence of hypertension, coronary heart disease, and stroke in Korean adults. *J. Ethn. Foods*, 2:92–96.

Ryu, M. R. 2015. *Easy Science Underlying Taste*, Seoul, Korea, Ministry of Science, ICT and Future Planning.

Shin, D. H. and D. Jeong. 2015. Korean traditional fermented soybean products: Jang. *J. Ethn. Foods*, 2:2–7.

Simini, B. 2000. Serge Renaud: From French paradox to Cretan miracle. *Lancet*, 355, 48.

Song, H. J. and H. J. Lee. 2014. Consumption of Kimchi, a salt fermented vegetable, is not associated with hypertension prevalence. *J. Ethn. Foods*, 1:8–12.

Song, J. H. 2009. A study on the diachronic change of temperature sensation words. PhD Thesis, Kyungbuk University.

Song, J. H. 2011. On an aspect of the meaning change of the "siwonhada." *Korean Language Literature*, 111:37–56.

Surh, Y. J. 2003. Cancer chemoprevention with dietary phytochemicals. *Nat. Rev. Cancer*, 3:768–780.

Willett, W. C., F. Sacks, A. Trichopoulou et al. 1995. Mediterranean diet pyramid: A cultural model for healthy eating. *Am. J. Clin. Nutr.*, 61:1402S–1406S.

Yang, H. J., D. J. Jang, K. R. Chung, K. S. Kim, and D. Y. Kwon. 2015. Origin names of gochu, kimchi, and bibimbap. *J. Ethn. Foods*, 2:162–172.

Yoon, S. S. 1999. *The Culture and History of Korean Foods*, Seoul, Korea, Shinkwang.

3

Kimchi and Its Health Benefits

Kun-Young Park and Jaehyun Ju

CONTENTS

3.1 Introduction 43
3.2 History 44
3.3 Classification 47
3.4 Raw Ingredients 49
3.5 Processing and Recipes 49
3.6 Fermentation and LAB 51
3.7 Functionalities 54
    3.7.1 Improvement of Colon Health 55
    3.7.2 Antioxidative and Antiaging Effects 58
    3.7.3 Cancer Preventive Effects 60
    3.7.4 Antiobesity Effect 66
    3.7.5 Hypolipidemic Effect and Control of Metabolic Syndrome 69
3.8 Conclusion 72
References 73

3.1 Introduction

Kimchi is a lactic acid bacteria (LAB) fermented vegetable food in Korea, where fermentation of salted vegetables was used as a food preservation method about 2,000 years ago (Cheigh, 2002). There are 161–187 kinds of kimchi in Korea (Son, 1991; Park et al., 1994a) depending on the raw materials, manufacturing method, and other characteristics. However, baechu kimchi, which is mainly prepared with baechu cabbage, is the major kimchi, accounting for more than 70% of kimchi intake in Korea.

During kimchi preparation, LAB naturally present in the main ingredients, especially in baechu cabbage, play a major role in fermentation; numbers of LAB rise while other bacteria involved in putrefaction decline. Microbes in spices are also involved in fermentation, but LAB in baechu cabbage are the predominant bacteria in the kimchi fermentation process (Yun et al., 2014). Taste, quality, and health functionality of kimchi are subject to changes in condition of fermentation such as temperature (kimchi LAB especially requires low-temperature fermentation), subingredients, microorganisms, material of the fermentation container, etc. Kimchi, which is LAB-based fermented food, contains 10^{7-9} colony-forming units (CFUs)/g of LAB, organic acids, vitamins, flavor compounds, phytochemicals, etc., resulting in a healthy fermented food product that is rich in numerous nutrients that are derived from vegetables and further modified by the fermentative bacteria (Park and Cheigh, 2004).

Kimchi has played an important role in supplying nutrition, including dietary fiber, vitamins, minerals, and health-beneficial phytochemicals to the majority of Koreans who have endured long harsh winters. The traditional Korean diet consists of steamed rice as a staple and other side dishes; daily consumption of kimchi used to be about 300 g/day (sufficient to be accompanied with steamed rice as a one to three side dish), although its daily consumption has fallen to 60–100 g/day recently. Kimchi has its own excellence not just because of its health functionalities due to its ingredients but also by fermentation products that contribute taste, texture, quality, and health functionality, owing to its special fermentation process, which increases the LAB in baechu cabbage from 10^4 CFUs/g to 10^9 CFUs/g. Kimchi, known as LAB-based functional food made of vegetables and spices, is regarded as a top-tier healthy food.

Considering nutrition and phytochemicals, kimchi demonstrates efficacies such as anticancer, antioxidation, antiaging, antiobesity, immunity promotion, etc. (Park et al., 2014). Kimchi-derived LAB showed numerous health-promoting efficacies as well (Park and Kim, 2012). Almost all kimchi was home-made in the past, but now nearly 50% of kimchi consumed is industrially manufactured. Heterofermentative LAB-based fermentation is the important factor in promoting the taste of kimchi (Kim et al., 2016). From nine brands of commercial kimchi available in South Korea, heterofermentative LAB such as *Weisella koreensis*, *Lactobacillus graminis*, *Lab. sakei*, *Leuconostoc gelidum*, and *Leu. mesenteroides* are found to be the most commonly used. Thus, many studies are in progress for improving the quality of kimchi-derived starter LAB (especially probiotic effects of kimchi LAB) as well as changes in functionality and quality of kimchi by using different starter LABs. In this chapter, we introduce the history, types, manufacturing process, microbe-based fermentation, and functionality of kimchi.

3.2 History

A primitive type of kimchi began with the simple brining of vegetables. This type of kimchi was consumed as a side dish in the Three Kingdom era (approximately 57 BC–AD 667). Salted vegetables were estimated to have been manufactured and consumed in the ancient time until the end of Samguksidae (meaning "Three Kingdom era"). Jeo, which means salted vegetable in Chinese character, is regarded as a precursor of kimchi and is estimated to have been consumed in the era of Gojoseon (approximately 300 BC), especially at the beginning of the Iron Age. Thus, kimchi is estimated to have originated at least 2,000 years ago (Cheigh, 2002). Kimchi was manufactured by using white radish as the main ingredient at the beginning and then baechu cabbage and red pepper powder; other vegetables began to be incorporated, eventually resulting in the current type of kimchi in the late seventeenth century.

Salt and spices for kimchi preparation were introduced in the Jeminyosul period (AD 540) according to the ancient Chinese agricultural manual, and appeared to have been used in Samguksidae and the unified Shilla dynasty. At that time, an ancient type of kimchi, called jeo, might have been widely consumed. A stone-based jar found in Beobju temple (located in the Sokri mountains of Chungcheong province) is estimated to be the kimchi jar used for fermentation in AD 720, giving a clue that the kimchi manufactured with salt and jeotgal (fermented fish) was widely consumed in that era. Watery kimchi, including nabak kimchi and dongchimi, was developed in the united Silla dynasty (AD 668–935). Consumption of such fermented food accompanied with staple foods was assumed to prevail and to have been developed in Samguksidae, even though records of its use have not survived over time. According to a Korean historical record called *Samguksagi*, published in AD 1145, fermented vegetables were prepared using a stone pickle jar, indicating that these foods were commonly available at that time.

During the early Goryeo dynasty (AD 936–1391), Buddhism accepted vegetarian diets while declining meat-based diets. The preparation and use of various added ingredients became more diverse with time. For example, the *Gapoyukyeong* (from the *Donggukyisanggukjip*, published in AD 1241) states that white radish leaves in soy paste were used to prepare summer vegetables and salt for winter vegetables, making these kimchi preparations different from the jangajji (vegetables pickled in soy paste or soy sauce).

The word "chimchae," the Chinese term for kimchi, appears for the first time in Yisaek's *Mogunjip* (1320–1396); the article also contains records about dongchimi and nabak kimchi. Until the Goryeo dynasty, the main vegetable used to make kimchi was radishes rather than Korean baechu cabbages. Records show that cucumber, eggplant, and green onions were also used to make vegetables at that time to radishes.

Many foreign vegetable species were introduced into Korean foods during the Chosun dynasty (1392–1910), specifically the early stage of the dynasty (1392–1600); thus, by introduction of such foreign vegetables, kimchi began to have more variety. *Gugupbyukon* (1518) introduced various vegetables, including cucumber, eggplant, leek, dropwart, baechu cabbage, burdock, bamboo shoot, mustard leaf, turnip, as well as garlic, ginger, and green onion, as subingredients. *SuwunJapbang* (1481–1552) recorded the subingredients and preparation method of kimchi of that period. Radish, cucumber, eggplant, and green onion were the main ingredients and garlic, ginger, and Chinese pepper were the subingredients.

Domundaejak (Hur Kyun, 1569–1618) was a record of the use of baechu cabbage. It was natural baechu cabbage (Chinese cabbage), and then a Korean variety was developed, with cabbage packed well with layers of leaves throughout the head, for the preparation of kimchi in the 1800s. *Jibongyusul* (Lee Su Kwang, 1614) imported and introduced various vegetables—especially red pepper for its characteristic pungency. *Sasichanyocho* (Kang Hee Maeng, 1655) reported the use of various spices and vegetables, but it did not introduce baechu cabbage and red pepper, which were not generally cultivated at that time.

Eumshikdimibang (1670), the first book of recipes written in Korean characters, also contains information about several types of kimchi and detailed descriptions of preparation methods. The *Jeungbosanlimgyeongje* (Yu Jung Im, 1760) introduces 50 kinds of vegetables and condiments, including baechu cabbage and red pepper, even though red pepper was cultivated and used before in Korea. The word for baechu kimchi appeared in speaking of using red pepper powder (RPP) in this book, and spices, especially red pepper, were strongly recommended for kimchi preparation. During this time, many types of kimchi recipes were introduced in written form tor the first time in history. *Gyuhapchongseo* (Binghurgak Lee, 1759–1824), the first cookbook for women, also described kimchi preparation in detail: types of main ingredients, use of jeotgal (fermented fish), salting method, and use of fish and meat. This record eventually contributed to development of the modern type of kimchi.

Developments of agricultural technology, especially of vegetable cultivation, led to additional varieties of kimchi in the eighteenth and nineteenth centuries. *Nonggawolryeongga* (1816), a poem-type agricultural manual written on a monthly basis, introduced over 35 types of vegetables, but put greatest emphasis on the cultivation of radish and baechu cabbage for kimchi preparation.

To summarize, white radish, cucumber, eggplant, and green onion were used for kimchi in the early Chosun dynasty, whereas the kimchi of the mid- and late Chosun dynasty can be characterized by active use of red pepper; use of white radish, eggplant, baechu cabbage, and cucumber as the main ingredients; and use of spices as subingredients. Lactic acid fermentation was maximized by adjustment of fermentation and lactic acid-based bacteriostatic action; it resulted from immersion of fresh vegetables into salty water, followed by preparation with other subingredients (including spices and fishes), all of which became common in the late Chosun dynasty. Tongbaechu kimchi, Bossam kimchi, dongchimi, seokbakji, and chonggak kimchi also prevailed at that time.

Buinpilji (1915), an improved version of *Guhapchongseo*, shows detailed preparation methods of kimchi. It introduces white radish and baechu cabbage as the main ingredients of kimchi, and emphasizes the importance

Kimchi and Its Health Benefits 47

of RPP and the use of jeotgal and jeotguk (soup of fermented fish). Also, it introduces other subingredients, including pine nut, oyster, glue plant, etc. *Joseonyorijebeob* (1913) is the modern recipe book after the Chosun dynasty, introducing diverse types of kimchi such as tongkimchi, seokbakji, jeotgukji, ssam kimchi, dongchimi, and kaktugi. *Joseonmussangshinsik yorijebeob* (Lee Yongki, 1924) is the standard recipe book up to the present time, and it summarizes a portion of *Imwonshipyukji*. It also introduces detailed processes of kimjang by the two phases of preparation (salting and preparation method), as well as burying the kimjang jar into the ground for maintaining proper fermentation temperature.

3.3 Classification

Various types of kimchi are now made in Korea, depending on the raw ingredients used, processing methods, harvest seasons, and geographical regions. Baechu cabbage and radish are the main ingredients used in making kimchi; however, other vegetables are used depending on seasonal availability in different regions. For example, people living near the sea naturally use more seafood products in kimchi. Jo and Nam (1979) reported 55 varieties of kimchi, 31 of baechu-derived and radish-derived kimchi, 8 of jangajji (sliced vegetables pickled in soy sauce), 4 of kaktugi (diced radish kimchi), 2 of dongchimi (whole-radish watery kimchi without red pepper powder), and 6 of other types in reviewing published data on kimchi in Korea from 1959 to 1976. Park et al. (1994) reported that a total of 187 types of kimchi are now consumed in Korea.

Table 3.1 shows 161 varieties of kimchi; eight different groups based on the main raw ingredients have been classified (Son, 1991). The first group comprises baechu cabbage kimchi (12 types), of which tongbaechu kimchi (two pieces of whole cabbage kimchi) is the most popular, followed by baek kimchi and bossam kimchi. In the second group are radish kimchis (17 types), with dongchimi and chonggak kimchi being the favorite. In the kaktugi group (25 types), radish kaktugi is the most popular. In the fourth group, comprising sokbakji and nabak kimchi, there are 20 varieties including sokbakji and nabak kimchi. Green and stem vegetables are in the fifth classification group of kimchi (27 types), which includes got (mustard leaf) kimchi and kodulbaegi kimchi. The sixth group includes fruit and root-vegetable kimchi (27 types); cucumber kimchi and burdock kimchi are favorites. The green onion, garlic, and leek group contains 14 varieties; green onion and leek kimchi are favorites, especially in the southern part of Korea. The final group has 19 varieties of kimchi composed of meat, fish, shellfish, and seaweed.

A survey on the preference of kimchi prepared in Korean households shows that baechu cabbage kimchi is the most frequently prepared, followed

48 *Korean Functional Foods*

TABLE 3.1

Classification of Kimchi by Raw Ingredients

Groups	Varieties
1. Baechu kimchi (baechu cabbage kimchi) (12 varieties)	Tongbaechu kimchi (whole cabbage kimchi), baek kimchi, bossam kimchi (wrapped-up kimchi), vegetables pickled right before eating, etc.
2. Radish kimchi (17 varieties)	Dongchimi (watery radish kimchi), chonggak dongchimi, mupinul kimchi (slit-cut radish kimchi, chonggak kimchi, sunmu kimchi (turnip kimchi), chae kimchi (julienne radish kimchi), muchung dongchimi (radish leaf kimchi) musobaegi (stuffed radish), pickled radish kimchi, musun kimchi (radish shoot kimchi), etc.
3. Kaktugi (25 varieties)	Radish kaktugi, radish and oyster kaktugi, radish and wild rocambole kaktugi, radish and leek kaktugi, radish and radish leaf kaktugi, cucumber kaktugi, chonggak kaktugi, radish and salted pollack guts kaktugi, parboiled radish kaktugi, yolmu kaktugi, radish and cod kaktugi, etc.
4. Sokbakji and nabak kimchi (20 varieties)	Sokbakji, wax gourd sokbakji, baby ginseng nabak kimchi, nabak kimchi (watery sliced cabbage and radish kimchi), chang kimchi, changzanji, etc.
5. Green vegetables and stem vegetables (27 varieties)	Shigumchi kimchi (spinach kimchi), gat kimchi (mustard leaf kimchi), kodulbaegi kimchi (wild lettuce kimchi), kongnamul kimchi (soybean sprout kimchi), minari kimchi (dropwort kimchi), doraji kimchi (broad bellflower kimchi), dolnamul kimchi (sedum kimchi), young mustard leaf kimchi, etc.
6. Fruit and root vegetable kimchi (27 varieties)	Oi kimchi (cucumber kimchi), oi sobagi (stuffed cucumber kimchi), pickled cucumber, hobak kimchi (pumpkin kimchi), gaji kimchi (eggplant kimchi), koguma kimchi (sweet potato kimchi), putgochu kimchi (green pepper kimchi), uong kimchi (burdock kimchi), cucumber kimchi, kam kimchi (persimmon kimchi), etc.
7. Green onion, garlic, and leek kimchi (14 varieties)	Green onion kimchi, leek kimchi, green onion zanji, dalrae kimchi (wild rocambole kimchi), etc.
8. Meat, fish, shellfish, and seaweed kimchi (19 varieties)	Meat kimchi, chicken kimchi, pheasant kimchi, earshell kimchi, green laver kimchi, oyster kimchi, codfish kimchi, dried pollack kimchi, squid kimchi, Alaska pollack kimchi, marine products kimchi, miyok kimchi (brown seaweed kimchi), etc.

Total: 161 varieties

Source: Son, K. H. 1991. *Korean J Diet Cult* 6:503–520.

by radish kaktugi, watery kimchi of dongchimi, and then miniature radish and stem chonggak kimchi (Cheigh and Park, 1994). Although both baechu kimchi and kaktugi are important kimchi, baechu kimchi is by far the most popular and represents what is commonly referred to as kimchi. Also, the most commercially marketed varieties of kimchi are baechu kimchi (more than 70%) and radish kimchi (around 20%).

3.4 Raw Ingredients

The main ingredients most frequently used to make kimchi are baechu cabbage, radish, miniature radish, cucumber, etc. However, the baechu cabbage (*Brassica compestris* sp. Pekinensis) or radish (*Raphabus satirus* L.) are the main ingredients. The quality and species of the ingredients may markedly affect the organoleptic characteristics of kimchi. For example, quality, cultivation method, and the kind and type of baechu resulted in different taste, texture, fermentation behavior, health function, etc.

Spices, seasoning, and other materials can be used as subgredients to increase taste, quality, and functionality of kimchi. The spices used to prepare kimchi are red pepper powder, garlic, ginger, green onion, leek, mustard, black pepper, onion, and cinnamon. Seasonings for kimchi are salt (various kinds of salt are used to increase taste and functionality), salted and fermented shrimp, fermented anchovies, soy sauce, vinegar, chemical seasoning agents (including monosodium glutamate), sweetening agents (cane sugar), sesame seed or its oil, and oysters; these are optionally added to kimchi to improve and vary flavor and taste depending on the type of kimchi. Additional kimchi ingredients are vegetables (watercress, carrot, parsley, mustard leaves, etc.), fruits and nuts (jujube, gingko nut, pine nut, chestnut, apple, orange, etc.), cereals (polished barley, glutinous rice, wheat flour, and malt), seafoods (oyster, squid, shrimp, Alaskan pollack, yellow croaker, scabbard fish), and meats (beef and pork). Fish and meats are added to improve the flavor and cereals are added to enhance lactic acid fermentation (Park and Cheigh, 2004).

3.5 Processing and Recipes

Methods of preparing kimchi differ depending on the ingredients used, family preference, regional customs, etc. The essential process consists of preparation and pretreatment of raw ingredients, mixing the ingredients, packaging, and fermentation. Pretreatments of raw ingredients include grading, washing, and cutting. Other ingredients are also graded, washed and cut, sliced, or chopped for proper mixing. Pretreated raw baechu cabbage or radish is brined at proper concentrations of dry salt, brine solution, or dry salt plus brine solution overnight. The cabbage is then rinsed and the water drained for 3 hours, and mixed together with a mixture of chopped or sliced subingredients (spices, seasonings, salt-pickled fishes, and other vegetables) and dry salt to make a final salt concentration of 2.5%; however, the overall salt level was lowered to 1.4%–1.8% recently.

As shown in Figure 3.1(a), baechu can be prepared by two major methods. One is used for tongbaechu kimchi, a more kimchi preparation using whole

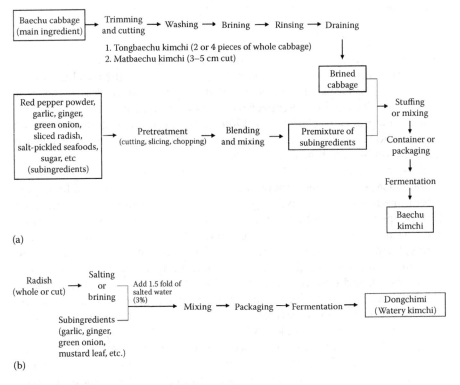

FIGURE 3.1
Flow charts for processing of (a) baechu kimchi and (b) watery kimchi (dongchimi).

cabbage, preserved for the long-term winter season, for kimjang, and that is typical of kimchi prepared at home. The other method used is to cut matbaechu kimchi, a common preparation style for commercial products, export, and daily, informal family eating (Park and Cheigh, 2004).

For the preparation of tongbaechu kimchi, baechu is slit lengthwise into two or four parts with a knife inserted through the bottom of the cabbage head. The cut cabbages are treated with dry salt (usually bittern-reduced solar salt) or with 10% brine overnight (10 hours). The brined cabbage is rinsed to remove excess salt and then drained. A premixture of spices and other subingredients, according to a recipe, is packed between the layers of the cabbage leaves. The stuffed cabbage is wrapped with outer leaves, which removes the oxygen, and then packed into a clay pot (traditionally onggi was used, but any containers can be used), which allows for a facultative anaerobic condition for the LAB fermentation. Cabbage is cut to 3–5 cm in length to make matbaechu kimchi and salted in salt solution (8%–15%) for 2–7 hours, rinsed with fresh water, and then drained. As an alternative salting method, a whole cabbage that is cut into two or four pieces is salted like tongbaechu kimchi before being cut into smaller sizes. Premixed subingredients are combined and then the same procedure as for tongbaechu kimchi is used.

Kimchi and Its Health Benefits　　　　51

Dongchimi is a representative watery kimchi, and the processing method is shown in Figure 3.1(b). A whole oriental radish (12–15 × 7 × 10 cm) kimchi requires a large quantity of seasoned water. Whole radishes are salted with dry salt and then rinsed. The rinsed uncut or cut radishes are mixed with other ingredients (Moon et al., 1995; Cheigh, 2002) in a large quantity of 3% to 4% brine solution and then fermented in a jar while completely immersed in the mixed ingredients and water. Garlic, ginger, and green onion are the main subingredients for dongchimi preparation; however, fermented green peppers, pears, and glue plant are frequently used. When serving, radishes are removed from the container and sliced. Because dongchimi liquid has a salty taste for storage, water can be added according to taste.

We have standardized the composition of baechu kimchi ingredients, from scientific papers, cookbooks, recipes from kimchi factories, family traditions, etc. (Cho et al., 1997; Cho, 1999), and the recipe is as follows: The brined baechu cabbage (100%) is mixed with 13.0% sliced radish, 3.5% red pepper powder, 1.4% crushed garlic, 0.6% crushed ginger, 2.2% fermented anchovy juice, 1.0% sugar, 2.0% green onion, and a final salt concentration of 2.5%. We have also developed kimchi recipes for improving anticancer function by adding some functional subingredients and then manipulating the recipes. The anticancer kimchi (ACK) or cancer-preventive kimchi (CPK) has been developed containing functional ingredients such as Chinese pepper (Cho, 1999; Han et al., 2011b), Korean mistletoe extract (Kil, 2004), mustard leaf (Choi, 2001; Kim et al., 2007), and different kinds of salt (Jung, 2000; Park et al., 2014). After interviewing cancer patients Kim (2002) used starter cultures (Han et al., 2011a; Bong et al., 2013). A recipe of ACK is as follows: The brined baechu cabbage (100%) is mixed with 2.5% red pepper powder, 2.8% crushed garlic, 0.6% crushed ginger, 11.0% sliced radish, 2.0% green onion, 1.0% sugar, 7.5% mustard leaf, 0.1% Chinese pepper, 2.8% pear, 5.0% mushroom (shiitake) and sea tangle juice, 0.05% mistletoe extract powder (Kil, 2004), *Lab. plantarum* (10^6 CFUs/g) as a starter, and a final salt content of 2.2% (Lee, 2016).

The recipe for dongchimi is 100% of salted small-sized whole radish, 1.0% crushed garlic, 0.3% crushed ginger, 3.3% green onion, 3.3% of fermented green pepper, and addition of 150% of water. The final salt content is 2.0%–3.0% (Moon et al., 1995; Park and Cheight, 2004).

3.6 Fermentation and LAB

Kimchi fermentation occurs naturally. The main endogenous microorganisms, LAB, ferment sugars such as glucose, fructose, etc. in the cabbage and subingredients. Various chemical, physical, and biological factors may also contribute directly to the growth of LAB and to the extent of fermentation. Several factors influence kimchi fermentation, kinds of microorganisms, salt concentration, fermentable carbohydrates, other available nutrients, the presence of inhibitory compounds, the absence of O_2, pH, and fermenting temperature. The temperature, salt concentration, and pH have a great effect on the rate and extent of the fermentation by LAB. It takes a shorter time when the temperature is increased and the salt concentration is decreased.

The microorganisms in kimchi fermentation should be tolerant to salt, acidity, anaerobic conditions, and endogenous antimicrobial compounds in the ingredients; thus, the final starters can be LAB and other bacteria are removed or killed during the processing. The brining process extracts the water from the cabbage by osmotic activity and suppresses the growth of undesirable aerobic bacteria. At the same time, it offers a relatively favorable environment for LAB under increased salinity (Choe et al., 1991). Fermentation is mainly carried out by the cabbage LAB after the brining process; other microorganisms present in ingredients other than the cabbage may also be involved in the fermentation, but LAB from the brined cabbage seems to be the main natural starters (Yun et al., 2014). It is important to keep anaerobic conditions to minimize the growth of aerobic microorganisms and to stimulate the growth of LAB during fermentation (Park et al., 1994b).

The kimchi fermentation process includes several distinct phases based on the changes in pH, acidity, CO_2 level, and sugar content. The first stage has a rapid decrease of pH and an increase in acidity and CO_2 levels. These changes are accompanied by a decrease in reducing sugars after the initial lag phase. With the decrease in the free sugars fructose and glucose, lactate, acetate, CO_2, and ethanol were detected as heterofermentative fermentation products, and a considerable amount of mannitol accumulated during the fermentation (Wisselink et al., 2002). Mannitol results in a refreshing taste and is a good replacement for sugars in diabetic foods. The changes in free sugars and fermentation products were closely correlated with pH changes and growth of the bacterial population (Jung et al., 2011). The next stage shows a gradual drop in pH, a further increase in acidity and CO_2 levels, and a rapid disappearance of reducing sugar. The final stage of fermentation proceeds with no or only slight change in pH, acidity, CO_2, and reducing sugar (Cheigh and Park, 1994). The pH and acidity of optimally ripened kimchi are 4.2% to 4.5% and 0.4% to 0.8% as lactic acid, respectively.

Kimchi fermentation can also be divided into four stages based on acidity: initial stage (acidity <0.2), immature stage (acidity 0.2–0.4), optimally ripened stage (acidity 0.4–0.9), and over-ripened stage (acidity >0.9) (CODEX, 2001). *Leu. mesenteroides* appeared at the immature stage and optimally ripened stage, *Lab. plantarum* and *Lab. sakei* at the initial stage until the over-ripened stage. *Wei. koreensis* appeared at the over-ripened stage and increased to the end of fermentation (Cho et al., 2009). Kimchi fermentation was governed by three genera: *Leuconostoc*, *Lactobacillus*, and *Weissella*. The genus *Leuconostoc* was most abundant during the kimchi fermentation, followed by *Lactobacillus* and *Weissella*. *Leuconostoc* dominated at the beginning stages of kimchi fermentation, but as the fermentation progressed, the abundance of *Lactobacillus* and *Weissella* increased. After the middle stages of fermentation, *Leuconostoc*, *Lactobacillus*, and *Weissella* became the predominant bacterial groups in the microbial community, and their cumulative abundance reached approximately 80% after day 23 at 4°C. *Lactobacillus* (29.3%) and *Weissella* (30.1%) levels significantly increased compared to *Leuconostoc* (21.8%) at day 23. However, after day 23, the abundance of *Leuconostoc* increased again, and that of *Lactobacillus* and *Weissella* gradually decreased until day 29 at 4°C (Jung et al., 2011).

Figure 3.2 shows the lactic acid bacterial communities in nine commercial kimchi samples from representative Korean kimchi companies. The pH values of the kimchi samples ranged from 4.3 to 4.7, and total LAB counts ranged from 1.3×10^7 to 1.6×10^9 CFUs/g (Kim et al., 2016). *Weissella*, *Lactobacillus*, and *Leuconostoc* were the dominant genera accounting for 52%, 28%, and 20%, respectively, of identified genera by a pyrosequencing method. *Wei. koreensis* (34.4%) was dominant followed by *Lab. graminis* (12.5%), *Wei. cibaria* (11.2%), *Lab. sakei* (9.2%), and *Leu. gelidum* (8.9%). The mean pH value of the nine studied samples was 4.4 and average total LAB count was 7.7×10^8 CFUs/g. All bacterial strains detected in the commercial kimchi were heterofermentative

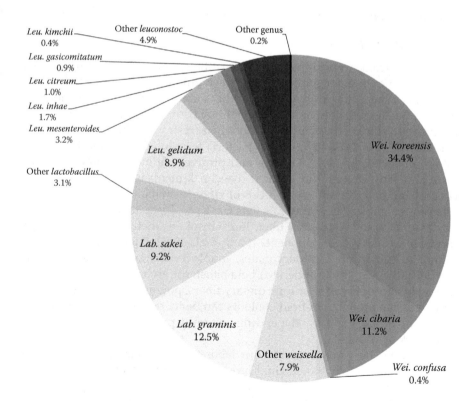

FIGURE 3.2
Lactic acid bacterial communities in nine commercial kimchi samples from representative Korean kimchi companies. (From Kim, H. Y. et al. 2016, *Food Sci Biotechnol* 25:541–545.)

LAB, which can produce various fermented products and grow actively at low temperature. Recently, LAB starters have been developed to produce consistently high-quality commercial kimchi products (Lee et al., 2015c). Representative kimchi LAB have been isolated for fermentation characteristics and studied for probiotic activities to improve the quality and bioactivity of kimchi. *Leu. citreum* (Chang and Chang, 2011), *Leu. mesenteroides* (Jung et al., 2012), and mixed cultures of *Leu. mesenteroides* and *Lab. plantarum* (Bong et al., 2013) that showed better probiotic activities were employed as starters to ferment kimchi. The mixed culture fermented kimchi showed higher free radical scavenging and anticancer effects than naturally fermented kimchi. *Weissella*, especially *Wei. koreensis*, was the most dominant species in the kimchi samples. Studies on bacteria composition in kimchi published before 2000 did not mention the genus *Weissella*. This was likely because it was considered to be a *Leuconostoc* subspecies before being reclassified by Collins and Gibson (1999).

3.7 Functionalities

The main ingredients of kimchi are baechu cabbage and radish. Subingredients are red pepper powder, garlic, ginger, green onion, etc. that are used as folk medicine. When kimchi is prepared, other subingredients can be added to improve taste, nutrition, and functionality. Historically, kimchi was a protective food during the winter season when fresh vegetables were unavailable to Koreans. It is a lactic acid bacteria-fermented probiotic food with LAB numbering up to 10^9 CFUs/g and produces fermented products with taste and long storage life. Kimchi (baechu kimchi) is a low-calorie food (18 kcal/100 g). It contains high levels of vitamins (vitamin C, beta-carotene, vitamin B complex, etc.), minerals (Na, Ca, K, Fe, P), dietary fibers (24% on a dry base; 7.8% soluble dietary fiber, 16.2% insoluble dietary fiber), and other fermented functional components (Park et al., 1996). Functional substances found in kimchi are isothiocyanates, indole-3-carbinol, allyl sulfur compounds (allicin, diallyl sulfide, etc.), beta-sitosterol, ascorbic acid, carotenoids, flavonoids, tocopherol, selenium, dietary fibers, polyunsaturated fatty acids, LAB, etc. The protein and lipid contents can be increased by the addition of fish, clam, oyster, and meat depending on family preference (Park and Rhee, 2005; Park et al., 2014).

Kimchi has been developed in our laboratory to enhance its functionalities, especially for such medicinal properties as anticancer and antiobesity effects. Various main ingredients and subingredients were employed to increase anticancer activity of kimchi while leaving the organoleptic properties unchanged or improved. Addition of Chinese pepper, mistletoe powder, mustard leaf, LAB powder, starter cultures or using organically cultivated

Kimchi and Its Health Benefits   55

baechu cabbage, different kinds of salts, etc. were attempted (Cho, 1999; Jung, 2000; Choi, 2001; Kil, 2004; Bong et al., 2013; Jeong et al., 2015; Lee, 2016). Also, fermentation conditions such as temperatures and types of containers were modified for quality optimization and promotion of functionality.

We have reported our and other research results on kimchi and its health benefits in review papers and other book chapters (Cheigh and Park, 1994; Park, 1995; Park and Cheigh, 2004; Park and Rhee, 2005; Park and Kim, 2012; Park et al., 2014; Park and Jeong, 2016; Park et al., 2017). The health benefits of kimchi thus far studied are

1. Food source of probiotics
2. Improvement of colon health
3. Cancer-preventive effect
4. Control and reduction of body weight
5. Control of lipid profiles and metabolic syndrome
6. Antioxidative and antiaging effects
7. Others (promotion of immune function and appetite, etc.)

Thus, we will introduce and discuss mainly new findings along with the important functional activities of kimchi and kimchi LAB.

3.7.1 Improvement of Colon Health

The effects of kimchi on colon health of young healthy subjects and IBS (irritable bowel syndrome) patients were investigated by Kim (2016). Twenty-eight subjects participated in a 4-week clinical test, divided into a standard kimchi (SK) group and functional (anticancer kimchi recipe) kimchi (FK) group; they were administered 210 g of kimchi per day. An average fecal pH per experimental groups was changed from 6.6 ± 0.9 (week 1) to 6.4 ± 0.7 (end of week 4) in the SK group and from 6.8 ± 0.7 to 6.3 ± 0.7 in the FK group. Eighty-seven IBS patients participated in another 12-week clinical test for the improvement of colon health, were divided into SK and FK groups, and were also administered 210 g of kimchi per day. An average fecal pH was changed from 7.1 ± 0.5 (week 1) to 6.7 ± 0.4 (end of week 12) in the SK group and from 7.1 ± 0.5 to 6.5 ± 0.4 in the FK group. Thus, administration of kimchi, SK or FK, reduced fecal pH in both normal subjects and IBS patients.

The harmful enzymes, β-glucosidase and β-glucuronidase, in the colon significantly decreased in both SK and FK groups (Figure 3.3). Fecal β-glucosidase in SK was reduced from 4.8 ± 0.4 units/g (week 1) to 2.1 ± 0.5 (end of week 4, $p < 0.01$), while β-glucosidase in FK was also reduced from 4.7 ± 0.9 units/g to 2.2 ± 0.3. Also, fecal β-glucuronidase in SK was significantly decreased from 8.7 ± 1.2 units/g (week 1) to 2.8 ± 1.5 (end of week 4, $p < 0.01$), while β-glucuronidase in

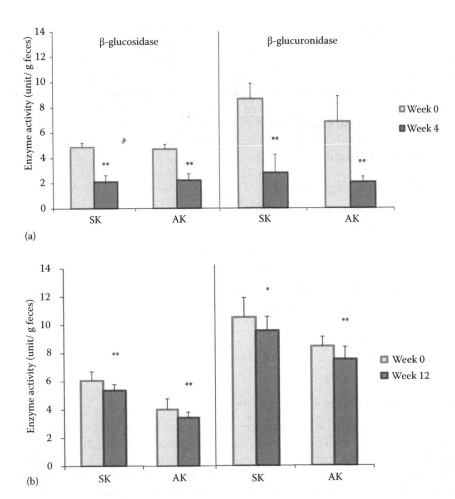

FIGURE 3.3
Fecal β-glucosidase- and β-glucuronidase activity changes of (a) normal healthy subjects and in (b) IBS patients who consumed standardized kimchi (SK) and functional kimchi (FK). Data represent mean ± SD. *Means significantly different from week 0 value ($p < 0.05$). **Means significantly different from week 0 value ($p < 0.01$). (From Kim, H. Y. 2016. Effects of kimchi intake on colon health of Korean young adults and irritable bowel syndrome patients. PhD diss., Pusan National University, Busan, Korea.)

FK was reduced from 6.8 ± 2.0 units/g to 2.1 ± 0.4 ($p < 0.01$). Among IBS patients, the fecal β-glucosidase in SK was significantly decreased from 6.1 ± 0.6 units/g (week 1) to 5.4 ± 0.4 (end of week 12, $p < 0.01$), and β-glucosidase in FK was significantly reduced from 4.4 ± 0.8 units/g to 3.7 ± 0.4 ($p < 0.01$). Fecal β-glucosidase activity among IBS patients was also reduced after a 12-week experiment in a similar manner; β-glucuronidase in SK was decreased from 10.3 ± 0.6 units/g (week 1) to 9.4 ± 0.1 (end of week 12, $p < 0.05$), and β-glucuronidase in FK was significantly reduced from 8.6 ± 0.5 units/g to 7.6 ± 0.7 ($p < 0.01$).

Kimchi and Its Health Benefits

Kimchi and kimchi LAB play important roles in decreasing the pH of the colon environment (Lee et al., 1996; Kil, 2004; Kil et al., 2004) and causing decreases in the harmful enzymes and helping maintain good colon health (Park and Kim, 2012). Decreases in fecal pH might have been the result of surviving kimchi LAB-producing acids; low pH in colon kills pathogenic and harmful microorganisms and reduces the intestinal absorption of potential toxic compounds (Martineau and Laflamme, 2002). Fermentation of dietary fiber by LAB can form short-chain fatty acid (SCFA), which is known to promote colon health resulting from immunomodulation, blood vessel dilation, increase in colon peristalsis, and wound healing. Butyrate, one of the SCFAs, is found to modulate inflammatory reactions in IBD patients. Bengmark (2001) indicated that *Lab. plantarum* can make SCFA from dietary fibers that can induce apoptosis of colon cancer cells and may help prevent colon cancer. β-glucosidase can make toxic aglycones from plant glucosides, and β-glucuronidase can hydrolyze glucuronic acid conjugate and promote enterohepatic circulation of toxic materials. β-glucuronidase, nitroreductase, and azoreductase are the well-known major enteric enzymes, most of which convert precarcinogens into carcinogens (Goldin and Gorbach, 1976). Koreans and Germans eat kimchi and sauerkraut, respectively, which may result in low activity of hazardous enteric enzymes and low fecal pH (Oh et al., 1993). We have also reported that dead kimchi LAB, *Lab. plantarum*, prevented colitis and colon cancer in animal studies, and it produced IgA, inhibited proinflammatory cytokines, and increased NK cell activation (Lee et al., 2015a, 2015b). Thus, administration of kimchi may be helpful for lowering fecal pH and deactivation of hazardous enteric enzymes, which may result in maintaining good colon health and suppressing the formation of carcinogens and eventually promote colon health and colorectal cancer prevention.

IBS patients have symptoms such as abdominal pain or discomfort, desperation for bowel movement, incomplete evacuation, and bloating. The changes in intensity scores of symptoms are presented in Table 3.2 and characterized on a scale of 1 (no symptoms) to 5 (extremely severe symptoms). Both groups (SK and FK) resulted in the same trend. Their symptoms were all significantly decreased (p < 0.001), from 2.2–2.6 to 1.3–1.4. It has been reported that probiotics could decrease IBS symptoms (Kajander et al., 2005). Capsaicin in RPP in kimchi can promote secretion of gastric juices, recovering gastric mucosa, sterile action, and colon peristaltic movement (Sohn, 2002; Choi, 2001). Proinflammatory cytokines of IL-1β, TNF-α, and IL-6 are positively related to IBS. TNF-α and IL-6 are associated with abdominal pain and inconvenience, etc. (Hughes et al., 2013). Kim (2016) reported that TNF-α significantly decreased (p < 0.001) after 12-week kimchi consumption; thus decreases in the cytokines are also related with the suppression of symptoms. The genera *Faecalibacterium*, *Roseburia*, and *Phascolarctobacterium*, and *Lactobacillus* and *Bifidobacterium* species that are beneficial microorganisms in the colon markedly increased, and *Escherichia* sp. levels decreased; therefore, kimchi consumption changed the microbial community in the colon.

TABLE 3.2

Comparison of Irritable Bowel Symptom Scores between IBS Patients Who Participated in Clinical Studies

	SK		FK	
	W-0	W-12	W-0	W-12
Abdominal pain or discomfort	2.4 ± 0.6	1.4 ± 0.5[a]	2.5 ± 0.6	1.4 ± 0.4[a]
Urgent feeling to have bowel movement	2.2 ± 0.9	1.3 ± 0.5[a]	2.2 ± 0.8	1.4 ± 0.5[a]
Incomplete evacuation	2.5 ± 0.8	1.4 ± 0.5[a]	2.4 ± 0.8	1.4 ± 0.6[a]
Bloating	2.6 ± 0.7	1.3 ± 0.5[a]	2.5± 0.6	1.4 ± 0.6[a]

Source: Kim, H. Y. 2016. PhD diss., Pusan National University, Busan, Korea.

Notes: Data represent mean ± SD. SK, IBS patients consumed standardized kimchi ($n = 30$); FK, IBS patients consumed functional kimchi ($n = 29$). IBS score was based on the intensity of symptoms rated from 1 to 5: 1 for no symptoms, 2 for light to moderate symptoms, 3 for moderate symptoms, 4 for severe symptoms, 5 for extremely severe symptoms.

[a] Means significantly different from week 0 value ($p < 0.001$).

Lactobacillus species increased from 0.11% to 3.38% in SK and FK groups. IBS patients showed increased *Bifidobacterium* species after kimchi consumption. One patient who consumed SK increased *Bifidobacterium* from 0.95% to 16.8% after 12 weeks (Kim, 2016).

3.7.2 Antioxidative and Antiaging Effects

Oxidative stress and nitrosative stress are known as precursors to chronic diseases such as cardiovascular diseases, diabetes, Alzheimer's disease, cancers, etc. (Kim et al., 2014a). Antioxidative compounds in kimchi may scavenge free radicals formed in the body by acting as hydrogen donors (Hwang and Song, 2000). Kimchi contains powerful antioxidants from ingredients, metabolites and LAB, including the natural free radical scavengers vitamin C, chlorophyll, phenols, carotenoids, dietary fibers, and other phytochemicals. Fermented metabolites with LAB can decrease or eliminate oxidants, pro-oxidants, and other free radicals, which might be direct or indirect causes of aging (Ryu et al., 2004).

DPPH radical scavenging activity and scavenging effects of kimchi on NO, O_2^-, and $\cdot$OH radicals were measured under different fermentation stages at different dose levels. At a concentration of 1000 μg/mL, fresh (Fr), optimally ripened (OptR), and over-ripened (OvR) kimchi, NO was scavenged by 24.9%, 64.8%, and 54.9%, respectively. O_2^- was scavenged by 30.1%, 52.8%, and 34.8%. $\cdot$OH radical scavenging effects were 42.2%, 53.8%, and 43.2%, respectively. Thus, kimchi showed the highest antioxidative capacity when optimally ripened (Kim et al., 2014a). Oxidative stress was induced by SNP (NO), pyrogallol $\left(O_2^-\right)$, and SW-1 (ONOO⁻) in LLC-PK$_1$ cells. Kimchi, especially OptR and OvR kimchi, effectively decreased the oxidative stresses. Kimchi also exerted anti-inflammatory effects by suppressing SIN-1 induced mRNA and protein expressions of COX-2, iNOS, NF-κB p65, and IκB. The COX-2 and iNOS expressions were elevated in SIN-1-treated LLC-PK$_1$ cells; however, 500 µg/mL of kimchi markedly decreased mRNA and protein expression of COX-2, iNOS, and NF-κB p65. OvR kimchi caused a marked decrease of the expressions (Kim et al., 2014a).

Antiaging effects of kimchi have also been studied. Free radical production and antioxidative enzyme activities in brains of senescence-accelerated mice (SAM) showed that kimchi moderated the increase in free radical production due to aging (Kim et al., 2002). Baechu kimchi containing both 30% mustard leaf and mustard leaf kimchi-fed groups showed greater inhibition of free-radical production in the brain than those receiving standard baechu kimchi. The antiaging activity of kimchi has also been evaluated by using the stress-induced premature senescence (SIPS) model (Kim et al., 2011a). WI-38 human fibroblasts challenged with H$_2$O$_2$ showed a loss of cell viability, an increase in lipid peroxidation, and a shortening of the cell life span, indicating the induction of SIPS. Kimchi, especially OptR kimchi, attenuated cellular oxidative stress by increasing cell viability and inhibition of lipid peroxidation. In addition, the life span of WI-38 cells was expanded, indicating a promising role of kimchi as an antiaging food.

Antiaging effects of kimchi were evaluated in hairless mice by adding kimchi to an AIN-76 diet for 20 weeks. Morphological changes in the epidermis and dermis were observed at week 16, and the antioxidant effects against UV-induced photoaging and the free radical scavenging effect were studied at week 20 (Ryu, 2000). The epidermal thickness of the hairless mice was found to be greater (22%–37%) in the kimchi (baechu, mustard leaf, and leek kimchi) fed groups, whereas the stratum corneum was thinner (58%–62%) relative to the control group, indicating that kimchi promoted healthy skin conditions. Collagen synthesis at the dermis increased with kimchi treatment as the activity of the rough endoplasmic reticulum of the fibroblast was greater than that of the control group. Type IV collagen, which supports matrices at the basement membrane, was present in greater amounts in the kimchi-fed groups than the control group, especially the group fed the mustard leaf kimchi (52% higher vs. control). Lipid oxidation (TBARS content) in the livers of the hairless mice fed a kimchi diet was retarded compared to the control, and the concentrations of superoxide anion, hydroxyl radical, and H$_2$O$_2$ were lower than in the control group, indicating greater free-radical scavenging capacity.

Choi et al. (2014) investigated the effect of kimchi against memory impairment induced by Aβ-25-35 in an *in vivo* Alzheimer's mouse model. The Aβ-25-35 was injected into the brains of ICR mice and then OptR kimchi was orally administered for 2 weeks. Objective cognitive ability, T-maze tests, and Morris water maze tests indicated that kimchi exerted strong protection against cognitive impairment induced by Aβ-25-35 ($p < 0.05$). Kimchi

60   *Korean Functional Foods*

exhibited a protective effect against lipid peroxidation in the brain by Aβ-25-35. Thus, kimchi has strong antioxidant properties that could be its basic mechanism for preventing chronic diseases.

3.7.3 Cancer Preventive Effects

We were the first to report that kimchi exhibits antimutagenicity against mutagens/carcinogens of aflatoxin B_1 and MNNG in the Ames test and the SOS chromotest *in vitro* (Park et al., 1995; Park, 1995). Optimally ripened (OptR) kimchi showed the highest antimutagenicity compared to freshly prepared (Fr) kimchi and over-ripened (OvR) kimchi (Park, 1995). The kimchi extract also exhibited antimutagenic activity in the *Drosophila* wing test *in vivo* (Hwang et al., 1997) and anticlastogenic activity in MMC-induced mice using the *in vivo* supravital staining micronucleus assay (Ryu and Park, 2001). Kimchi extracts inhibited the growth of human cancer cells (AGS gastric cancer cells, HT-29 colon cancer cells, MG-63 osteocarcinoma cells, HL-60 leukemia cells, and Hep3B liver cancer cells) in the SRB and MTT assays. Furthermore, kimchi induced apoptosis in various human cancer cells (Cho, 1997, 1999; Park and Rhee, 2005). β-sitosterol and a linoleic acid derivative were the main active compounds that showed anticancer activity in kimchi (Cho, 1997; Cho et al., 2004). The dichloromethane fraction and β-sitosterol, an active compound in the fraction, arrested the cancer cell cycle in the G2/M phase and induced apoptosis of HL-60 human leukemia cells (Cho, 1999).

Methanol extracts from kimchi samples and the dichloromethane (DCM) fraction were used to treat Rat2 fibroblast normal cells and HO6 H-Ras^{v12} transformed Rat2 cells (Park et al., 2003). The kimchi samples from commercial baechu cabbage kimchi (CK), organically cultivated baechu cabbage kimchi (OK), and the DCM fraction from CK inhibited the proliferation of HO6 transformed cells more effectively than the Rat2 normal cells. The DCM fraction showed greater effect than CK and OK, but OK exerted a greater effect than CK. The survival rates of Ras^{v12}-transformed Rat2 cells were very low (i.e., 23%, 18%, and 9% after treatment with CK, OK, and the DCM fraction, respectively); however, survival rate of normal Rat2 fibroblasts was about 70% following treatment with any of the three kimchi samples. Thus, kimchi can suppress cell growth and increase apoptosis in cancer cells, but not normal cells. Jeong et al. (2015) recently indicated that kimchi did not show cytotoxicity in nontransformed RGM-1 gastric mucosal cells, but it exhibited significant cytotoxicity in AGS cancer cells. Kimchi induced selective cytotoxicity of transformed AGS cancer cells. Cell viability with different doses (1.0–7.5 mg/mL) of S kimchi (standardized kimchi) and CP kimchi (cancer-preventive kimchi) was studied. Doses of 5 and 7.5 mg/mL of kimchi extracts showed significant cytotoxicity in AGS cancer cells ($p < 0.05$); however, it did not show any toxicity in nontransformed gastric mucosal cells (Figure 3.4a). They checked the expression of heme oxygenase-1 (HO-1), which is a cytoprotective

Kimchi and Its Health Benefits

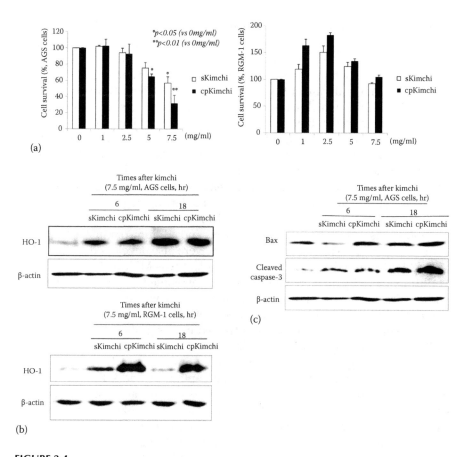

FIGURE 3.4
Biological actions of standard kimchi (sKimchi) and cancer-preventive kimchi (cpKimchi); comparison in an *in vitro* H. pylori cell model. (a) Cell survival by MTT assay. MTT assay was done in AGS cells (left) and RGM-1 cells (right) treated with 1, 2.5, 5, and 7.5 mg/mL concentration of sKimchi and cpKimchi soluble extracts, respectively. (b) Western blot of HO-1 after each kimchi extract. (c) Western blot for Bax and cleaved caspase-3. (From Jeong, M. et al. 2015, *Oncotarget* 6:29513–29526.)

gene, to validate the selective cytotoxicities of CP kimchi in cancer cells only. The expression of HO-1 was more prominent in RGM-1 cells (Figure 3.4b). The expressions were greatly increased in CP kimchi. The cytotoxicities of CP kimchi were blunted in RMG-1 cells through strong induction of the cytoprotective gene, HO-1. CP kimchi showed selective apoptotic action in AGS cancer cells, increased expression of Bax, and cleaved caspase-3 compared to S kimchi (Figure 3.4c); however, CP kimchi did not show any increased expression of Bax in noncancer cells (Data not shown). Thus, kimchi may selectively act against cancer cells, but not nonmalignant cells.

We have endeavored to increase the anticancer function of kimchi. Various types of kimchi were developed by adding different subingredients (Cho,

1999). Adding Chinese pepper increased the anticancer effect. Using organically cultivated baechu cabbage (Obc) instead of general baechu cabbage significantly increased its anticancer effect. The Obc has more nutrients and phytochemicals such as vitamin C, carotenoids, chlorophyll, total dietary fibers, etc. (Choi and Park, 1998). We also added 0.05% of Korean mistletoe powder (Kil, 2004), which caused morphological changes in A 549 human lung carcinoma cells; Bax, especially, significantly increased but Bcl-2 decreased. The kinds of salt used in kimchi preparation are also very important for increasing taste, quality, and functionality of kimchi (Jung, 2000; Choi, 2001; Kil, 2004). Traditionally, natural sea salt without bittern (NS-B removed brined water from the natural sea salt) was used. Cancer-preventive or anticancer kimchi was developed by considering the opinions of cancer patients and other related experiments (Kim, 2002). Kimchis with increased concentrations of red pepper powder, garlic, and addition of mustard leaf and Chinese pepper (A-kimchi) and MI kimchi were also developed, A-kimchi + 2.5% RPP (decreased RPP) + 7.5% mustard leaf was MI kimchi (Choi, 2001). Antitumor activity in sarcoma-180 cell-transplanted BALB/c mouse was studied. Standardized (S) kimchi inhibited tumor weight by 21%; however, A and MI kimchi resulted in tumor weight suppression rates of 35% and 42%. NK cell activities of the kimchi-treated mice significantly increased in A (40%) and MI (60%) kimchi ($p < 0.05$). We also employed different kinds of salt for brining the cabbage. The NS-B, Guwun (baked) salt, and bamboo salt showed better taste and overall acceptability and killed pathogenic and spoilage microorganisms and increased antioxidative and anticancer activities etc. (Choi, 1998; Jung et al., 2001; Han et al., 2009). Using Guwun salt + KCl or bamboo salt (nine times baked; 9×) significantly increased antitumor activities and increased NK cell activity (Jung et al., 2001). We isolated *Leu. mesenteroides* PNU and *Lab. plantarum* PNU from kimchi and used them as starter cultures. The starter (10^6 CFUs/g) added kimchi significantly increased anticancer activity (Bong et al., 2013; Lee et al., 2016).

Fermentation conditions also affect anticancer activities of kimchi. Cho (1999) revealed that lower temperature fermentation was better than high temperature for increasing anticancer activity of kimchi. The fermentation container is also important for improving taste and anticancer effects of kimchi. Onggi with or without glaze, polypropylene containers that are usually used for kimchi refrigeration, plastic containers, stainless steel containers, and glass bottles were studied (Kim, 2010; Jeong et al., 2011). Onggi without glaze, especially, was most beneficial for facilitating facultative anaerobic conditions for LAB, and resulted in the best taste and antioxidative and anticancer effects; the glass bottles showed the worst result.

Added ingredients and different fermentation times were evaluated for their impacts on anticancer effects in human HT-29 colon cancer cells. As shown in Figure 3.5, anticancer kimchi (AK) with added or adjusted ingredients compared to SK (standardized kimchi) showed better anticancer effects. The fermentation time was also an important factor in anticancer

Kimchi and Its Health Benefits

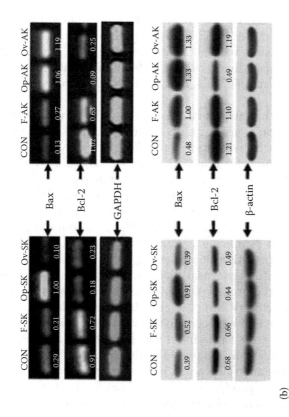

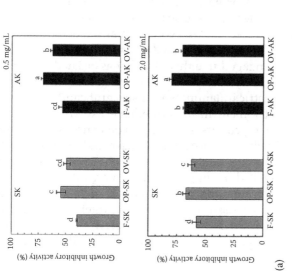

FIGURE 3.5
Inhibitory effects of kimchi on growth of HT-29 human colon cancer cells based on an MTT assay (a). Effects of standardized kimchi and anticancer kimchi varieties on mRNA and protein expressions of Bax and Bcl-2 in HT-29 human colon carcinoma cells (b). SK = standardized kimchi; F-SK = fresh SK; Op-SK = optimally ripened SK; Ov-SK = over-ripened SK; AK = anticancer kimchi; F-AK = fresh AK; Op-AK = optimally ripened AK; Ov-AK = over-ripened AK. Data were reported as a mean ± SD. [a–d]Mean values with different letters above bars are significantly different ($p < 0.05$) based on Duncan's multiple range test. The number below bands is the band intensity of the factor divided by the band intensity of the housekeeping gene (GAPDH and β-actin). The GAPDH and β-actin band is shown to confirm equal loading of mRNA and protein and the 2 mg/mL of each sample treated with kimchi, respectively. (From Kim, B. K. et al. 2015, *Food Sci Biotechnol* 24:629–633.)

activity. Especially, Op-AK kimchi showed higher cancer cell growth inhibitory effects than F-AK or Ov-AK (Figure 3.5a). The fermentation process seemed to increase the anticancer effect. Op-AK significantly increased Bax mRNA and protein expression, while Bcl-2 expressions were significantly decreased (Figure 3.5b). Thus, kimchi exhibited the highest anticancer and other functionality (Kim et al., 1997, 2011, 2014, 2015) at an optimally ripened stage.

Recently we have found that functional kimchi showed anticancer effects on *Helicobacter pylori*-associated gastric cancer (Jeong et al., 2015). The cancer-preventive kimchi (CP kimchi) was studied in C57BL/6 mice with chronic *H. pylori*-initiated gastric tumorigenesis and a high-salt diet for 36 weeks. Erythematous and nodular changes, mucosal ulcerations, and erosive lesions in the stomach were noted at the 24th week, but CP kimchi administration significantly ameliorated the tumor development. Figure 3.6 shows that long-term intake of CP kimchi prevented the *H. pylori*–induced gastric tumorigenesis. It produced significant gastric tumors as well as a severe degree of chronic atrophic gastritis at 36 weeks (Figure 3.6a, b) and presented with findings including nodular mucosal changes, thinned gastric mucosa, adenomatous polyps, and tumorous lesions with central ulcerations. These gross lesions were severe chronic atrophic gastritis, gastric ulcer, gastritis cystica profunda, adenoma, and adenocarcinoma as revealed by pathological observation. The whole gross lesion index was significantly increased in the control group, but significantly decreased in the group with CP kimchi ($p < 0.05$; Figure 3.6a). Similar results noted in gross appearance were also drawn from pathological analysis ($p < 0.01$, Figure 3.6a). Figure 3.6(b) shows significant tumorigenesis on gross observation in the control group that was proven to be gastric adenoma or gastric adenocarcinoma, but CP kimchi administration significantly decreased gastric tumorigenesis ($p < 0.01$). CP kimchi also significantly reduced COX-2 expression and macrophage infiltration. Macrophage-related inflammatory mediators, including IL-1β, VEGF, IL-6, and MMP-2, that are engaged in either *H. pylori*-associated gastritis or carcinogenesis were significantly decreased by CP kimchi. Transcription factors STAT3 and NF-κB in gastric inflammations also significantly decreased.

The anticancer effects of kimchi in azoxymethane (AOM) and dextran sulfate sodium (DSS) inducing colitis-associated colon cancer in mice were also studied (Kim et al., 2014b). Increased colon length and decreased colon weight/length ratio and tumor numbers in colon were observed in the kimchi-treated group, especially ACK (kimchi prepared with an anticancer kimchi recipe). Kimchi decreased proinflammatory cytokines, such as TNF-α, IL-6, IFN-γ, etc., in serum and colon tissues, and mRNA; protein expressions of proinflammatory genes such as iNOS and COX-2 were also significantly reduced, but p53 and p21 expression significantly increased, especially in ACK. Thus, kimchi can show anticancer effects, but cancer-preventive or anticancer kimchi that we prepared from various experiments significantly increased the anticancer effect in human cancer cells and *in vivo* model

Kimchi and Its Health Benefits

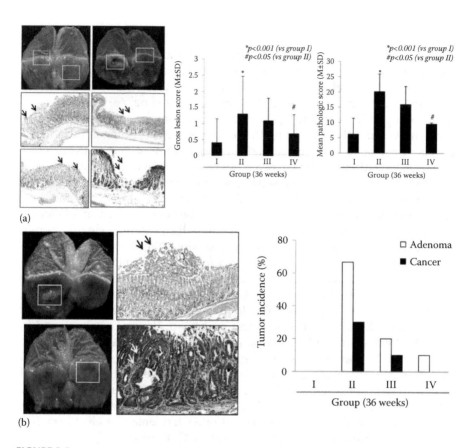

FIGURE 3.6
Prevention of *H. pylori*–induced gastric tumorigenesis with long-term intake of cpKimchi (36 weeks after *H. pylori* infection). (a) Gross and pathological pictures and index according to group. On gross evaluation of resected stomach, the following findings were obtained; nodular mucosal changes, thinned gastric mucosa, adenomatous polyps, and tumorous lesion with central ulcerations. The whole gross lesion index was significantly increased in the control group, but significantly decreased in the group administered with cpKimchi ($p < 0.05$). Severe chronic atrophic gastritis, gastric ulcer, gastritis cystica profunda, adenoma, and adenocarcinoma were shown in control group (×100). The mean pathological scores were significantly increased in control group, but significantly decreased in group administered with cpKimchi ($p < 0.05$). (b). The gastric cancer occurrence rate, according to group gastric adenoma, and cancer occurrence were significantly increased in the control group, but significantly decreased in the group administered with cpKimchi (×100) ($p < 0.05$). (From Jeong, M. et al. 2015, *Oncotarget* 6:29513–29526.)

systems of gastric cancer and colon cancer in mice. The kimchi inhibited expressions of proinflammatory cytokines, inflammation, and macrophage infiltration. It selectively induced apoptosis, increased expressions of p53 and p21, etc.; however, kimchi can protect normal cells by strongly increasing the expression of OH-1 genes and did not affect apoptosis and inflammation in the normal cells.

3.7.4 Antiobesity Effect

Kimchi has been shown to control body weight and related genes in the liver and adipocytes in epididymal fat tissues of diet-induced obese (DIO) mice (Choi, 2001; Yoon et al., 2005; Ahn, 2007; Kim et al., 2011b; Choi et al., 2013; Cui et al., 2015; Lee et al., 2015; Lee, 2016). Capsaicin in red pepper powder, one of the main ingredients of kimchi, can remove fats from the body by stimulating spinal nerves and thus activating the release of catecholamine in the adrenal glands. It promotes metabolism and the expenditure of energy (Kim, 1998). However, kimchi showed a better weight-loss effect than RPP itself (Choi, 2001). Rats fed kimchi containing the same level of RPP plus a high-fat diet showed an even further decrease in body weight ($p < 0.05$) and perirenal fat pad compared to the RPP diet group after 4 weeks. The decrease in fat accumulation by kimchi is due to combined effects of other ingredients, including garlic, radish, ginger, ginger with RPP, and/or fermented products (Yoon et al., 2005).

Antiobesity effects were shown not only for kimchi with RPP but also whitish baechu kimchi without RPP (baek kimchi). Baek kimchi exerted more effective antiobesity properties than baechu kimchi in a high-fat diet induced obesity animal model, probably due to the higher content of radish and pear used in baek kimchi. RPP, garlic, and ginger are the main spices used in kimchi. These spices and radish significantly decreased weight gain in the mice, but garlic and ginger showed greater effects on reducing body weight gain than RPP (Yoon et al., 2005). The garlic and ginger diet group exhibited significantly lower weights of liver, epididymal, and perirenal fat pads, and also decreased the levels of triacylglycerol (TG) and total cholesterol (TC) in serum, liver, and the fat pads. LAB and other fermented products are also found to decrease body weight (Moon et al., 2012; Kang et al., 2015).

In our studies, kimchi also showed antiobesity effects in humans. A group of obese women who were supplemented with kimchi capsules (3 and 6 g of freeze-dried kimchi/day) and exercised (1 hour, once per week) exhibited a remarkable decrease in body weight and body mass index (BMI) compared with the group that was not supplemented with the kimchi capsules. The visceral fat area and serum TG and low-density lipoprotein (LDL) levels were also significantly decreased, but high-density lipoprotein (HDL) increased in the kimchi-supplemented group compared with the group not supplemented with kimchi (Ahn, 2007). Kim et al. (2011b) reported that consumption of kimchi, especially fermented kimchi, leads to a reduction in body weight, BMI, and percentage of body fat in overweight and obese subjects. We again confirmed the antiobesity effect of kimchi in high-fat diet-induced obese C57BL/6 mice. As shown in Table 3.3. the weight of normal mice was 24.7 ± 0.9 g; however, the HFD, S kimchi (standardized kimchi) group and the D kimchi (Korean commercial D kimchi with inoculation of *Leu. mesenteroides*) group were 29.1 ~ 29.5 g after being fed a high-fat diet for 4 weeks. Mice became obese by feeding them HFD for another 4 weeks. However, when HFD containing 10% of freeze-dried S kimchi or D kimchi was used for 4 more weeks, the body weight gains

Kimchi and Its Health Benefits

TABLE 3.3

Body Weights, Food Intakes, Food Efficiency Ratios, and Tissue Weights in DIO (Diet-Induced Obese) Mice

		ND[a]	HFD[b]	S Kimchi[c]	D Kimchi[d]
Body weight (g)	Initial	23.4 ± 1.3[e]	23.3 ± 1.3[f]	23.5 ± 0.6	23.4 ± 0.6
	Fourth week	24.7 ± 0.9 (1.3)[g]	29.5 ± 1.1 (6.2)	29.1 ± 0.7 (5.6)	29.3 ± 0.7 (5.9)
	Eighth week	27.2 ± 1.2 (2.5)	43.0 ± 3.4 (13.5)	32.8 ± 2.5 (3.7)[h]	32.6 ± 2.3 (3.3)[h]
Body weight gain (g/d)		0.1 ± 0.1	0.5 ± 0.1	0.1 ± 0.1	0.1 ± 0.1
Food intake (g/d)		3.4 ± 0.1[e]	3.5 ± 0.2	3.4 ± 0.1	3.5 ± 0.1
Food efficiency ratio (FER[i]; %)		2.7 ± 0.8	13.9 ± 1.7	3.9 ± 0.1[h]	3.5 ± 0.5[h]

Source: Cui, M. et al., *J Ethnic Foods*, 2, 137–144, 2015.

[a] ND: normal diet
[b] HFD: high-fat diet
[c] S kimchi: standardized kimchi
[d] D kimchi: Korean commercial kimchi
[e] Not significant
[f] Results are presented as means ± SDs.
[g] Numbers in parentheses mean increase in body weight.
[h] Significantly different ($p < 0.05$) in the same raw compared to HFD.
[i] FER is total weight gain/total food intake.

significantly decreased; body weight of the HFD group was 43.0 ± 3.4 g, which was an increase of 13.5 g, but the body weights of S kimchi and D kimchi were significantly lower at 32.8 ± 2.5 g and 32.6 ± 2.3 g, and increased only 3.7 and 3.3g, respectively. Food efficiency ratio (FER) in the HFD group was 13.9% ± 1.7%; however, FERs in S kimchi and D kimchi were significantly reduced to 3.9% ± 0.1% and 3.5% ± 0.5%, respectively (Table 3.3). The body weight markedly increased after an additional 4 weeks of high-fat feeding; however, kimchi feeding with the high-fat diet significantly inhibited body fat gain. The D kimchi group exhibited significantly decreased serum levels of TG, TC, LDL-C, insulin, and leptin and increased HDL-C and adiponectin with reduction of the body weight (Cui et al., 2015). Kimchi treatment also significantly reduced HFD-induced lipid formation in liver. Hepatic mRNA expressions of adipogenesis-related genes of C/EBP-α, PPAR-γ, SREBP-1c, and FAS were significantly lower than those in the HFD group, but fatty acid oxidation-related gene, CPT-1 expression was higher. In epididymal fat tissues, mean adipocyte sizes in epididymal fat were 7.5 ± 2.6 units in the HFD, 3.4 ± 0.8 in S kimchi, 1.8 ± 0.7 in D kimchi, and 2.0 ± 0.7 in the normal diet (ND). Kimchi treatment significantly decreased the size of adipocytes in epididymal fat when using D kimchi and was similar to that in the ND group. The MCP-1 mRNA expression (an important mediator of macrophage activity and promotor of inflammatory response in adipose tissues) and IL-6 expression (an inflammatory cytokine) were significantly reduced compared to HFD after 8 weeks of the experiment.

We have worked to develop functional antiobesity kimchi (FK). The FK kimchi was prepared by adding 5% green tea leaves, 0.1% Chinese pepper, pear, and mushroom and sea tangle juice, and bamboo salt was used instead of solar salt (Lee, 2016). MSFK was used as the starter cultures (*Leu mesenteroides* + *Lab. plantarum*) + FK, to make mixed starter culture fermented FK. As shown in Figure 3.7, FK and MSFK significantly decreased body weight gain compared to the HFD and standardized kimchi (SK) group during 8 weeks of high-fat diet feeding. The weight gain results were statistically the same as for the normal group. SK decreased body weight gain and was statistically different from FK from day 28 to day 56. Our observations also included pathological analyses from liver and adipose tissue after 8 weeks (day 56). Severe accumulation of lipid in liver tissue was found in the HFD group, and lipid accumulation accompanied by slight inflammation was found in the SK group; liver tissues from FK and MSFK groups showed the same condition as that in the normal group. Also, enlarged adipocytes and inflammation were observed in adipose tissue from the HFD group in comparison with that in the normal group, while adipose tissues from the MSFK group showed the same condition as that in the normal group. Serum levels of TG, TC, LDL, and leptin were all increased in the HFD group, but FK and MSFK groups showed decreases in these factors similar to that in the normal group. HDL and adiponectin concentration of the FK and MSFK groups were increased in comparison with those from the HFD group, whereas the MSFK group

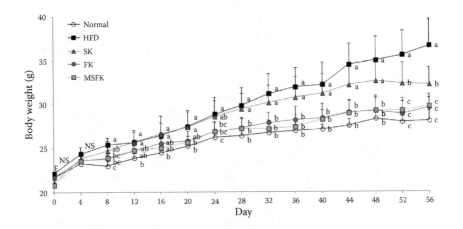

FIGURE 3.7
Effects of standardized kimchi (SK), functional kimchi (FK) and mixed starter-fermented functional kimchi (MSFK) on changes in body weight in HFD-induced obesity in mice. Symbols: normal = normal diet; HFD = high-fat diet; SK= high-fat diet + standardized kimchi; FK = high-fat diet + functional kimchi; MSFK = high-fat diet + mixed starter fermented functional kimchi. [a-c]Means with different letters on the same day are significantly different ($p < 0.05$) by Duncan's multiple range test. (From Lee, K. H. 2016. Lactic acid bacteria starter fermented kimchi inhibits obesity and colitis-associated colon cancer in C57BL/6J mice. Ph.D. diss., Pusan National University, Busan, Korea.)

showed the most prominent promotion of the factors. Hepatic expressions of lipogenesis-related genes including SREBP-1c, C/EBP-α, and PPAR-γ were promoted in HFD group, but were significantly lower in the FK and MSFK groups. Green tea leaves in the FK and MSFK groups played an important role in suppressing lipid accumulation, owing to caffeine and theamine (Zheng et al., 2004), and bamboo salt used to prepare the FK decrease obesity (Ju, 2016). Thus, manipulation of ingredients could increase the antiobesity effect of kimchi. Custom-made kimchi could be developed for the prevention of obesity and decrease of body fat for obese subjects.

3.7.5 Hypolipidemic Effect and Control of Metabolic Syndrome

Kimchi showed a hypolipidemic effect in various animal and human studies (Kwon et al., 1997, 1999; Ahn, 2007; Kim et al., 2011b; Kim, 2016; Lee, 2016). Plasma TG and cholesterol levels were lower in rats fed on a kimchi diet. Kimchi consumption decreased VLDL-C and LDL-C, but significantly increased HDL-C. The levels of hepatic cholesterol, TG, total lipids, and apolipoproteins B decreased, but fecal total fat, cholesterol, TG, and apoliprotein A-1 levels were significantly increased (Kwon et al., 1997). Fermented kimchi was more effective for lowering total lipids, cholesterol, and TG levels of the epididymal fat pad than fresh kimchi (Kim et al., 2011b). The TG concentration of feces from the kimchi groups was higher than that of the control group, indicating that kimchi stimulates lipid mobilization from the epididymal fat pad as well as lipid excretion via feces. High levels of dietary fiber in kimchi may also contribute to the capture and excretion of cholesterol and TG via the feces.

Ray and Bhunia (2008) reported that LAB metabolize dietary cholesterol and deconjugate bile salt in the colon while also preventing their reabsorption in the liver, decreasing cholesterol levels in the serum. Kimchi has 10^{7-9} CFUs/g of LAB. Thus, LAB in kimchi may also decrease serum cholesterol after kimchi consumption. We have recently conducted clinical studies of kimchi effects on serum lipids. Kimchi intake (210 g/d) changed serum lipid profiles and some markers of dyslipidemia in young healthy subjects for 4 weeks. As shown in the Table 3.4, the serum levels of TG, TC, and LDL decreased, but HDL increased. Functional kimchi especially showed significant changes ($p < 0.05$, $p < 0.01$; Table 3.4). Adiponectin levels were significantly increased in both kimchi-treated groups. IL-6 and MCP-1 were also significantly decreased. Thus, it is certain that lipid profile can be improved when kimchi is consumed; FK that has more functional ingredients especially showed better results.

Metabolic syndrome is defined as having three or more of the five of the following symptoms: high blood glucose concentrations (diabetes or prediabetes), obesity, high serum triglycerides, high blood pressure, and decreased HDL-C (Kaur, 2014). Kim et al. (2011b) reported that fermented kimchi (matured for 5 hours at room temperature, then stored at 5°C–10°C for 10 days, pH 4.3 ± 0.02) had more beneficial effects compared with those of fresh

70   *Korean Functional Foods*

TABLE 3.4

Changes in Serum Lipid, Metabolic, and Inflammatory Markers in Healthy Subjects Consuming Baechu Kimchi for 4 Weeks

	SK		FK	
	W-0	**W-4**	**W-0**	**W-4**
TG (mg/dL)	72.6 ± 23.5	67.0 ± 17.3	82.0 ± 34.8	62.3 ± 21.8[a]
TC (mg/dL)	167.5 ± 30.5	164.1 ± 25.8	171.2 ± 21.8	153.3 ± 16.3[a]
LDL (mg/dL)	104.9 ± 22.4	82.1 ± 13.4[a]	104.0 ± 25.2	84.7 ± 13.5[a]
HDL (mg/dL)	48.5 ± 8.1	58.1 ± 8.8[a]	50.9 ± 7.8	67.3 ± 11.2[b]
Adiponectin (µg/mL)	6.6 ± 1.1	8.8 ± 2.3[a]	6.5 ± 1.0	9.0 ± 2.9[a]
IL-6 (pg/mL)	1.4 ± 0.9	1.3 ± 0.3	1.9 ± 1.0	0.7 ± 0.2[a]
MCP-1 (pg/mL)	313.5 ± 68.0	294.0 ± 55.0	254.1 ± 64.9	232.8 ± 34.7

Source: Kim, H. Y. 2016. PhD diss., Pusan National University, Busan, Korea.

Notes: Results are presented as means ± SDs. FK: functional kimchi; SK: standardized kimchi.

[a] Significantly different ($p < 0.05$) compared to that in W-0.

[b] Significantly different ($p < 0.01$) compared to that in W-0.

kimchi (1-day-old kimchi-stored at 1°C, pH 6.0 ± 0.01) on metabolic parameters that are related to cardiovascular disease and metabolic syndrome risks in overweight and obese subjects. Obese patients with a BMI above 25 kg/m^2 were assigned to two 4-week diet phases separated by a 2-week washout period. The subjects consumed either fresh or fermented kimchi, 300 g/day. Table 3.5 shows significant decreases in body weight, BMI, and body fat in groups that consumed fresh kimchi and fermented kimchi, and especially the fermented kimchi group showed significant decreases in the WHR (waist–hip ratio) and fasting blood glucose. Net differences in blood pressure, percentage of body fat, fasting glucose, and total cholesterol in the fermented kimchi group were significantly greater than those in the fresh kimchi group. Fasting insulin levels, which are closely related to insulin resistance and are higher in patients with metabolic syndrome, were significantly decreased in the fermented kimchi group. MCP-1 and other proinflammatory cytokines including CRP, TNF-α, and IL-6 are positively related to development of atherosclerosis; the fermented kimchi group had significantly reduced levels of MCP-1. Leptin production in obese cells plays an important role in controlling the pituitary system to suppress appetite and increase energy expenditure to control body weight. Serum leptin levels are higher in obese subjects, indicating leptin resistance. Ruige et al. (1999) reported that leptin secretion increases in direct proportion to the amount of body fat. Leptin levels can also be associated with insulin resistance because body fat is positively related to insulin resistance. Leptin decreased significantly after consumption of the fermented kimchi. The fermented kimchi group exhibited beneficial effects on various factors associated with metabolic syndrome, including blood pressure, percentage of body fat, fasting

Kimchi and Its Health Benefits

TABLE 3.5
Changes in Metabolic Parameters Related to Metabolic Syndrome in Obese Subjects by Kimchi Intake

	Fresh kimchi (n = 22)		Fermented kimchi (n = 22)	
	Initial[a]	Final[b]	Initial[c]	Final[d]
Body weight (kg)	72.9 ± 9.6	71.7 ± 9.4[e]	73.0 ± 10.1	71.5 ± 9.7[e]
BMI (kg/m²)	27.4 ± 2.2	27.0 ± 2.2[e]	27.5 ± 2.2	26.9 ± 2.2[e]
WHR	0.86 ± 0.05	0.85 ± 0.06	0.86 ± 0.06	0.84 ± 0.06[e]
Body fat (%)	31.9 ± 4.0	31.6 ± 4.0[e]	32.1 ± 4.3	31.4 ± 4.4[e,f]
Blood pressure, systolic (mmHg)	125.8 ± 10.7	122.1 ± 7.9	126.1 ± 12.1	121.3 ± 6.9[f]
Blood pressure, diastolic (mmHg)	76.1 ± 9.9	74.7 ± 8.5	76.9 ± 9.7	72.7 ± 7.4[f]
Glucose, fasting (mg/dL)	101.0 ± 11.1	96.6 ± 10.5	100.0 ± 10.2	94.1 ± 11.3[e,f]
Insulin, fasting (μIU/mL)	15.0 ± 6.9	13.4 ± 5.3	14.9 ± 6.2	11.0 ± 5.6[e]
Total cholesterol (mg/mL)	176.0 ± 29.5	172.0 ± 31.6	171.0 ± 25.7	161.0 ± 29.9[e,f]
MCP-1 (pg/mL)	170.0 ± 59.4	157.0 ± 48.9	167.0 ± 50.9	154.0 ± 41.0[e]
Leptin (ng/mL)	21.0 ± 6.6	19.3 ± 7.0	20.2 ± 1.3	15.7 ± 11.4[e]

Source: Kim, E. K. et al. 2011b. *Nutr Res* 31:436–443.

[a] Initial data of fresh kimchi group were the means of data on week 0 of group 2 and week 6 of group 1.

[b] Final data of fresh kimchi group were the means of data on week 4 of group 2 and week 10 of group 1.

[c] Initial data of fresh kimchi group were the means of data on week 0 of group 1 and week 6 of group 2.

[d] Final data of fresh kimchi group were the means of data on week 4 of group 1 and week 10 of group 2.

[e] Significantly different from initial value ($p < 0.05$).

[f] Significantly different between fresh and fermented kimchi groups ($p < 0.05$).

glucose, and total cholesterol compared with the fresh kimchi group. Thus, kimchi, especially fermented kimchi, has a positive effect on obesity, lipid metabolism, inflammatory processes, and metabolic syndrome-related factors.

In a human study, 100 volunteers were assigned to low (15 g/d, $n = 50$) and high (210 g/d, $n = 50$) kimchi intake, and were housed together in a dormitory for 7 days. Identical meals except with different amounts of kimchi were provided and volunteers were instructed to maintain their normal physical activity (Choi et al., 2013). The levels of fasting blood glucose (FBG), total glucose, total cholesterol, and LDL-C significantly decreased in both groups after 7 days of kimchi consumption. FBG significantly decreased in the group with high kimchi intake rather than in low kimchi intake group. The levels of TG and total cholesterol significantly decreased in both groups ($p < 0.05$) during the 7-day intervention trial in young healthy subjects. Serum total antioxidant status (TAS mmol/L) in both groups significantly increased by 5.2% in the low-consumption group and 7.5% in the high-consumption group. In another study, kimchi exhibited blood glucose-lowering and antidiabetic effects (Islam and Choi, 2009). Administration of freeze-dried baechu kimchi to high fat diet–fed, streptozotocin (STZ)-induced type-2 diabetic rats resulted in increased serum insulin concentrations and pancreatic β-cell function after 4 weeks as well as decreased blood glycated Hb levels. Lowered FBG and better glucose tolerance were observed in the kimchi-fed group. These findings suggested that baechu kimchi has antidiabetic effects even when administered with a high fat diet. If the kimchi preparation method and the amount of kimchi consumed are controlled, with both normal and low-fat diets, antidiabetic effects and control of metabolic syndrome will be much improved.

3.8 Conclusion

Kimchi is a fermented vegetable probiotic food. The main ingredients are cruciferous vegetables (baechu cabbage and radish), and subingredients are red pepper powder, garlic, ginger, green onions, fermented fishes, etc. In traditionally prepared kimchi, the naturally present microorganisms, especially LAB in the cabbage and subingredients, are the starters for fermentation. Brining the cabbage with different kinds of salt has been shown to affect taste, fermentation characteristics and functionality of kimchi. The use of high-quality ingredients, the predominant LAB, whether using ambient bacteria or adding starters; low-temperature fermentation; and facultative anaerobic conditions (using onggi as a container) for the fermentation are important factors for preparing kimchi with better taste and functionality. The predominant LAB genera are *Leuconostoc*, *Lactobacillus* and *Weissella* in kimchi fermentation. The representative species are *Leu. mesenteroides*, *Leu. citrium*, *Lab. plantarum*, *Lab. sakei*, and *Wei. koreensis*. The heterofermentation becomes dominant and provides better taste and uniform quality to the kimchi. The biochemical changes of kimchi are influenced by the predominant LAB, quality and amount of ingredients, fermentation conditions, etc. Fermentation metabolites from ingredients and action of LAB and their combined effects produce the kimchi taste, quality, and functionality.

Kimchi, especially optimally fermented kimchi, has various health benefits such as control of colon health, antioxidation, antiaging, cancer preventive, and antiobesity effects, control of dyslipidemia and metabolic syndrome, etc. due to presence of LAB and various nutraceuticals and metabolites from the ingredients, which also impact the taste of kimchi. The LAB concentrations significantly increase up to 10^9 CFUs/mL or g after fermentation. The kimchi LAB are good probiotics, exhibiting antimicrobial activity and antimutagenic andanticancer, immunomodulatory, anti-inflammatory, antiobesity, and cholesterol- and lipid-lowering effects (see Chapter 4). Thus, kimchi ingredients, LAB, fermentation, and metabolites are important factors that modulate various functionalities. Kimchi can also be developed as

Kimchi and Its Health Benefits

custom-made foods for different needs, race, age-adjusted kimchi, and specific disease prevention such as anticancer, antiobesity, antiallergy, etc., by changing the ingredients, LAB starters, and other fermentation conditions.

References

Ahn, S. J. 2007. The effect of kimchi powder supplement on the body weight reduction of obese adult women. MS thesis, Pusan National University, Busan, Korea.

Bengmark, S. 2001. Use of prebiotics, probiotics, and synbiotics in clinical immunonutrition. Seoul, Korea: *Proceedings of International Symposium on food nutrition and health for 21st century*, 187–213.

Bong, Y. J., J. K. Jeong, and K. Y. Park. 2013. Fermentation properties and increased health functionality of kimchi by kimchi lactic acid bacteria starters. *J Korean Soc Food Sci Nutr* 42:1717–1726.

Chang, J. Y., and H. C. Chang. 2011. Growth inhibition of foodborne pathogens by kimchi prepared with bacteriocin-producing starter culture. *J Food Sci* 76:M72–78.

Cheigh, H. S. 2002. History of kimchi. In: *Kimchi culture and scientific technology*, Series I. 147–270.

Cheigh, H. S., and K. Y. Park. 1994. Biochemical, microbiological, and nutritional aspects of kimchi (Korean fermented vegetable products). *Crit Rev Food Sci Nutr* 34:175–203.

Cho, E. J. 1999. Standardization and cancer chemopreventive activities of Chinese cabbage kimchi. PhD diss., Pusan National University, Busan, Korea.

Cho, E. J., J. S. Choi, S. H. Kim et al. 2004. *In vitro* anticancer effect of active compounds from Chinese cabbage kimchi. *J Kor Assoc Cancer Prev* 9:98–103.

Cho, E. J., K. Y. Park, and S. H. Rhee. 1997. Standardization of ingredient ratios of Chinese cabbage kimchi. *Korean J Food Sci Technol* 29:1228–1235.

Cho, K. M., R. K. Math, S. M. Islam et al. 2009. Novel multiplex PCR for the detection of lactic acid bacteria during kimchi fermentation. *Mol Cell Probes* 23:90–94.

Choe, S. M., Y. S. Jun, K. Y. Park et al. 1991. Changes in the contents of moisture, reducing sugar, microorganisms, NO_2 and NO_3 during salting in various varieties of Chinese cabbage for kimchi fermentation. *Res. Bull. Coll. Home Econ. Pusan Natl. Univ.* 17:25–30.

Choi, I. H., J. S. Noh, J. S. Han et al. 2013. Kimchi, a fermented vegetable, improves serum lipid profiles in healthy young adults: Randomized clinical trial. *J Med Food* 16:223–229.

Choi, J. M., S. H. Lee, K. Y. Park et al. 2014. Protective effect of kimchi against Aβ-25-35-induced impairment of cognition and memory. *J Korean Soc Food Sci Nutr.* 43:360–365.

Choi, S. M. 2001. Antiobesity and anticancer effects of red pepper powder and kimchi. PhD diss., Pusan National University, Busan, Korea.

Choi, W. Y., and K. Y. Park. 1998. Brining property and antimutagenic effects of organic Chinese cabbage kimchi. *J Food Sci Nutr* 3:287–291.

CODEX (Codex Alimentarius Commission). 2001. Codex standard for kimchi. Codex Stan 223. Food and Agriculture Organization of the United Nations, Rome, Italy.

Collins, M. D., and G. R. Gibson. 1999. Probiotics, prebiotics, and synbiotics: Approaches for modulating the microbial ecology of the gut. *Am J Clin Nutr* 69:1052S–1057S.

Cui, M., H. Y. Kim, K. H. Lee et al. 2015. Antiobesity effects of kimchi in diet-induced obese mice. *J Ethnic Foods* 2:137–144.

Goldin, B. R., and S. L. Gorbach. 1976. The relationship between diet and rat fecal bacterial enzymes implicated in colon cancer. *J Natl Cancer Inst* 57:371–375.

Han, G. J., A. R. Son, S. M. Lee et al. 2009. Improved quality and increased *in vitro* anticancer effect of kimchi by using natural sea salt without bittern and baked (guwun) salt. *J Korean Soc Food Sci Nutr* 38:996–1002.

Han, G. J., H. S. Choi, S. M. Lee et al. 2011b. Addition of starters in pasteurized brined baechu cabbage increased kimchi quality and health functionality. *J Korean Soc Food Sci Nutr* 40:110–115.

Han, W., W. Hu, and Y. M. Lee. 2011a. Anticancer activity of human cancer (HT-29) cell line from different fraction of *Zanthoxylum schnifolium* fruits. *Kor J Pharmacol* 42:282–287.

Hughes, P. A., H. Zola, I. A. Penttila et al. 2013. Immune activation in irritable bowel syndrome: Can neuroimmune interactions explain symptoms? *Am J Gastroenterol* 108:1066–1074.

Hwang, J. W., and Y. O. Song. 2000. The effect of solvent fractions of kimchi on plasma lipid concentration of rabbit fed high cholesterol diet. *J Korean Soc Food Sci Nutr* 29:204–210.

Hwang, S. Y., Y. M. Hur, Y. H. Choi et al. 1997. Inhibitory effect of kimchi extracts on mutagenesis of aflatoxin B1. *Environ Mut Carcino* 17:133–137.

Islam, M. S., and H. Choi. 2009. Antidiabetic effect of Korean traditional baechu (Chinese cabbage) kimchi in a type 2 diabetes model of rats. *J Med Food* 12:292–297.

Jeong, J. K., Y. W. Kim, H. S. Choi et al. 2011. Increased quality and functionality of kimchi when fermented in Korean earthenware (onggi). *Int J Food Sci Biotechnol* 46:2015–2021.

Jeong, M., J. M. Park, Y. M. Han et al. 2015. Dietary prevention of *Helicobacter pylori*-associated gastric cancer with kimchi. *Oncotarget* 6:29513–29526.

Jo, J. S., and C. W. Nam. 1979. Standardization of kimchi and related products. *Bull Dongduk Women's University* 9:199–212.

Ju, J. 2016. Inhibitory effects on obesity and colon cancer by solar salt and bamboo salt in C57BL/6J mice. PhD diss., Pusan National University, Busan, Korea.

Jung, J. Y., S. H. Lee, J. M. Kim et al. 2011. Metagenomic analysis of kimchi, a traditional Korean fermented food. *Appl Environ Microbiol* 77:2264–2274.

Jung, J. Y., S. H. Lee, H. J. Lee et al. 2012. Effects of *Leuconostoc mesenteroides* starter cultures on microbial communities and metabolites during kimchi fermentation. *Int J Food Microbiol* 153:378–387.

Jung, K. O. 2000. Studies on enhancing cancer chemopreventive (anticancer) effects of kimchi and safety of salts and fermented anchovy. PhD diss., Pusan National University, Busan, Korea.

Jung, K. O., S. M. Lee, S. H. Rhee et al. 2001. Reduced comutagenic and antimutagenic effects of bamboo salt prepared with KCl and NaCl. *J Korean Cancer Prev* 6:140–147.

Kajander, K., K. Hatakka, T. Poussa et al. 2005. A probiotic mixture alleviates symptoms in irritable bowel syndrome patients: A controlled 6-month intervention. *Aliment Pharmacol Ther* 22:387–394.

Kang, B. K., M. S. Cho, T. Y. Ahn et al. 2015. The influence of red pepper powder on the density of *Weissella koreensis* during kimchi fermentation. *Sci Rep* 5:15445. doi: 10.1038/srep15445.

Kaur, J. 2014. A comprehensive review on metabolic syndrome. *Cardiol Res Pract* 2014:943162. doi: 10.1155/2014/943162.

Kil, J. H. 2004. Studies on development of cancer preventive and anticancer kimchi and its anticancer mechanism. PhD Diss. Pusan National University, Busan, Korea.

Kil, J. H., K. O. Jung, H. S. Lee et al. 2004. Effects of kimchi on stomach and colon health of *Helicobacter pylori*-infected volunteers. *J Food Sci Nutr* 9:161–166.

Kim, B. K., J. M. Choi, S. A. Kang et al. 2014a. Antioxidative effects of kimchi under different fermentation stage on radical-induced oxidative stress. *Nutr Res Pract.* 8:638–643.

Kim, B. K., K. Y. Park, H. Y. Kim et al. 2011a. Anti-aging effects and mechanisms of kimchi during fermentation under stress-induced premature senescence cellular system. *Food Sci Biotechnol* 20:643–649.

Kim, B. K., J. L. Song, J. H. Ju et al. 2015. Anticancer effects of kimchi fermented for different times and containing added ingredients in HT-29 human colon carcinoma cells. *Food Sci Biotechnol* 24:629–633.

Kim, E. K., S. Y. An, M. S. Lee et al. 2011b. Fermented kimchi reduces body weight and improves metabolic parameters in overweight and obese patients. *Nutr Res* 31:436–443.

Kim, H. Y. 2016. Effects of kimchi intake on colon health of Korean young adults and irritable bowel syndrome patients. PhD diss., Pusan National University, Busan, Korea.

Kim, H. Y., Y. J. Bong, J. K. Jeong et al. 2016. Heterofermentative lactic acid bacteria dominate in Korean commercial kimchi. *Food Sci Biotechnol* 25:541–545.

Kim, H. Y., J. L. Song, H. K. Chang et al. 2014b. Kimchi protects against azoxymethane/dextran sulfate sodium-induced colorectal carcinogenesis in mice. *J Med Food.* 17:833–841.

Kim, J. H., M. J. Kwon, S. Y. Lee et al. 2002. The effect of kimchi on production of free radicals and antioxidative enzyme activities in the brain of SAM. *J Korean Soc Food Sci Nutr* 31:117–123.

Kim, K. M. 1998. Increase in swimming endurance capacity of mice by capsaicin. PhD diss., Kyoto University, Kyoto, Japan.

Kim, S. H. 2002. The study of preference on kimchi by the cancer patients and the development of cancer preventive kimchi. MS thesis, Pusan National University, Busan, Korea.

Kim, Y. T., B. K. Kim, and K. Y. Park. 2007. Antimutagenic and anticancer effects of leaf mustard and leaf mustard kimchi. *J Food Sci Nutr* 12:84–88

Kim, Y. W. 2010. Studies on excellent qualities of kimchi fermented on onggi. MS thesis, Pusan National University, Busan, Korea.

Kwon, M. J., J. H. Chun, Y. S. Song et al. 1999. Daily kimchi consumption and its hypolipidemic effect in middle-aged men. *J Korean Soc Food Sci Nutr* 28:1144–1150.

Kwon, M. J., Y. O. Song, and Y. S. Song. 1997. Effects of kimchi on tissue and fecal lipid composition and apoprotein and thyroxine levels in rats. *J Korean Soc Food Sci Nutr* 26:507–513.

Lee, H. A., Y. J. Bong, H. Kim et al. 2015a. Effect of nanometric *Lactobacillus plantarum* in kimchi on dextran sulfate sodium-induced colitis in mice. *J Med Food* 18:1073–1080.

Lee, H. A., H. Kim, K. W. Lee et al. 2015b. Dead nano-sized *Lactobacillus plantarum* inhibits azoxymethane/dextran sulfate sodium-induced colon cancer in BALB/c mice. *J Med Food.* 18:1400–1405.

Lee, K. E., U. H. Choi, and G. E. Ji. 1996. Effect of kimchi intake on the composition of human large intestinal bacteria. *Korean J Food Sci Technol* 28:981–986.

Lee, K. H. 2016. Lactic acid bacteria starter fermented kimchi inhibits obesity and colitis-associated colon cancer in C57BL/6J mice. Ph.D. diss., Pusan National University, Busan, Korea.

Lee, K. H., Y. J. Bong, H. A. Lee et al. 2016. Probiotic effects of *Lactobacillus plantarum* and *Leuconostoc mesenteroides* isolated from kimchi. *J Korean Soc Food Sci Nutr* 45:12–19.

Lee, K. H., J. L. Song, E. S. Park et al. 2015d. Antiobesity effects of starter fermented kimchi on 3T3-L1 adipocytes. *Prev Nutr Food Sci* 20:298–302.

Lee, M. E., J. Y. Jang, J. H. Lee et al. 2015c. Starter cultures for kimchi fermentation. *J Microbiol Biotechnol* 25:559–568.

Martineau, B., and D. P. Laflamme. 2002. Effect of diet on markers of intestinal health in dogs. *Res Vet Sci* 72:223–227.

Moon, S. W., D. W. Cho, W. S. Park et al. 1995. Effects of salt concentration on tongchimi fermentation. *Korean J Food Sci Technol* 27:11–18.

Moon, Y. J., J. R. Soh, J. J. Yu et al. 2012. Intracellular lipid accumulation inhibitory effect of *Weissella koreensis* OK1-6 isolated from kimchi on differentiating adipocyte. *J Appl Microbiol* 113:652–658.

Oh, Y. J., I. J. Hwang, and C. Leitzmann. 1993. Regular intake of kimchi prevents colon cancer. *Kimchi Sci Ind* 2:9–22.

Park, K. Y. 1995. The nutritional evaluation, and antimutagenic and anticancer effects of kimchi. *J Korean Food Sci Nutr* 24:169–182

Park, K. Y., K. A. Baek, S. H. Rhee et al. 1995. Antimutagenic effect of kimchi. *Foods Biotech* 4:141–145

Park, K. Y., and H. S. Cheigh. 2004. Kimchi. In: *Handbook of food and beverage fermentation technology,* ed. Y. H. Hui, I. M. Goddik, A. S. Hansen, J. Josephsen, W. K. Nip, P. S. Stanfield and F. Toldra, 621–655. New York: Marcel Dekker Inc.

Park, K. Y., E. J. Cho, S. H. Rhee et al. 2003. Kimchi and an active component, beta-sitosterol, reduce oncogenic H-Ras[v12]-induced DNA synthesis. *J Med Food* 6:151–156.

Park, K. Y., J. O. Ha, and S. H. Rhee. 1996. A study on the contents of dietary fibers and crude fiber in kimchi ingredients and kimchi. *J Korean Food Sci Nutr* 25:69–75

Park, K. Y., and J. K. Jeong. 2016. Kimchi (Korean fermented vegetable) as a probiotic food. In: *Probiotics, prebiotics, and synbiotics.* ed. R. R. Watson, V. R. Preedy, 391–408. London, United Kingdom: Elsevier.

Park, K. Y., J. K. Jeong, Y. E. Lee et al. 2014. Health benefits of kimchi (Korean fermented vegetables) as a probiotic food. *J Med Food.* 17:6–20.

Park, K. Y., and B. K. Kim. 2012. Lactic acid bacteria in vegetable fermentations. In: *Lactic acid bacteria–Microbiological and functional aspects.* ed. S. Lahtinen, S. Salminen, A Ouwehand, A. von Wright, 187–211. Boca Raton, FL: CRC Press Inc.

Park, K. Y., H. Y. Kim, and J. K. Jeong. 2017. Ch. 20. Kimchi and its health benefits. In: *Fermented foods in health and disease prevention*. ed. J. Frías, C. Martínez-Villaluenga, E. Peñas, 477–502. London, United Kingdom: Elsevier.

Park, K. Y., and S. H. Rhee. 2005. Functional foods from fermented vegetable products: Kimchi (Korean fermented vegetables) and functionality. In: *Asian functional foods*. ed. J. Shi, C. T. Ho, F. Shahidi, 341–380. Boca Raton, FL: CRC Press Inc.

Park, W. S., M. J. Koo, B. H. Ahn et al. 1994a. Standardization of kimchi-manufacturing process. Report of Korean Food Research Institute, Seoul, Korea.

Park, W. S., I. S. Lee, Y. S. Han et al. 1994b. Kimchi preparation with brined Chinese cabbage and seasoning mixture stored separately. *Korean J Food Sci Technol* 26:231–238.

Ray, B., and A. Bhunia. 2008. *Fundamental Food Microbiology*, 165–168. Boca Raton, FL, CRC Press Inc.

Ruige, J. B., J. M. Dekker, W. F. Blum et al. 1999. Leptin and variables of body adiposity, energy balance, and insulin resistance in a population-based study. The Hoorn study. *Diabetes Care* 22:1097–1104.

Ryu, B. M. 2000. Effect of kimchi on inhibition of skin aging of hairless mouse. PhD diss., Pusan National University, Busan, Korea.

Ryu, B. M., S. H. Ryu, Y. S. Lee et al. 2004. Effect of different kimchi diets on oxidation and photooxidation in liver and skin of hairless mice. *J Korean Soc Food Sci Nutr* 33:291–298.

Ryu, J. C., and K. Y. Park. 2001. Anticlastogenic effect of baechu (Chinese cabbage) kimchi and buchu (leek) kimchi in mitomycin C-induced micronucleus formations by supravital staining of mouse peripheral reticulocytes. *Environ Mut Carcino* 21:51–56.

Sohn, C. I. 2002. Selected summary: The treatment of functional dyspepsia with red pepper. *J Neurogasteroenterol Motil* 8:208–209.

Son, K. H. 1991. Variety and use of kimchi. *Korean J Diet Cult* 6:503–520.

Wisselink, H. W., R. A. Weusthuis, G. Eggink et al. 2002. Mannitol production by lactic acid bacteria: A review. *Int Dairy J* 12:151–161.

Yoon, J. Y., K. O. Jung, J. H. Kil et al. 2005. Antiobesity effect of major Korean spices (red pepper powder, garlic, and ginger) in rats fed high fat diet. *J Food Sci Nutr* 10:58–63.

Yun, J. Y., J. K. Jeong, S. H. Moon et al. 2014. Effects of brined cabbage and seasoning on fermentation of kimchi. *J Korean Soc Food Sci Nutr* 43:1081–1087.

Zheng, G., K. Sayama, T. Okubo et al. 2004. Anti-obesity effects of three major components of green tea, catechins, caffeine and theanine, in mice. *In Vivo* 18:55–62.

4

Lactic Acid Bacteria in Kimchi

Hak-Jong Choi, Jieun Lee, and Ja-Young Jang

CONTENTS

4.1 Introduction 79
4.2 Antimicrobial Activities 80
    4.2.1 Antifungal Activities...80
    4.2.2 Bacteriocin Production..83
        4.2.2.1 Bacteriocins Produced by Genus *Lactococcus*...............83
        4.2.2.2 Bacteriocins Produced by Genus *Lactobacillus* 83
        4.2.2.3 Bacteriocins Produced by Genus *Leuconostoc*
                and Other Genera...84
    4.2.3 Anti-*Helicobacter pylori* Effects...85
4.3 Antimutagenic and Anticancer Effects...85
4.4 Immunomodulatory Effects 88
4.5 Anti-Inflammatory Effects 91
4.6 Allergic Alleviatory Effects 91
4.7 Antiobesity and Cholesterol- and Lipid-Lowering Effects....................92
4.8 Kimchi LAB Degrade NO_2 and Insecticide...93
4.9 Other Physiological Functions...94
4.10 Conclusion 95
References...96

4.1 Introduction

Kimchi is a traditional Korean vegetable product that is fermented by various lactic acid bacteria (LAB) at low temperatures, ensuring proper ripening and preservation. More than high levels (about 10^7–10^9 colony-forming units [CFUs]/g) and 100 different species of LAB are involved in kimchi fermentation, such as genera *Lactococcus*, *Lactobacillus*, *Leuconostoc*, *Weissella*, and *Pediococcus*. There are several potential health or nutritional benefits possible from some species of LAB. LAB produce various compounds, including mannitol, γ-aminobutyric acid (GABA), ornithine, conjugated linoleic acids, and oligosaccharides; these components contribute to the fermentation characteristics and health functionality. Compared with LAB isolated from dairy products, whose various functional properties are well known, the functionality of kimchi LAB has become of interest only in the last few decades. Accumulating evidence has shown that kimchi LAB confer probiotic properties, as well as antimicrobial, anticancer, antioxidative, antiobesity, and immunomodulatory benefits (Park et al., 2014b; Choi et al., 2015). In addition, LAB as biopreservation organisms are of particular interest; they have been used for centuries as starter cultures in the food industry and are able to produce different kinds of bioactive molecules, such as organic acids, fatty acids, hydrogen peroxide, and bacteriocins (Lindgren and Dobrogosz, 1990; Dodd and Gasson, 1994; Stiles, 1996; Schnurer and Magnusson, 2005). In this chapter, we will discuss the current knowledge on how kimchi LAB can influence host physiology and their potential therapeutic use in alleviating imbalances in the host's metabolism.

4.2 Antimicrobial Activities

During kimchi fermentation, LAB generate various organic acids, such as lactic acid and acetic acid. They also produce CO_2, ethanol, diacetyl, H_2O_2, and bacteriocins, all of which have an antimicrobial activity (Table 4.1).

4.2.1 Antifungal Activities

A number of studies have shown that kimchi LAB produce antimicrobial compounds against various fungi. In an early study, approximately 120 LAB were isolated from kimchi. Of these, five isolates, identified as *Lactobacillus casei, Lactobacillus lactis,* and *Lactobacillus pentosus,* revealed strong antagonistic activity against *Aspergillus fumigatus* as well as *Aspergillus flavus, Fusarium moniliforme, Penicillium commune,* and *Rhizopus oryzae* (Kim et al., 2005). The antifungal compounds produced by *Lactobacillus plantarum* strain AF1 from kimchi were shown to be active against *A. flavus, A. fumigatus, Aspergillus ochraceus, Aspergillus nidulans, Aspergillus petrakii, Epicoccum nigrum,* and *Cladosporium gossypiicola.* The compounds were purified from culture supernatant and identified as 2,5-piperazinedione, 3,6-bis(2-methylpropyl), and δ-dodecalactone, with molecular weights of 226 and 198.3 kDa, respectively. These antifungal compounds were highly heat stable, and their activity was not destroyed following proteolytic enzymatic treatment (Yang and Chang, 2010; Yang et al., 2011).

In addition, this strain was also capable of inhibiting the growth of various Gram-positive and Gram-negative bacteria. *Lb. plantarum* YML007 was isolated from kimchi and produced a proteinaceous antifungal compound active against *A. flavus, A. oryzae,* and *Fusarium oxysporum;* its molecular mass was determined as 1256.617 Da by matrix-assisted laser desorption/ ionization time-of-flight (MALDI-TOF) analysis (Ahmad Rather et al., 2013). The antifungal activity was completely inactivated by proteinase K and

TABLE 4.1

Antimicrobial Activities of Lactic Acid Bacteria Isolated from Kimchi

Characteristics	Antimicrobial Spectra	Kimchi Lactic Acid Bacteria	Ref.
Antifungal activity	Antagonistic activity against *A. fumigatus, A. flavus, Fusarium moniliforme, Penicillium commune, Rhizopus oryzae*	*Lb. casei, Lb. lactis, Lb. pentosus*	Kim et al., 2005
	Antifungal activities against *A. flavus, A. fumigatus, A. ochraceus, A. nidulans, A. petrakii, Epicoccum nigrum,* and *Cladosporium gossypiicola*	*Lb. plantarum* strain AF1	Yang and Chang, 2010; Yang et al., 2011
	Antifungal activities against *A. flavus, A. oryzae,* and *F. oxysporum*	*Lb. plantarum* YML007	Ahmad Rather et al., 2013
	Antifungal activities against *Pen. brevicompactum* strain FI02	*Lb. sakei* ALI033	Huh and Hwang, 2016
	Preventing overgrowth of fermenting strains and delaying postacidification during storage	*Lb. sakei* ALI033	Choi et al., 2016
Bacteriocin production	Antimicrobial activity against *Listeria monocytogenes* and *Staphylococcus aureus*	*Lc. lactis* subsp. *lactis* H-559	Lee et al., 1999
	Antimicrobial activity against *L. monocytogenes, S. aureus,* and *Salmonella typhimurium*	*Lc. lactis* subsp. *lactis* A164	Choi et al., 2000
	Producing lacticin YH-10 active against *Pseudomonas synxantha* and *Acetobacter aceti*	*Lc. lactis* subsp. *lactis* YH-10	Choi et al., 2004
	Antimicrobial activity against spore-forming *Alicyclobacillus*	*Lactococcus* sp. CU216	Park et al., 2004
	Producing bacteriocin KC24 active against *L. monocytogenes*	*Lc. lactis* subsp. *lactis* KC24	Han et al., 2013
	Antimicrobial activity against some LAB and *L. monocytogenes.*	*Lb. sakei* P3-1	Kim et al., 2004a
	Producing sakacin P active against *Streptococcus mutans*	*Lb. sakei* K7	Moon et al., 2011
	Antimicrobial activity against *Salmonella typhimurium* and *E. coli* KCTC1467	*Lb. sakei* B16	Ahn et al., 2012
	Antimicrobial activity against *Lb. plantarum, Lb. pentosus, Lb. delbrueckii* subsp. *lactis,* and *E. faecalis*	*Lb. paraplantarum* C7	Lee et al., 2007
	Antimicrobial activity against *Lactobacillus, Enterococcus, Streptococcus, Bacillus,* and *Listeria*	*Lb. brevis* 925A	Ehrmann et al., 2000; Wada et al., 2009

(Continued)

TABLE 4.1 (CONTINUED)

Antimicrobial Activities of Lactic Acid Bacteria Isolated from Kimchi

Characteristics	Antimicrobial Spectra	Kimchi Lactic Acid Bacteria	Ref.
	Antimicrobial activity against *B. cereus*	*Lb. plantarum* KK3	Chung et al., 2010
	Bactericidal activity against some LAB and *E. coli* O157:H7	*Lb. plantarum* K11	Lim and Im, 2007
	Bacteriocin active against *S. aureus*	*Leuconostoc* sp. J2	Choi et al., 1999
	Unknown bacteriocin inducer	*Leu. mesenteroides* B7	Yang et al., 2002
	Antimicrobial activity against *L. monocytogenes* and *S. aureus* Producing pediocin K23-2	*P. pentosaceus* K23-2	Shin et al., 2008
Anti-*H. pylori* effects		*W. confusa* PL9001	Nam et al., 2002
		Lb. paraplantarum KNUC25	Ki et al., 2010
		Lb. plantarum NO1	Lee and Chang, 2008

Lactic Acid Bacteria in Kimchi

trypsin treatment. *Lactobacillus sakei* ALI033 isolated from kimchi exhibited antifungal activity against *Penicillium brevicompactum* strain FI02. In this case, the putative antifungal compounds were not stable at high pH and retained their activity after proteinase K treatment, suggesting that they were not proteins (Huh and Hwang, 2016). In addition, treatment with cinnamon ethanol extract and *Lb. sakei* ALI033 successfully improved the quality of yogurt by preventing overgrowth of fermenting strains and delaying postacidification during storage (Choi et al., 2016).

4.2.2 Bacteriocin Production

A number of studies have reported that LAB isolated from kimchi produce bacteriocins against several food spoilage and food-borne pathogens (Lee et al., 2014a).

4.2.2.1 Bacteriocins Produced by Genus Lactococcus

Lactococcus lactis subsp. *lactis* H-559 was isolated and identified from kimchi. This strain presented strong antimicrobial activity against *Listeria monocytogenes* and *Staphylococcus aureus*. The strain's bacteriocin was heat stable and retained its activity at pH 2.0–10.0. The molecular weight of the bacteriocin was calculated as 3343.7 Da (Lee et al., 1999). *Lc. lactis* subsp. *lactis* A164 isolated from kimchi was found to produce a nisin-like bacteriocin, which was active against closely related LAB and some food-borne pathogens, such as *L. monocytogenes*, *S. aureus*, and *Salmonella typhimurium*.

Analysis of the bacteriocin-encoding gene showed that strain A164 was a nisin Z-producer (Choi et al., 2000). *Lc. lactis* subsp. *lactis* YH-10 isolated from kimchi produced lacticin YH-10, which is active against some LAB and Gramnegative bacteria, such as *Pseudomonas synxantha* and *Acetobacter aceti*. The molecular weight of the bacteriocin appeared to be 14 kDa, and its antimicrobial activity was completely inactivated by amylase treatment (Choi et al., 2004). *Lactococcus* sp. CU216 isolated from kimchi produced a highly heat- and acid-stable bacteriocin, active against Gram-positive bacteria such as sporeforming *Alicyclobacillus* (Park et al., 2004). A bacteriocin KC24-producer, *Lc. lactis* subsp. *lactis* KC24, was isolated from kimchi. This strain's bacteriocin was shown to be more active against *L. monocytogenes* than nisin (Han et al., 2013).

4.2.2.2 Bacteriocins Produced by Genus Lactobacillus

Lb. sakei P3-1 isolated from kimchi produced a bacteriocin active against some LAB and *L. monocytogenes*. The activity was lost following proteinase K treatment. Its molecular weight was determined by sodium dodecyl sulfate-polyacrylamide gel electrophoresis (SDS-PAGE) to be about 4.0 kDa (Kim et al., 2004a). *Lb. sakei* K7, which was isolated and identified from kimchi, produced an antimicrobial compound effective against *Streptococcus mutans*, the causative agent of dental caries. The compound's activity remained unaltered at 60°C–100°C, but was inactivated by protease treatment, suggesting that it was a bacteriocin (Moon et al., 2011). Analysis of the bacteriocin-encoding gene revealed that *Lb. sakei* K7 was a sakacin P producer. *Lb. sakei* B16 produced a bacteriocin with a very wide antimicrobial spectrum, including *Salmonella typhimurium* and *Escherichia coli* KCTC 1467 (Ahn et al., 2012).

The bacteriocin produced by *Lactobacillus paraplantarum* C7 from kimchi was active against *Lb. plantarum*, *Lb. pentosus*, *Lb. delbrueckii* subsp. *lactis*, and *Enterococcus faecalis*. Based on its amino acid sequence, the compound was classified as a class II bacteriocin, characterized by a Gly–Gly motif. In addition, the bacteriocin-encoding gene was located on chromosomal DNA (Lee et al., 2007). *Lactobacillus brevis* 925A isolated from kimchi released a bacteriocin active against several species of *Lactobacillus*, *Enterococcus*, *Streptococcus*, *Bacillus*, and *Listeria*. A plasmid curing study showed that the corresponding bacteriocin gene was located on a 65-kb plasmid, and its amino acid sequence was identical to that of *Lb. plantarum* TMW1.25 (Ehrmann et al., 2000; Wada et al., 2009).

Lb. plantarum KK3 was isolated from gochunipkimchi (red pepper leaf kimchi). This strain showed tannase activity and was highly effective against some food pathogens including *Bacillus cereus*. Its activity was sensitive to proteinase K treatment, indicating its proteinaceous nature (Chung et al., 2010). *Lb. plantarum* K11 isolated from dongchimi (watery kimchi) showed bactericidal activity against some LAB and *E. coli* O157:H7. The bacteriocin activity was retained at pH 3.0–9.0 and was stable at 70°C for 60 min or 100°C for 30 min (Lim and Im, 2007).

4.2.2.3 *Bacteriocins Produced by Genus* Leuconostoc *and Other Genera*

Leuconostoc sp. J2 from kimchi produced a bacteriocin active against *S. aureus*. The molecular weight of the bacteriocin was determined by tricine-SDS-PAGE analysis as 2.5 kDa. A 2.5-kb *Eco*RI fragment from a *Leuconostoc* sp. J2 plasmid was cloned into *E. coli*, where it was successfully expressed as a recombinant bacteriocin with antimicrobial activity against *S. aureus* (Choi et al., 1999). *Leuconostoc mesenteroides* B7 was isolated from kimchi; the corresponding bacteriocin was heat and pH stable, was active against *Lb. plantarum*, and had a molecular weight of 3.5 kDa. Interestingly, production of the bacteriocin was enhanced by coculturing with *Lb. plantarum* KFRI 464, indicating that the latter might contain a presently unknown bacteriocin inducer (Yang et al., 2002). A kimchicin GJ7-producer, *Leuconostoc citreum* GJ7, was isolated from kimchi and, again, production of the bacteriocin increased upon coculture with *Lb. plantarum* KFRI 464 (Chang et al., 2007). *Pediococcus pentosaceus* K23-2 isolated from kimchi-released pediocin K23-2, which is active against *L. monocytogenes* and *S. aureus*. This strain's bacteriocin was heat and pH stable, insensitive to organic solvent treatment, and presented a molecular weight of about 5 kDa (Shin et al., 2008). However, its amino acid sequence has not been determined.

4.2.3 Anti-*Helicobacter pylori* Effects

As a pathological agent, *H. pylori* causes gastritis and gastric carcinoma. *Weissella confusa* PL9001 isolated from kimchi was shown to inhibit the binding of *H. pylori* to the stomach epithelium, thus reducing its colonization by *H. pylori* (Nam et al., 2002). *Lb. paraplantarum* KNUC25 was isolated from overfermented kimchi. After *H. pylori* and the cell-free supernatant of *Lb. paraplantarum* KNUC25 were cocultured, *H. pylori* failed to adhere on to gastric epithelial AGS cells (Ki et al., 2010). *Lb. plantarum* NO1 isolated from kimchi also revealed strong antibacterial activity against *H. pylori*. Specifically, the culture supernatant of *Lb. plantarum* NO1 decreased the urease activity of *H. pylori* by 40% ~ 60%. Additionally, *Lb. plantarum* inhibited the binding of *H. pylori* to human gastric cells by more than 33% (Lee and Chang, 2008). Collectively, these reports suggest that the administration of *Lb. plantarum* and *Lb. paraplantarum* might reduce *H. pylori* infection, although further studies are required to investigate the efficacy of kimchi LAB for treating and/or preventing *H. pylori* infections.

4.3 Antimutagenic and Anticancer Effects

The antimutagenic activity of several kimchi LAB has been reported (Park et al., 1998; Son et al., 1998). The mutagenic properties of 4-NQO (4-nitroquinolone-1-oxide), MelQ (2-amino-3,4-dimethylimidazo[4,5-f]quinoline), and Trp-P-2 (3-amino-1-methyl-5H-pyrido[4,3-b]indole) were significantly suppressed by kimchi LAB when using the Ames test and the SOS chromotest (Son et al., 1998). The cell body of *Leu. mesenteroides* showed a comparable antimutagenic activity against 4-NQO, MelQ, and MNNG (*N*-methyl-*N'*-nitro-*N*-nitrosoguanidine) as that exhibited by dairy LAB such as *Lactobacillus acidophilus*. Interestingly, this antimutagenic activity was present in the cell wall fraction, rather than in the cytosolic fraction and was thus retained irrespective of whether the cells were dead or alive (Park et al., 1998). The culture supernatant of *Lb. plantarum* KLAB21 isolated from kimchi showed antimutagenic effect against MNNG and 4-NQO in the Ames test using *Salmonella typhimurium* TA100 and TA98 (Park and Rhee, 2001). In addition, three different glycoproteins responsible for the antimutagenic properties of kimchi LAB were identified (Rhee and Park, 2001) (Table 4.2).

The glycopeptide fragments of the LAB cell wall have been found to be responsible for the strains' antitumor activity (Bogdanov et al., 1975; Friend and Shahani, 1984). In the cell wall, peptidoglycan is combined with muramyl peptide. Muramyl dipeptide and its derivatives have been known to stimulate cell-mediated immune function by increasing production of superoxide anion and H_2O_2 in macrophages and inhibiting growth of tumor cells

TABLE 4.2

Health Benefits of Lactic Acid Bacteria Isolated from Kimchi

Characteristics	Functionalities	Kimchi Lactic Acid Bacteria	Ref.
Antimutagenic and anticancer effects	Antimutagenic activity against 4-NQO, MelQ, and MNNG	*Leu. mesenteroides*	Park et al., 1998
	Antimutagenic effect against MNNG and 4-NQO	*Lb. plantarum* KLAB21	Park and Rhee, 2001
	Antiproliferative effect on tumor cells, suppressing proliferation of human colon cancer cells	Cytoplasmic fraction of strain KFRI342	Chang et al., 2012
	Decrease of tumor formation on lung	Heat-inactivated and lyophilized *Lb. plantarum* and *Leu. mesenteroides*	Kim et al., 1991
	Reduction of colorectal tumor formation	Dead nano-sized *Lb. plantarum*	Lee et al., 2016
Immunomodulatory effects	Regulation of both systematic and mucosal immunity	Administration of the homogenate of *Lb. plantarum*	Chae et al., 1998
	Induction of macrophage and complement activation	Cellular fractions of *Lb. brevis* FSB-1	Kim et al., 2004b
	Increase of the proliferation of murine Peyer's patch cells	Cellular fractions of *Lb. acidophilus* DDS-1	Seo and Lee, 2007
	Mitogenic activity, stimulating the proliferation of Peyer's patch cells	*Lb. plantarum* PS-21	Lee et al., 2006
	Enhancement of Th1 activity	*Lb. plantarum*	Won et al., 2011a
	Enhancement of Th1 response	*Lb. sakei* WIKIM-100	Park et al., 2013
	Enhancement of cytokine production	Oral administration of *Lb. sakei* K101 and *Lb. plantarum* K55-5	Lee et al., 2016
	Modulation of T-cell-related immune responses	*Lb. brevis* G-101	Jang et al., 2013b
	Modulation of Treg-cell response	*W. cibaria* WIKIM28	Lim et al., 2017
	Regulation of the function of natural killer (NK) cells	Oral administration of *Lb. plantarum* HY7712	Jang et al., 2013a

(Continued)

TABLE 4.2 (CONTINUED)

Health Benefits of Lactic Acid Bacteria Isolated from Kimchi

Characteristics	Functionalities	Kimchi Lactic Acid Bacteria	Ref.
Anti-inflammatory effects	Amelioration of inflammatory bowel disease	Lb. brevis G-101	Jang et al., 2013b
	Amelioration of inflammatory bowel disease	Lb. sakei K17	Eun et al., 2016
	Amelioration of inflammatory bowel disease	Lb. curvatus WiKim38	Jo et al., 2016
	Amelioration of inflammatory bowel disease	Lc. paracasei LS2	Park et al., 2017a
Allergic alleviatory effects	Alleviation of atopic dermatitis-like symptoms	Intake of Lb. plantarum K8 extracts	Lee et al., 2008
	Alleviation of atopic dermatitis-like symptoms	Oral administration of Lb. sakei proBio65	Park et al., 2008; Kim et al., 2013
	Alleviation of atopic dermatitis-like symptoms	W. cibaria WIKIM28	Lim et al., 2017
	Suppression of airway hyper-responsive reactions in asthma model	Lb. plantarum or Lb. curvatus	Hong et al., 2010
Antiobesity, cholesterol- and lipid-lowering effects	Reduction of body weight and lowered lipid levels	Supplementation of kimchi LAB powder	Kwon et al., 2004
	Decrease of adipogenesis and lipogenesis-related gene expression	Cytoplasmic fraction and culture supernatant of W. koreensis OK1-6	Moon et al., 2012
	Decrease of adipogenesis and lipogenesis-related gene expression	Leu. mesenteroides KCCM11353P, Lb. plantarum KCCM11352P	Lee et al., 2015c
	Antihyperglycemic and antiobesity effects	Lb. sakei OK67	Lim et al., 2016
	Reduction of mesenteric adipose depot	Lb. plantarum HAC01	Park et al., 2017b
	Hypocholesterolemic and antiobesity effects	Leuconostoc kimchii GJ2	Jo et al., 2015

(Bogdanov et al., 1975). *Lb. acidophilus* KFRI342 showing probiotic properties (resistance to acid and bile salts) was isolated from kimchi. The cytoplasmic fraction of strain KFRI342 exhibited a strong antiproliferative effect on tumor cells, suppressing proliferation of human colon cancer cells by 38%, while inhibiting only 10% of normal cells. In addition, strain KFRI342 augmented quinone reductase activity and immunostimulating activities through an increased secretion of nitric oxide (NO) and interleukin (IL)-1α, respectively (Chang et al., 2012).

Administration of heat-inactivated and lyophilized *Lb. plantarum* and *Leu. mesenteroides* to sarcoma-180-induced ICR mice decreased tumor formation by 57% and 39%, respectively. In C57BL/6 mice with Lewis lung carcinoma, the same LAB suppressed cancer growth by 42% and 44%, respectively (Kim et al., 1991). Another study has shown that intake of the cell lysate of *Lb. plantarum* markedly decreased the formation of ascites tumors in BALB/c mice, and the expected life span of the animals was extended by 60% (the average life span was 34.2 days) (Shin et al., 1998). Recently, dead nano-sized *Lb. plantarum* (nLp) have been reported to inhibit azoxymethane/dextran sulfate sodium (DSS)-induced colon cancer in mice. Animals fed nLp showed fewer colonic tumors and reduced expression of inflammatory markers (Lee et al., 2015b). In particular, combined intake of nLp and kimchi markedly induced tumor-cell apoptosis and cell cycle arrest, resulting in reduced colorectal tumor formation (Lee et al., 2016).

4.4 Immunomodulatory Effects

A number of studies have reported that LAB isolated from kimchi possess immunomodulatory effects in various immunological settings (Choi et al., 2015). Administration of the homogenate of *Lb. plantarum* isolated from kimchi increased the proliferation of splenocytes and Peyer's patch cells, the production of NO by macrophages, serum levels of tumor necrosis factor (TNF)-α and IL-2, and levels of intestinal IgA. This suggests that *Lb. plantarum* homogenate regulates both systematic and mucosal immunity in mice (Chae et al., 1998). Cellular fractions of *Lb. brevis* FSB-1 isolated from kimchi have been reported to induce macrophage and complement activation; however, they could not stimulate the proliferation of bone marrow cells (Kim et al., 2004b). In a similar study, cellular fractions of *Lb. acidophilus* DDS-1 isolated from kimchi increased the proliferation of murine Peyer's patch cells. Interestingly, the cell wall fraction of *Lb. acidophilus* DDS-1 only weakly stimulated macrophage activation (Seo and Lee, 2007). Lee et al. (2006) have reported that *Lb. plantarum* PS-21, characterized by strong mitogenic activity, stimulated the proliferation of Peyer's patch cells. In particular, a peptidoglycan fraction of *Lb. plantarum* PS-21

Lactic Acid Bacteria in Kimchi

was responsible for enhancing production of the cytokines TNF-α and IL-6 in RAW 264.7 macrophage cells.

Several studies have shown that many kimchi LAB are capable of regulating the T-helper (Th)1/Th2 balance. Addition of *Lb. plantarum* strains isolated from kimchi to ovalbumin (OVA)-sensitized splenocytes appeared to promote Th1 activity but suppressed Th2 activity (Won et al., 2011a). *Lb. sakei* WIKIM-100 isolated from kimchi displayed a similar effect, markedly increasing production of interferon (IFN)-a Th1 cytokine, in OVA-sensitized mouse splenocytes. Interestingly, this bacterium potently inhibited the secretion of interleukin (IL)-4, a Th2 cytokine (Park et al., 2013). However, a recent study has shown that not all LAB modulate the Th1/Th2 balance in a similar manner (Hong et al., 2014). Accordingly, a strain of *Lb. plantarum* isolated from kimchi increased IL-4 and OVA-specific IgE production in OVA-immunized mice (Hong et al., 2014). Oral administration of *Lb. sakei* K101 and *Lb. plantarum* K55-5 isolated from kimchi enhanced cytokine production in the splenocytes and blood of immunosuppressed mice, whereas *Lb. plantarum* K8 from kimchi failed to do so (Lee et al., 2016).

Modulation of T-cell-related immune responses, following treatment with kimchi LAB, depends on an altered function of antigen-presenting cells. *Lb. brevis* G-101 isolated from kimchi induced IL-10 production in lipopolysaccharide (LPS)-stimulated peritoneal macrophages, but lowered the secretion of TNF-α, IL-1β, IL-6, and IL-10; decreased the phosphorylation of interleukin-1 receptor-associated kinase 1 (IRAK1) and AKT serine/threonine kinase (AKT); or activated nuclear factor-kappa beta (NF-κB) and mitogen-activated protein kinases (MAPKs). Moreover, the strain was capable of polarizing M1 macrophages to M2-like macrophages (Jang et al., 2013b).

A recent study has reported that *Weissella cibaria* WIKIM28 isolated from gatkimchi (a subtype of kimchi made from mustard leaves) regulated dendritic cell function (Lim et al., 2017). WIKIM28-treated mouse bone marrow–derived dendritic cells (DCs) showed enhanced TNF-α, IL-12, and IL-10 production, as well as increased surface expression of inducible T-cell costimulator ligand (ICOS-L) and programmed death ligand-1 (PD-L1), two tolerogenic dendritic cell markers. The authors further demonstrated the function of WIKIM28-treated dendritic cells in regulating T-cell immunity. Coculturing WIKIM28-treated dendritic cells and naïve CD4+ T-cells induced the generation of CD4+CD25+Foxp3+ regulatory T (Treg)-cells. This indicates that *W. cibaria* WIKIM28 first induces tolerogenic dendritic cells, which, in turn, promote the generation of CD4+CD25+Foxp3+ Treg-cells (Figure 4.1).

Kimchi LAB have been reported to regulate the function of natural killer (NK) cells. Oral administration of *Lb. plantarum* HY7712 isolated from kimchi restored the cytotoxicity of NK and cytotoxic T-cells in immunosuppressed mice (Jang et al., 2013a). In addition, this strain enhanced NK cell function by activating the toll-like receptor (TLR)2/NF-κB signaling pathway in a γ-irradiated aging mouse model (Lee et al., 2014b). Figure 4.2 summarizes the immunomodulatory effects of kimchi LAB.

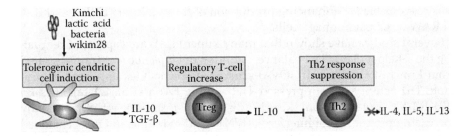

FIGURE 4.1
Weissella cibaria WIKIM28 isolated from gatkimchi induces the generation of tolerogenic DCs, which promote Treg differentiation. TGF = transforming growth factor; IL = interleukin; Th = T-helper; Treg = regulatory T-cell.

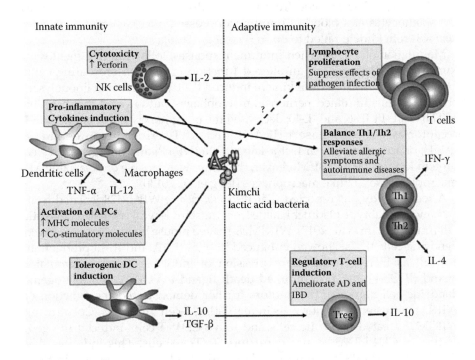

FIGURE 4.2
Immunomodulatory effects of kimchi LAB. LAB modulate immune responses by inducing either innate or adaptive immunity. APCs = antigen-presenting cells; MHC = major histocompatibility complex; TGF = transforming growth factor; TNF = tumor necrosis factor; IL = interleukin; IFN = interferon; Th = T-helper; Treg = regulatory T-cell; DC = dendritic cell; AD = atopic dermatitis; IBD = inflammatory bowel disease.

4.5 Anti-Inflammatory Effects

Kimchi LAB possessing anti-inflammatory activity have been successfully applied for the treatment of inflammatory bowel disease (IBD) as they are capable of enhancing the frequency and function of Tregs, which then suppress hypersensitive immune responses. Intake of nano-sized nLp has been shown to protect against colitis in a dextran sulfate sodium (DSS)-induced mouse colitis model (Lee et al., 2015a). Similarly, *Lb. brevis* G-101, which induces IL-10 production in macrophages, ameliorated the effect of colitis in a 2,4,6-trinitrobenzenesulfonic acid (TNBS)-induced mouse colitis model. Intake of *Lb. brevis* G-101 inhibited the production of inflammatory cytokines, such as IL-1β, IL-6, and TNF-α (Jang et al., 2013b). Similarly, oral administration of *Lb. sakei* K17, which induces IL-10 expression in dendritic cells and peritoneal macrophages, was found to suppress colon shortening and myeloperoxidase activity, as well as increase IL-10 production in TNBS-induced colitis mice.

Furthermore, this bacterium enhanced the expression of tight junction proteins in the colon (Eun et al., 2016). *Lactobacillus curvatus* WiKim38, which also induces IL-10 production in dendritic cells, was similarly isolated from kimchi. Its oral administration to DSS-induced colitis mice augmented the survival rate and improved disease scores as well as histopathological severity of the colon (Jo et al., 2016). Another study has shown that *Lactobacillus paracasei* LS2 isolated from kimchi also ameliorated inflammatory bowel disease. Mice fed LS2 exhibited increased survival, fewer disease symptoms, and more CD4$^+$Foxp3$^+$ Treg-cells than control mice (Park et al., 2017a). The anti-inflammatory effect of kimchi LAB has been studied extensively. Oral administration of *Lb. brevis* OW38 from kimchi to aged mice (18 months old) inhibited the expression of inflammatory markers, such as myeloperoxidase, TNF, and IL-1β, as well as NF-κB activation. In addition, OW38 treatment increased the expression of genes involved in colonic tight junctions, such as zonula occludens-1, occludin, and claudin-1, and the expression of senescence markers p16, p53, and SAM domain- and HD domain-containing protein 1 (SAMHD1) in the colon and the hippocampus of aged mice (Jeong et al., 2016).

4.6 Allergic Alleviatory Effects

Several LAB have been described as ameliorating allergies, such as atopic dermatitis and asthma, in animal models by decreasing the allergenic IgE level. Intake of *Lb. plantarum* K8 extracts alleviated atopic dermatitis-like symptoms by reducing IgE secretion in serum and the production of Th2 cytokines in a mouse model of atopic dermatitis (Lee et al., 2008). Oral administration of *Lb. sakei* proBio65 isolated from kimchi also resulted in prompt recovery from atopic dermatitis by reducing the levels of both IgE and Th2 cytokines (Park et al., 2008; Kim et al., 2013). Similar studies have shown that three strains of *Lb. plantarum* isolated from kimchi suppress house-dust mite-induced dermatitis in NC/Nga mice by activating Th1 immune responses and the function of Treg-cells (Won et al., 2011b, 2012). Another study has shown that *Lb. plantarum* SY11 and SY12 have antiallergic effects as they decreased the levels of NO, Th2 cytokines, cyclooxygenase-2, and inducible NO synthase (Lee et al., 2014c). A recent study has reported that oral administration of *W. cibaria* WIKIM28 isolated from gatkimchi reduced atopic dermatitis-like skin lesions, epidermal thickening, and serum IgE levels by inducing Treg responses (Lim et al., 2017).

Asthma is a hyper-responsive immune reaction in the airways. Disease symptoms are accompanied by the accumulation of various inflammatory cells and increased production of Th2 cytokines and IgE. Administration of *Lb. plantarum* or *Lb. curvatus* from kimchi suppressed airway hyper-responsive reactions by potentially enhancing the frequency and function of Treg-cells in a murine asthma model. Thus, kimchi *Lactobacillus* strains exert suppressive effects on allergic diseases characterized by airway hyper-responsiveness by modulating the function of intestinal immune cells (Hong et al., 2010).

4.7 Antiobesity and Cholesterol- and Lipid-Lowering Effects

A number of studies have reported antiobesity and lipid-lowering effects of kimchi LAB in a diet-induced obese mouse model. Supplementation of kimchi LAB powder (KL) in high-fat diet (HFD)-fed SD rats over a period of 8 weeks reduced body weight and lowered lipid levels. Rats fed 10% and 20% kimchi LAB displayed 13% and 15% body weight loss and 42% and 48% visceral fats reduction, respectively. In addition, kimchi LAB intake decreased the levels of plasma triglyceride, cholesterol, and low-density lipoprotein (LDL). Finally, kimchi LAB facilitated the excretion of triglyceride and cholesterol, indicating that the bacteria might have a similar role to dietary fiber (Kwon et al., 2004).

Cytoplasmic fraction and culture supernatant of *Weissella koreensis* OK1-6 isolated from kimchi inhibited intracellular lipid accumulation in differentiating 3T3-L1 cells. Expression of adipogenesis/lipogenesis-related genes, such as CCAAT enhancer-binding protein (C/EBP)-α, aP2, fatty acid synthase (FAS), and sterol regulatory element-binding protein 1 (SREBP1), decreased upon treatment with both the spent culture medium extract and cytoplasmic fraction of *W. koreensis* OK1-6 (Moon et al., 2012). In addition, intake of kimchi fermented with this strain as a starter culture for 12 weeks reduced body and epididymal fat pad weight in HFD-induced obese mice (Park et al., 2012). A similar study has shown that kimchi fermented with starter consisting of *Leu. mesenteroides* KCCM 11353P and *Lb. plantarum* KCCM 11352P exerted an antiobesity effect in 3T3-L1 adipocytes. The levels of lipid, triglyceride, and glycerol accumulation in differentiating adipocytes were significantly reduced following treatment with kimchi extracts, in line with down-regulation of peroxisome proliferator-activated receptor (PPAR)-γ, C/EBP-α, and FAS (Lee et al., 2015c).

Lb. sakei OK67 isolated from kimchi exerted antihyperglycemic and anti-obesity effects in HFD-induced obese mice. Oral administration of OK67 reduced the elevated lipopolysaccharide levels in the blood and colonic fluid induced by an HFD, and the expression of PPAR-γ, FAS, and TNF-α in adi-pose tissue (Lim et al., 2016). A recent study has reported that intragastric feeding of *Lb. plantarum* HAC01 isolated from kimchi in diet-induced obese mice lowered the mesenteric adipose depot. Interestingly, next-generation sequencing analysis of gut microbiota revealed that HAC01 increased the relative abundance of the Lachnospiraceae family while decreasing that of the Ruminococcaceae family in the intestine (Park et al., 2017b). These results indicate that kimchi LAB may modulate obesity-associated gut microbiota and thus alleviate obesity.

Lb. plantarum KCTC 3928 isolated from kimchi displayed hypocholester-olemic effects in C57BL/6 mice. Mice fed double-coated *Lb. plantarum* with protein and polysaccharide, along with an HFD, exhibited decreased levels of LDL cholesterol and plasma triglyceride by 42% and 32%, respectively, whereas fecal bile acid excretion was increased by 45%. The live *Lb. plantarum* showed hypocholesterolemic effects in mice due to induction of fecal bile acid secretion followed by increased degradation of hepatic cholesterol into bile acids. The same was observed following intake of kimchi fermented with a starter culture of *Leuconostoc kimchii* GJ2. In this case, rats fed a high-fat and high-cholesterol diet showed significantly reduced serum total cho-lesterol, triglyceride, and LDL cholesterol levels (Jo et al., 2015).

4.8 Kimchi LAB Degrade NO₂ and Insecticide

Kimchi LAB are capable of removing nitrite during kimchi fermentation. All sodium nitrite was depleted following an initial incubation (1–2 days) at 30°C and 36°C; however, it should be noted that the depletion rate was slower at lower temperatures. Similarly, *Leu. mesenteroides* isolated from kimchi depleted less than 20% of NO_2 after 10 days at 5°C, 86% ~ 93% after 7 days at 15°C, and more than 90% after 5 days at 20°C or 2 days at 30°C and 36°C (Oh et al., 2004). Several other strains of kimchi LAB were also capable of depleting nitrite. *Leuconostoc mesenteroides* subsp. *dextranicum* and *Leuconostoc lactis* actively depleted nitrite without prior adaptation in nitrite at 15°C–25°C (Ko et al., 2009). *Lb. brevis* KGR3111, *Lb. curvatus* KGR2103, *Lb. plantarum* KGR5105, and *Lb. sakei* KGR4108 isolated from kimchi showed tolerance against nitrate or nitrite and reduced the amount of NO_2 in fermented sausages to 58.46–75.80 mg/L (Paik and Lee, 2014).

Some kimchi LAB have also been shown to degrade insecticides. The organophosphorus (OP) insecticide, chlorpyrifos (CP) (30 mg/L), was degraded rapidly by day 3 (83.3%) and completely by day 9 at 8°C during kimchi (yeulmu-mulkimchi) fermentation (Cho et al., 2009). Four chlorpyrifos-degrading LAB were isolated from kimchi and identified as *Leu. mesenteroides* WCP907, *Lb. sakei* WCP902, *Lb. plantarum* WCP931, and *Lb. sakei* WCP904. The results showed that chlorpyrifos could be utilized by the bacteria as the sole source of carbon and phosphorus.

4.9 Other Physiological Functions

The antioxidant activity of *Lb. plantarum* KCTC3099 isolated from kimchi was determined by measuring resistance to reactive oxygen species (ROS). Intact cells and cell-free extracts of *Lb. plantarum* exhibited strong antioxidant activity against lipid peroxidation. This strain was able to survive even after 8 h in the presence of both 1 mM H_2O_2 and 0.4 mM hydroxyl radicals, and in the presence of a paraquat-generated superoxide anion (Lee et al., 2005).

Several LAB have been shown to produce bioactive γ-aminobutyric acid (GABA). GABA is generated by glutamic acid decarboxylase (GAD), which catalyzes the α-decarboxylation of L-glutamic acid. GABA exhibits several physiologically beneficial functions, such as hypotensive and diuretic effects, as well as regulation of neurological disorders. A strong GABA-producing LAB strain, *Lactobacillus buchneri* MS, was isolated from kimchi. The optimal condition for GABA production was achieved by growing the MS strain in MRS broth containing 5% monosodium glutamate, 1% NaCl, and 1% glucose, with an initial pH of 5.0 at 30°C for 36 h. This resulted in 251 mM GABA and a 94% conversion rate.

Furthermore, *Lb. buchneri* MS displayed neuroprotective effects against neuronal cell death induced by H_2O_2, retonone, sodium nitroprussade, paraquat, dieldrin, or $MnCl_2$ (Cho et al., 2007). Another kimchi LAB strain, *Lb. brevis* K203, was optimized for GABA production in medium containing 6% L-glutamic acid, 4% maltose, 2% yeast extract, 1% NaCl, 1% $CaCl_2$, 2 g Tween 80, and 0.02 mM pyridoxal 5'-phosphate at an initial pH of 5.25. After 72 h of cultivation at 37°C, GABA production reached 44.4 g/L (Binh et al., 2014). Novel GAD genes have been characterized from kimchi LAB. A GAD gene from *Lb. brevis* OPK-3 showing high GABA productivity (84.3 mg/L/h) was cloned and characterized. Open reading frame analysis showed that the gene encoded a protein of 467 amino acid residues with 83%, 71%, and 60% similarity to GAD of *Lb. plantarum*, *Lc. lactis*, and *L. monocytogenes*, respectively (Park and Oh, 2007). Another study on 3,000 kimchi isolates identified *Lactobacillus zymae* GU240 as the highest GABA-producing strain; its GAD gene was cloned and overexpressed in *E. coli*. Using recombinant GAD protein, the authors determined that maximum GAD activity was at pH 4.5 and 41°C and was dependent on pyridoxal 5′-phosphate. In the presence of glutamate, the enzyme's K_m and V_{max} were 1.7 and 0.01 mM/min, respectively (Park et al., 2014a).

4.10 Conclusion

Kimchi is a traditional Korean vegetable product that is naturally fermented by various LAB present in its raw materials and fermented for a certain period of time at ambient temperature. Natural fermentation with unsterilized raw materials leads to the growth of various LAB. They are the main component and occur with in high numbers ($10^8 \sim 10^9$ CFUs/g) in kimchi and produce various compounds, including organic acids, ethanol, mannitol, bacteriocins, γ-amino butyric acid, ornithine, conjugated linoleic acids, and oligosaccharide, which contribute to the fermentation characteristics and health functionality of kimchi.

Many studies have been conducted using bacteriocin-producing kimchi LAB from the genera *Lactococcus*, *Lactobacillus*, *Leuconostoc*, and other genera. These studies mainly focused on antimicrobial activity inhibiting the growth of harmful microorganisms including *Listeria monocytogenes*, *Staphylococcus aureus*, *Salmonella typhimurium*, etc. In addition, small organic compounds' antifungal peptides produced by LAB are mainly associated with antifungal activity.

The physiological effects of kimchi LAB have been extensively studied. Kimchi LAB exhibited antitumor, antimutagenic, and anti-inflammatory effects. These LAB revealed the preventive effect of mutation induced by 4-NQO, MeIQ, and Trp-p2. Their cellular components, such as glycopeptide fragments of cell wall and cell lysates, increased the anticancer effect in human colon and lung carcinoma cells by inhibiting the growth and proliferation of tumor cells and regulating immune-stimulating factors. They also ameliorated the symptoms of allergy-related diseases such as atopic dermatitis and asthma by suppressing inflammation and modulating the Th1/Th2 balance and function of Treg-cells.

Recent studies have been reported that LAB exhibited antiadipogenic and lipolytic effects in adipocytes as well as possessing weight-controlling and antioxidant effects in an obesity mouse model. They also reduced levels of serum cholesterol, triglycerides, and LDL cholesterol in a high-fat and high-cholesterol diet animal model. In addition, kimchi LAB are capable of producing bioactive compounds such as GABA and degrading insecticides.

References

Ahmad Rather, I., B. J. Seo, V. J. Rejish Kumar et al. 2013. Isolation and characterization of a proteinaceous antifungal compound from *Lactobacillus plantarum* YML007 and its application as a food preservative. *Lett Appl Microbiol* 57:69–76.

Ahn, J. E., J. K. Kim, H. R. Lee, H. J. Eom, and N. S. Han. 2012. Isolation and characterization of a bacteriocin-producing *Lactobacillus sakei* B16 from kimchi. *J Korean Soc Food Sci Nutr* 41:721–726.

Binh, T. T., W. T. Ju, W. J. Jung, and R. D. Park. 2014. Optimization of γ-amino butyric acid production in a newly isolated *Lactobacillus brevis*. *Biotechnol Lett* 36:93–98.

Bogdanov, I. G., P. G. Dalev, A. I. Gurevich et al. 1975. Antitumor glycopeptides from *Lactobacillus bulgricus* cell wall. *FEBS Lett* 57:259–261.

Chae, O., K. Shin, H. Chung, and T. Choe. 1998. Immunostimulation effects of mice fed with cell lysate of *Lactobacillus plantarum* isolated from kimchi. *KSBB J* 13:424–430.

Chang, J. H., Y. Y. Shim, S. K. Cha, M. J. T. Reaney, and K. M. Chee. 2012. Effect of *Lactobacillus acidophilus* KFRI342 on the development of chemically induced precancerous growths in the rat colon. *J Med Microbiol* 61:361–368.

Chang, J. Y., H. J. Lee, and H. C. Chang. 2007. Identification of the agent from *Lactobacillus plantarum* KFRI464 that enhances bacteriocin production by *Leuconostoc citreum* GJ7. *J Appl Microbiol* 103:2504–2515.

Cho, K. M., R. K. Math, S. M. Islam et al. 2009. Biodegradation of chlorpyrifos by lactic acid bacteria during kimchi fermentation. *J Agric Food Chem* 57:1882–1889.

Cho, Y. R., J. Y. Chang, and H. C. Chang. 2007. Production of γ-aminobutyric acid (GABA) by *Lactobacillus buchneri* isolated from kimchi and its neuroprotective effect on neuronal cells. *J Microbiol Biotechnol* 17:104–109.

Choi, E. M., Y. H. Kim, S. J. Park, Y. I. Kim, Y. M. Ha, and S. K. Kim. 2004. Characterization of bacteriocin, lacticin YH-10, produced by *Lactococcus lactis* subsp. *lactis* YH-10 isolated from kimchi. *J Life Sci* 14:683–688.

Choi, H. J., C. I. Cheigh, S. B. Kim, and Y. R. Pyun. 2000. Production of a nisin-like bacteriocin by *Lactococcus lactis* subsp. *lactis* A164 isolated from kimchi. *J Appl Microbiol* 88:563–571.

Choi, H. J., H. S. Lee, S. Her, D. H. Oh, and S. S. Yoon. 1999. Partial characterization and cloning of leuconocin J, a bacteriocin produced by *Leuconostoc* sp. J2 isolated from the Korean fermented vegetable Kimchi. *J Appl Microbiol* 86:175–181.

Choi, H. J., N. K. Lee, and H. D. Paik. 2015. Health benefits of lactic acid bacteria isolated from kimchi, with respect to immunomodulatory effects. *Food Sci Biotechnol* 24:783–789.

Choi, Y. J., H. Y. Jin, H. S. Yang, S. C. Lee, and C. K. Huh. 2016. Quality and storage characteristics of yogurt containing *Lactobacillus sakei* ALI033 and cinnamon ethanol extract. *J Anim Sci Technol* 58:16.

Chung, J. H., Y. Bae, Y. Kim, and J. H. Lee. 2010. Characteristics of bacteriocin produced by a *Lactobacillus plantarum* strain isolated from kimchi. *Korean J Microbiol Biotechnol* 38:481–485.

Dodd, H. M., and M. J. Gasson. 1994. Bacteriocins of lactic acid bacteria. In *Genetics and Biotechnology of Lactic Acid Bacteria*, ed. M. J. Gasson, and W. M. de Vos. 211–251. London: Blackie Academic and Professional

Ehrmann, M. A., A. Remiger, V. G. H. Eijsink, and R. F. Vogel. 2000. A gene cluster encoding plantaricin 1.25b and other bacteriocin-like peptides in *Lactobacillus plantarum* TMW1.25. *Biochim Biophy Acta* 1490:355–361.

Eun, S. H., S. M. Lim, S. E. Jang, M. J. Han, and D. H. Kim. 2016. *Lactobacillus sakei* K17, an inducer of IL-10 expression in antigen-presenting cells, attenuates TNBS-induced colitis in mice. *Immunopharm Immunotoxicol* 38:447–454.

Friend, B. A., and K. M. Shahani. 1984. Antitumor properties of lactobacilli and dairy products fermented by lactobacilli. *J Food Prot* 47:717–723.

Han, E. J., N. K. Lee, S. Y. Choi, and H. D. Paik. 2013. Short communication: Bacteriocin KC24 produced by *Lactococcus lactis* KC24 from kimchi and its antilisterial effect in UHT milk. *J Dairy Sci* 96:101–104.

Hong, H. J., E. Kim, D. Cho, and T. S. Kim. 2010. Differential suppression of heat-killed lactobacilli isolated from kimchi, a Korean traditional food, on airway hyper-responsiveness in mice. *J Clin Immunol* 30:449–458.

Hong, Y. F., H. Kim, H. R. Kim, M. G. Gim, and D. K. Chung. 2014. Different immune regulatory potential of *Lactobacillus plantarum* and *Lactobacillus sakei* isolated from kimchi. *J Microbiol Biotechnol* 24:1629–1635.

Huh, C. K., and T. Y. Hwang. 2016. Identification of antifungal substances of *Lactobacillus sakei* subsp. ALI033 and antifungal activity against *Penicillium brevicompactum* strain FI02. *Prev Nutr Food Sci* 21:52–56.

Jang, S. E., E. H. Joh, H. Y. Lee et al. 2013a. *Lactobacillus plantarum* HY7712 ameliorates cyclophosphamide-induced immunosuppression in mice. *J Microbiol Biotechnol* 23:414–421.

Jang, S. E., S. R. Hyam, M. J. Han et al. 2013b. *Lactobacillus brevis* G-101 ameliorates colitis in mice by inhibiting NF-κB, MAPK and AKT pathways and by polarizing M1 macrophages to M2-like macrophages. *J Appl Microbiol* 115:888–896.

Jeong, J. J., K. A. Kim, Y. J. Hwang, M. J. Han, and D. H. Kim. 2016. Anti-inflammaging effects of *Lactobacillus brevis* OW38 in aged mice. *Benef Microbes* 7:707–718.

Jo, S. G., E. J. Noh, J. Y. Lee et al. 2016. *Lactobacillus curvatus* WiKim38 isolated from kimchi induces IL-10 production in dendritic cells and alleviates DSS-induced colitis in mice. *J Microbiol* 54:503–509.

Jo, S. Y., E. A. Choi, J. J. Lee, and H. C. Chang. 2015. Characterization of starter kimchi fermented with *Leuconostoc kimchii* GJ2 and its cholesterol-lowering effects in rats fed a high-fat and high-cholesterol diet. *J Sci Food Agric* 95:2750–2756.

Ki, M. R., S. Y. Ghim, I. H. Hong et al. 2010. In vitro inhibition of *Helicobacter pylori* growth and of adherence of cagA-positive strains to gastric epithelial cells by *Lactobacillus paraplantarum* KNUC25 isolated from kimchi. *J Med Food* 13:629–634.

Kim, H. T., J. Y. Park, G. G. Lee, and J. H. Kim. 2004a. Isolation of a bacteriocin-producing *Lactobacillus sakei* strain from kimchi. *J Korean Soc Food Sci Nutr* 33:560–565.

Kim, H. Y., H. S. Bae, and Y. J. Baek. 1991. *In vivo* antitumor effects of lactic acid bacteria on Sarcoma 180 and mouse Lewis lung carcinoma. *J Korean Cancer Assoc* 23:188–196.

Kim, J. Y., B. K. Park, H. J. Park, Y. H. Park, B. O. Kim, and S. Pyo. 2013. Atopic dermatitis-mitigating effects of new *Lactobacillus* strain, *Lactobacillus sakei* probio 65 isolated from kimchi. *J Appl Microbiol* 115:517–526.

Kim, S. Y., K. S. Shin, and H. Lee. 2004b. Immunopotentiating activities of cellular components of *Lactobacillus brevis* FSB-1. *J Korean Soc Food Sci Nutr* 33:1552–1559.

Ko, J. L., C. K. Oh, M. C. Oh, and S. H. Kim. 2009. Depletion of nitrite by lactic acid bacteria isolated from commercial kimchi. *J Korean Soc Food Sci Nutr* 38:892–901.

Kwon, J. Y., H. S. Cheigh, and Y. O. Song. 2004. Weight reduction and lipid lowering effects of kimchi lactic acid powder in rats fed high fat diets. *J Korean Soc Food Sci Nutr* 36:1014–1019.

Lee, H., H. J. Choi, and M. J. Seo. 2014a. Characteristics of bacteriocins by lactic acid bacteria isolated from kimchi. *Curr Top LAB Probiotics* 2:1–6.

Lee, H. A., Y. J. Bong, H. Kim et al. 2015a. Effect of nanometric *Lactobacillus plantarum* in kimchi on dextran sulfate sodium-induced colitis in mice. *J Med Food* 18:1073–1080.

Lee, H. A., H. Kim, K. W. Lee, and K. Y. Park. 2015b. Dead nano-sized *Lactobacillus plantarum* inhibits azoxymethane/dextran sulfate sodium-induced colon cancer in BALB/c mice. *J Med Food* 18:1400–1405.

Lee, H. A., H. Kim, K. W. Lee, and K. Y. Park. 2016. Dietary nanosized *Lactobacillus plantarum* enhances the anticancer effect of kimchi on azoxymethane and dextran sulfate sodium-induced colon cancer in C57BL/6J mice. *J Environ Pathol Toxicol Oncol* 35:147–159.

Lee, H. Y., T. Ahn, S. H. Park et al. 2014b. *Lactobacillus plantarum* HY7712 protects against the impairment of NK-cell activity caused by whole-body γ-irradiation in mice. *J Microbiol Biotechnol* 24:127–131.

Lee, H. J., Y. J. Joo, C. S. Park et al. 1999. Purification and characterization of a bacteriocin produced by *Lactococcus lactis* subsp. *lactis* H-559 isolated from kimchi. *J Biosci Bioeng* 88:153–159.

Lee, I. H., S. H. Lee, I. S. Lee, Y. K. Park, D. K. Chung, and R. Choue. 2008. Effects of probiotic extracts of kimchi on immune function in NC/Nga mice. *Korean J Food Sci Technol* 40:82–87.

Lee, J., K. T. Hwang, M. S. Heo, J. H. Lee, and K. Y. Park. 2005. Resistance of *Lactobacillus plantarum* KCTC 3099 from Kimchi to oxidative stress. *J Med Food* 8:299–304.

Lee, J. H., D. H. Kweon, and S. C. Lee. 2006. Isolation and characterization of an immunopotentiating factor from *Lactobacillus plantarum* in kimchi: Assessment of immunostimulatory activities. *Food Sci Biotechnol* 15:877–883.

Lee, K. H., J. Y. Park, S. J. Jeong et al. 2007. Characterization of paraplantaricin C7, a novel bacteriocin produced by *Lactobacillus paraplantarum* C7 isolated from Kimchi. *J Microbiol Biotechnol* 17: 287–296.

Lee, K. H., J. L. Song, E. S. Park, J. Ju, H. Y. Kim, and K. Y. Park. 2015c. Anti-obesity effects of starter fermented kimchi on 3T3-L1 adipocytes. *Prev Nutr Food Sci* 20:298–302.

Lee, N. K., S. Y. Kim, K. J. Han, and H. D. Paik. 2014c. Probiotic potential of *Lactobacillus* strains with anti-allergic effects from kimchi for yogurt starters. *LWT-Food Sci Technol* 58:130–134.

Lee, Y., and H. C. Chang. 2008. Isolation and characterization of kimchi lactic acid bacteria showing anti-*Helicobacter pylori* activity. *J Microbiol Biotechnol* 36:106–114.

Lee, Y. D., Y. F. Hong, B. Jeon, B. J. Jung, D. K. Chung, and H. Kim. 2016. Differential cytokine regulatory effect of three *Lactobacillus* strains isolated from fermented foods. *J Microbiol Biotechnol* 26:1517–1526.

Lim, S. K., M. S. Kwon, J. Lee et al. 2017. *Weissella cibaria* WIKIM28 ameliorates atopic dermatitis-like skin lesions by inducing tolerogenic dendritic cells and regulatory T-cells in BALB/c mice. *Sci Rep* 7:40040.

Lim, S. M., and D. S. Im. 2007. Bactericidal effect of bacteriocin of *Lactobacillus plantarum* K11 isolated from dongchimi on *Escherichia coli* O157. *J Food Hyg Safety* 22:151–158.

Lim, S. M., J. J. Jeong, K. H. Woo, M. J. Han, and D. H. Kim. 2015. *Lactobacillus sakei* OK67 ameliorates high-fat diet-induced blood glucose intolerance and obesity in mice by inhibiting gut microbiota lipopolysaccharide production and inducing colon tight junction protein expression. *Nutr Res* 36:337–348.

Lindgren, S. E., and W. J. Dobrogosz. 1990. Antagonistic activities of lactic acid bacteria in food and feed fermentations. *FEMS Microbiol Rev* 7:149–163.

Moon, J. S., J. E. Ahn, A. R. Han et al. 2011. Anticariogenic activities of *Lactobacillus sakei* K-7 isolated from kimchi. *KSBB J* 26:513–516.

Moon, Y. J., J. R. Soh, J. J. Yu, H. S. Sohn, Y. S. Cha, and S. H. Oh. 2012. Intracellular lipid accumulation inhibitory effect of *Weissella koreensis* OK1-6 isolated from kimchi on differentiating adipocyte. *J Appl Microbiol* 113:652–658.

Nam, H., M. Ha, O. Bae, and Y. Lee. 2002. Effect of *Weissella confusa* strain PL9001 on the adherence and growth of *Helicobacter pylori*. *Appl Environ Microbiol* 68:4642–4645.

Oh, C. K., M. C. Oh, and S. H. Kim. 2004. The depletion of sodium nitrite by lactic acid bacteria isolated from kimchi. *J Med Food* 7:38–44.

Paik, H. D., and J. Y. Lee. 2014. Investigation of reduction and tolerance capability of lactic acid bacteria isolated from kimchi against nitrate and nitrite in fermented sausage condition. *Meat Sci* 97:609–614.

Park, C. W., M. Youn, Y. M. Jung et al. 2008. New functional probiotic *Lactobacillus sakei* probio 65 alleviates atopic symptoms in the mouse. *J Med Food* 11:405–412.

Park, H. D., and C. H. Rhee. 2001. Antimutagenic activity of *Lactobacillus plantarum* KLAB21 isolated from kimchi Korean fermented vegetables. *Biotechnology Lett* 23:1583–1589.

Park, J. A., P. B. Tirupathi Pichiah, J. J. Yu, S. H. Oh, J. W. Daily, III, and Y. S. Cha. 2012. Anti-obesity effect of kimchi fermented with *Weissella koreensis* OK1-6 as starter in high-fat diet-induced obese C57BL/6J mice. *J Appl Microbiol* 113:1507–1516.

Park, J. S., I. Joe, P. D. Rhee, C. S. Jeong, and G. Jeong. 2017a. A lactic acid bacterium isolated from kimchi ameliorates intestinal inflammation in DSS-induced colitis. *J Microbiol* 55:304–310.

Park, J. Y., S. J. Jeong, and J. H. Kim. 2014a. Characterization of a glutamate decarboxylase (GAD) gene from *Lactobacillus zymae*. *Biotechnology Lett* 36:1791–1799.

Park, K. B., and S. H. Oh. 2007. Cloning, sequencing and expression of a novel glutamate decarboxylase gene from a newly isolated lactic acid bacterium, *Lactobacillus brevis* OPK-3. *Bioresour Technol* 98:312–319.

Park, K. Y., J. K. Jeong, Y. E. Lee, and J. W. Daily 3rd. 2014b. Health benefits of kimchi (Korean fermented vegetables) as a probiotic food. *J Med Food* 17:6–20.

Park, K. Y., S. H. Kim, and T. J. Son. 1998. Antimutagenic activities of cell wall and cytosol fraction of lactic acid bacteria isolated from kimchi. *J Food Sci Nutr* 3:329–333.

Park, S., Y. Ji, H. Y. Jung et al. 2017b. *Lactobacillus plantarum* HAC01 regulates gut microbiota and adipose tissue accumulation in a diet-induced obesity murine model. *Appl Microbiol Biotechnol* 101:1605–1614.

Park, S. S., M. H. Kim, K. S. Han, and S. Oh. 2004. Use of bacteriocin produced by *Lactococcus* sp. CU216 with pH sensitive liposome entrapment. *Korean J Food Sci Anim Resour* 24:97–102.

Park, S. Y., H. M. Jin, H. J. Lim et al. 2013. Immunomodulatory effects of lactic acid bacteria isolated from kimchi on the function of mouse T cells. *Curr Top LAB Probiotics* 1:133–137.

Rhee, C. H., and H. S. Park. 2001. Three glycoproteins with antimutagenic activity identified in *Lactobacillus plantarum* KLAB21. *Appl Environ Microbiol* 67:3445–3449.

Schnurer, J., and J. Magnusson. 2005. Antifungal lactic acid bacteria as biopreservatives. *Trends Food Sci Technol* 16:70–78.

Seo, J., and H. Lee. 2007. Characteristics and immunomodulating activity of lactic acid bacteria for the potential probiotics. *Korean J Food Sci Technol* 39:681–687.

Shin, K. S., O. W. Chae, I. C. Park, S. K. Hong, and T. B. Choe. 1998. Antitumor effects of mice fed with cell lysate of *Lactobacillus plantarum* isolated from kimchi. *Korean J Biotechnol Bioeng* 13:357–363.

Shin, M. S., S. K. Han, K. S. Kim, and W. K. Lee. 2008. Isolation and partial characterization of a bacteriocin produced by *Pediococcus pentosaceus* K23-2 isolated from kimchi. *J Appl Microbiol* 105:331–339.

Son, T. J., S. H. Kim, and K. Y. Park. 1998. Antimutagenic activities of lactic acid bacteria isolated from kimchi. *J Korean Assoc Cancer Prev* 3:65–74.

Stiles, M. E. 1996. Biopreservation by lactic acid bacteria. *Antonie Van Leeuwenhoek* 70:331–345.

Wada, T., M. Noda, F. Kashiwabara et al. 2009. Characterization of four plasmids harbored in a *Lactobacillus brevis* strain encoding a novel bacteriocin, brevicin 925A, and construction of a shuttle vector for lactic acid bacteria and *Escherichia coli*. *Microbiology* 155:1726–1737.

Won, T. J., B. Kim, Y. Lee et al. 2012. Therapeutic potential of *Lactobacillus plantarum* CJLP133 for house-dust mite-induced dermatitis in NC/Nga mice. *Cell Immunol* 277:49–57.

Won, T. J., B. Kim, Y. T. Lim et al. 2011b. Oral administration of *Lactobacillus* strains from kimchi inhibits atopic dermatitis in NC/Nga mice. *J Appl Microbiol* 110:1195–1202.

Won, T. J., B. Kim, D. S. Song et al. 2011a. Modulation of Th1/Th2 balance by *Lactobacillus* strains isolated from kimchi via stimulation of macrophage cell line J774A.1 *in vitro*. *J Food Sci* 76:H55–H61.

Yang, E. J., and H. C. Chang. 2010. Purification of a new antifungal compound produced by *Lactobacillus plantarum* AF1 isolated from kimchi. *Int J Food Microbiol* 139:56–63.

Yang, E. J., J. Y. Chang, H. J. Lee et al. 2002. Characterization of the antagonistic activity against *Lactobacillus plantarum* and induction of bacteriocin production. *Korean J Food Sci Technol* 34:311–318.

Yang, E. J., Y. S. Kim, and H. C. Chang. 2011. Purification and characterization of antifungal δ-dodecalactone from *Lactobacillus plantarum* AF1 isolated from kimchi. *J Food Prot* 74:651–657.

5

Health Benefits of Doenjang (Soybean Paste) and Kanjang (Soybean Sauce)

Kun-Young Park and Eui-Seong Park

CONTENTS

5.1 Introduction 102
5.2 History 103
5.3 Processing Methods and Microorganisms Used in Fermentation 104
    5.3.1 Traditional Doenjang and Kanjang 105
    5.3.2 Modified Commercial Doenjang 108
    5.3.3 Modified Commercial Kanjang 109
5.4 Nutritional and Functional Components 110
    5.4.1 Doenjang 110
    5.4.2 Kanjang 112
5.5 Health Benefit Effects of Doenjang 113
    5.5.1 Antioxidative Effects 113
    5.5.2 Anticancer Effects of Doenjang 115
        5.5.2.1 Antimutagenic Effect 115
        5.5.2.2 Anticancer Effect 116
        5.5.2.3 Increasing Anticancer Effects of Doenjang 117
    5.5.3 Antiobesity Effects of Doenjang 120
    5.5.4 Prevention of Cardiovascular Diseases 123
    5.5.5 Other Functions 125
        5.5.5.1 Promotion of Immune Function 125
        5.5.5.2 Probiotic Function of *Bac. subtilis* 125
        5.5.5.3 Diabetes 126
5.6 Functionality of Kanjang 126
    5.6.1 Antioxidative Effects of Kanjang 126
    5.6.2 Anticancer Properties of Kanjang 129
    5.6.3 Other Functions 132
        5.6.3.1 Immunomodulation 132
        5.6.3.2 Anti-Inflammation 133
        5.6.3.3 Antihypertension 134
5.7 Conclusion 134
References 135

5.1 Introduction

The Korean Gallup Polls (2004) reported that of the top five favorite foods for Koreans, doenjang stew was ranked first, followed by kimchi stew and then kimchi, bulgogi (boiled beef) and bibimbap (cooked rice with assorted vegetables and other ingredients). Doenjang and kanjang (also designated as ganjang) have a long history and are the most basic foods for Koreans. Manchuria, which was an old territory of Goguryeo, and the Korean peninsula were the homes of the soybeans (Park, 2006). The Chinese book Samkukji AD 3 indicated that Koreans developed soybean fermented foods and spread their technology to neighboring countries. Korean ancestors regarded doenjang as a folk medicine as well as a seasoning for adding flavor to foods (Park et al., 2004). Doenjang and kanjang were traditionally used to treat gonorrhea, eye disease, toxification, inflammation, etc. (Park, 2009a).

Traditional jang (doenjang and kanjang) is fermented first by making meju used as a starter culture and the main ingredient of the jang and then the meju is further fermented in brine (salt + water). The fermented liquid part (kanjang) is separated from the fermented paste (doenjang) after the fermentation. Thus, soybeans, salt, and water are the main ingredients to make doenjang and kanjang. Soybeans contain nutritive and non-nutritive components. Soybean has approximately 40% protein, 20% lipid, and 30% carbohydrate, and phytochemicals. Cooked rice is the main staple for the Korean diet (Kim et al., 2000). Rice contains approximately 7% protein, 1% lipid, and more than 80% carbohydrate. Thus, soybean foods make up for the weak points of eating rice only, balancing the three major nutrients; also, the essential amino acids present in the rice and soy foods complement each other, providing a complete protein. Isoflavones (genistin, daidzin, glycetin), lecithin, saponin, phytic acid, inositol, trypsin inhibitor, anthocyanin, and phenol compounds are the main non-nutritive phytochemcial components found in soybeans (Isanga and Zhang, 2008). The isoflavone aglycones (genistein and daidzein) increase during the fermentation. The phytoestrogens, genistein and daidzein, can have various health benefits, including prevention of cancers such as breast cancer, prostate cancer and colon cancer, as well as cardiovascular diseases, osteoporosis, obesity, menopausal syndrome, etc. (Sirotkin and Harrath, 2014).

Soybean proteins and amino acids, polyunsaturated fatty acids, various fermented metabolites, microorganisms, and melanoidins are other functional components found after the soybean fermentation. Soybean itself has the lowest glycemic index, which helps in lowering blood glucose levels and is a good food for diabetic patients (Kim et al., 2012).

Black soybeans have anthocyanins from the soybean coats, which have anticancer, antiobesity, antioxidative activities, etc. (Cheigh et al., 1990; Kwon et al., 2008; Lim et al., 2009; Park et al., 2015a). The type of salt used for the preparation of doenjang and kanjang is also an important factor to increase

Health Benefits of Doenjang (Soybean Paste) and Kanjang (Soybean Sauce) 103

the functionality of the soybean foods. Use of bamboo salt for the preparation of the soy-fermented foods increased anticancer and antiobesity activities (Hwang et al., 2007; Kim et al., 2007; Hwang et al., 2008; Lee et al., 2008, 2011a; Song, 2012; Jeong et al., 2013; Shim et al., 2015). Doenjang and kanjang have more benefits due to the fermentation products than unfermented soybeans, which are the raw materials. Taste, preservation ability, and functionality are markedly increased as a result of fermentation.

5.2 History

Jang was originally used as the name of the liquid phase of kanjang, with a narrow meaning; today, it has a broader meaning that includes doenjang, cheongkukjang (Chungkukjang), kochujang, chunjang, mixed jang, etc. Doenjang was an important source of protein for ancient Koreans, who were deficient in meat intake; it also served as a basic seasoning for Korean foods. Soybeans, whose wildtype species derived from Manchuria and the Korean peninsula, have been cultivated in northeastern China, Korea, Japan, and far eastern Russia. Thus, there are many soybean-derived foods and dishes in Korean diets. *Samgukji*, the historical novel written by Jinsu (AD 233–297), reported that people in Goguryeo used to develop a variety of fermented foods. Thus, it may be inferred that salt-based fermented foods began to be manufactured and consumed at that time. Old archives, such as *Jeyijeon*, written by Yangseo (AD 557–637), and *Dongyijeon*, written by Namsa (unidentified), reported that people in the Goguryeo dynasty (37 BC–AD 668) had already developed various fermented foods such as soybeans, fish, liquor and vegetables. Also, there existed a record that jang and shi were used for a wedding dinner in AD 683 (King Sinmun of the Shilla dynasty); *Samgukyusa*, one of the Korean archives written by Il Yeon (AD 1206–1289), contained a record that jang was used as a wound-healing remedy as well as a food.

Haedongyeoksa, a history book from the Balhae empire, refers to another soybean-derived product called shi. It is made by fermenting soybeans in a dark place with a mixture of salt, sharing the same concept as chunggukjang. Shi was born in the northern part of Korea and migrated to the Han empire of China; dujang was developed in the southern part of Korea, which was later called maljang (currently it is called meju in modern Korea) and migrated to Japan to be called miso (Park, 2009a). Maljang is made by long-term fermentation of soybean in salted water. Miso, the Japanese style soybean paste, was derived from maljang; it migrated to Japan during the era of the Nara empire. *Daeboyulryong* (AD 701) of Japan also introduced jang, shi, and maljang, which is referred to as miso. *BangunJipyeok* (AD 1778) indicated that jang was known as jiang in China and Mongolia, misoon in Manchuria, and miso in Japan. The goryobangeon section in the book, *Gyerimyusa*, referred to it as miljo. Thus, the Korean soybean paste named jang became misoon, miljo, myojo, and then miso when the soybean paste was brought to Japan.

Sasisanyocho (AD 1590), written by Kang Hee Maeng, referred to kanjang, doenjang, and some variations of doenjang called pojang and jeupjeo. One royal record written about the first year of King Danjong referred to jinjang as fermented jang, which may imply that fermented jang became available at that time. *Hunmongjahoe* (AD 1527) contained a record that kanjang was classified as chomjang, danjang and jangyu; also, shi was alternately referred to as jeonguk-shi, jeongukjang, or dushi. *Dongeuibogam* (AD 1613), written by Hurjun, which is a famous Korean medicine book, described how to make medicinal doenjang from soybeans and how to fix the sour doenjang as well as special types of jang such as fermented fish (dujang and hae), yukjang, and nomaekjang.

Many records from the mid-Chosun dynasty have also described jang. *Guhwangboyubang* (AD 1660) and *Gyugonsieuibang* (AD 1670) mentioned a new type of term related to jang. *Sanjungilgi*, written by Jung Si Han (AD 1625–1707), introduced the terms jeonjeongjang and jeonjang, referring to the jang that underwent specific processing such as baking and fermentation. All jang manufacturing methods were compiled in *Sanlimgyeongje*, written by Hong Man Seon (AD 1643–1715). *Jungbosanlimkyungji* (AD 1760) described maljang and read meyjo and, then meju. It also indicated 45 different processing methods for soybean products, the appropriate day for making jang, selection of water, salt quality, how to handle the pottery container, and how to fix the off-taste of jang. *Gosasinseo* (AD 1771) also introduced types and manufacturing methods of jang.

The modern versions of doenjang and kanjang were first manufactured during the era of Japanese occupation (1909–1945), when Japanese jang plants were built on the Korean peninsula. After liberation in 1945, the abandoned jang plants were acquired by the Koreans, which was the milestone for the beginning of the industrialized version of jang. Manufacturing methods of jang became standardized after 1962, when the Union of the Korean Soybean Industry was established. In spite of industrialization, some homemade traditional doenjang and kanjang is still manufactured on a small scale, and considerable research has focused on the reformation of the manufacturing process after the superiority of traditionally made doenjang and kanjang was discovered.

5.3 Processing Methods and Microorganisms Used in Fermentation

Hwang (2004) standardized the doenjang processing method from collected methods found in 80 scientific papers, cookbooks, and commercial factories in Korea, classifying them by traditional method and modified commercial methods using koji (*Aspergillus oryzae*) as the starter. The traditional method, using the old traditional ways of fermenting soybeans, used natural fermentation by ambient microorganisms in the environment; however, modified commercial methods use only *Asp. oryzae* and other starters with carbohydrate sources and soybeans. Grain-type meju has also been developed for use as a starter, when meju is prepared, by inoculating *Asp. oryzae*. *Bacillus subtilis* naturally exists in soybeans for meju fermentation instead of natural fermentation as a modified traditional method.

5.3.1 Traditional Doenjang and Kanjang

Soybeans (especially larger sizes), salt (usually solar salt without bittern), and water are the main ingredients used to prepare doenjang and kanjang. Soybeans are washed and soaked in water at 15°C for 12 hours. The soybeans are cooked for 4 hours or autoclaved at 121°C for 30 minutes, and then cooled to 45°C–50°C. The cooked soybeans are crushed and molded into a brick shape (8–12 × 12–18 × 15–25 cm^3) to make meju, which can be fermented naturally. Meju will be the starter and main raw material for the preparation of doenjang and kanjang. The rectangular, brick-shaped meju is dried for 2–3 days in the air; traditionally, meju is tied up with rice straw and hung at the edge of an eave to allow natural fermentation for 30 days. The naturally present bacteria, molds, and yeasts from soybeans, rice straw, air, etc., participate in the meju fermentation of traditionally prepared meju (Figure 5.1a). Modified meju preparations are shown in Figure 5.1b (Hwang, 2004). *Asp. oryzae* is used as a fermentation starter. Koji is made of wheat flour or rice by inoculation with *Asp. oryzae* and is widely used to produce doenjang. Using koji is more convenient than the traditional natural fermentation. The soybean grains inoculated with *Asp. oryzae* (0.2%) and naturally present *Bac. subtilis* in soybeans ferment at 30°C for 36 hours and are then dried at 40°C. This can be a koji-fermented grain type meju; however,

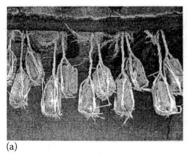
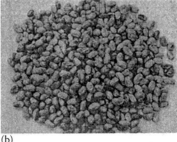

(a)   (b)

FIGURE 5.1
(a) Traditional rectangular shaped meju blocks fermented naturally and (b) grain-type meju fermented with starters.

during grain-type meju fermentation, other microorganisms can still participate in the fermentation.

We isolated representative microorganisms from the traditional meju samples and identified microorganisms that actively participate in the meju fermentation to take advantage of using both traditional and industrial processing methods; one such method was used as an effective and beneficial microorganism for starter cultures of meju fermentation. The grain-type meju was prepared with inoculation of well characterized starter cultures for doenjang and kanjang preparation. Using beneficial mixed starter cultures can improve the quality and functionality of meju and doenjang (Jeong, 2012).

For the second fermentation, the meju is mixed with salt and water as shown in Figure 5.2. The mixing ratio for the traditional method is approximately 1:1:4 (18.4 ± 4.4: 14.6 ± 2.1: 67.0 ± 4.4, w/w/w; Park et al., 2002; Hwang, 2004), and the modified method of grain meju is 1:0.46:1.7 (w/w/w), for meju (only doenjang prepared without separating kanjang), salt, and water, respectively (Jeong, 2012). Then they are usually fermented for 60 days in a clay pot. Some dried red pepper and pieces of charcoal are placed on top of the mixture and fermented for 2–3 months in the clay pot. The liquid part of the meju brine mixture is separated and filtered after the fermentation and is kanjang (soy sauce), which is boiled to destroy harmful microorganisms and to remove off-flavors, etc. While the solid part of the mixture becomes doenjang, the crushed solid part is put into another pot. The doenjang undergoes an additional 2–6 months of fermentation. The longer the fermentation time, more than 1–6 years, gives high quality and better functionality to doenjang (Hwang, 2004; Shim et al., 2015). The water (Ham et al., 2008; Park, 2009b) and kinds of salt could also affect the quality and functionality of doenjang and kanjang (Lee et al., 2008).

Yu (1998) isolated 70 microorganisms—36 molds, 18 yeasts, and 16 bacteria—from traditional meju. Representative molds were genera *Aspergillus, Mucor, Penicillium,* and *Rhizopus. Saccharomyces, Candida, Hansenula,* and *Zygosaccharomyces* were the major yeasts. However, the genus *Bacillus* was the dominant bacteria with *Pediococcus* as lactic acid bacteria (LAB). Kim et al. (2009) found that *Bacillus subtilis, Bac. licheniformis,* and LAB such as *Leu. mesenteroides, Tetragenococcus halophilus,* and *Enterococcus faecium,* as well as *Mucor plumbeus, Asp. oryzae,* and *Debaryomyces hansenii* were the main fungi in doenjang samples. Kim (1976) reported that *Asp. oryzae, Penicillium* sp., *Mucor* sp., and *Rhizopus* sp. were the predominant fungi. *Bac. subtilis* was the predominant bacteria species detected. Major microorganisms of meju are *Bacillus* sp., as the ratio of *Bacillus* sp. to molds is approximately 100:1. Yeasts such as *Saccharomyces* sp. and LAB along with molds and the *Bacillus* sp. participate in the ripening of meju in brine (Yu, 1998). *Bacillus* sp. is the major bacteria during meju, doenjang, and kanjang fermentation.

Mucor hiemalis and *Rhizopus stolonifer* were used as starters to prepare grain-type meju (Kim and Kim, 1999) and showed better sensory evaluation

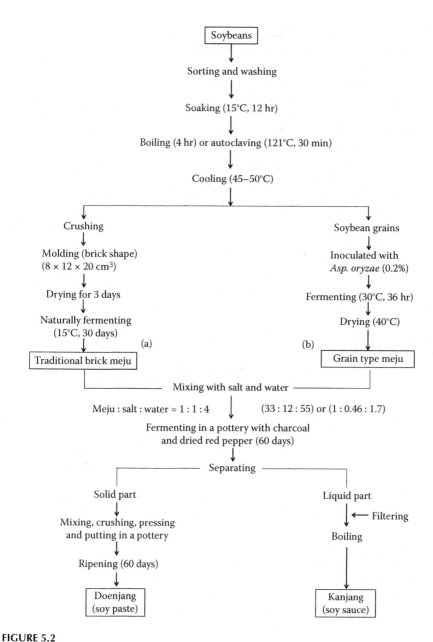

FIGURE 5.2
Processing of meju and meju-derived fermented Korean traditional soybean paste (doenjang) and soybean sauce (kanjang); (a) traditional method and (b) modified method using koji. (From Hwang, K. M. 2004. Studies on the enhancement of chemopreventive and anticancer effects of doenjang. Ph.D. diss., Pusan National Univ., Busan, Korea.)

than using *Aspergillus* and *Bacillus* as starters. Kim et al. (2002a) developed a three-step fermentation method for the preparation of grain-type traditional meju with starters. Lactic acid bacteria were inoculated first to inhibit wild *Bacillus* that produce bad odors, but produce lactic acid, H_2O_2, and bacteriocin; they were then inoculated with *Asp. oryzae* for the second fermentation, and *Bac. subtilis* as the third step to enzymatically hydrolyze proteins and produce amino acids that contribute the characteristic savory flavors. Various microorganisms were isolated from traditional meju samples. The total counts of aerobic bacteria, lactic acid bacteria, and yeasts and molds were 10^{7-8} colony-forming units (CFUs)/g, 10^{6-8} CFUs/g, and 10^{7-8} CFUs/g, respectively. LAB counts were similar to bacteria, yeast, and mold counts. *Lab. plantarum*, *Leu. mesenteroides*, and *Lac. lactis* were isolated from the meju. *Bac. subtilis* was the predominant strain found in the meju. *Asp. oryzae* and *Mucor racemosus* were the representative molds. However, three microorganisms, *Bac. subtilis*, *Asp. oryzae*, and *Lac. lactis*, that showed the highest enzyme activities and functionality from the isolates were selected as starters (Jeong, 2012). Grain-type meju was prepared with the inoculation of this mixed starter culture. 10^6 CFUs/g of *Bac. subtilis* and 0.2% *Asp. oryzae* were inoculated first and fermented at 30°C for 48 hours, 10^6 CFUs/g of *Lac. lactis* was inoculated and fermented at 37°C for 24 hours, and then doenjang was manufactured with this meju. This doenjang showed excellent fermentation characteristics, organoleptic qualities, and health functionalities, compared to industrial doenjang, and was comparable to traditional ones (Jeong, 2012).

5.3.2 Modified Commercial Doenjang

The preparation method for modified commercial doenjang is shown in Figure 5.3. Rice, wheat flour, or barley as a carbohydrate source is washed, soaked, and drained and then steamed or cooked for 40 minutes and cooled. 0.2% of *Asp. oryzae* by the weight of starch source is inoculated and cultivated at 30°C–35°C for 3 days; this becomes koji. As koji starters, *Asp. sojae*, *Bac. subtilis*, *Bac. lichiniformis*, *Rhi. delemar*, etc., can also be used (Hwang, 2004). Defatted or imported soybeans are washed and soaked in water overnight (8–9 hours) and drained for 1 hour, and then autoclaved (1 kg/cm^2) for 1 hour and cooled. The cooled soybeans and koji are mixed and crushed. After water and salt are added, the mixture is fermented at 30°C for 30 days. To imitate Korean traditional doenjang, traditional meju and soybeans are mixed and pasteurized at 60°C for 30 minutes and then packaged. The standardized ingredient ratio of the commercial doenjang is 39.8 ± 7.7% soybeans, 22.6 ± 4.4% starch source, 12.5 ± 1.4% salt, and 25.1 ± 9.0% water (Hwang, 2004). The taste of modified commercial doenjang was comparable to both miso and traditional doenjang, since it was fermented with both *Asp. oryzae* and *Bac. subtilis*. Vitamins B_1 and B_2 formation significantly increased three times after 3 months of fermentation. Since the fermented soybean products have been industrially developed by the Japanese, the Japanese style of jang has

Health Benefits of Doenjang (Soybean Paste) and Kanjang (Soybean Sauce)

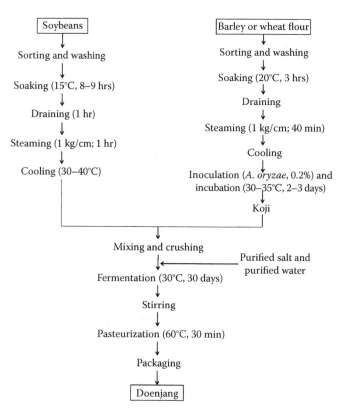

FIGURE 5.3
Processing method of modified commercial soybean paste (doenjang).

been manufactured in jang plants in Korea. *Asp. oryzae* is used as the koji mold for production of hydrolytic enzymes of raw materials and *Bac. subtilis* or *Bac. licheniformis* is for the flavor production of traditional jang (Park, 2009a).

5.3.3 Modified Commercial Kanjang

Defatted soybeans are sorted, water is added, and the mixture is cooked or autoclaved at 1 kg/cm^2 for 60 minutes and cooled. Wheat grains are roasted, become a brown color on the surface, and are gelatinized; the grain breaks into four or five pieces and *Asp. oryzae* or *Asp. sojae* is added and mixed with the cooked and cooled defatted soybeans to make koji. The ratio of defatted soybean and wheat is 55:45 and the mixture is fermented at 30°C–35°C for 2–3 days. 100%–130% of brined water (18%–20% salt) is added to the koji volume in the tank, mixed, and fermented (Park, 2009a). The fermentation is carried out for 6–12 months, stirring once a day at the initial stage, and then once every 2–3 days. It is fermented at 10°C–15°C for the first month and then

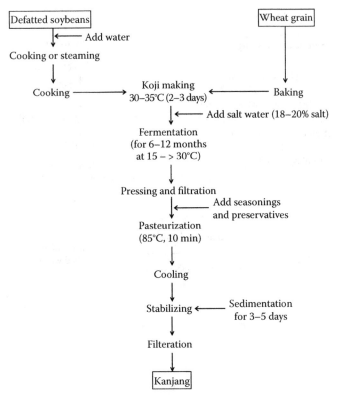

FIGURE 5.4
Processing method of manufacturing modified commercial soy sauce (kanjang).

at 25°C–30°C. The levels of *Bacillus* sp. decrease; however, *Pediococcus halophilus* and *Zygosaccharomyces rouxii* start to grow after 1 month of fermentation. The fermented product is pressed and filtered, preservatives and seasonings are added, and then it is pasteurized (80°C–85°C for 10–30 minutes). Then it is cooled and allowed to stand for 3–5 days in the tank to remove sediments, filtered, and packaged, and thus becomes the kanjang product (Figure 5.4).

5.4 Nutritional and Functional Components

5.4.1 Doenjang

Soybeans, which are the major component of doenjang and kanjang, are called "animal meat produced in the field" in Korea because of the high content and quality of the protein they provide. Soybeans contains 9.7% water, 36.2% protein, 17.8% lipid, 30.7% carbohydrate, 5.0% fiber, 5.6% ash, and some

Health Benefits of Doenjang (Soybean Paste) and Kanjang (Soybean Sauce)   111

functional phytochemicals (*Food Composition Table*, 2006). The contents of three major nutrients—proteins, lipids, and carbohydrates—are 33%–47%, 11%–23%, and 21%–28%, respectively, depending on the variety.

When 15 traditionally prepared doenjang samples were analyzed, they averaged 54.7% water, 13.8% crude protein, 8.0% crude lipid, 14.4 mL titratable acidity, and 11.8% salt. The level of free amino acid was 3.81%, of which glutamic acid was 25%, the highest level; leucine, alanine, histidine, lysine, proline, and valine were also found in relatively high concentrations (Park et al., 2000a). Doenjang also contains oligosaccharides and 3.1% dietary fiber. The digestibility of raw soybean is approximately 55% and that of cooked soybean is 65%, but doenjang is 85% digestible (Lee, 2003). Lactic acid was the predominant organic acid present, and acetic, malic, citric, and oxalic acids were also detected. Linoleic acid (52.2%), oleic acid (20.7%), and linolenic acid (8.7%) were the most abundant unsaturated fatty acids, comprising 81.6% of the total fatty acids (Park et al., 2000a).

The functional compounds found in doenjang include the followings: protease inhibitor, amino acids and peptides from proteins, oligosaccharides of raffinose, and stachyose and dietary fiber from carbohydrates; free fatty acids include linoleic, oleic, and linolenic acids and vitamin E and lecithin were identified in the lipid fraction. The minerals in doenjang included P, Ca, Mg, and S. Phytochemicals include phytic acid, saponins, squalene, β-sitosterol, isoflavones (daidzein, genistein), phenolic acids (syringic, vanillic, chlorogenic, ferulic, cinnamic acids, etc.), browning products, lignan, carotenoids(lutein, α- and β-carotenes), etc. (Park et al., 2003; Isanga and Zhang, 2008). The contents of the isoflavone bioactive compounds (daidzein and genistein) from soybean, meju and doenjang were determined (Kim and Yoon, 1999). The daidzein and genistein aglycones significantly increased with the fermentation by the microorganisms. The free daidzein level was 106 ± 7 mg/kg in soybeans; however, the levels increased to 269 ± 38 and 578 ± 70 mg/kg in meju and doenjang, respectively (Table 5.1).

TABLE 5.1

Daidzein and Genistein Contents of Soybeans, Meju, and Doenjang[a]

	Soybeans	Meju	Doenjang
Daidzein, free	106 ± 7	269 ± 38	578 ± 70
Daidzein, total	406 ± 29	433 ± 41	538 ± 59
Daidzein aglycones (%)	26.0 ± 0.1	62.0 ± 3.3	107.7 ± 10.3
Genistein, free	95 ± 20	137 ± 16	455 ± 10
Genistein, total	484 ± 86	200 ± 7	538 ± 57
Genistein, aglycones (%)	19.5 ± 1.1	68.5 ± 6.6	85.3 ± 8.7
D/G ratio[b]	0.85 ± 0.01	2.2 ± 0.2	1.0 ± 0.1

Source: Kim, J. S., and S. Yoon. 1999. *Korean J Food Sci Technol* 31:1405–1409.
[a] Milligrams per kilogram, dry basis.
[b] Total daidzein content/total genistein content ratio.

The free genistein content was 95 ± 20 mg/kg in soybean; however, the levels also increased to 137 ± 16 and 455 ± 10 mg/kg in meju and doenjang, respectively. Total daidzein/total genistein content ratio was 1.0 ± 0.1 mg/kg in doenjang. Thus, the aglyconed isoflavone levels were significantly increased during the fermentation to become doenjang (five or six times). The microbial community participating in doenjang fermentation resulted in different metabolites. The *Aspergillus* population was linked to sugar metabolism and *Bacillus* sp. was that of fatty acids, but *Teragenococcus* and *Zygosaccharomyces* were associated with amino acids. Thus, microbial assortment in the doenjang process determined the quality of doenjang (Lee et al., 2017).

Taste components of traditional and commercial doenjang are free amino acids, nucleotides, and their related compounds. The amount of glutamic acid was the highest, followed by aspartic acid, leucine, lysine, and alanine (Kim and Rhee, 1988). In commercial doenjang, prepared with soybean and starch sources, glycine was the amino acid present in the highest concentration, followed by glutamic acid, valine (Kim and Lee, 1985). The levels of glutamic and aspartic acids were markedly increased during 60–80 days of fermentation. The amounts of phenylalanine, leucine, and arginine increased considerably compared to those of other amino acids, and proline specifically increased after 180 days of fermentation (Kim and Rhee, 1990). Guanosine monophosphate (GMP) was the nucleic acid that related to the taste of commercial and traditional doenjang (Kim and Rhee, 1988). Inosine monophosphate (IMP) and GMP markedly increased with a prolonged fermentation period (Kim and Rhee, 1990). The taste of Korean traditional soybean paste (doenjang) tends to be a palatable blend of sweet, salty, bitter, and sour flavors, with relative contributions of each judged to be approximately 26.0%, 17.8%, 8.6%, and 3.1%, respectively (Yang et al. 1992).

5.4.2 Kanjang

Kanjang has 19%–26% salt content, 0.55%–1.22% of total nitrogen, and lactic acid as the highest concentration of organic acids. The total nitrogen content is composed of 50%–70% of free amino acids, 15%–35% peptides, 11%–15% ammonia nitrogen, and low levels of nucleic acids, Maillard reaction products, and amines. Glutamic acid is the major flavor compound that contributes the savory taste in kanjang. There are about 300 kinds of fermented metabolites, but other major flavor compounds include ethanol, lactic acid, glycerol, acetic acid, 4-hydroxy-2,5-dimethyl-3(2H)-furanone (HDMF), 4-hydroxy-2(or 5)-ethyl-5(or 2)-methyl-3(2H)-furanone (HEMF), 2,3-butandiol, etc. (Kataoka, 2005). The major components of kanjang are amino acids, sugars, and metabolites from fermentation such as alcohols, organic acids, and salt; it has a savory flavor and characteristic taste and flavor that combine sweet and salty flavors to the savory taste, and thus it is a natural seasoning. Traditional kanjang had a less sweet taste, organic acids, and sugars and thus the taste was not better than that of commercial kanjang. The composition from high to low of organic acid levels is as follows: butyric acid > propionic acid > acetic acid > formic acid. The high levels of butyric acid may cause the unique smell of traditional kanjang (Park, 2009a).

Commercial kanjang has especially high concentrations of acetic acid, which forms from bacteria, but the growth is inhibited by the high levels of salt. Thus, traditional kanjang has lower levels of acetic acid compared to commercial kanjang. The traditional kanjang has less flavor, taste, and color; higher turbidity and total nitrogen content; extracted components; organic acids; and sugars than the commercially fermented kanjang, but it is saltier. However, traditional kanjang has a more savory taste from amino acids of soybeans, a salty taste, and specific flavors and color from the organic acids and combined traditional flavoring. Thus, traditional kanjang can be used to give a good salty taste in soup and stew; however, commercial kanjang has a sweeter taste, and it can be used for increasing taste for side dishes and flavoring, and it is preferred when used for hard-boiled foods and chapchae (Kim and Kim, 1996).

5.5 Health Benefit Effects of Doenjang

5.5.1 Antioxidative Effects

Doenjang has various antioxidative compounds, including isoflavones, phenolic acids, phytic acid, saponin, trypsin inhibitor, tocopherol, amino acid, peptides, etc. (Choi et al., 1993a; Kim et al., 2005a). Both lipid-soluble and water-soluble extracts from doenjang exhibited strong antioxidative activity (Cheigh et al., 1990). The TBA (thiobarbituric acid) values measured at low temperature (6°C) for 5 weeks in ground cooked meat (GCM) with doenjang are shown in Figure 5.5. The TBA value of the control (GCM, 10 g) increased over the incubation time. However, the group with GCM and doenjang (1.2 g salt content in 10 g of doenjang) showed no change in TBA value over time and there was no evidence that oxidative reactions occurred. However, the group treated with salt (1.2 g) in GCM showed higher TBA value than the group with GCM only. Salt enhanced the oxidation reaction, but salt (12% content) in doenjang did not cause an increase in TBA value, although it showed strong antioxidative activity. Thus, the negative action of salt can be prevented when it is in doenjang (Cheigh et al., 1990).

As the fermentation progresses, the antioxidant effect of doenjang is increased, due to the elevated phenolic compound levels during the fermentation (Song 2012). Genistin decreased to $59.6 \pm 1.2 \, \mu g/g$, when fermentation reached 60 days, from $550.7 \pm 27.1 \, \mu g/g$ in the beginning of fermentation. However, genistein increased from $11.1 \pm 0.7 \, \mu g/g$ before the fermentation to $283.8 \pm 11.7 \, \mu g/g$ at

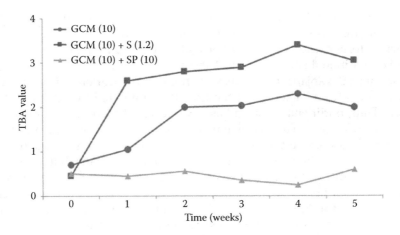

FIGURE 5.5
Changes in thiobarbituric acid (TBA) values of ground cooked meat (GCM) with the addition of soybean paste (SP; 1.2 g salt content in 10 g doenjang) and salt (S; 1.2 g) during storage for 5 weeks at 6°C. (From Cheigh, H. S. et al., 1990, *J Korean Soc Food Nutr* 19:163–167.)

60 days of fermentation (Lee and Cheigh, 1997a). Crude phenolic compounds from doenjang significantly decreased the levels of peroxide and conjugated diene contents, inhibited lipoxygenase (LOX) activity in the LOX–linoleic acid system and showed almost the same effect of α-tocopherol; metal (FeCl$_3$) chelation and free radical scavenging activities were also increased (Lee and Cheigh, 1997b). Both phenolic acid and isoflavone fraction exhibited an identical antioxidative effect against the oxidation of linoleic acid (Kim et al., 1994). The hydrophilic fraction of browning products from meju exhibited much higher antioxidant activity than the lipophilic fraction, and the former fraction was dramatically increased at the early stage of fermentation. Hydrophilic browning products (Kim et al., 2002b) and phenolic compounds in doenjang showed strong antioxidative activity against linoleic acid peroxidation (Lee et al., 1991).

Isoflavones, phenolic acid, tocopherol, and anthocyanin in black soybeans showed antioxidative activity. Genistein among isoflavones, gentisic acid among phenolic acids, γ-tocopherol, and anthocyanin showed the highest antioxidative activity; anthocyanin showed the strongest synergistic effect. The antioxidant activity of doenjang prepared with black soybean was higher than that of doenjang fermented with yellow soybean because of anthocyanin contents in the black soybeans. In particular, the seed coat of the black beans contained 1.42 mg/g of delphinidin-3-glucoside, 5.77 mg/g of cyanidin-3-glucoside, and 0.3 mg/g of petunidin-3-glucoside (Kim et al., 2005a).

Free amino acids formed during fermentation of doenjang also exhibited antioxidative activities. Doenjang contains high levels of glutamic acid, lysine, tryptophan, histidine, and tyrosine. Histidine, tryptophan, tyrosine, and methionine all showed strong antioxidative activity (Moon and Cheigh, 1987). Peptides can also exert antioxidant activity; His-containing peptides such as His–His show antioxidative activity by acting as metal ion chelates, active-oxygen quenchers, and hydroxyl radical scavengers (Chen et al., 1998; Muramoto and Hatakeyama, 2003). Soy saponin extracts and saponins inhibit lipid peroxidation (Jeon, 1998; Yoshiki et al., 1998). Soy saponins decreased malondialdehyde formation, and the activity was significantly higher than that of ascorbate or α-tocopherol in HepG2 cells. It also increased both the glutathione peroxide and glutathione S-transferase levels (Sung, 2000; Jun et al., 2002). One-year fermented doenjang showed increased contents of phenolics and isoflavone aglycones, and exhibited strong antioxidant and anti-inflammatory activities (Kwak et al., 2015).

5.5.2 Anticancer Effects of Doenjang

5.5.2.1 Antimutagenic Effect

Strong antimutagenic effects against aflatoxin B_1(AFB$_1$) were first observed in a doenjang methanol extract (Moon, 1990; Park et al., 1990). The AFB$_1$-mediated mutagenesis was completely blocked at the level of 25 mg/plate of the traditional doenjang extract in *Salmonella typhimurium* TA100 strain Ames test (Figure 5.6). Commercial doenjang, chungkookjang, and miso also exhibited lower antimutagenic activities, probably due to the smaller portion of soybean used and shorter fermentation time (Park, 2003). Doenjang extract further showed antimutagenicity toward other mutagens/carcinogens of benzo(a)pyrene(B(a)P), N,N-dimethylnitrosamine (DMN), N-methyl-N-nitro-N-nitroguanidine (MNNG), 4-nitroquinoline-1-oxide (4-NQO), etc.

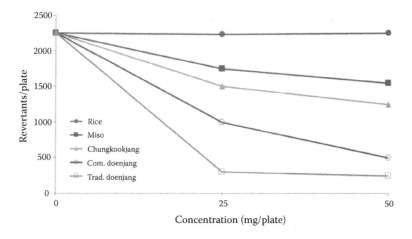

FIGURE 5.6
Effect of methanol extracts of various fermented soybean foods on the mutagenesis of aflatoxin B_1 in *Salmonella typhimurium* TA100 strain. (From Park, K. Y. et al., 1990, *J Korean Soc Food Nutr* 19:156–162.)

in different experimental systems of the SOS chromotest, *Drosophila* wing spot test (Park et al., 1995, 1996a; 1996b; Lim, 1997; Park et al., 1997, 1999; Yun et al., 1999, 2000; Park, 2003). Genistein, linoleic acid, β-sitosterol glucoside, soya saponin, trypsin inhibitor, etc. were the active compounds that showed antimutagenic activities in doenjang; however, genistein and linoleic acid were the major ones (Lim, 1997; Park et al., 2003).

5.5.2.2 Anticancer Effect

The growth of human cancer cells such as AGS gastric adenocarcinoma cells, Hep3B hepatocellular cancer cells, HT-29 colon cancer cells, and MG-63 osteosarcoma cells was significantly inhibited by doenjang methanol extract (Lim, 1997; Choi et al., 1999; Lim et al., 1999; Park et al., 2000b). The doenjang hexane fraction (DHF) from the methanol extract showed the highest growth inhibitory effect on HT-29 cells (Park et al., 2000b). The DHF suppressed the growth of various tumor cells, and was evaluated for its effects on cell cycle progression in MCF-7 human breast carcinoma cells (Choi et al., 2001). DHF induced a G1 phase arrest of the cell cycle, which correlated with the accumulation of the hypophosphorylated form of pRB (retinoblastoma protein) and enhanced association of pRB with the transcription factor E2F-1. The expression of D-type cyclins was decreased by DHF in a time-dependent manner, but DHF did not affect the expressions of cyclin E and A. The p53 (tumor suppressor gene) and p21 (cyclin-dependent kinase [Cdk] inhibitor), which is a known downstream effector of p53, and association of p21 with Cdk2 were markedly induced in DHF-treated cells. Thus, DHF arrested the G1 phase of the cell cycle by inhibiting pRB phosphorylation, decreasing expression of D-type cyclins and increasing Cdk inhibitor p21.

Linoleic acid (LA) was the main free fatty acid found in the hexane fraction of the doenjang methanol extract and was identified as an active compound (Moon, 1990). LA decreased the growth of various human cancer cells (Lim, 1997; Park et al., 2000b) and delayed tumor growth in transplanted sarcoma-180 ascites tumor cells in BALB/c mice (Zhu et al., 1989; Hah et al., 1992; Rhew et al., 1992). LA enhanced the phagocytic activity and natural killer cell activity *in vitro* and *in vivo* (Kim et al., 1992; Jeong et al., 1993). It also showed a capacity to differentiate Caco-2 cells and F9 teratocarcinoma cells (Lim, 1997; Llor et al., 2003).

The other major active compound in doenjang was genistein, which induced G2/M arrest in MCF-7 and MDA-MB-231 human breast cancer cells by inhibiting Cdc2 and Cdk2 kinase activities and decreasing cyclin B1 expression (Choi et al., 1998). Genistein induces p21 in PC-3-M human prostate carcinoma cells, which inhibits the threshold kinase activities of Cdk inhibitors and associated cyclins, leading to a G2/M arrest in the cell cycle progression (Choi et al., 1998, 2000). Genistein is also known to inhibit angiogenesis and metastasis *in vitro* (Fotsis et al., 1993; Rauth et al., 1997) and to suppress tumorigenesis and carcinogenesis *in vivo* (Steele et al., 1995; Cai and Wei, 1996). The low incidence of prostate cancer in Asian men, especially from China, Japan, and Korea, is probably due to the consumption of genestein in soy foods (Hong, 2000). The soy peptides derived from soy paste, soy hydrolysates, and soy sauce showed anticancer effects in cancer cell lines. Peptide fractions from doenjang that contained the hydrophobic amino acids glycine, alanine, proline, valine, leucine, isoleucine, and phenylalanine showed anticancer effects on SNUF-12 and SWF-12 human cancer cells (Lee, 1998).

Doenjang greatly inhibited solid tumor growth of transplanted sarcoma-180 tumor cells in BALB/c mice (Park et al., 1999). The tumor growth was inhibited by 64.0%, 79.3%, and 39.7% when 5 mg/kg of the hexane, methanol, and hot water (5 minutes, 15 minutes) extracts from doenjang were administered to the BALB/c mice, respectively; survival time (life span) of the mice increased by 58.2%, 66.3%, and 38.9%, respectively, demonstrating that the methanol extract was the most effective. Doenjang is usually consumed as doenjang soup or stew in Korea. Antitumor effects of doenjang thus are still active even when boiled or cooked. Antimutagenicity of doenjang was still stable (95%) against MNNG and AFB_1, after 60 minutes at 100°C heat treatment (Yoon et al., 1996). The active isoflavone compounds are also heat stable (Aguiar et al., 2012). The methanol extract of traditional doenjang, miso (Maruseng, Co., Japan), and cooked soybeans extended the life span of BALB/c mice with transplanted sarcoma-180 tumor cells by 68%, 41%, and 11%, respectively. Doenjang exhibited the greatest effect, indicating that the soybean content and fermentation process are important factors for mediating the anticancer effect (Kim et al., 1999).

5.5.2.3 Increasing Anticancer Effects of Doenjang

Fermentation time: Prolonging the fermentation time of doenjang production was found to increase the anticancer effect of doenjang (Park et al., 2003; Jung et al., 2006; Shim et al., 2015). A 2-year fermented doenjang showed higher antimutagenic, anticancer, antitumor, and antimetastatic effects compared to 3- and 6-month fermented doenjangs. Increased browning products, aglycone isoflavones, free fatty acids, and peptides formed during longer fermentation times are the major reasons for the increased bioactivities. The antimutagenicity against AFB_1 and anticancer effects against AGS gastric cancer cells and HT-29 colon cancer cells were also greatly increased when doenjang was ripened for 2 years. The 2-year-old doenjang resulted in a two- to five-fold increase in antitumor effects on sarcoma-180 tumor cell-injected mice (Table 5.2). Natural killer cell activities and antimetastastic effects against colon 26-M3.1 cells implanted in mice were also significantly increased compared to the 3- or 6-month fermented doenjang (Jung et al., 2006).

Salt type: Salt is another important factor that affects anticancer activity of doenjang (Ha and Park, 1998; Hwang, 2004; Hwang et al., 2007; Lee et al., 2008;

TABLE 5.2

Antitumor Activities of Methanol Extracts from Doenjang Prepared with Different Fermentation Times in Tumor-Bearing BALB/c Mouse with Sarcoma-180 Cells

Sample	Tumor (Weight, g)	Inhibition Rate (%)
S-180 + PBS	5.8 ± 0.3^a	–
S-180 + 3 MD	5.4 ± 0.2^a	7
+ 6 MD	4.7 ± 0.3^b	19
+ 24 MD	3.6 ± 0.2^c	38

Notes: S-180 = sarcoma-180 tumor cells; PBS = phosphate buffered saline; 3 MD = 3-month fermented doenjang; 6 MD = 6-month fermented doenjang; 24 MD = 24-month fermented doenjang.

[a-c] Means with different letters are significantly different ($p < 0.05$) by Duncan's multiple range test.

Shim et al., 2015). Purified salt (PS) is generally used for making doenjang commercially. Solar salt (SS) without bittern from the salt ponds of Korea is traditionally used to make doenjang. Bamboo salt (BS)—solar salt packed in a bamboo container plugged with mud on the open side and then heated one to nine times at more than 1000°C—is also used to make doenjang. BS is used as a folk medicine for chronic disease, especially cancer, in Korea (Zhao, 2011). BS1-D and BS9-D (once-baked BS (1 × BS)-used and nine-times-baked BS (9 × BS)-used doenjangs, respectively) showed higher antimutagenic effects that are induced by AFB_1, MNNG, and 4-NQO. BS1-D exerted a greater suppressive effect on chromosome aberrations in mitomycin C-induced micronucleus in mice than SDS-D (sun-dried salt-used doenjang) and PS-D (purified salt-used doenjang) (Hwang et al., 2008). The antimetastasis activity of doenjang samples made with different kinds of salt was also studied. The BALB/c mice were injected with colon 26-M3.1 cells and then treated with doenjang extracts prepared with PS, commercial salt (CS), and BS1-D and BS9-D at concentrations of 0.5 and 1.0 mg/mouse. As shown in Table 5.3, The control number of lung metastasis was 87 ± 13. PS-doenjang showed 31%–57% inhibition of the metastatic numbers to the lung, and CS-doenjang increased to 40%–63% inhibition, but BS9-D exhibited 97%–98%, the highest inhibition rate. BS1-D also exhibited a high rate of antimetastatic activity (75%–85%) in the BALB/c mice (Hwang, 2004).

Another study prepared doenjang with different bamboo salts and different fermentation times (Shim et al., 2015), from 3Y3B-D (3-year fermentation using 3 × BS-used doenjang) to 6Y9B-D (six-year fermentation using 9 × BS-used doenjang). 6Y9B-D showed the highest total polyphenol content and the highest antioxidative and anticancer effects against HT-29 colon cancer cells. Proinflammatory cytokines of TNF-α and IL-6 and COX-2 and iNOS

TABLE 5.3

Inhibitory Effect of Methanol Extracts from Doenjang Made with Various Kinds of Salt on Tumor Metastasis Produced by Colon 26-M3.1 Cells

Treatment	No. of Lung Metastasis (Inhibition, %)			
	0.5 (mg/mouse)		1.0 (mg/mouse)	
	Mean ± SD	Range	Mean ± SD	Range
Control	87 ± 13[a]	68 ~ 98	87 ± 13[a]	68 ~ 98
PS-doenjang	60 ± 17[b] (31)	45 ~ 78	37 ± 7[b] (57)	29 ~ 42
CS-doenjang	52 ± 8[b] (40)	45 ~ 61	32 ± 4[b] (63)	29 ~ 37
BS1-doenjang	22 ± 9[c] (75)	12 ~ 29	13 ± 2[c] (85)	11 ~ 14
BS9-doenjang	3 ± 1[d] (97)	2 ~ 5	2 ± 2[d] (98)	0 ~ 6

Source: Hwang, K. M. 2004. PhD diss., Pusan National Univ., Busan, Korea.
Notes: PS = purified salt; CS = commercial salt; BS = bamboo salt.
[a-d] Means with different letters in the same column are significantly different ($p < 0.05$) by Duncan's multiple range test.

inflammation gene expressions were the lowest in the cancer cells treated with 6Y9B-D; doenjang with long fermentation time and using 9 × BS was most effective.

Starter cultures used for fermenting doenjang: We isolated probiotic starter cultures from meju samples and studied enzyme activities and probiotic effects when using starter cultures for the preparation of meju and doenjang (Jeong, 2012). Colon carcinogenesis was induced by AOM and DSS in C57BL/6 mice and the meju and doenjang made with probiotic starters were orally administered for 4 weeks. The administration of meju and doenjang prepared with the mixed starter cultures (*Lac. lactis, Asp. oryzae,* and *Bac. subtilis*) ameliorated symptoms of colon cancer. The doenjang made with probiotic starter cultures decreased the number of neoplasia and decreased serum proinflammatory cytokine levels and iNOS and COX-2 expression levels in colon tissues of the mice. It increased Bax, but decreased Bcl-2 levels, and increased p21 and p53 expressions in the colon tissues compared to other samples (Jeong et al., 2012, 2014). Thus, meju and doenjang prepared with starter cultures exhibited better results for cancer prevention by ameliorating the symptoms of colon cancer, reducing the tumor numbers, regulating proinflammatory cytokines levels and expressions of inflammation and apoptosis-related genes in the colon tissues, and was safer, without the risk of contaminations with pathogenic microorganisms.

Others: Black soybeans improved doenjang's anticancer effects (Bae et al., 2007; Lim et al., 2009, Park et al., 2015a). Black soybeans of var. *Seoritae* (big size, 25 g/100 grains) significantly inhibited the growth of AGS human gastric cancer cells. Doenjang made with var. *Seoritae* showed the highest anticancer effect on the AGS cells compared to yellow soybeans (large size, 25 g/100 grains) and seomoctae (black soybeans; small size, 10 g/100 grains) (Bae et al., 2007). Adding ginger or garlic (Park et al., 2005), Japanese apricot, mushrooms (Lee et al., 2001; Lee, 2002), sea tangle (Choi et al., 2002; Ham et al., 2008), mushroom (Kim et al., 2003), and *Surcuma longa* L. (Jung et al., 2007) can increase the anticancer effect of doenjang. Doenjang prepared with ginger, 5% sea tangle, *Phellinus linteus*, and *Ganoderma lucidum* showed higher antimutagenic and anticancer effects than the control doenjang. We also tried to prepare doenjangs by adding bamboo salt, isoflavones, green tea, mistletoe extract powder, etc. to increase the anticancer effect of doenjang (Hwang, 2004; Hwang et al., 2007; Hwang and Park 2007).

5.5.3 Antiobesity Effects of Doenjang

An active compound in doenjang—genistein—also exerts strong antiobesity effects by inhibiting the uptake of glucose; stimulating lipolysis, including fatty acid accumulation through PPARα; inhibiting liver TG accumulation; improving lipid profiles and hepatic steatosis; and attenuating the increase in body weight and visceral fat in HFD-fed mice (Choi et al., 2005; Kim et al., 2005b; Park et al., 2006). Genistein reduced body weight, mobilized body fat, and induced apoptosis of adipose tissue in ovariectomized female mice (Kim et al., 2005b).

The antiobesity properties of doenjang have been the subject of considerable research (Kwon et al., 2006; Kwak et al., 2012; Bae et al., 2013). Doenjang showed the highest antiobesity effect among Korean fermented soybean foods (Kwon et al., 2006). SD rats were fed for 4 weeks on a normal diet (ND), high-fat diet (HFD, 12% lard in the ND), or diets containing 10% freeze-dried doenjang, chungkukjang, kochujang, or samjang (obtained from MoonOkRae Co., Soonchang, Jeollabukdo, Korea). Body weight (BW), food efficiency ratio (FER), and adipose tissue weight were significantly decreased (especially final BW) by the consumption of doenjang and were significantly decreased to 251.3 ± 22.3 g, the same BW of ND (259.0 ± 16.1 g). The doenjang sample used was traditionally fermented for 2 years (Table 5.4).

Samjang (261.1 ± 17.0 g), kochujang (270.5 ± 5.4 g), and chungkukjang (277.1 ± 13.8 g) also decreased BW compared to HFD (295.1 ± 11.6 g; Table. 5.4). The TG and cholesterol concentrations in liver and perirenal fat pad showed similar trends to those of the body weights. Doenjang showed the highest weight reduction and lipid-lowering activities, similarly to ND, of the rats fed with a high-fat diet. Fermented soybean foods exhibited antiobesity effects; however, soybean-fermented traditional doenjang resulted in the greatest effects.

Kwak et al. (2012) reported that doenjang decreased visceral fat accumulations and adipocyte size of epididymal adipocytes, as well as fat accumulation in liver of SD rats fed with high-fat diet. The rats were fed basal (BA, 5% fat), high-fat (HF, 30% fat), HF + cooked soybean (soy), and HF + doenjang (DJ) diets for 8 weeks. The HF group increased body weight, liver weight, hepatic TG and cholesterol levels, and epididymal fat pad weight compared to BA. The doenjang group gained significantly less visceral fat weight and epididymal adipocyte size, and the soy group experienced a mild reduction without significance compared to HF (Figure 5.7a). Fat accumulation

TABLE 5.4

Changes of Body Weight, Food Intake, and Food Efficiency Ratio (FER) of Rats Fed Various Soybean Fermented Food-Added Diets for 30 Days

	ND[a]	HFD[b]	HFD + Doenjang	HFD + Chungkukjang	HFD + Kochujang	HFD + Samjang
Body weight						
Initial weight (g)	143.7 ± 3.9[c]	143.7 ± 3.9	143.8 ± 4.1	143.7 ± 3.9	143.9 ± 4.5	143.7 ± 5.0
Final weight (g)	259.0 ± 6.1[e,f]	295.1 ± 11.6[d]	251.3 ± 22.3[f]	277.1 ± 3.8[d,e]	270.5 ± 5.4[e,f]	261.1 ± 17.0[e,f]
Weight gain (g/day)	3.9 ± 0.6[e]	4.8 ± 0.4[d]	3.8 ± 0.3[e]	4.2 ± 0.5[e]	4.2 ± 0.1[e]	4.0 ± 0.2[e]
Food intake (g/day)	18.3 ± 1.6[c]	18.9 ± 2.9	17.5 ± 0.8	18.1 ± 0.5	17.3 ± 1.3	17.4 ± 0.7
FER[g]	0.20 ± 0.04[f]	0.26 ± 0.02[d]	0.21 ± 0.01[e,f]	0.24 ± 0.02[d,e]	0.24 ± 0.01[d,e]	0.23 ± 0.01[d,e,f]

Source: Kwon, S. H., K. B. Lee, K. S. Im et al., 2006. *J Korean Soc Food Sci Nutr* 35:1194–1199.

[a] Normal diet is based on the AIN-93M diet.

[b] Contains 12% lard oil added to the normal diet.

[c] Not significant.

[d-f] Means with different letters in the same row are significantly different (p < 0.05) by Duncan's multiple range test.

[g] Food efficieny ratio.

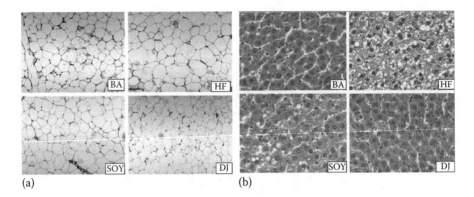

FIGURE 5.7
Light microscopic observation of (a) epididymal adipocytes and (b) fat accumulation in hematoxylin and eosin-stained liver tissue. Magnification × 100. (From Kwak, C. S. et al., 2012, *J Med Food* 15:1–9.)

droplets could not be found in livers of rats fed DJ, similarly to the BA group; however, accumulation of lipid droplets was found in HF and soy groups (Figure 5.7b). The body weight gain of DJ for up to 8 weeks was the same as that in BA. The DJ group also had significantly lower levels of TG, TC, AI (atherogenic index), and leptin in serum, and DJ lowered FAS (fatty acid synthase) and elevated CPT (carnitine palmitoyltransferase)-1 activity in liver tissue compared to BA, HF, and soy groups. It was suggested that these antiobesity effects may be partly due to the isoflavone aglycones in doenjang.

Lee and Kim (2002) studied the effects of dietary supplementation of 6-month fermented traditional doenjang on the changes in serum biochemical components and histopathological changes of organs of rats fed a high-fat and a high-cholesterol diet. The rats consumed a control diet, high-fat diet (40% of the total calories), and doenjang diet (0.5%, 1%, and 5%). The feeding of the 0.5% doenjang diet reduced the adverse effects of the high-fat and high-cholesterol diets on the food efficiency ratio (FER), weight gain, relative organ weights, fecal lipid levels, and improved serum lipid component levels. Especially significant reductions in TG, total lipid, total cholesterol, LDL cholesterol, and AI (atherogenic index) were observed, but a significant increase was found in the level of HDL cholesterol ($p < 0.05$). It also reduced the severe histopathological lesions of livers. The feeding of 1% and 5% doenjang diets showed even better lowering of the risk factors. These results demonstrated that doenjang may protect against the dyslipidemia induced by a high-fat and/or a high-cholesterol diet. Cha et al. (2012) indicated that doenjang supplementation (9.9 g dry/day) for 12 weeks in overweight adults significantly reduced body weight, body fat mass, and body fat compared to a control group.

We conducted some interesting studies demonstrating that doenjang has a potent antiobesity effect compared with exercise. A high-fat diet (HFD) containing 23% lard alone or with 10% black soybean doenjang (BSD) or 10% yellow soybean doenjang (SD) was administered for 8 weeks in C57BL/6 mice. The mice

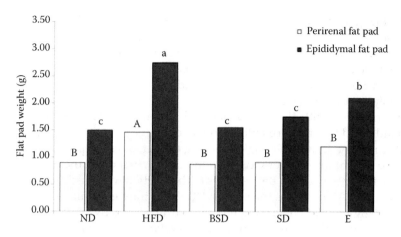

FIGURE 5.8
Lipid weight in perirenal fat pad and epididymal fat pad of mice fed with doenjang samples and after exercise (1h/day) in C57BL/6 mice.

in the exercise group (E) were given HFD + 1 hour of swimming exercise/day. The HFD group had body weights of 40.4 ± 3.3 g after 8 weeks. ND was 31.3 ± 2.3 g. The body weights of the BSD group, SD group, and exercise group were 32.9 ± 2.0 g, 34.3 ± 4.0 g, and 32.8 ± 3.1 g, respectively. However, TG and total cholesterol levels were lowest in the BSD group. As shown in Figure 5.8, fat pad weights were the lowest in BSD, similar to levels of ND, and the exercise group had higher fat pad weights than BSD and SD. The expression of mRNA and protein for PPARγ and SREBP1c in the mouse liver was significantly lower in BSD compared to the exercised group. That means doenjang intake, especially black soybean doenjang, was the same as or better than the exercise for decreasing body weight and fat, even though doenjang consumption plus exercise may be a better way to prevent or treat obesity.

5.5.4 Prevention of Cardiovascular Diseases

Cardiovascular diseases (CVDs) such as hypertension, heart attack, or stroke are well known to occur from atherosclerosis, thrombosis, fibrinolytic activity, high levels of TG, TC, LDL, and VLDL in serum, LDL oxidation, etc. Soybeans and soybean foods have been recommended to control cardiovascular diseases (Park, 2009a). The amino acid distribution of soy protein, peptides, unsaturated fatty acids, isoflavones, saponins, plant sterols, phytic acids, and dietary fiber in doenjang confer potential cardiovascular protection (Chung et al., 1999; Park, 2009a). Asian populations with diets high in soybean food consumption have lower CHD (coronary heart disease) rates than Western populations, which have a low intake of soybeans and soybean products (Beaglehole, 1990). High soybean intakes reduce the incidence of cardiovascular diseases (Beaglehole, 1990; Erdman, 2000).

Doenjang showed fibrinolytic activity. The activity was 10 times higher in traditional doenjang samples than in the commercial doenjang samples due to the soybean contents. *Bacillus* sp. isolated from doenjang exhibited a strong fibrinolytic effect (Kim, 1998). *Bac. amyoliquefaciens, Bac. pantotheticus,* and *Bac. subtilis* were isolated from doenjang and identified. They also showed strong fibrinolytic activity. Thus, the isolated *Bacillus* sp., culture media, and doenjang fermented with the *Bacillus* sp. had fibrinolytic activities. Shon (1996) also indicated that the fermented product of peptides from doenjang showed antithrombotic activity. Though doenjang extract and its peptide fractions all showed antithrombotic activity, fraction number 16 showed the highest activity. The major residues in the peptides of the fraction were histidine, arginine, and alanine. Alanine was the highest (40.5%) of the free amino acids.

ACE (angiotensin converting enzyme) inhibitory activity was also found in doenjang (Shin et al., 1995). *Bacillus subtilis* SCB-3 isolated from meju of Soonchang, Jeollabukdo province in Korea exhibited the highest ACE inhibitory activity (Hwang, 1997). Changes in general components and ACE inhibitory activity of doenjang fermented by *Bac. subtilis* were examined for 90 days. The maximum protease activity of the doenjang was reached after 60 days of fermentation at 30°C, at which time the ACE inhibitor rate was also the highest. The fermented doenjang had significantly higher ACE inhibitory effects compared to the nonfermented soy beans. Long fermented doenjang produced ACE inhibitory peptides as part of the protease activity; this might have been due to fermented products such as peptides, aglyconed isoflavones, etc. (Shin et al., 1995).

Various peptides from doenjang were isolated and identified as ACE inhibitors. Suh et al. (1996) reported that an ACE inhibitor was isolated and the purified inhibitor showed competitive inhibition of ACE. The amino acid profile of the peptides consisted of alanine, phenylalanine, leucine, glutamic acid, glycine, serine, and aspartic acid. The amino acids that were present at the highest concentrations were 55.5% alanine, 39.8% phenylalanine, and 2.1% leucine. The active ACE inhibitory peptide was isolated from traditional doenjang (Suh et al., 1996) and the active compound was identified as a dipeptide, Arg-Pro with ACE IC_{50} of 92 μM. Shin et al. (1995) also isolated ACE inhibitory peptide from doenjang through ultrafiltration and ion exchange prep high-performance liquid chromatography (HPLC). The peptide contained high levels of histidine with small amounts of other amino acids. His-His-Leu isolated from doenjang exhibited ACE inhibitory activity and antihypertensive activity *in vitro* and *in vivo* (Shin et al., 2001).

Ser-Trp was a peptide that showed ACE inhibitory activity from miso (Shimakage et al., 2012). Soybean peptides from soybean hydrolysate lowered plasma levels of TG and LDL-c. ACE activities in aorta and kidney decreased compared to control. These peptides have beneficial effects on hypertension and atherosclerosis (Chung et al., 1999). In several human trials, soy protein isolate with the isoflavones has been shown to lower diastolic and systolic blood pressure (Beaglehole, 1990; Welty et al., 2007). Isoflavones in doenjang

Health Benefits of Doenjang (Soybean Paste) and Kanjang (Soybean Sauce) 125

can lower serum cholesterol concentration, and decrease oxidation of LDL cholesterol due to polyphenolic structure (Jenkins, 2000). It is reported that isoflavones via estrogenic effects (high affinity for the β-estrogen receptor), independently of cholesterol-lowering effects, inhibit LDL oxidation, enhance vascular reactivity, and inhibit platelet aggregation; phytosterols can also decrease cholesterol absorption, and MUFA and PUFA in doenjang may also reduce serum cholesterol levels, LDL-c, etc. (Nydahl et al., 1994).

5.5.5 Other Functions

5.5.5.1 Promotion of Immune Function

Traditional doenjang and its active fraction (Mw >100 kDa) stimulated the growth of mouse spleen lymphocytes. The immunomodulatory effect was not found in cooked soybeans. The BMR (biological response modifier) level in the traditional doenjang was significantly higher than in commercial doenjang and miso (Lee, 1999). It was stable at heat treatment (100°C for 30 minutes) and selectively stimulated the expansion of B lymphocytes. The BRM of doenjang was suggested to be protein or glycoprotein by precipitation using ammonium sulfate. The fraction increased TNF-α and IL-12 production from peritoneal macrophages, and IL-6 and IFN-γ from splenic lymphocytes. The active fraction decreased IgE production and thus could possibly be used for allergy treatment (Lee et al., 1997).

Doenjang can also promote the systemic immune activity of the body by improving the mucosal immune response and blood circulation in the GI tract. One group of mice fed with a basal diet plus 5% doenjang, in comparison with the control group without doenjang, was found to have significantly higher CD4+ and CD8+ lymphocyte density, immunoreactivity of universal nitric oxide synthase (uNOS), and colon immunoreactive density of protein kinase C-α (PKC-α). These morphological and immunological results indicated that the intake of doenjang could improve the mucosal immune response, blood circulation in the GI tract, and the immune activity of the body (Lee et al., 2011b). Two-year fermented doenjang significantly increased natural killer cell activity (two to three times) of BALB/c mouse compared to those of the sarcoma-180 cell-transplanted control group (Jung et al., 2006). The intake of doenjang enhances the immune function of natural killer cells, and thus it is thought to exhibit cancer preventive and anticancer effects.

5.5.5.2 Probiotic Function of Bac. subtilis

Bac. subtilis is a main microorganism in doenjang fermentation, and it is considered to be a probiotic (Meroni et al., 1983; Mazza, 1994; Sorokulova et al., 1997; Green et al., 1999; Pinchuk et al., 2001). In European countries, *Bac. subtilis* is used for oral bacteriotherapy and bacterioprophylaxis of gastrointestinal disorder that may cause diarrhea, and thus *Bac. subtilis* is sold as a probiotic (Green et al., 1999). *Bac. subtilis* acts as an immunostimulatory agent in various diseases (Meroni et al., 1983) and as an *in vitro* and *in vivo* stimulant of secretory IgA. *Bac. subtilis* intake is thought to restore normal microflora following extensive antibiotic use or illness (Mazza, 1994). *Bac. subtilis* 3 also secretes antibiotics and inhibits *Helicobacter pylori* activity and showed antagonistic properties against species of the family Enterobacteriaceae. *Bac. subtilis* 3 produced antibiotics, amicoumacin A, and showed anti-inflammatory effects and antibacterial activity against *H. pylori*. It inhibited growth of aflatoxigenic molds of *Asp. flavus* and *Asp. parasiticus* (Kim and Roh, 1998; Kang et al., 2000). In one clinical test, administering subjects aged 60–74 with *Bac. subtilis* CU1 at a concentration of 2.0×10^9 CFUs/day for 4 months resulted in fewer symptoms of common infectious diseases. Especially, biological samples (stool and saliva) from subjects administered the probiotic *Bac. subtilis* showed increased fecal and salivary secretory IgA concentrations compared to the placebo. Thus, the administration of *Bac. subtilis* induced immune stimulation and provided elderly persons with resistance against common infectious diseases (CIDs) (Lefevre et al., 2015).

5.5.5.3 Diabetes

Doenjang along with chungkukjang and soybean supplemented diet groups decreased blood glucose levels and improved lipid metabolism (decreased total cholesterol and LDL-c, increased HDL-c) and attenuated the progression of diabetes in streptozotocin-induced diabetic rats (Kim et al., 2012). Some commercial doenjangs promote glucose uptake into muscle cells in C2C12 myoblast cells, suggesting that doenjang could be an antidiabetic food (Lee et al., 2012). Soybean oligosaccharide (Kim et al., 2001), soybean fiber (Nuttall, 1993), isoflavone (Wiseman, 2000), water-soluble carbohydrate (Anderson, 1980), pinitol (Davis et al., 2000), and browning products (Seok, 2000) are known to lower blood glucose. These components seem to improve the sensitivity of insulin to glucose and perhaps restore the function of damaged pancreatic β-cells (Kim et al., 2012). Soy protein associated with isoflavones improves glucose control and insulin resistance. Isoflavones modulate pancreatic insulin secretion (Bhathena and Volasquez, 2002). Thus, doenjang may improve diabetic symptoms by controlling blood glucose and serum lipid metabolism in diabetic rats.

5.6 Functionality of Kanjang

5.6.1 Antioxidative Effects of Kanjang

Fermented soy sauce (kanjang) has free amino acids, peptides, reducing sugars, organic acids, phenolic substances, flavor compounds, maillard browning products, and other fermentation products. Kanjang has antioxidant activity with the ability to scavenge free radicals *in vitro* and *in vivo* (Moon, 1987; Moon and Cheigh, 1990; Moon, 1991; Choi et al., 1993b; Kataoka, 2005; Kwon et al., 2014; Song et al., 2014; Lee et al., 2015). Commercially prepared fermented kanjang with cooked soybeans, parched wheat, and salt solution showed strong antioxidant effects. Cooked ground meat (CGM), CGM-water, CGM-brine, and CGM-kanjang were prepared and stored at 6°C for 5 weeks, and the kanjang showed antioxidation effects against lipid oxidation in CGM. The activity significantly increased with the length of fermentation time. The maillard browning product was the major antioxidative substance, especially lower molecular weight; melanoidin exhibited a strong antioxidative activity, mainly due to hydroxy and double bonds of the melanoidin (Moon, 1987). The furanones of 4-hydroxy-2(or 5)-ethyl-5(or 2)-methyl-3(2H)-furanone (HEMF), 4-hydroxy-2,5-dimethyl-3(2H)-furanone (HDMF), and 4-hydroxy-5-methyl-3(2H)-furanone (HMF) that formed from the maillard reaction during fermentation may be related to the active compounds (Kataoka, 2005). Shao (2009) studied antioxidative activity of kanjang according to the fermentation time. The antioxidant effect of fermented kanjang significantly increased with fermentation time (Figure 5.9). Thus, fermentation of soybeans and wheat played an important role in the the antioxidant effect.

DPPH radical scavenging activity was measured using six commercial kanjangs from Korea. As shown in Figure 5.10, soybean-fermented commercial kanjang (SFK) and Korean traditional kanjangs (KK) showed strong antioxidative effects; however, acid-hydrolyzed kanjang (AHK) showed much lower activity than the fermented kanjangs. The mixed kanjang (fermented kanjang + AHK, JK, JK-SP) showed lower activity, but higher than AHK. JK (jin kanjang) is SFK + AHK with a different ratio. AHK, also called

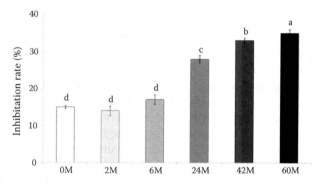

FIGURE 5.9
Electron-donating abilities of kanjang (soy sauces) with different fermentation times. 0M: Unfermented, fresh soy sauce; 2M: fermented for 2 months; 6M: fermented for 6 months; 24M: fermented for 2 years, 42M: fermented for 3.5 years; 60M: fermented for 5 years. a–d: Means with the different letters on the bars are significantly different (p < 0.05) by Duncan's multiple range test. (From Shao, L. 2009, Studies on physicochemical changes and cancer preventive effects of fermented soy sauces during ripening period, MS thesis. Pusan National Univ. Busan, Korea.)

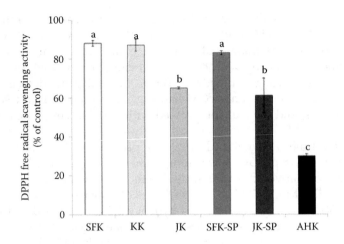

FIGURE 5.10
DPPH free radical scavenging activities of six kinds of soy sauces. SFK: soy sauce fermented with soybean (D Co.); KK: Korean traditional kanjang; JK: mixed soy sauce (fermented soy sauce mixed with acid hydrolyzed soy sauce, 50:50, D Co.); SFK-SP: soy sauce sample fermented with soybean, S Co.); JK-SP: mixed soy sauce sample (50:50), S Co; AHK: acid hydrolyzed soy sauce. a–c: Means with different letters on the bars are significantly different ($p < 0.05$) by Duncan's multiple range test. (From Song, J. L. 2012, Anticancer effects of fermented sesame sauce. Ph.D. diss., Pusan National Univ., Busan, Korea.)

chemical soy sauce, is manufactured with defatted soybeans and/or other protein-enriched materials, which are hydrolyzed with HCl for 8–10 hours at high temperature, and the hydrolysate is neutralized with NaOH or Na_2CO_3 (Song, 2012). Thus, AHK that is nonfermented kanjang did not have effective antioxidation activity.

Lee et al. (2015) studied traditionally fermented Korean kanjang. Seventeen samples of the traditional kanjang were obtained from six provinces in Korea. The antioxidant activity ranged from 8.96% to 63.39% for DPPH radical scavenging activity, from 0.12 to 2.41 antiradical efficiency (AE) mg/mL for ferric reducing antioxidant power (FRAP) value, and from 8.42 to 115.69 Trolox equivalent (TE) mg/mL for oxygen radical absorbance capacity (ORAC). Protease activity and polyphenol contents were also correlated with antioxidant activities ($R = 0.97$). The amino nitrogen also correlated with DPPH radical scavenging activity. Thus, protease activity, total polyphenol, and amino nitrogen are well correlated with the activity. This indicates that the fermentation process can affect the antioxidant activity of kanjang. The fermentation container can also affect antioxidant activity of the traditional kanjang (Lee, 2011; Park et al., 2015b). Kanjang prepared in onggi (traditional pottery that has been used for making Korean fermented foods) showed much higher antioxidant effects and better sensory evaluation than that made in glass or stainless-steel containers.

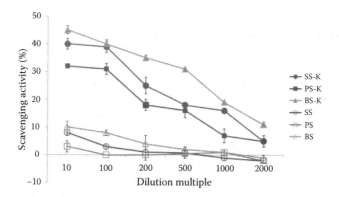

FIGURE 5.11
Hydroxyl radical (·OH) scavenging activity. SS: solar salt, PS: purified salt, BS: bamboo salt (1×); SS-K: soy sauce fermented with solar salt; PS-K: soy sauce fermented with purified salt; BS-K: soy sauce fermented with bamboo salt (1×).

Regional onggi can affect the quality of kanjang in color, protease activity, and antioxidant activity. Thus, the container used in fermentation was another influencing factor (Park et al., 2015b). LLC-PK1 cells (porcine renal tubule cells) that are used for studying ROS-induced renal damage were challenged with H_2O_2 and treated with kanjang extracts for studying the effects on oxidative stress (Song et al., 2014). Fermented sesame sauce (FseS) was introduced along with acid-hydrolyzed soy sauce (AHSS) and fermented soy sauce (FSS). The fermented sauces (FSS and FseS) exhibited strong antioxidant activities. They scavenged DPPH and significantly inhibited H_2O_2-induced oxidative damage in the LLC-PK1 cells compared to AHSS. FSS and FseS significantly increased cellular CAT (catalase), SOD (superoxide dismutase), and GSH-Px (glutathione peroxidase) activities and their mRNA expressions.

We also compared the different kinds of salt (purified salt, PS; solar salt, SS; and bamboo salt, 1xBS) and the soy sauce prepared with these different salts. As shown in Figure 5.11 kanjangs showed much better hydroxy radical scavenging activities than salts. Kanjang prepared with the different salts showed much different antioxidant activity. Kanjang prepared with BS exhibited the highest hydroxy radical scavenging activity, followed by SS kanjang and PS kanjang. Thus, fermentation with soybean and different kinds of salt, especially with BS, can increase the antioxidative activity of kanjang.

5.6.2 Anticancer Properties of Kanjang

The antimutagenic effects of Korean traditional fermented soybean products have been studied in kanjang, doenjang, kochujang, and chungkukjang. Kanjang, like other soybean products, showed antimutagenic protection against 4-NQO, MNNG, and AFB1 in the SOS chromotest (Yoon et al., 1996).

Typical kanjang and kanjang made with deep-sea water exhibited antimutagenicity against MNNG and 4-NQO in the Ames test (*Salmonella typhimurium* TA100 and TA98). The kanjang samples also showed *in vitro* anticancer effects in human cancer cells (AGS human stomach adenocarcinoma, A549 human lung carcinoma, MCF-7 human breast adenocarcinoma, Hep3B human hepatocellular carcinoma, HeLa human cervical adenocarcinoma) (Ham et al., 2008). Kanjang (25 mg/kg body weight) also inhibited the growth of sarcoma-180 tumor cells transplanted in BALB/c mice by 29.5 ± 7.3% and 40.9 ± 7.0% in typical kanjang and deep-sea water kanjang, respectively.

Song (2012) studied colon cancer preventive effects of kanjang *in vitro* and *in vivo*. Fermented soy sauce (FSS) inhibited the growth of HCT-116 cancer cells. However, acid hydrolyzed soybean sauce (AHSS) exhibited no or a weak inhibitory activity on the growth of HCT-116 human colon cancer cells. The apoptosis-related gene expression was also studied (Figure 5.12a, b). Induction of apoptosis in cancer cells is an important anticancer mechanism (Milligan and Schwartz, 1997) and the Bcl-2 family plays an important regulatory role in cellular apoptosis. The antiapoptosis proteins form ion channels in cell membrane, and these ion channel activities may control apoptosis by influencing the permeability of intracellular membranes, cytochrome c release from mitochondria, and then activation of caspase (Hengartner, 2000).

Cytochrome c released in cytoplasm induces the apoptosis protease-activating factor 1 (APAF-1) and ATP/dATP to assemble the apoptosome so that caspase-9 can undergo proteolytic maturation for activation. Active caspase-9, in turn, cleaves and activates the effector caspases, which finally leads to the apoptotic phenotype including DNA fragmentation and chromatin condensation (Kroemer et al., 2007). FSS was found to decrease mRNA and protein expression of Bcl-2 and Bcl-xL and increase proapoptotic protein Bax gene expression; however, AHSS showed only weak induction of apoptosis. The caspase family also plays an important role in driving apoptosis in both extrinsic and intrinsic pathways. Activation of caspase-3 has been observed to exert effects that are either dependent or independent of mitochondrial cytochrome c release and caspase-9 function (Deveraux and Reed, 1999). During the caspase cascade, however, caspase-3 functions to inhibit XIAP activity by

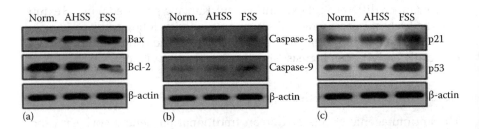

FIGURE 5.12
Effects of soy sauce extracts on protein expression of Bax, Bcl-2, caspase-3, caspase-9, p21, and p53 in HCT-116 cells. AHSS: acid hydrolyzed soy sauce; FSS: fermented soy sauce.

cleaving caspase-9 at a specific site, preventing XIAP from being able to bind to inhibit caspase-9 activity (Denault et al., 2007). Caspase-3 is required for some typical hallmarks of apoptosis. FSS effectively increased mRNA and protein expressions of caspase-3 and caspase-9 compared to AHSS (Figure 5.12b).

The Cdk inhibitors, p21 and p27, and p53, were studied in HCT-116 colon cancer cells. The expression levels of p21 and p53 significantly increased; however, AHSS lowered their expressions compared to FSS in HCT-116 cells. Thus, fermented kanjang can induce apoptosis and expression of Cdk inhibitors of p21 and p53. The anticancer effect of FSS was further studied *in vivo* (Song, 2012). FSS showed anticancer effects on AOM/DSS-induced colitis-associated colon cancer in BALB/c mice. Colon length increased with FSS extract administration, but AHSS decreased colon length, even compared with the control, in mice treated with AOM/DSS. The proinflammatory cytokines, TNF-α, and IL-6, in serum significantly decreased in the FSS group, but not AHSS. The tumor numbers formed in colon tissue were significantly lower with FSS treatment (Figure 5.13a). The gene expression of COX-2 and iNOS, and Bcl-2 and Bcl-xL also decreased in the FSS group; however, p53

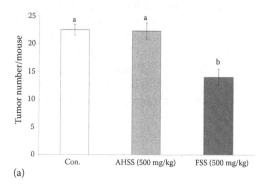

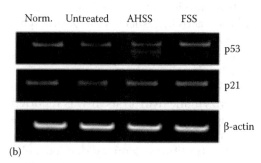

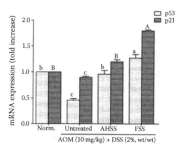

FIGURE 5.13
(a) Tumor numbers in the colon tissues and (b) mRNA expression of p53 and p21 in colon tissue of colitis-associated colon cancer mice treated with soy sauce extracts. a–c: Means with the different letters are significantly different (p < 0.05) by Duncan's multiple range tests. Con: control; AHSS: acid hydrolyzed soybean sauce; FSS: fermented soybean sauce. (From Song, J. L. 2012, Anticancer effects of fermented sesame sauce. Ph.D. diss., Pusan National Univ., Busan, Korea.)

132 Korean Functional Foods

and p21 expressions significantly increased (Figure 5.13b). The fermentation process is important, and thus fermented soy sauce has preventive effects against colon cancer.

Katoaka (2005) reviewed the anticancer effects of Japanese-style fermented soy sauce (shoyu). With or without nitrite, shoyu administered to mice in the tumor initiation stage inhibited benzo(a)pyrene (BP)-induced forestomach neoplasia. Both the number of neoplasms per animal and the incidence of neoplasia were decreased by the feeding amount of soy sauce used in the study (Benjamin et al., 1991). Diets containing 10% soy sauce or 10% miso were fed to mice for 13 months. They both significantly decreased the frequency and multiplicity of liver tumors in mice (Ito et al., 1993). Soy sauce does not contain high amounts of water-insoluble isoflavones, genistein, and daidzein, with concentrations of only about 5 ppm (Katoaka, 2005). 4-Hydroxy-3($2H$)-furanone derivatives and shoyu flavones, which are present at about 60 ppm, may affect the tumorigenesis in male C3H mice. HEMF is one of the active antioxidants and anticarcinogen compounds (Nagahara et al., 1992). Other flavor compounds of 4-hydroxy-5-methyl-3($2H$)-furanone (HMF) and 4-hydroxy-2,5-dimethyl-3(2H)-furanone (HDMF) showed similar activities. Soy sauce contains 10 ppm and 100–300 ppm of HDMF and HMF, respectively. The furanons in soy sauce are formed chemically by the Maillard reaction between sugars and amino acids during fermentation (Hodge et al., 1972; Hicks and Feather, 1975). The IC_{50} values for HDMF, 4-hydroxy-2(or 5)-ethyl-5(or 2)-methyl-3(2H)-furanone (HEMF), and HMF are 39, 44, and 55 μM, respectively. Anticarcinogen activity against BP-induced mouse forestomach neoplasia was correlated with the concentrations of furanones in the same order.

5.6.3 Other Functions

5.6.3.1 Immunomodulation

Polysaccharides, which are derived from foods and other edible materials, are reported to have immunomodulatory activities such as increasing lymphocyte proliferation and complement activation (Bao et al., 2002; Zhu et al., 2008; Zhao et al., 2010). Thus, there have been several reports about the effects of kanjang, especially kanjang-derived polysaccharides, on immunomodulation (Park et al., 2012; Lee and Shin, 2013, 2014). Polysaccharides from the cell wall of soybeans are resistant to enzymatic hydrolysis. It was reported that the polysaccharides remain in kanjang even after fermentation and are called kanjang polysaccharides (Ko et al., 2013).

Lee and Shin (2013) reported that the traditional kanjang-derived polysaccharides (TKP) and commercial kanjang-derived polysaccharides (CKP) significantly augmented NO and ROS production by RAW 264.7 cells in a dose-dependent manner. mRNA expressions of IL-6 and TNF-α by TKP at 1000 μg/mL were 63 and 73 times higher than negative controls, and 32 and 5 times higher than those of CKP, respectively. TKP also increased the expression of mRNA of FcRI, but CKP did not. Thus, TKP increased macrophage activation in the RAW 264.7 cells. The polysaccharide derived from TK contains rhamnogalacturonan II (RG-II) including 1.1% of the monosaccharide 2-keto-3-deoxy-D-manno-2-octulosonic acid (KDO). Anticomplement activities were higher in TKP (65%) than CKP (56%) at 1000 µg/mL. TKP caused complement activation via both alternative and classical pathways, but CKP caused the activation via only the classical pathway. TKP increased secretions of IL-6 and IL-12 at 40 µg/mL in macrophages. Therefore, it was concluded that the immunostimulatory activity of TKP was greater than that of CKP based on the anticomplement activity (Park et al., 2012).

Polysaccharide fractions from TK and CK were obtained, and intestinal immunomodulating activities were examined (Lee and Shin, 2014). They increased IL-6 production in culture supernatants of Peyer's patch cells. However, only TKP increased *in vitro* IgA production by Peyer's patch cells, as well as greater stimulation of bone marrow cell proliferation through Peyer's patch cells than in the CKP group. Oral administration of TKP induced IL-6 and IgA productions by Peyer's patch cells and increased IgA excretion into mouse stools; however, oral administration of polysaccharides from TK was much more effective than those from CK. The CK is prepared by the Japanese method, using a carbohydrate source and soybean and koji (*Aspergillus oryzae*) fermentation; however, TK is prepared by using soybean only, is separated from soy paste after fermentation, and is fermented with mixed cultures such as *Bac. subtilis*, molds, yeasts, etc. in meju. It seems that different raw material and fermentation microorganisms result in different metabolites, flavor, and qualities. Fermented polysaccharides from soybeans during TK fermentation may cause these strong immunomodulation effects.

5.6.3.2 Anti-Inflammation

Twenty kanjang samples were obtained, and polysaccharides from kanjang (KPS) were extracted. The KPS showed anti-inflammatory effects as assessed by proinflammatory cytokine release, and mRNA expression in mast cells. The amount of histamine and β-hexosaminidase release was markedly decreased by KPS in RBL-2H3 cells. KPS also decreased mRNA expression and release of the proinflammatory cytokines: IL-6, IL-8, and TNF-α in PMACI-stimulated human mast cells (HMC-1). The fermented kanjang showed significant anti-inflammatory effects on mast cells compared to acid-hydrolyzed kanjang samples. Thus, the KPS might also suppress allergic inflammatory reactions (Ko et al., 2013). Kim et al. (2016) reported that kanjang extracts and fractionated compounds decreased TNF-α and IL-1β levels in BV2 microglial cells with lipopolysaccharide (LPS)-induced inflammation. Seven indole alkaloid derivatives were isolated from kanjang methanol extract. These compounds inhibited the production of nitric oxide and prostaglandin E2 in the BV-2 cells. The 3-indole acetic acid and flazine from kanjang showed antineuroinflammatory action, suppressed iNOS and COX-2 protein expression in LPS-stimulated BV2 cells, and significantly inhibited the NF-κB pathway.

5.6.3.3 Antihypertension

It is generally known that salt intake increases blood pressure. Thus, kanjang, which is about 20% salt, may cause hypertension. Mun et al. (2017) indicated that Korean traditional kanjang showed antihypertensive effects. Kanjang was fed to Sprague–Dawley rats along with the same levels of salt only. The group receiving only the salt showed a significant increase in systolic blood pressure compared to the control group, but the group receiving the kanjang did not experience increased blood pressure. It seems that even though the kanjang has the same salt content as given to the salt group, it inhibited the increase in blood pressure, probably due to the metabolites produced from soybeans during the fermentation.

Japanese researchers studied the antihypertensive effect of fermented soy sauce, shoyu. Kinoshita et al. (1993) obtained two major fractions of high molecular weight (Hmw) and low molecular weight (Lmw) from shoyu by using gel filtration chromatography. The fractions were administered to spontaneously hypertensive rats (SHRs) and two-kidney Goldblantt hypertensive (2KGH) rats, and their blood pressures were measured. Blood pressure decreased 1–8 hours after administration of the Hmw fraction and returned to the baseline level within 24 hours. The active compound was nicotianamine (N-[N-(3-amino-3-carboxypropyl)-3-amino-3-carboxypropyl]-azetidine-2-carboxylic acid) from the purification of the Hmw fraction by HPLC, which is an angiotensin converting enzyme (ACE) inhibitor. It was suggested that the antihypertensive effect of shoyu might have resulted from suppression of ACE activity. The nicotianamine seemed to come from the soybeans in soy sauce. More studies are needed to better characterize the antihypertensive effect of kanjang and the mechanisms, active compounds, salt effect, etc.

5.7 Conclusion

Doenjang and kanjang have long histories of traditional and industrial production, are almost universally consumed in Korea, and have had a great impact on Korean culinary arts. The main raw materials are soybeans, salt, water, and natural microorganisms. They have been manufactured at home traditionally as an annual event. Japanese-style manufacturing methods of soybean fermented foods was accepted industrially during the Japanese occupation of the Korean peninsula. The three major companies that manufacture Korean fermented soybean food are CJ CheilJedang, Daesang, and Sempyo Co. They are producing commercial doenjang and kanjang along with new, related products of mixed jang, flavored jang, and sauces, in addition to traditional jang for the new generation and worldwide customers.

Although Korean traditional soybean foods have been developed, modified, and researched, the industry is still a small-scale one. New and better starters should be isolated, and determination of their characteristics and functionality as probiotics must follow with appropriate methods for preparation of meju. Traditional doenjang and kanjang need to be manufactured by using high-quality raw materials, starters, and fermentation methods industrially. Traditional manufacturing methods have been replaced by more convenient and hygienic modified methods. Doenjang has anticancer, antiobesity, and antioxidant effects, etc., and it has been used as a seasoning for enhancing the taste of foods. Kanjang has been used in foods as a replacement for table salt, it mainly is used as a seasoning for enhancing the flavor of foods. Kanjang has better antioxidative, anticancer, and immunomodulatory effects with longer fermentation times in its preparation. It seems that soybeans, fermented products, participating microorganisms in the fermentation, and fermentation time are important factors to increase health benefits of doenjang and kanjang. Additional research is needed to optimize meju, starters, fermentation, manufacturing methods, etc. for soybean fermented foods. Improvements in maintaining consistent quality while increasing flavor and functionality are still needed in the Korean fermented soybean food industry.

References

Aguiar, C. L., R. Haddad, M. N. Eberlin et al. 2012. Thermal behavior of malonyl-glucoside isoflavones in soybean flour analyzed by RPHPLC/DAD and eletrospray ionization mass spectrometry. *LWT-Food Sci Technol* 48:114–119.

Anderson, J. W. 1980. Dietary fiber and diabetes. In *Medical Aspects of Dietary Fiber*, 193–221. New York: Springer.

Bae, C. R., D. Y. Kwon, and Y. S. Cha. 2013. Anti-obesity effects of salted and unsalted doenjang supplementation in C57BL/6J mice fed with high fat diet. *J Korean Soc Food Sci Nutr* 42:1036–1042.

Bae, M. S., S. S. Bak, S. H. Moon, and K. Y. Park. 2007. Increased *in vitro* anticancer effects of black soybean (Seoritae) meju on AGS human gastric cancer cells. *Cancer Prev Res* 12:281–286.

Bao, X., Z. Wang, J. Fang, and X. Li. 2002. Structural features of an immunostimulating and antioxidant acidic polysaccharide from the seeds of *Cuscuta chinensis*. *Planta Med* 68:237–243.

Beaglehole, R. 1990. International trends in coronary heart disease mortality morbidity and risk factors. *Epidemiol Rev* 12:1–15.

Benjamin, H., J. Storkson, A. Nagahara, and M. W. Pariza. 1991. Inhibition of benzo(a)pyrene-induced mouse forestomach neoplasia by dietary soy sauce. *Cancer Res* 51:2940–2942.

Bhathena, S. J., and M. T. Velasquez. 2002. Beneficial role of dietary phytoestrogens in obesity and diabetes. *Am J Clin Nutr* 76:1191–1201.

Cai, Q., and H. Wei. 1996. Effect of dietary genistein on antioxidant enzyme activities in SENCAR mice. *Nutr Cancer* 25:1–7.

Cha, Y. S., J. Yang, H. I. Back et al. 2012. Visceral fat and body weight are reduced in overweight adults by the supplementation of doenjang, a fermented soybean paste. *Nutr Res Pract* 6:520–526.

Cheigh, H. S., K. S. Park, G. S. Moon, and K. Y. Park. 1990. Antioxidative characteristics of fermented soybean paste and its extracts on the lipid oxidation. *J Korean Soc Food Nutr* 19:163–167.

Chen, H. M., K. Muramoto, F. Yamauchi et al. 1998. Antioxidative properties of histidine-containing peptides designed from peptide fragments found in the digests of a soybean protein. *J Agric Food Chem* 46:49–53.

Choi, C. B., E. Y. Lee, D. S. Lee, and S. S. Ham. 2002. Antimutagenic and anticancer effects of ethanol extract from Korean traditional doenjang added sea tangle. *J Korean Soc Food Sci Nutr* 31:322–328.

Choi, H. S., J. S. Lee, and C. Y. Lee. 1993b. Antioxidative characteristics of melanoidin related products fractionated from fermented soybean sauce. *J Korean Soc Food Nutr* 22:570–575.

Choi, H. S., J. S. Lee, K. Y. Park, and G. S. Moon. 1993a. Antioxidative activity of browning products fractionated from fermented soybean sauce. *J Korean Soc Food Nutr* 22:565–569.

Choi, M. S., U. J. Jung, M. J. Kim et al. 2005. Effect of genistein and daidzein on glucose uptake in isolated rat adipocytes; comparison with respective glycones. *J Food Sci Nutr* 3:52–57.

Choi, S. Y., M. J. Cheigh, J. J. Lee et al. 1999. Growth suppression effect of traditional fermented soybean paste (doenjang) on the various tumor cells. *J Korean Soc Food Sci Nutr* 28:458–463.

Choi, Y. H., B. T. Choi, W. H. Lee et al. 2001. Doenjang hexane fraction-induced G1 arrest is associated with the inhibition of pRB phosphorylation and induction of Cdk inhibitor p21 in human breast carcinoma MCF-7 cells. *Oncol Rep* 8:1091–1096.

Choi, Y. H., S. J. Lee, M. Kim et al. 1998. Genistein induced inginition of cell proliferation and programmed cell death in the human cancer cell lines. *J Korean Cancer Assoc* 30:800–808.

Choi, Y. H., W. H. Lee, K. Y. Park, and L. Zhang. 2000. p53-Independent induction of p21 (WAF1/CIP1), reduction of cyclin B1 and G2/M arrest by the isoflavone genistein in human prostate carcinoma cells. *Japanese J Cancer Res* 91:164–173.

Choi, Y. H., L. Zhang, W. H. Lee, and K. Y. Park. 1998. Genistein-induced G2/M arrest is associated with the inhibition of cyclin B1 and the induction of p21 in human breast carcinoma cells. *Int J Oncology* 13:391–396.

Chung, S. W., M. A. Choi, J. S. Park et al. 1999. Effect of dietary soybean hydrolysate on plasma lipid profiles, select biochemical indexes, and histopathological changes in spontaneously hypertensive rats. *Korean J Food Sci Technol* 31:1101–1108.

Davis, A., M. Christiansen, J. F. Horowitz et al. 2000. Effects of pinitol treatment on insulin action in subjects with insulin resistance. *Diabetes Care* 23:1000–1005.

Denault, J. B., B. P. Eckelman, H. Shin et al. 2007. Caspase 3 attenuates XIAP (X-linked inhibitor of apoptosis protein)–mediated inhibition of caspase 9. *Biochem J* 405:11–19.

Deveraux, Q. L., and J. C. Reed. 1999. IAP family proteins—Suppressors of apoptosis. *Genes Develop* 13:239–252.

Erdman, J. W. 2000. Soy protein and cardiovascular disease: A statement for health-care professionals from the nutrition committee of the AHA (American Heart Association). *Circulation* 102:2555–2559.

Food Composition Table. 2006. Seventh revised edition. 2006. National rural resources development institute, R.D.A., 78–79. Suwon, Korea: Sammi Publishing Co.

Fotsis, T., M. Pepper, H. Adlercreutz et al. 1993. Genistein, a dietary-derived inhibitor of *in vitro* angiogenesis. *Proceed Nat Acad Sci* 90:2690–2694.

Gallup Korea. 2004. The favorite foods of Korean. Gallup Korea. http://www.gallup.co.kr/gallupdb/reportContent.asp?seqNo=56&pagePos=2&selectYear=0&search=1&searchKeyword=%C0%BD%BD%C4.

Green, D. H., P. R. Wakeley, A. Page et al. 1999. Characterization of two *Bacillus* probiotics. *Appl Environ Microbiol* 65:4288–4291.

Ha, J. O., and K. Y. Park. 1998. Comparison of mineral contents and external structure of various salts. *J Korean Soc Food Sci Nutr* 27:413–418.

Hah, J. C., T. H. Rhew, E. S. Choe et al. 1992. Antitumor effect of linoleic acid against sarcoma-180 detected by the use of protein A-gold complex in mice. *J Korean Cancer Assoc* 24:783–789.

Ham, S. S., S. H. Kim, S. J. Yoo et al. 2008a. Antimutagenicity and cytotoxic effects of methanol extract from deep sea water salt and sea tangle added soybean paste (doenjang). *J Korean Soc Food Sci Nutr* 37:416–421.

Ham, S. S., S. H. Kim, S. J. Yoo et al. 2008b. Biological activities of soybean sauce (kanjang) supplemented with deep sea water and sea tangle. *Korean J Food Preserv* 15:274–279.

Hengartner, M. O. 2000. The biochemistry of apoptosis. *Nature* 12:770–776.

Hicks, K. B., and M. S. Feather. 1975. Mechanism of formation of 4-hydroxy-5-methyl-3(2H)-furanone, a component of beef flavor, from *Amadori* products. *J Agric Food Chem* 23:957–960.

Hodge, J. E., F. D. Mills, and B. E. Fisher. 1972. Compounds of browned flavor derived from sugar-amine reactions. *Cereal Sci Today* 17:34–40.

Hong, S. J. 2000. Health potential of genistein against prostate diseases. *Proceedings of International Symposium on Soybean Human Health*, 13–24. Seoul, Korea.

Hwang, J. H. 1997. Angiotensin I converting enzyme inhibitory effect of doenjang fermented by *Bac. subtilis* SCB-3 isolated from meju, Korean traditional food. *J Korean Soc Food Sci Nutr* 26:775–783.

Hwang, K. M. 2004. Studies on the enhancement of chemopreventive and anticancer effects of doenjang. Ph.D. diss., Pusan National Univ., Busan, Korea.

Hwang, K. M., K. O. Jung, C. H. Song, and K. Y. Park. 2008. Increased antimutagenic and anticlastogenic effects of doenjang (Korean fermented soybean paste) prepared with bamboo salt. *J Med Food* 11:717–722.

Hwang, K. M., S. H. Oh, and K. Y. Park. 2007. Increased antimutagenic and *in vitro* anticancer effects by adding green tea extract and bamboo salt during doenjang fermentation. *J Korean Soc Food Sci Nutr* 36:1–7.

Hwang, K. M., and K. Y. Park. 2007. Increased antimutagenic and *in vitro* anticancer effects by adding isoflavone and mistletoe extracts during doenjang fermentation. *Cancer Prev Res* 12:68–74.

Isanga, J., and G. N. Zhang. 2008. Soybean bioactive components and their implications to health—A review. *Food Rev Int* 24:252–276.

Ito, A., A. H. Watanabe, and N. Basaran. 1993. Effects of soy products in reducing risk of spontaneous and neutron-induced liver tumors in mice. *Int J Oncology* 2:773–776.

Jenkins, D. J., C. W. Kendall, M. Garsetti et al. 2000. Effect of soy protein foods on low-density lipoprotein oxidation and *ex vivo* sex hormone receptor activity—A controlled crossover trial. *Metabolism* 49:537–543.

Jeon, H. S. 1998. Effect of soybean saponins and major antioxidants on aflatoxin B_1-induced mutagenicity and DNA adduct formation. MS thesis. Sookmyung Women's Univ., Seoul, Korea.

Jeong, J. H., K. H. Kim, M. W. Chang et al. 1993. The influence of linoleic acid and ursolic acid on mouse peritoneal macrophage activity. *Korean J Immunol* 15:53–60.

Jeong, J. K. 2012. Improvement of quality and probiotic effect of meju and doenjang prepared with mixed starter cultures. Ph.D. diss., Pusan National Univ., Busan, Korea.

Jeong, J. K., H. K. Chang, and K. Y. Park. 2012. Inhibitory effects of meju prepared with mixed starter cultures on azoxymethane and dextran sulfate sodium-induced colon carcinogenesis in mice. *J Carcinogenesis* 11:13.

Jeong, J. K., H. K. Chang, and K. Y. Park. 2014. Doenjang prepared with mixed starter cultures attenuates azoxymethane and dextran sulfate sodium-induced colitis-associated colon carcinogenesis in mice. *J Carcinogenesis* 13:9.

Jeong, M. W., J. K. Jeong, S. J. Kim, and K. Y. Park. 2013. Fermentation characteristics and increased functionality of doenjang prepared with bamboo salt. *J Korean Soc Food Sci Nutr* 42:1915–1923.

Jun, H. S., S. E. Kim, and M. K. Sung. 2002. Protective effect of soybean saponins and major antioxidants against aflatoxin B_1-induced mutagenicity and DNA-adduct formation. *J Med Food* 5:235–240.

Jung, H. K., S. S. Bak, and K. Y. Park. 2007. Increased *in vitro* anticancer effects of doenjang block by the addition of *Curcuma longa* L. *Cancer Prev Res* 12:220–224.

Jung, K. O., S. Y. Park, and K. Y. Park. 2006. Longer aging time increases the anticancer and antimetastatic properties of doenjang. *Nutrition* 22:539–545.

Kang, K. J., J. H. Jeong, and J. I. Cho. 2000. Inhibition of aflatoxin-producing fungi with antifungal compound produced by *Bacillus subtilis*. *J Food Hyg Safety* 15:122–127.

Kataoka, S. 2005. Functional effects of Japanese-style fermented soy sauce (shoyu) and its components. *J Biosci Bioeng* 100:227–234.

Kim, A. R., J. J. Lee, S. S. Cha et al. 2012. Effect of soybeans, chungkukjang, and doenjang on blood glucose and serum lipid profile in streptozotocin-induced diabetic rats. *J Korean Soc Food Sci Nutr* 41:621–629.

Kim, D. C., T. H. Quang, C. S. Yoon et al. 2016. Anti-neuroinflammatory activities of indole alkaloids from kanjang (Korean fermented soy source) in lipopolysaccharide-induced BV2 microglial cells. *Food Chem* 213:69–75.

Kim, D. H., and S. H. Kim. 1999. Biochemical characteristics of whole soybean cereals fermented with *Mucor* and *Rhizopus* strains. *Korean J Food Sci Technol* 31:176–182.

Kim, I. J., J. O. Lee, M. H. Park et al. 2002a. Preparation method of meju by three step fermentation. *Korean J Food Sci Technol* 34:536–539.

Kim, H. J., K. H. Sohn, S. H. Chae et al. 2002b. Brown color characteristics and anti-oxidizing activity of doenjang extracts. *Korean J Soc Food Cookery Sci* 18:644–654.

Kim, J. G., and W. S. Roh. 1998. Changes of aflatoxins during the ripening of Korean soy paste and soy sauce and the characteristics of the changes—Part 1. *J Food Hyg Safety* 13:313–317.

Kim, J. S., and S. Yoon. 1999. Isoflavone contents and beta-glucosidase activities of soybeans, meju and doenjang. *Korean J Food Sci Technol* 31:1405–1409.

Kim, K. H., M. W. Chang, and Y. I. Sunwoo. 1992. Effects of linoleic acid and ursolic acid on the natural killer cell activity in the mice. *J Kosin Med College* 8:25–45.

Kim, K. H., K. Y. Park, S. H. Lee, and S. Y. Lim. 2007. Effect of solvent fractions from doenjang on antimutagenicity, growth of tumor cells and production of interleukin-2. *J Life Sci* 17:791–797.

Kim, M. C. 1976. The microbiological studies on Korean jang. *J Gyeongsang National Univ* 15:1–26.

Kim, M. H., S. S. Im, Y. B. Yoo et al. 1994. Antioxidative materials in domestic meju and doenjang-(4)-separation of phenolic compounds and their antioxidative activity. *J Korean Soc Food Nutr* 23:792–798.

Kim, M. H., H. Y. Kim, W. K. Kim et al. 2001. Effects of soy oligosaccharides on blood glucose and lipid metabolism in streptozotocin-induced diabetic rats. *Korean J Nutr* 34: 3–13.

Kim, M. J., and H. S. Rhee. 1988. The contents of free amino acids nucleotides and their related compounds in soy paste made from native and improved meju and soy paste product. *J Korean Soc Food Sci Nutr* 17:69–72.

Kim, M. J., and H. S. Rhee. 1990. Studies on the changes of taste compounds during soy paste fermentation. *Korean J Food Cookery Sci* 6:1–8.

Kim, M. K., S. H. Moon, J. W. Park, and K. Y. Park. 1999. The effect of doenjang (Korean soy paste) on the liver enzyme activities of the sarcoma-180 cell transplanted mice. *Prev Nutr Food Sci* 4:260–264.

Kim, S., S. Moon, and B. M. Popkin. 2000. The nutrition transition in South Korea. *Am J Clinic Nutr* 71:44–53.

Kim, S., I. Sohn, Y. S. Lee, and Y. S. Lee. 2005b. Hepatic gene expression profiles are altered by genistein supplementation in mice with diet-induced obesity. *J Nutr* 135:33–41.

Kim, S. H. 1998. New trends of studying on potential activities of doenjang. *Korea Soybean Digest* 15:8–15.

Kim, S. H., T. W. Kwon, Y. S. Lee et al. 2005a. A major antioxidative components and comparison of antioxidative activities in black soybean. *Korean J Food Sci Technol* 37:73–77.

Kim, S. H., and H. J. Lee. 1985. Characteristics of bitter peptides from cheese and soybean paste. *Korean J Food Sci Technol* 17:276–282.

Kim, S. J., C. W. Park, S. J. Park et al. 2003. Enhanced antitumorigenicity and antimutagenicity of doenjang prepared from mushroom mycelia-cultured traditional mejus. *J Korean Soc Food Sci Nutr* 32:143–148.

Kim, T. W., J. H. Lee, S. E. Kim et al. 2009. Analysis of microbial communities in doenjang, a Korean fermented soybean paste, using nested PCR-denaturing gradient gel electrophoresis. *Int J Food Microbiol* 131:265–271.

Kim, Y. A., and H. S. Kim. 1996. Consumption pattern and sensory evaluation of Korean traditional soy sauce and commercial soy sauce. *Korean J Soc Food Sci* 12:280–290.

Kinoshita, E., J. Yamakoshi, and M. Kikuchi. 1993. Purification and identification of an angiotensin I-converting enzyme inhibitor from soy sauce. *Biosci Biotech Biochem* 57:1107–1110.

Ko, Y. J., G. R. Lee, and C. H. Ryu. 2013. Anti-inflammatory effect of polysaccharide derived from commercial kanjang on mast cells. *J Life Sci* 23:569–577.

Kroemer, G., L. Galluzzi, and C. Brenner. 2007. Mitochondrial membrane permeabilization in cell death. *Physiol Rev* 87:99–163.

Kwak, C. S., S. C. Park, and K. Y. Song. 2012. Doenjang, a fermented soybean paste, decreased visceral fat accumulation and adipocyte size in rats fed with high fat diet more effectively than nonfermented soybeans. *J Med Food* 15:1–9.

Kwak, C. S., D. Son, Y. S. Chung, and Y. H. Kwon. 2015. Antioxidant activity and anti-inflammatory activity of ethanol extract and fractions of doenjang in LPS-stimulated Raw 264.7 macrophages. *Nutr Res Pract* 9:569–578.

Kwon, H. J., H. S. Kim, Y. H. Choi et al. 2014. Antioxidant activity and quality characteristics on the maturation period of the soy sauce with *Gastrodia elata* and oak mushroom (*Lentinus edodes*). *Korean J Food Preserv* 21:231–238.

Kwon, J. I., G. Y. Kim, K. Y. Park et al. 2008. Induction of apoptosis by linoleic acid is associated with the modulation of Bcl-2 family and Fas/FasL system and activation of caspases in AGS human gastric adenocarcinoma cells. *J Med Food* 11:1–8.

Kwon, S. H., K. B. Lee, K. S. Im et al. 2006. Weight reduction and lipid lowering effects of Korean traditional soybean fermented products. *J Korean Soc Food Sci Nutr* 35:1194–1199.

Lee, B. K. 1999. The physiological activity function of traditional soy fermented products. Ch. 3. Reinforcement of immunization of doenjang. *International Symposium*. 77–100. Yeungnam University Jang Research Center.

Lee, B. K., Y. S. Jang, S. Y. Yi et al. 1997. Immunomodulators extracted from Korean-style fermented soybean paste and their function. 1. Isolation of B cell mitogen from Korean-style fermented soybean paste. *Korean J Immunol* 19:559–570.

Lee, C. H., Y. Youn, G. S. Song, and Y. S. Kim. 2011b. Immunostimulatory effects of traditional doenjang. *J Korean Soc Food Sci Nutr* 40:1227–1234.

Lee, H. J. 1998. Anticancer activity of soybean peptides. *Proceedings of International Symposium on Soybean Peptides and Human Health*, 13–21. Seoul, Korea.

Lee, J. H. 2003. *65 Doenjang cooking recipes for good health*, 10. Seoul, Korea: Lee's Com.

Lee, J. H. 2011. Increased qualities and *in vitro* anticancer effects of doenjang and kanjang that fermented in onggi. MS thesis. Pusan National Univ., Busan, Korea.

Lee, J. H., M. H. Kim, and S. S. Im. 1991. Antioxidative materials in domestic meju and doenjang-(1)-lipid oxidation and browning during fermentation of meju and doenjang. *J Korean Soc Food Nutr* 20:148–155.

Lee, J. S., and H. S. Cheigh. 1997a. Antioxidative characteristics of isolated crude phenolics from soybean fermented foods (doenjang). *J Korean Soc Food Nutr* 26:376–382.

Lee, J. S., and H. S. Cheigh. 1997b. Composition and antioxidative characteristics of phenolic fractions isolated from soybean fermented food. *J Korean Soc Food Sci Nutr* 26:383–389.

Lee, I. K., and J. K. Kim. 2002. Effects of dietary supplementation of Korean soybean paste (Doenjang) on the lipid metabolism in rats fed a high fat and/or a high cholestrol diet. *J Koran Public Health Assoc* 28:282-305.

Lee, K. I., R. J. Moon, S. J. Lee, and K. Y. Park. 2001. The quality assessment of doenjang added with Japanese apricot, garlic and ginger, and samjang. *Korean J Soc Food Cookery Sci* 17:472-477.

Lee, K. I., K. Y. Park, and H. K. Ahn. 2011a. The anticancer effects of doenjang made with various kinds of salt. *Korean J Culinary Res* 17:241-252.

Lee, M. S., and K. S. Shin. 2013. Macrophage activation by polysaccharides from Koreans commercial and traditional soy sauces. *Korean J Food Nutr* 26:797-805.

Lee, M. S., and K. S. Shin. 2014. Intestinal immune-modulating activities of polysaccharides isolated from commercial and traditional Korean soy sauces. *J Korean Soc Food Sci Nutr* 43:9-15.

Lee, S., Y. Jeong, S. B. Yim, and S. Yu. 2015. Antioxidant activity of Korean traditional soy sauce. *J Korean Soc Food Sci Nutr* 44:1399-1406.

Lee, S., S. Lee, D. Singh et al. 2017. Comparative evaluation of microbial diversity and metabolite profiles in doenjang, a fermented soybean paste, during the two different industrial manufacturing processes. *Food Chem* 221:1578-1586.

Lee, S. J. 2002. Studies on the enhancement of cancer preventive effects of doenjang. MS thesis. Pusan National Univ., Busan, Korea.

Lee, S. J., K. I. Lee, S. H. Moon, and K. Y. Park. 2008. Antimutagenic effects on methanol extracts of doenjang made with various kinds of water or salt. *J Korean Soc Food Sci Nutr* 37:691-695.

Lee, S. Y., I. S. Kim, S. L. Park et al. 2012. Antidiabetic activity and enzymatic activity of commercial doenjang certified for traditional foods. *Korean Soc Biotechnol Bioeng J* 27:361-366.

Lefevre, M., S. M. Racedo, G. Ripert et al. 2015. Probiotic strain *Bacillus subtilis* CU1 stimulates immune system of elderly during common infectious disease period: A randomized, double-blind placebo-controlled study. *Immun Ageing* 12:24.

Lim, S. Y. 1997. Studies on the antimutagenic and anticancer activities of doenjang. Ph.D. diss., Pusan National Univ., Busan, Korea.

Lim, S. Y., K. Y. Park, M. S. Bae, and K. H. Kim. 2009. Effect of doenjang with black soybean on cytokine production and inhibition of tumor metastasis. *J Life Sci* 19:264-270.

Lim, S. Y., K. Y. Park, and S. H. Rhee. 1999. Anticancer effect of doenjang *in vitro* sulforhodamine B (SRB) assay. *J Korean Soc Food Sci Nutr* 28:240-245.

Llor, X., E. Pons, A. Roca et al. 2003. The effects of fish oil, olive oil, oleic acid and linoleic acid on colorectal neoplastic processes. *Clin Nutr* 22:71-79.

Mazza, P. 1994. The use of *Bacillus subtilis* as an antidiarrhoeal microorganism. *Boll Chim Farm* 133:3-18.

Meroni, P. L., R. Palmieri, and W. Barcellini. 1988. Effect of long-term treatment with *Bacillus subtilis* on the frequency of urinary tract infections in older patients. *Chemioterapia* 2:142-144.

Milligan, C. E., and L. M. Schwartz. 1997. Programmed cell death during animal development. *Brit Med Bull* 53: 570-590.

Moon, G. S. 1987. Antioxidative characteristics of fermented soybean sauce in lipid oxidation. Ph.D. diss., Pusan Natioanl Univ., Busan, Korea.

Moon, G. S. 1991. Comparison of various kinds of soybean sauces on their antioxidative activities. *J Korean Soc Food Nutr* 20:582-589.

Moon, G. S., and H. S. Cheigh. 1987. Antioxidative characteristics of soybean sauce in lipid oxidation process. *Korean J Food Sci Technol* 19:537–542.

Moon, G. S., and H. S. Cheigh. 1990. Separation and characteristics of antioxidative substances in fermented soybean sauce. *Korean J Food Sci Technol* 22:461–465.

Moon, S. H. 1990. Antimutagenic effect of doenjang (Korean soy paste). MS thesis. Pusan National Univ., Busan, Korea.

Mun, E. G., H. S. Sohn, M. S. Kim, and Y. S. Cha. 2017. Antihypertensive effect of ganjang (traditional Korean soy sauce) on Sprague-Dawley rats. *Nutr Res Prac* 11:388–395.

Muramoto, K., and E. Hatakeyama. 2003. Structures and properties of antioxidative peptides derived from food protein digests. *Food Ingred J Japan* 208:52–58.

Nagahara, A., H. Benjamin, J. Storkson et al. 1992. Inhibition of benzo[a]pyrene-induced mouse forestomach neoplasia by a principal flavor component of Japanese-style fermented soy sauce. *Cancer Res* 52:1754–1756.

Nuttall, F. Q. 1993. Dietary fiber in the management of diabetes. *Diabetes* 42:503–508.

Nydahl, M. C., I. B. Gustafsson, and B. Vessby. 1994. Lipid-lowering diets enriched with monounsaturated or polyunsaturated fatty acids but low in saturated fatty acids have similar effects on serum lipid concentrations in hyperlipidemic patients. *Am J Clinic Nutr* 59:115–122.

Park, E. S., J. Y. Lee, K. Y. Park. 2015a. Anticancer effects of black soybean doenjang in HT-29 human colon cancer cells. *J Korean Soc Food Sci Nutr* 44:1270–1278.

Park, H. R., M. S. Lee, S. Y. Jo et al. 2012. Immuno-stimulating activities of polysaccharides isolated from commercial soy sauce and traditional Korean soy sauce. *Korean J Food Sci Technol* 44:228–234.

Park, H. W., M. S. Yang, J. H. Lee et al. 2006. Long term feeding with soy isoflavone and L-carnitine synergistically suppresses body weight gain and adiposity in high-fat diet induced obese mice. *Nutr Sci* 9:179–189.

Park, K. H. 2006. A study of esthetic consciousness of the earthenware revealed in Goguryeo mural painting. *Korean Soc Oriental Art Studies* 11:29–46.

Park, K. Y. 2009a. *The sciences and health functionality of jangs* (Korea traditional soybean fermented foods). Korea Jang Cooperative. Dongseunambuk Publishing Co., Seoul, Korea.

Park, K. Y., K. M. Hwang, K. O. Jung, and K. B. Lee. 2002. Studies on the standardization of doenjang (Korean soybean paste): 1. Standardization of manufacturing method of doenjang by literatures. *J Korean Soc Food Sci Nutr* 31:343–350.

Park, K. Y., K. O. Jung, S. H. Rhee, and Y. H. Choi. 2003. Antimutagenic effects of doenjang (Korean fermented soy paste) and its active compounds. *Mutation Res/ Fundamental Mole Mechanisms Mutagen* 523:43–53.

Park, K. Y., S. Y. Kim, and S. H. Rhee. 1996a. Antimutagenic and anticarcinogenic effects of doenjang. *J Korean Assoc Cancer Prev* 1:99–107.

Park, K. Y., J. M. Lee, S. H. Moon, and K. O. Jung. 2000b. Inhibitory effect of doenjang (fermented Korean soy paste) extracts and linoleic acid on the growth of human cancer cell lines. *Prev Nutr Food Sci* 5:114–118.

Park, K. Y., S. J. Lee, K. I. Lee, and S. H. Rhee. 2005. The antitumor effect in sarcoma-180 tumor cell of mice administered with Japanese apricot, garlic or ginger doenjang. *Korean J Food Cookery Sci* 21:599–606.

Park, K. Y., S. H. Moon, H. S. Baik, and H. S. Cheigh. 1990. Antimutagenic effect of doenjang (Korean fermented soy paste) toward aflatoxin. *J Korean Soc Food Nutr* 19:156–162.

Park, K. Y., S. H. Moon, H. S. Cheigh, and H. S. Baik. 1996b. Antimutagenic effects of doenjang (Korean soy paste). *J Food Sci Nutr* 1:151–158.

Park, K. Y., M. H. Son, S. H. Moon, and K. H. Kim. 1999. Cancer preventive effects of doenjang *in vitro* and *in vivo*. 1. Antimutagenic and *in vivo* antitumor effects of doenjang. *J Korean Assoc Cancer Prev* 4:68–78.

Park, S., S. Lee, S. Park et al. 2015b. Antioxidant activity of Korean traditional soy sauce fermented in Korean earthenware, onggi, from different regions. *J Korean Soc Food Sci Nutr* 44:847–853.

Park, S. K., H. J. Jeong, S. H. Kim et al. 2004. Quality properties of traditional doenjang supplemented with extracts of Korean herb medicines. *J Life Sci* 14:553–559.

Park, S. K., K. I. Seo, S. H. Choi et al. 2000a. Quality assessment of commercial doenjang prepared by traditional method. *J Korean Soc Food Sci Nutr* 29:211–217.

Park, S. S. 2009b. Antiobese and antiinflammatory effect of bioceramic stone water and its application to doenjang. Ph.D. diss., Pusan Natinaol Univ., Busan, Korea.

Park, S. Y. 2003. The manufacture of cancer preventive doenjang and anticancer effects of doenjang. MS thesis, Pusan National Univ., Busan, Korea.

Pinchuk, I. V., P. Bressollier, B. Verneuil et al. 2001. *In vitro* anti-*Helicobacter pylori* activity of the probiotic strain *Bacillus subtilis* 3 is due to secretion of antibiotics. *Antimicrob Agents Chemother* 45:3156–3161.

Rauth, S., J. Kichina, and A. Green. 1997. Inhibition of growth and induction of differentiation of metastatic melanoma cells *in vitro* by genistein: Chemosensitivity is regulated by cellular p53. *British J Cancer* 75:1559–1566.

Rhew, T. H., S. M. Park, H. Y. Chung et al. 1992. Antitumorigenic activities of linoleic acid detected by in situ hybridization on transplanted tumors in mice. *Cancer Res Treatment* 24:493–503.

Seok, H. M. 2000. The brown pigment of doenjang; expectation of anti-diabetic- and anti-cancer efficacy. *Bull Food Technol* 13:122–126.

Shao, L. 2009. Studies on physicochemical changes and cancer preventive effects of fermented soy sauces during ripening period, MS thesis. Pusan National Univ. Busan, Korea.

Shim, J. H., E. S. Park, I. S. Kim, and K. Y. Park. 2015. Antioxidative and anticancer effects of doenjang prepared with bamboo salt in HT-29 human colon cancer cells. *J Korean Soc Food Sci Nutr* 44:524–531.

Shimakage, A., M. Shinbo, S. Yamada. 2012. ACE inhibitory substances derived from soy foods. *J Biol Macromol* 12:72–80.

Shin, Z. I., C. W. Ahn, H. S. Nam et al. 1995. Fractionation of angiotensin converting enzyme (ACE) inhibitory peptides from soybean paste. *Korean J Food Sci Technol* 27:230–234.

Shin, Z. I., R. Yu, S. A. Park et al. 2001. His-His-Leu, an angiotensin I converting enzyme inhibitory peptide derived from Korean soybean paste, exerts antihypertensive activity *in vivo*. *J Agric Food Chem* 49:3004–3009.

Shon, D. H., K. Lee, S. H. Kim et al. 1996. Screening of antithrombotic peptides from soybean paste by the microplate method. *Korean J Food Sci Technol* 28:684–688.

Sirotkin, A. V., and A. H. Harrath. 2014. Phytoestrogens and their effects. *European J Pharmacol* 741:230–236.

Song, J. L. 2012. Anticancer effects of fermented sesame sauce. Ph.D. diss., Pusan National Univ., Busan, Korea.

Song, J. L., J. H. Choi, J. H. Seo et al. 2014. Antioxidative effects of fermented sesame sauce against hydrogen peroxide-induced oxidative damage in LLC-PK1 porcine renal tubule cells. *Nutr Res Pract* 8:138–145.

Sorokulova, I., B., V. A. Beliavskaia, V. A. Masycheva, and V. V. Smirnov. 1997. Recombinant probiotics: Problems and prospects of their use for medicine and veterinary practice. *Vestn Ross Akad Med Nauk* 3:46–49.

Steele, V. E., M. A. Pereira, C. C. Sigman, and G. J. Kelloff. 1995. Cancer chemoprevention agent development strategies for genistein. *J Nutr* 125:713–716.

Suh, H. J., Y. S. Kim, S. H. Chung et al. 1996. Functionality and inhibitory effect of soybean hydrolysate on angiotensin converting enzyme. *Korean J Food Nutr* 9:167–175.

Sung, M. K. 2000. Soy saponins as a cancer prevention agent. *Proceedings of International Symposium on Soybean and Human Health*, 47–63. Seoul, Korea.

Welty, F. K., K. S. Lee, N. S. Lew, and J. R. Zhou. 2007. Effect of soy nuts on blood pressure and lipid levels in hypertensive, prehypertensive, and normotensive postmenopausal women. *Archives Internal Med* 167:1060–1067.

Wiseman H. 2000. The therapeutic potential of phytoestrogens. *Expert Opin Investig Drugs Aug* 9:1829–1840.

Yang, S. H., M. R. Choi, J. K. Kim, and Y. G. Chung. 1992. Optimization of the taste components composition in traditional Korean soybean paste. *J Korean Soc Food Nutr* 21:449–453.

Yoon, K. D., D. J. Kwon, S. S. Hong et al. 1996. Inhibitory effect of soybean and fermented soybean products on the chemically induced mutagenesis. *Korean J Appl Microbiol Biotechnol* 24:525–528.

Yoshiki, Y., S. Kudou, and K. Okubo. 1998. Relationship between chemical structures and biological activities of triterpenoid saponins from soybean. *Biosci Biotechnol Biochem* 62:2291–2299.

Yu, J. Y. 1998. Characteristics of meju and microorganisms for traditional soybean fermented foods. *The First Symposium and Expo for Soybean-Fermented Foods*, 31–87. The Research Institute of Soybean-Fermented Foods. Yeungnam Univ., Kyungsan, Korea.

Yun, H. S., K. Y. Park, and W. H. Lee. 2000. Antimutagenic effects of genistein in *Drosophila* somatic mutation assaying system. *J Korean Assoc Cancer Prev* 5:135–143.

Yun, H. S., M. A. Yoo, K. Y. Park, and W. H. Lee. 1999. Antimutagenic effect of genistein toward environmental mutagen. *J Korean Environ Sci Soc* 8:569–574.

Zhao L., Y. Dong, G. Chen, and Q. Hu. 2010. Extraction, purification, characterization and antitumor activity of polysaccharides from *Ganoderma lucidum*. *Carbohyd Polym* 80:783–789.

Zhao, X. 2011. Anticancer and anti-inflammatory effects of bamboo salt and *Rubus coreanus Miquel* bamboo salt, Ph.D. diss., Pusan National Univ., Busan, Korea.

Zhu, H., Y. Zhang, J. Zhang, and D. Chen. 2008. Isolation and characterization of an anti-complementary protein-bound polysaccharide from the stem barks of *Eucommia ulmoides*. *Int Immunopharmacol* 8: 1220–1230.

Zhu, Y. P., Z. W. Su, and C. H. Li. 1989. Growth-inhibition effects of oleic acid, linoleic acid, and their methyl esters on transplanted tumors in mice. *J Nat Cancer Institute* 81:1302–1306.

6

Cheongkukjang

Sunmin Park and James W. Daily

CONTENTS

6.1 History 145
6.2 Food Processing 147
6.3 Food Composition 148
    6.3.1 Changes in Soybean Composition in Cheongkukjang 148
    6.3.2 Metabolite Profiling of Cheongkukjang 151
6.4 Health Benefits 153
    6.4.1 Health Benefits of Cheongkukjang 153
    6.4.2 Bioactive Compounds 154
    6.4.3 Poly-γ-Glutamic Acid 154
    6.4.4 Isoflavone Glucosides and Aglycones 155
    6.4.5 Peptides and Proteins 156
    6.4.6 Polysaccharides and Lipopeptides 157
    6.4.7 Vitamins K and B_{12} 157
    6.4.8 Cheongkukjang as a Whole Food 158
    6.4.9 Human Research 158
6.5 Conclusions on Health Benefits of Cheongkukjang 160
References 161

6.1 History

Soybean (*Glycine max* Merill) has long been an important protein source to complement grain protein in Asian countries. Soybean products contain various functional components including peptides, isoflavonoids and more (Dastmalchi and Dhaubhadel, 2015). Fermentation is one of the major processes used in preparing soybeans for consumption. Fermented soybean paste is an indigenous food for use in cooking in East and Southeast Asia (Han et al., 2011). Korea developed and used its own traditional fermented foods 2000 years ago (Chettri and Tamang, 2015). Among various fermented soybean products, cheongkukjang has some unique characteristics, such as short-term fermentation without salt, and the fermentation has been mainly conducted with bacilli (Kwon et al., 2010).

The origin of cheongkukjang is not clearly known. Because of the Korean name cheongkukjang, people think it came from the Chung dynasty, which began in 1616. However, a version of cheongkukjang named goguryeojang has been used from the Goguryeo dynasty, which spanned from 37 BC to AD 668, and is recorded in *Samkooksagi* (the history of three kingdoms). *Samkooksagi* is the written history of the Goguryeo, Baekje, and Silla dynasties and was completed in 1145. A possible scenario for the origin of cheongkukjang is that soybeans fermented when the cavalry soldiers and nomads put cooked soybeans in the bags made with rice straw underneath their horses in Mongol areas, and they found the fermented soybeans eatable; this is cheongkukjang. However, soybeans did not grow on the Mongol prairies, so they were obtained from Manchuria, the part of the Goguryeo dynasty where soybeans were cultivated. In the Silla dynasty, cheongkukjang was called yeomsi and si and was used in cooking dishes in the Goguryeo, Baekje, and Silla dynasties; this use was recorded several times in *Samkooksagi*. In 1715, the household manual, "Sallymkeongje," was written by Banseon Hong and described proper methods for agriculture, housing, eating, and health. It included references to jeonkookjang, or cheongkukjang; in 1766, the method for making cheongkukjang was written in detail in the extended "Sallymkeongje" written by Joomlym (Figure 6.1). Thus, cheongkukjang probably originated from the Goguryeo dynasty and versions of it have been distributed into Nepal, Indonesia, Vietnam, and Southwest Asia.

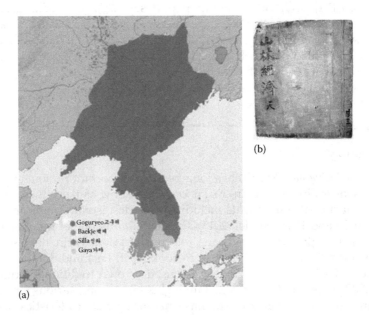

FIGURE 6.1
(a) Map of Korea during the Goguryeo dynasty. (b) Sallymkeongje, ancient book of Korean history.

Natto is the only fermented soybean food that is very similar to cheongkukjang. The origin of natto is controversial. There are two competing hypotheses from Japanese historians: One is that natto was encountered inside rice straw in the eastern area of Japan and the other is that it came from China. However, there is no food similar to cheongkukjang or natto in China. Although dubuchi is a fermented soybean without salt in China, it is fermented with different bacteria compared to cheongkukjang and at lower temperature. Thus, the origins of natto may be linked to those of cheongkukjang during the Baekje dynasty. Cheongkukjang may be the original unsalted, short-term, fermented soybean food.

6.2 Food Processing

When preparing cheongkukjang, dried soybeans are sorted, washed, and soaked in water for 12 h at 15°C and boiled for 4 h at 100°C. The cooked soybeans are cooled to 40°C and fermented with rice straw in a fermentation chamber at 30°C for 24–72 h according to the contents of the *Bacillus*. The optimal fermentation time is 48 h in most cases. The traditionally made cheongkukjang contains several kinds of bacilli (Yang et al., 2013). The *Bacillus* species are different in cheongkukjang according to the areas and seasons during fermentation due to the different environments where bacteria live. Since rice straw containing local ambient bacilli is traditionally used as a fermentation starter, cheongkukjang is predominantly fermented with *Bacillus* species and also some other bacteria such as *Enterococcus*, *Pseudomonas*, and *Rhodococcus* (Hong et al., 2012). Many different *Bacillus* strains have been identified by rRNA gene sequencing or recA sequencing using the randomly amplified polymeric DNA-PCR method (Kwon et al., 2009), *Bacillus subtilis*, *B. amyloliquenfaciens*, *B. licheniformis*, and *B. thuringiensis* are found in traditionally made cheongkukjang. *B. subtilis* is the predominant strain in traditional cheongkukjang (Yang et al., 2013).

Since the components of cheongkukjang made in a traditional manner (TFC) are different according to areas and seasons and different environmental bacteria, the functionality of cheongkukjang is also different. TFC made in Sunchang (Chonnam, Korea) is known to have good quality. Cheongkukjang is made commercially with specific bacilli such as *B. subtilus* and *B. licheniformis*—called modernized cheongkukjang (Yang et al., 2013). This cheongkukjang has consistent quality and functionality. Modernized cheongkukjang is fermented (SFC) with *B. licheniformis* SCD 111067P obtained from the Institute of Sunchang Fermented Soybean Research Institutes (Sunchang, Korea). *Bacillus* is cultivated in Luria–Bertani broth at 37°C with shaking (128 rpm, Jeio Tech, Daejeon, Korea) to expand the number of *Bacillus* spp. Soaked soybeans are steamed at 121°C for 1 h, cooled to 40°C, and inoculated with 1% (v/w) *Bacillus* at concentrations of 10^7–10^8 CFU • mL^{-1}. The inoculated soybean preparation

148 *Korean Functional Foods*

is then fermented at 42°C for 48 h. Research on the *Bacillus* species has shown them to have superior efficacy for alleviating metabolic diseases and to have a better taste than traditionally made cheongkukjang (Kwon et al., 2007; Park et al., 2016).

In Korea, cheongkukjang has been traditionally used to make soup with vegetables, but people recently have been consuming it raw with milk or yogurt.

6.3 Food Composition

6.3.1 Changes in Soybean Composition in Cheongkukjang

The major components of soybeans are isoflavonoids, dietary fiber, unsaturated fatty acids, and proteins—all of which have functionality and contribute to modulate metabolism in their original states. However, after fermentation, they are changed into different forms. For example, isoflavonoids exist as glycated forms in soybeans, but fermentation changes them into isoflavonoid aglycones (Kwon et al., 2006). Dietary fibers and proteins are changed into smaller sized polysaccharides and peptides. Isoflavonoid aglycones and smaller pieces of dietary fiber and peptides increase bioavailability. The nature of the changes in components is influenced by bacteria species and fermentation periods.

Fermentation improves the nutritional and functional properties of soybeans by increasing contents of small bioactive compounds. Soybeans contain 0.1 to 5 mg total isoflavones per gram, primarily as a form of β-glucosides, genistin, daidzin, and glycitin, containing 50% to 55%, 40% to 45%, and 5% to 10% of the total isoflavone content, respectively (Murphy et al., 2002). Raw soybeans contain about 3000 mg total isoflavone/kilogram and total isoflavone contents decrease by about 50% during cooking prior to their fermentation to make cheongkukkjang (Jang et al., 2006). The total isoflavone contents of cheongkukjang slightly decrease during 45 h of fermentation. However, the profiles of isoflavonoids are greatly modified during fermentation: The contents of isoflavone glycosides, mainly including daizein, glycitin, and genistin, decrease by about 40% during 45 h of fermentation, whereas the contents of isoflavonoid aglycones consisting of deizein, glycitein, and genistein exhibit a marked increase by 2.9-, 54.0-, and 20.6-fold, respectively (Jang et al., 2006) (Table 6.1).

Amino acid and peptide concentrations were markedly changed among the various small metabolites derived from macromolecules (Tables 6.2 and 6.3). Some amino acids increased and others remained almost constant with increased fermentation periods. Glutamate, the richest amino acid in soybean, is obviously decreased by fermentation, suggesting that microorganisms might use it as a preferred nitrogen source (Kada et al., 2013).

TABLE 6.1

Isoflavone Contents in 70% Methanol Extracts of Traditionally Fermented Cheongkukjang and Cheongkukjang Fermented with Different *Bacillus* Species for 48 Hours

	CSB	TFC	BS	BL	BA
Daidzin	489.2 ± 17.4[d]	150.6 ± 20.0[c]	85.9 ± 5.3[b]	61.8 ± 5.1[a]	103.7 ± 5.1[b]
Glycitin	156.8 ± 18.6[d]	75.2 ± 11.4[c]	48.2 ± 2.3[b]	32.6 ± 0.5[a]	55.3 ± 3.5[b]
Genistin	844.4 ± 22.2[d]	254.0 ± 37.1[c]	118.3 ± 7.7[ab]	104.9 ± 11.3[a]	145.5 ± 8.8[b]
Malonyl daidzin	125.1 ± 7.5[a]	162.3 ± 27.1[b]	310.2 ± 26.9[d]	211.0 ± 10.3[c]	291.5 ± 8.9[d]
Malonyl glycitin	24.2 ± 6.4[a]	32.7 ± 3.8[b]	80.6 ± 7.3[d]	61.2 ± 3.9[c]	68.1 ± 4.1[c]
Malonyl genistin	149.7 ± 12.8[c]	32.9 ± 9.3[a]	78.8 ± 18.2[b]	93.5 ± 20.7[b]	85.3 ± 19.6[b]
Acetyl daidzin	103.3 ± 7.6[d]	17.6 ± 2.5[a]	38.8 ± 3.9[b]	42.1 ± 3.7[bc]	48.3 ± 6.4[c]
Acetyl glycitin	60.2 ± 3.3[a]	Trace	Trace	Trace	Trace
Acetyl genistin	150.7 ± 3.8[c]	12.7 ± 2.2[a]	15.7 ± 0.4[ab]	17.2 ± 2.1[b]	19.2 ± 2.0[b]
Total glycosides	*1,952 ± 29.3[c]*	*737.9 ± 98.7[ab]*	*776.6 ± 59.0[b]*	*624.3 ± 55.9[a]*	*816.9 ± 41.9[b]*
Daidzein	25.0 ± 6.5[a]	170.3 ± 49.9[c]	78.7 ± 5.0[b]	138.3 ± 9.2[c]	72.9 ± 2.6[b]
Glycitein	12.6 ± 3.9[a]	66.3 ± 9.0[c]	41.3 ± 3.3[b]	74.3 ± 5.4[c]	37.4 ± 1.2[b]
Genistein	25.9 ± 4.8[a]	122.5 ± 17.8[d]	48.9 ± 2.0[b]	85.0 ± 5.0[c]	39.3 ± 0.9[b]
Total aglycones	*63.5 ± 8.0[a]*	*359.1 ± 76.1[c]*	*168.8 ± 10.0[b]*	*297.5 ± 19.5[c]*	*149.6 ± 4.4[b]*
Total isoflavones	*1,413 ± 98.0[b]*	*1,097 ± 174.2[a]*	*945.4 ± 67.5[a]*	*921.8 ± 74.4[a]*	*966.5 ± 45.2[a]*

Notes: Micrograms per gram of dry matter. TFC = traditionally fermented cheongkukjang; BS = cheongkukjang fermented with *B. subtilus;* BL = cheongkukjang fermented with *B. licheniformis;* BA = cheongkukjang fermented with *B. amyloliquefaciens.* Values are the means ± SD (*n* = 3).

[a,b,c,d] Values on the same row with different superscripts were significantly different by Tukey's test at p < 0.05.

Cheongkukjang has a characteristic flavor that is generally acceptable to Koreans, but the flavor is not tolerable to some people from other countries. The major compounds contributing to the peculiar odor of cheongkukjang are volatile organic acids such as acetic acid, propionic acid, 2-methylpropanoic acid, butanoic acid, and 3-methylbutanoic acid, as identified by gas chromatography-mass spectrometry (GC-MS) (Park et al., 2007). The contents of volatile organic acids in cheongkukjang are highly dependent on the fermentation period. The branched-chain organic acids (2-methypropionic acid and 3-methylbutanoic acid) are abundantly formed during the fermentation and are determinants of the characteristic flavor of cheongkukjang (Yang et al., 2011).

Cheongkukjang also contains poly-γ-glutamic acid (γ-PGA), an anionic polypeptide in which D- and/or L-glutamate is polymerized via γ-amide linkages (Bae et al., 2010; Choi et al., 2015). γ-PGA is produced in soybean fermentation with some strains of *Bacillus* species, including *B. subtilus, B. licheniformis,* and *B. natto.* γ-PGA is the main component of the extracellular mucilage. According to its molecular weight and the ratios of D- and L-glutamate, γ-PGA has different applications and functionality as functional foods and cosmetics (Bae et al., 2010; Choi et al., 2015).

TABLE 6.2

Free Amino Acid Content of Cheongkukjang Fermented in the Traditional Manner or with Different *Bacillus* Species for 48 Hours

	Sample				
	CSB	**TFC**	**BS**	**BL**	**BA**
Asp	21.2 ± 2.7[b]	14.3 ± 1.6[a]	13.9 ± 2.6[a]	17.8 ± 3.7[a]	14.5 ± 1.2[a]
Ser	14.0 ± 2.1	14.8 ± 1.7	8.8 ± 0.5	12.0 ± 6.2	12.0 ± 0.6
Glu	34.3 ± 5.4	82.1 ± 6.9	74.5 ± 17.4	90.7 ± 18.5	81.3 ± 7.1
Gly	16.3 ± 1.4[a]	32.7 ± 3.8[b]	26.2 ± 2.1[b]	36.5 ± 14.4[b]	21.8 ± 0.4[b]
His	122.6 ± 12.7[ab]	159.8 ± 28.8[b]	108.7 ± 11.8[a]	104.4 ± 34.2[a]	124.9 ± 12.3[ab]
Arg	97.8 ± 2.5[b]	103.1 ± 1.4[b]	65.8 ± 6.0[a]	66.2 ± 1.4[a]	63.6 ± 2.1[a]
Thr	17.0 ± 1.5	16.8 ± 6.6	15.5 ± 0.3	21.7 ± 9.8	23.6 ± 6.1
Ala	33.3 ± 0.8[a]	45.5 ± 2.7[b]	42.3 ± 1.3[b]	42.6 ± 7.3[b]	33.6 ± 1.1[a]
Pro	183.5 ± 5.9[c]	34.9 ± 0.9[a]	39.2 ± 2.0[b]	33.7 ± 3.1[a]	34.5 ± 0.9[a]
Tyr	13.2 ± 0.4[a]	110.1 ± 13.2[c]	35.9 ± 28.1[b]	47.8 ± 10.4[b]	41.0 ± 1.5[b]
Val	28.1 ± 1.8[a]	50.5 ± 7.4[b]	45.7 ± 4.5[b]	48.2 ± 5.9[b]	50.6 ± 4.0[b]
Met	8.2 ± 0.5[a]	28.4 ± 1.8[b]	25.8 ± 4.1[b]	29.5 ± 1.3[b]	26.4 ± 0.6[b]
Lys	19.0 ± 4.3[a]	103.7 ± 11.1[b]	81.0 ± 9.7[b]	88.3 ± 20.2[b]	91.6 ± 3.8[b]
Ile	4.6 ± 2.1[a]	46.0 ± 7.2[b]	38.0 ± 6.0[b]	39.9 ± 3.3[b]	36.4 ± 2.8[b]
Leu	9.2 ± 1.1[a]	69.0 ± 4.1[c]	45.3 ± 4.8[b]	49.9 ± 2.4[b]	48.1 ± 4.6[b]
Phe	25.3 ± 4.1[a]	62.4 ± 1.5[c]	42.9 ± 5.7[b]	45.9 ± 3.5[b]	43.3 ± 4.0[b]
Total	647.6 ± 11.4[a]	974.1 ± 20.1[c]	709.3 ± 19.8[b]	775.1 ± 18.6[b]	747.4 ± 21.4[b]

Notes: Milligrams per 100 g. TFC = traditionally fermented cheongkukjang; BS = cheongkukjang fermented with *B. subtilus*; BL = cheongkukjang fermented with *B. licheniformis*; BA = cheongkukjang fermented with *B. amyloliquefaciens*. Values are the means ± SD (n = 3).

[a,b,c] Values on the same row with different superscripts were significantly different by Tukey's test at p < 0.05.

TABLE 6.3

Peptide Content of Cheongkukjang Fermented in the Traditional Manner or with Different *Bacillus* Species for 48 Hours

Sample	Peptides (mg/g)
CSB	48.0 ± 6.0[a]
TFC	109.6 ± 6.0[b]
BS	117.6 ± 11.7[b]
BL	113.9 ± 9.4[b]
BA	116.7 ± 1.3[b]

Notes: CSB = cooked soybeans; TFC = traditionally fermented cheongkukjang; BS = cheongkukjang fermented with *B. subtilus*; BL = cheongkukjang fermented with *B. licheniformis*; BA = cheongkukjang fermented with *B. amyloliquefaciens*. Values are the means ± SD (n = 3).

[a,b] Values in the same column with different superscripts were significantly different by Tukey's test at p < 0.05.

6.3.2 Metabolite Profiling of Cheongkukjang

The metabolic profiles of cooked soybean (CSB), TFC made in Sunnchang, and SFC made with *B. licheniformis* were analyzed by UPLC–Q–TOF mass according to the fermentation time. In metabolic profiling of cheongkukjang, fructose, glucose, mannose, sucrose, succinic acid, malonic acid, and most amino acids mainly contribute to the differentiation of the different cheongkukjangs (traditionally made versus cheongkukjang fermented with *B. subtilus*, *B. amyloliquenfaciens*, and *B. licheniformis*) according to fermentation time. The levels of most amino acids decreased in the early stage of fermentation and increased in the late stage with *B. subtilis* (Yang et al., 2015). The amounts of fatty acids generally increase throughout the fermentation process, but most organic acids, except for tartaric acids, decrease. The metabolomes of cheongkukjang are discriminated by fermentation periods and inoculated *Bacillus* strains (Figure 6.2, Table 6.4). The profiles of cheongkukjangs with different fermentation periods are discriminated mainly by tryptophan, citric acid, β-alanine, itaconic acid, 2-hydroxyglutaric acid, γ-aminobutyric acid, leucine, malic acid, and tartaric acid. Cheongkukjang fermented for 48 h produces metabolomes; the most occur among cheongkukjang with different fermentation periods. The profiles of cheongkukjangs fermented by inoculating with different *Bacillus* strains are differentiated by mannose, xylose, glutamic acid, and proline (Bae et al., 2010). Cheongkukjang fermented with *B. licheniformis* produces more polyglutamate than TFC, BA, and BS.

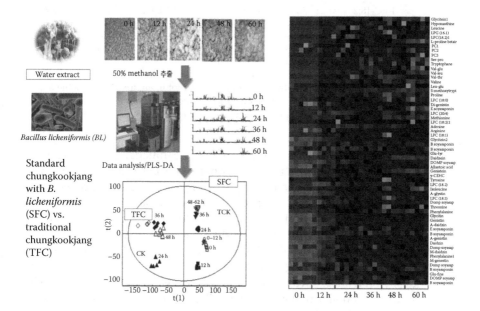

FIGURE 6.2
Process of metabolomic analysis of cheongkukjang.

152   *Korean Functional Foods*

TABLE 6.4

Metabolomic Profiles of Different Kinds of Cheongkukjang

			Normalized Intensity		
NO.*	Identification	VIP**	CSB	TFC	SFC (BL)
1	Proline	1.27	1.4 ± 1.9^a	0.7 ± 1.3^a	25.0 ± 5.7^b
2	Adenine	2.45	67.9 ± 33.1^a	147.0 ± 15.0^b	96.6 ± 30.4^a
3	Tyrosine	2.59	71.3 ± 16.5^a	222.3 ± 38.2^b	66.4 ± 8.2^a
4	Leucine/isoleucine	3.73	121.9 ± 28.2^a	188.3 ± 47.9^a	502.5 ± 249.6^b
5	Phenylalanine	4.27	271.1 ± 90.0^a	1429.5 ± 229.9^b	2127.2 ± 635.9^c
6	Ser-Pro	1.45	0.0 ± 0.0^a	0.0 ± 0.0^a	153.7 ± 64.2^b
7	Val-Glu	1.02	0.0 ± 0.0^a	0.0 ± 0.0^a	75.0 ± 47.4^b
8	Val-Leu	1.3	0.0 ± 0.0^a	22.1 ± 9.3^b	167.5 ± 13.7^c
9	Glu-Phe	6.64	1739.3 ± 106.6^c	58.5 ± 13.9^a	365.3 ± 22.8^b
10	Daidzin	4.08	$545.6 \pm 95.8b$	$100.2 \pm 17.1a$	$79.1 \pm 7.6a$
11	Genistin	4.94	460.1 ± 162.7^c	179.1 ± 21.0^b	106.1 ± 11.3^a
12	Acetylgenistin	3.31	328.8 ± 78.0^b	3.4 ± 3.4^a	13.8 ± 2.6^a
13	Daidzein	1.28	191.6 ± 126.8^a	1837.0 ± 111.2^c	1074.6 ± 120.2^b
14	Genistein	6.64	181.2 ± 113.8^a	1633.5 ± 132.6^c	891.5 ± 113.0^b
15	B soyasaponin Bb'	1.46	37.5 ± 20.1^{ab}	53.0 ± 13.3^b	26.3 ± 16.0^a
16	E soyasaponin Be	3.76	51.4 ± 40.2^a	133.3 ± 50.8^a	602.7 ± 190.5^b
17	DDMP soyasaponin βg	1.83	2021 ± 1245^c	210 ± 252^a	1185 ± 750^b
18	LPC***-18:3	7.18	295 ± 194^b	3.7 ± 5.1^a	1253 ± 678^c
19	LPC-18:2	7.29	201.5 ± 151.5^b	2.1 ± 4.7^a	747.7 ± 426.0^c
20	LPC-18:0	1.05	5.6 ± 4.0^a	0.0 ± 0.1^a	22.2 ± 10.5^b

Notes: CSB = cooked soybeans; TFC = traditionally fermented cheongkukjang; SFC(BL) = cheongkukjang fermented with *B. licheniformis*.

[a,b,c] Values on the same row with different superscripts were significantly different at $p < 0.05$.
*A number of metabolites marked in the PLS-DA loadings plot in Figure 6.3; **Variable importance in the projection and the value of over 1.0 indicated high relevance for explaining the difference of sample groups; ***Lysoposphatidylcholines containing indicated fatty acid.

In the metabolic profiles of CSB, TFC made in Sunnchang, and SFC made with *B. licheniformis*, the first two-component PLS-DA score plots of these metabolites show that the three samples were clearly discriminated from one another by the primary component t(1) or the secondary component t(2) based on the good model quality factors for fitness and predictability ($R_2X = 0.9115$, $R_2Y = 0.987$, and $Q_2Y = 0.975$) along with good cross validation characteristics (R_2 intercept = 0.383; Q_2 intercept = –0.474; P-value = 6.87e-15) (Figure 6.3) (Yang et al., 2015). Twenty metabolites, including amino acids, dipeptides, isoflavones, soyasaponins, and lysoposphatidylcholines (LPCs), were identified as major metabolites contributing to the differences among the CSB, TFC, and SFC. All except Glu-Phe and DDMP soyasaponin βg were formed during fermentation. In particular, it was observed that their levels

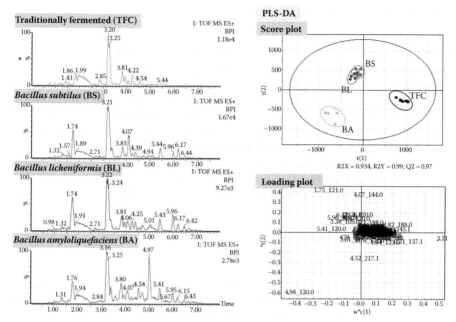

UPLC profile of traditionally fermented cheongkukjang and cheongkukjang fermented with different *bacillus* spp.

FIGURE 6.3
Results of metabolomic analysis of cheongkukjang.

in SFC, except isoflavone aglycones, were higher than those in TFC. In addition, γ-PGA, a viscous and sticky substance characteristic of cheongkukjang, was generated during fermentation and was highest in SFC (5.3% ± 0.2% of the total contents) as compared to TFC (2.2% ± 0.3% of the total contents) by about two fold.

6.4 Health Benefits

6.4.1 Health Benefits of Cheongkukjang

Cheongkukjang is distinguished from other fermented foods, including most fermented soy foods, by short fermentation time, different fermentative microorganisms, and low salt content. This results in a unique set of probiotic microbes as well as different bioactive compounds produced during fermentation. These differences result in a uniquely characteristic flavor and aroma, as well as in different functional compounds with health-promoting activities.

6.4.2 Bioactive Compounds

During the fermentation process of making cheongkukjang, numerous compounds are modified or synthesized by the bacteria. The sticky mucilaginous coating on the outside of the cheongkukjang is composed of γ-PGA, which is a polypeptide polymer of D- and L-glutamate residues joined together by γ-amide bonds, which appear to make γ-PGA resistant to proteolytic enzymes (Choi et al., 2015). Organic acids, including acetic acid, propionic acid, butanoic acid, and their metabolites, contribute to the characteristic flavor of cheongkukjang (Park et al., 2007). Soy isoflavone glycosides are hydrolyzed to form aglycones during fermentation, and proteins are broken down into smaller peptides and free amino acids (Kwon et al., 2010). All of these compounds, and many more, may also contribute to the health benefits of cheongkukjang.

6.4.3 Poly-γ-Glutamic Acid

The presence of γ-PGA is one of the defining characteristics of cheongkukjang, so it is not surprising that it contributes some of its most important benefits. The available research indicates that γ-PGA has potent immunomodulatory properties. Oral administration of a high molecular mass γ-PGA made by a *Bacillus subtilis* subspecies "cheongkukjang" was shown to inhibit the growth of MHC class 1-deficient tumor cells injected into C57BL/6 mice and to improve the survival time of the mice. In that study, the effect of γ-PGA was shown to be mediated by increases in the production of natural killer cells and interferon-γ (Kim et al., 2007a). Moon et al. (2012) also found that interferon production was increased by γ-PGA, and it provided mice protection against influenza A virus in their study. Furthermore, Kim et al. (2015) found that the antiviral activity of internal administration of γ-PGA protected mice against H1N1 (swine flu) influenza by increasing interferon-β and interleukin-12, and enhancing activation of natural killer cells and specific cytotoxic T-cells.

Interestingly, γ-PGA not only stimulates immune activation against pathogens, but also suppresses harmful immune activity by exerting anti-inflammatory actions by decreasing cyclooxygenase-2 expression in human colorectal cells, which also induced apoptosis in those cells (Shin et al., 2015). The anti-inflammatory effects of orally administered γ-PGA from cheongkukjang have also been demonstrated to be effective for treating atopic dermatitis in mice (Lee et al., 2014a) and when administered topically to promote corneal wound healing after burn injury in rabbits (Bae et al., 2010). Cheongkukjang-derived γ-PGA is also known to chelate calcium, forming a highly soluble complex in water (Bae et al., 2010). Chronic administration of γ-PGA to rats improved calcium absorption, calcium balance, and bone calcium content (Tanimoto et al., 2007; Yang et al., 2008). γ-PGA

Cheongkukjang 155

was also shown to improve calcium absorption in postmenopausal Japanese women, especially those with lower intakes of calcium, thus suggesting the possibility that γ-PGA could be useful for helping to prevent osteoporosis in postmenopausal women. Finally, a high molecular weight γ-PGA from cheongkukjang was shown to block the hypertriglyceridemic effects of eating a high-fructose diet in rats. The effect was mediated by the inhibition of lipogenic enzymes such as hepatic malic enzyme; glucose-6-phospantate dehydrogenase was also associated with lower circulating concentrations of cholesterol and nonesterified fatty acids (Jeon et al., 2013).

6.4.4 Isoflavone Glucosides and Aglycones

Isoflavones (considered to be phytoestrogens) are among the best characterized of the bioactive compounds of fermented soybean foods. Isoflavones in raw soybeans occur mostly as the glycosides genistin, daidzin, and glycitin; however, during the fermentation of cheongkukjang and other fermented soy foods, they are converted to the aglycones genistein, daidzein, and glycitein. Isoflavones in the aglycone form (Yang et al., 2009) have been found to be much better absorbed in humans than their corresponding glycosides. Interestingly, the most efficient bacterial species for producing isoflavone aglycones was *Lactobacillus acidophilus* KCTC 3925, a very common probiotic bacterium (Kim et al., 2016). This suggests that the functionality of cheongkukjang may be greatly influenced by the choice of bacteria used when making cheongkukjang by inoculation with bacteria rather than the traditional method of using naturally occurring bacteria from rice straw.

As with γ-PGA, soy isoflavones from cheongkukjang appear to have potent immunostimulatory properties. Choi et al. (2014) showed that cheongkukjang had much greater isoflavone (both glycosylated and aglycone) contents than two other Korean fermented soy foods, kochujang and doenjang. In their study, isoflavone-rich ethanol extracts were used to test responses by human immune cells; cheongkukjang extracts resulted in the greatest cell proliferation and nitric oxide production among extracts of cheongkukjang, kochujang, and doenjang. The ethanol extract from cheongkukjang has also been shown to improve immunity by suppressing apoptosis of mouse spleen and thymus cells (Kim, H.B. et al., 2007). However, although isoflavones are found in ethanol fractions of soy extracts, there may be other bioactive compounds in those fractions as well, and the bioactivities of the ethanol extracts may not be due exclusively to the isoflavones. Ghaemi et al. (2012) demonstrated that genistein treatment of mice (a cervical cancer mouse model) significantly increased lymphocyte proliferation, cytosol LDH release, and IFN-γ, thereby inhibiting tumor growth.

The ethanol extracts of cheongkukjang have also been shown to exert anti-inflammatory effects, although by somewhat different mechanisms than those demonstrated by γ-PGA. The ethanol extract of cheongkukjang has been shown to inhibit 5-lipoxygenase and to exert *in vivo* anti-inflammatory effects by suppressing arachidonic acid-induced mouse ear edema (Choi et al., 2008). Bae et al. (2014) demonstrated that the ethanol extract of cheongkukjang can help alleviate mast cell-dependent anaphylaxis, suppress ovalbumin-induced asthma-like symptoms, down-regulate the amount of eosinophil and monocytes infiltration in the lungs, and decrease mast cell degranulation and histamine release.

Antidiabetic actions of isoflavones, especially aglycones, have also been described. Yang et al. (2013) demonstrated that isoflavone-rich methanolic extracts of cheongkukjang fermented with *B. licheniformis* for 48 h and 72 h increased insulin secretion in MIN-6 cells and also protected the viability of pancreatic β-cells. In a type 2 diabetes model using 90% pancreatectomized diabetic rats, cheongkukjang enhanced insulin secretion and insulin/IGF-1 signaling by inducing insulin receptor substrate-2 expression. Cheongkukjang also increased pancreatic β-cell hyperplasia by promoting proliferation and suppressing apoptosis. (Kwon et al., 2007). However, that study used cheongkukjang itself and not just isoflavones or other components extracted from cheongkukjang. However, another *in vitro* study (Kwon et al., 2006) found that isoflavonoid fractions of cheongkukjang obtained from extraction and chromatographic separation enhanced insulin signaling and peroxisome proliferator–activator receptor-γ activation in cell studies. Cheongkukjang may be the ideal soy food for obtaining dietary isoflavones. Although longer term fermented soy pastes such as kochujang and doenjang convert glucosides to aglycones, they also appear to decrease in total isoflavones due to fermentative degradation. Choi et al. (2014) reported that cheongkukjang had much higher concentrations of both the glucosides and aglycones than did kochujang and doenjang. Furthermore, although some evidence supports the possibility that much of the glycosylated isoflavones may be absorbed after being converted to aglycones in the gut, the absorption is delayed (King et al., 1996; Zubik and Meydani, 2003). Therefore, the mixture of glucosides and aglycones in cheongkukjang may have the advantage of providing a time-released absorption.

6.4.5 Peptides and Proteins

A more recent area of interest is the soy peptides formed during fermentation of peptides. The savory flavor of fermented soy foods is largely due to the small peptides and free amino acids that are released by fermentative digestion and/or acid hydrolysis of the soybean proteins (Kwon et al., 2010). Lunasin is a 43-amino acid soy-derived peptide with numerous bioactivities, including anticancer and anti-inflammatory activities (Galvez et al., 2001a, 2011b). A study of peptides produced by cheongkukjang identified two peptides (Ala-Phe-Pro-Gly and Gly-Val-Ala-Trp-Trp-Met-Tyr) with potent anti-inflammatory properties. Both peptides inhibited lipopolysaccharide-induced nitric oxide production and iNOS mRNA expression (Lee et al., 2014b).

They further confirmed that the 30 mg/L of the two peptides inhibited the transcriptional induction of both TNF-α and IL-6 *in vitro*, which strongly suggested that the peptides may contribute to the anti-inflammatory properties of cheongkukjang. Other bioactive peptides have been identified in doenjang and miso, which are fermented for much longer than cheongkukjang (Kwon et al., 2010), but it is not known if those peptides are present in cheongkukjang. Cheongkukjang has also been reported to contain a fibrinolytic enzyme (similar to nattokinase) that may have potential for treating or preventing thrombosis (Jeong et al., 2015). The possibility of an antithrombotic enzyme in cheongkukjang is intriguing, but needs to be confirmed *in vivo* and eventually in human clinical trials.

6.4.6 Polysaccharides and Lipopeptides

Some lactic acid bacteria that ferment cheongkukjang form less commonly known substances including polysaccharides and lipoproteins (Kim et al., 2016). The polysaccharides that are formed include those composed only of single monosaccharide chains and those including various different monosaccharides. In contrast to some of the other components of cheongkukjang (γ-PGA, isoflavones, peptides), the polysaccharides appear only to stimulate immunity, including inflammatory processes stimulated by lipopolysaccharide (Lee et al., 2013; Cho et al., 2015). The immunostimulatory effects comprised a broad range of effects, including increased production of nitric oxide and tumor necrosis factor-α, increased activation of nuclear factor κB in macrophages, increased production of IL-2 and IFN-γ, and enhanced natural killer cell activity.

Lipopeptides with antimicrobial properties have also been demonstrated to be formed during the fermentation process of cheongkukjang preparation. A *Bacillus* species identified as *Bacillus* sp. LM7 that was shown to be a wild-type bacterium was shown to produce the broad spectrum antimicrobial lipopeptide(s) that inhibited pathogenic bacteria and fungi (Lee et al., 2016). The preservative properties of the lipopeptide may be important for the safety profile of traditionally made cheongkukjang since other fermented soy foods typically have a high salt content that helps control the growth of pathogenic bacteria. The authors also suggested that the lipopeptides from cheongkukjang might have value as a preservative for other natural products.

6.4.7 Vitamins K and B$_{12}$

Although cheongkukjang is rich in numerous essential nutrients, two vitamins stand out as more unique to fermented soy products, especially cheongkukjang. Vitamin K is produced as a product of bacterial fermentation and is often difficult to find in adequate amounts in many diets. Wu et al.

(2014) demonstrated that both vitamin K_2 and equal amounts of vitamin K_2 in cheongkukjang protected ovariectomized rats against bone mineral loss. Furthermore, cheongkukjang with doses standardized to equivalent doses of vitamin K was significantly more effective at maintaining femur bone mineral density than was isolated vitamin K_2 (menaquinone-7), suggesting that either the vitamin K from cheongkukjang is more effective or that it acts synergistically with other components of cheongkukjang.

Cheongkukjang and some other fermented foods may contain vitamin B_{12}. A report by Kwak et al. (2010) investigated why very old Koreans (centenarians) had better than expected vitamin B_{12} status compared to their Western counterparts, who consume many more animal products and would be expected to have consumed more vitamin B_{12}. They reported that low but relevant amounts of the vitamin were present in traditional fermented foods and seaweed and supplied roughly 30% of the vitamin B_{12} intake in that population. There were insufficient amounts to fully meet vitamin B_{12} requirements in the foods; nevertheless, if it can be confirmed that vitamin B_{12} is present in the amounts reported, fermented foods like cheongkukjang would be an important new source of vitamin B_{12} for those people who do not consume animal foods.

6.4.8 Cheongkukjang as a Whole Food

Although it is important to examine the functionalities of the bioactive compounds in cheongkukjang, it is normally consumed as a whole food. Freeze-dried cheongkukjang was shown to have profound antidiabetic effects at 5% of the diet in C75BL/KsJ-db/db mice (Kim et al., 2008). The cheongkukjang significantly lowered blood glucose and glycosylated hemoglobin and improved insulin sensitivity. However, fermentation of soybeans increases the concentrations of some bioactive compounds at the expense of others. Chai et al. (2012) showed that, with increasing fermentation time, the antioxidant capacity of soybean foods increased but estrogenic activity decreased. The decreased estrogenic activity was probably due to the loss of isoflavones over time and would suggest that cheongkukjang (short-term fermented soybeans) would be the preferable fermented product for helping such conditions as menopausal symptoms and osteoporosis. However, human studies are required to confirm specific benefits in people.

6.4.9 Human Research

Most of the human research evaluating the health-promoting properties of cheongkukjang has focused on metabolic effects such as obesity and diabetes. A clinical trial (Back et al., 2013; Byun et al., 2016) in young Korean adults (men and women, ages 19–29) who were overweight or obese by Korean standards (BMI > 23 kg/m^2 or waist circumferences over 80 or 90 cm for men and women) was conducted. This was a randomized, double-blind, placebo-controlled crossover study with 120 subjects at the beginning. Each subject was give 35 g of freeze-dried 24 h fermented cheongkukjang pills or an isocaloric placebo per day for 12 weeks and then crossed over after a washout period. Female, but not male, subjects taking cheongkukjang in the study had decreased body fat percentage, waist circumference, and waist-to-hip circumference, as well as increased lean body mass. Women also had lower C-reactive protein levels after consuming cheongkukjang, indicating chronic inflammation was suppressed. Most factors related to cardiovascular health and blood sugar regulation were not affected by cheongkukjang, which might have been due to the relatively young population, which had mostly normal levels at the beginning of the study.

In another 12-week study, 26 g/day of cheongkukjang or placebo for 12 weeks was given to 60 subjects aged 19–65 (Back et al., 2011). The subjects were evaluated for fat loss by computerized tomography (CT), and blood parameters and pressure were measured. The apolipoprotein-B concentration was lower in the cheongkukjang group after 12 weeks, but there were no other significant differences. However, there was a tendency for the cheongkukjang-supplemented group to have less visceral fat as measured by the CT scans. It seems likely that the two studies were of insufficient duration to adequately assess the effects of long-term use of cheongkukjang as a food, and they are suggestive of possible metabolic benefits, especially for weight loss.

Another study evaluated the effects of cheongkukjang with or without red ginseng on plasma lipids and fasting glucose (Shin et al., 2011). Forty-five subjects were divided into three groups of 15 subjects each and took either 2 g of starch placebo or 20 g of dried cheongkukjang with or without added ginseng for 8 weeks. In general, the cheongkukjang appeared to be similarly effective with or without ginseng, although the cheongkukjang alone seemed to be more effective for lowering fasting blood glucose. Cheongkukjang significantly lowered total cholesterol, apoliporotein-B, erythrocyte thiobarbituric acid-reactive substances (TBARS), and fasting blood glucose.

An epidemiological study by Park and Bae (2016) using Korean NHANES data also demonstrated possible anti-inflammatory activity of fermented foods including cheongkukjang. In their study, high consumption of fermented foods including cheongkukjang was associated with almost half the risk of atopic dermatitis after adjusting for possible confounders.

Taken together, the available human studies are highly suggestive that cheongkukjang can help prevent or reverse obesity, lower atherosclerotic risk factors, improve blood sugar regulation, and suppress inflammation. However, much of the data shows only modest effects, possibly due to the short durations of the studies. Larger long-term studies are needed to evaluate the putative effects of cheongkukjang on metabolic disorders and obesity.

6.5 Conclusions on Health Benefits of Cheongkukjang

Although the reductionist approach to studying health benefits of single bioactive compounds in cheongkukjang is important, there are numerous compounds produced during fermentation that may have additive or synergistic effects, as well as antagonistic effects. Synergistic or additive effects might include the combined action of isoflavones and vitamin K2 for preventing or treating osteoporosis. However, competing effects could include the immunostimulatory effects of polysaccharides in cheongkukjang. which appear to be proinflammatory but may be offset by anti-inflammatory effects of γ-PGA, isoflavones, and peptides. Therefore, more human trials using whole cheongkukjang as a food are needed to evaluate the overall effects of consuming cheongkukjang in humans. Although cheongkukjang has many potential health benefits (Table 6.5), the research to date would suggest that the major overall effects of cheongkukjang would be to reduce chronic inflammation and possibly to improve glucose metabolism and help maintain normal body weight.

TABLE 6.5

Potential Medicinal Functions of Cheongkukjang and Its Compounds

Function	Bioactive Compounds	Research Models	Ref.
Anticancer	PGA	Mice	Kim, T.W. et al., 2007
	Peptide (lunasin)	Human prostate cells	Galvez et al., 2011a
Immunostimulatory	PGA	Mice	Kim, T.W. et al., 2007
	Isoflavones	Human immune cells	Moon et al., 2012
	Polysaccharides	Macrophages	Choi et al., 2014
			Cho et al., 2015
Antiviral (swine flu)	PGA	Mice	Kim et al., 2015
Anti-inflammatory	PGA	Human colorectal cells	Shin et al., 2015
	Isoflavones	Mice (dermatitis)	Lee et al., 2014a
	Peptides	Mice (ear edema)	Choi et al., 2008
		Rats	Lee et al., 2014b
Bone loss	PGA	Human	Tanimoto et al., 2007
	Vitamin K	Rats	Wu et al., 2014
Antidiabetic	Isoflavones	Rats	Kwon et al., 2007
	Chungkookjang	MIN-6 cells	Yang et al., 2013
		Mice	Kim et al., 2008
Antithrombotic	Enzyme	Fibrin plate	Jeong et al., 2015
Antimicrobial	Lipoprotein	Bacterial and fungal cultures	Lee et al., 2016
Obesity	Chungkookjang	Humans	Byun et al., 2016
Dyslipidemia	Chungkookjang	Humans	Shin et al., 2009

Note: PGA = poly-γ-glutamic acid.

References

Back, H.I., K.C. Ha, H.M. Kim et al. 2013. The influence of the Korean traditional cheonggukjang on variables of metabolic syndrome in overweight/obese subjects: Study protocol. *BMC Complement Altern Med* 13:297.

Back, H.I., S.R. Kim, J.A. Yang, M.G Kim, S.W. Chae, and Y.S. Cha. 2011. Effects of cheonggukjang supplementation on obesity and atherosclerotic indices in overweight/obese subjects: A 12-week, randomized, double-blind, placebo-controlled clinical trial. *J Med Food* 14:532–537.

Bae, M.J., H.S. Shin, H.J. See, O.H. Chai, and D.H. Shon. 2014. Cheonggukjang ethanol extracts inhibit a murine allergic asthma via suppression of mast cell-dependent anaphylactic reactions. *J Med Food* 17:142–149.

Bae, S.R., C. Park, J.C. Choi, H. Poo, C.J. Kim, and M.H. Sung. 2010. Effects of ultra high molecular weight poly-gamma-glutamic acid from *Bacillus subtilis* (cheonggukjang) on corneal wound healing. *J Microbiol Biotechnol* 20: 803–808.

Byun, M.S., O.K. Yu, Y.S. Cha, and T.S. Park. 2016. Korean traditional cheonggukjang improves body composition, lipid profiles and atherogenic indices in overweight/obese subjects: A double-blind, randomized, crossover, placebo-controlled clinical trial. *Eur J Clin Nutr* 70:1116–1122.

Chai, C., Ju, H.K., Kim, S.C. et al. 2012. Determination of bioactive compounds in fermented soybean products using GC/MS and further investigation of correlation of their bioactivities. *J Chromatogr B Analyt Technol Biomed Life Sci* 880:42–49.

Chettri, R., and J.P. Tamang. 2015. *Bacillus* species isolated from tungrymbai and bekang, naturally fermented soybean foods of India. *Int J Food Microbiol* 197:72–76.

Cho, C.W., C.J. Han, Y.K. Rhee et al. 2015. Cheonggukjang polysaccharides enhance immune activities and prevent cyclophosphamide-induced immunosuppression. *Int J Biol Macromol* 72:519–525.

Choi, J.C., H. Uyama, C.H. Lee, and M.H. Sung. 2015. *In vivo* hair growth promotion effects of ultra-high molecular weight poly-γ-glutamic acid from *Bacillus subtilis* (cheonggukjang). *J Microbiol Biotechnol* 25:407–412.

Choi, J.H., M.J. Chung, D.Y. Jeong, and D.H. Oh. 2014. Immunostimulatory activity of isoflavone-glycosides and ethanol extract from a fermented soybean product in human primary immune cells. *J Med Food* 17:1113–1121.

Choi, Y.H., H. Lim, M.Y. Heo, D.Y. Kwon, and H.P. Kim. 2008. Anti-inflammatory activity of the ethanol extract of chungkukjang, Korean fermented bean: 5-lipoxygenase inhibition. *J Med Food* 11:539–543.

Dastmalchi, M. and S. Dhaubhadel. 2015. Proteomic insights into synthesis of isoflavonoids in soybean seeds. *Proteomics* 15:1646–1657.

Galvez, A.F., N. Chen, J. Macasieb, and B.O. de Lumen. 2001a. Chemopreventive property of a soybean peptide (lunasin) that binds to deacetylated histones and inhibits acetylation. *Cancer Res* 61:7473–7478.

Galvez, A.F., L. Huang, M.M. Magbanua, K. Dawson, and R.L. Rodriguez. 2011b. Differential expression of thrombospondin (THBS1) in tumorigenic and non-tumorigenic prostate epithelial cells in response to a chromatin-binding soy peptide. *Nutr Cancer* 63:623–636.

Ghaemi, A., H. Soleimanjahi, S. Razeghi et al. 2012. Genistein induces a protective immunomodulatory effect in a mouse model of cervical cancer. *Iran J Immunol* 9:119–127.

Han, B.Z., F.M. Rombouts, and M.J. Nout. 2001. A Chinese fermented soybean food. *Int J Food Microbiol* 65:1–10.

Hong, S.W., J.Y. Choi, and K.S. Chung. 2012. Culture-based and denaturing gradient gel electrophoresis analysis of the bacterial community from cheonggukjang, a traditional Korean fermented soybean food. *J Food Sci* 77:M572–578.

Jang, C.H., J.K. Lim, J.H. Kim et al. 2006. Change of isoflavone content during manufacturing of Cheonggukjang, a traditional Korean fermented soyfood. *Food Sci Biotechnol* 15:643–646.

Jeon, Y.H., M.S. Kwak, M.H. Sung, S.H. Kim, M.H. Kim, and M.J. Chang. 2013. High-molecular-weight poly-gamma-glutamate protects against hypertriglyceridemic effects of a high-fructose diet in rat. *J Microbiol Biotech* 23:785–793.

Jeong, S.J., K. Heo, J.Y. Park et al. 2015. Characterization of AprE176, a fibrinolytic enzyme from *Bacillus subtilis* HK176. *J Microbiol Biotechnol* 25:89–97.

Kada, S., A. Ishikawa, Y. Ohshima, and K. Yoshida. 2013. Alkaline serine protease AprE plays an essential role in poly-γ-glutamate production during natto fermentation. *Biosci Biotechnol Biochem* 77:802–809.

Kim, D.J., Y.J. Jeong, J.H. Kwon et al. 2008. Beneficial effect of chungkukjang on regulating blood glucose and pancreatic beta-cell functions in C75BL/KsJ-db/db mice. *J Med Food* 11:215–223.

Kim, E.H., Y.K. Choi, C.J. Kim, M.H. Sung, and H. Poo. 2015. Intranasal administration of poly-gamma glutamate induced antiviral activity and protective immune responses against H1N1 influenza-A virus infection. *Virol J* 12:160.

Kim, H.B., H.S. Lee, S.J. Kim et al. 2007a. Ethanol extract of fermented soybean, cheonggukjang, inhibits the apoptosis of mouse spleen, and thymus cells. *J Microbiol* 4:256–261.

Kim, J.S., J.H. Lee, J. Surh, S.A. Kang, and K.H. Jang. 2016. Aglycone isoflavones and exopolysaccharides produced by *Lactobacillus acidophilus* in fermented soybean paste. *Prev Nutr Food Sci* 21:117–123.

Kim, T.W., T.Y. Lee, H.C. Bae et al. 2007b. Oral administration of high molecular mass poly-gamma-glutamate induces NK cell-mediated antitumor immunity. *J Immunol* 179:775–780.

King, R.A., J.L. Broadbent, and R.J. Head. 1996. Absorption and excretion of the soy isoflavone genistein in rats. *J Nutr* 126:176–182.

Kwak, C.S., M.S. Lee, S.I. Oh, and S.C. Park. 2010. Discovery of novel sources of vitamin B_{12} in traditional Korean foods from nutritional surveys of centenarians. *Curr Gerontol Geriatr Res* 2010:374897.

Kwon, D.Y., J.W. Daily, H.J. Kim, and S. Park. 2010. Antidiabetic effects of fermented soybean products on type 2 diabetes. *Nutr Res* 30:1–13.

Kwon, D.Y., J.S. Jang, S.M. Hong et al. 2007. Long-term consumption of fermented soybean-derived cheonggukjang enhances insulinotropic action unlike soybeans in 90% pancreatectomized diabetic rats. *Eur J Nutr* 46:44–52.

Kwon, D.Y., J.S. Jang, J.E. Lee, Y.S. Kim, D.H. Shin, and S. Park. 2006. The isoflavonoid aglycone-rich fractions of cheonggukjang, fermented unsalted soybeans, enhance insulin signaling and peroxisome proliferator-activated receptor-gamma activity *in vitro*. *Biofactors* 26:245–258.

Kwon, G.H., Lee, H.A., Park, J.Y. et al. 2009. Development of a RAPD-PCR method for identification of Bacillus species isolated from Cheonggukjang. *Int J Food Microbiol* 129:282–287.

Lee, M.H., J. Lee, Y.D. Nam, J.S. Lee, M.J. Seo, and S.H. Yi. 2016. Characterization of antimicrobial lipopeptides produced by *Bacillus* sp. LM7 isolated from cheonggukjang, a Korean traditional fermented soybean food. *Int J Food Microbiol* 16:12–18.

Lee, S.J., H.K. Rim, J.Y. Jung et al. 2013. Immunostimulatory activity of polysaccharides from cheonggukjang. *Food Chem Toxicol* 59:476–484.

Lee, T.Y., D.J. Kim, J.N. Won, I.H. Lee, M.H. Sung, and H. Poo. 2014a. Oral administration of poly-γ-glutamate ameliorates atopic dermatitis in Nc/Nga mice by suppressing Th2-biased immune response and production of IL-17A. *J Invest Dermatol* 134:704–711.

Lee, W.H., H.M. Wu, C.G. Lee, I.H. Lee, M.H. Sung, and H. Poo. 2014b. Specific oligopeptides in fermented soybean extract inhibit NF-κB-dependent iNOS and cytokine induction by toll-like receptor ligands. *J Med Food* 17:1239–1246.

Moon, H.J., J.S. Lee, Y.K. Choi et al. 2012. Induction of type I interferon by high-molecular poly-γ-glutamate protects B6.A2G-Mx1 mice against influenza A virus. *Antiviral Res* 94:98–102.

Murphy, P.A., K. Barua, and C.C. Hauck. 2002. Solvent extraction selection in the determination of isoflavones in soy foods. *J Chromatogr B Analyt Technol Biomed Life Sci* 777:129–138.

Park, M.K., H.I. Choi, D.Y. Kwon, and Y.S. Kim. 2007. Study of volatile organic acids in freeze-dried cheonggukjang formed during fermentation using SPME and stable-isotope dilution assay (SIDA). *Food Chem* 105:1276–1280.

Park, S. and J.H. Bae. 2016. Fermented food intake is associated with a reduced likelihood of atopic dermatitis in an adult population (Korean National Health and Nutrition Examination Survey 2012–2013). *Nutr Res* 36:125–133.

Park, S., D.S. Kim, S. Kang, and B.R. Moon. 2016. Fermented soybeans, cheonggukjang, prevent hippocampal cell death and β-cell apoptosis by decreasing proinflammatory cytokines in gerbils with transient artery occlusion. *Exp Biol Med* 241:296–307.

Shin, E.J., M.J. Sung, J.H. Park et al. 2015. Poly-γ-glutamic acid induces apoptosis via reduction of COX-2 expression in TPA-induced HT-29 human colorectal cancer cells. *Int J Mol Sci* 16:7577–7586.

Shin, S.K., J.H. Kwon, Y.J. Jeong, S.M. Jeon, J.Y. Choi, and M.S. Choi. 2011. Supplementation of cheonggukjang and red ginseng cheonggukjang can improve plasma lipid profile and fasting blood glucose concentration in subjects with impaired fasting glucose. *J Med Food* 14:108–113.

Tanimoto, H., T. Fox, J. Eagles et al. 2007. Acute effect of poly-gamma-glutamic acid on calcium absorption in post-menopausal women. *J Am Coll Nutr* 26:645–649.

Wu, W.J., H.Y. Lee, G.H. Lee, H.J. Chae, and B.Y. Ahn. 2014. The antiosteoporotic effects of cheonggukjang containing vitamin K2 (menaquinone-7) in ovariectomized rats. *J Med Food* 17:1298–1305.

Yang, H.J., D.Y. Kwon, H.J. Kim et al. 2015. Fermenting soybeans with *Bacillus licheniformis* potentiates their capacity to improve cognitive function and glucose homeostasis in diabetic rats with experimental Alzheimer's type dementia. *Eur J Nutr* 54:77–88.

Yang, H.J., D.Y. Kwon, and N.R. Moon. 2013. Soybean fermentation with *Bacillus licheniformis* increases insulin sensitizing and insulinotropic activity. *Food Funct* 4:1675–1684.

Yang, H.J., S. Park, V. Pak, K.R. Chung, and D.Y. Kwon. 2011. Fermented soybean products and their bioactive compounds. *Soybeans Health* 2:21–58.

Yang, L.C., J.B. Wu, G.H. Ho, S.C. Yang, Y.P. Huang, and W.C. Lin. 2008. Effects of poly-gamma-glutamic acid on calcium absorption in rats. *Biosci Biotechnol Biochem* 72:3084–3090.

Yang, S.O., M.S. Kim, K.H. Liu et al. 2009. Classification of fermented soybean paste during fermentation by 1H nuclear magnetic resonance spectroscopy and principal component analysis. *Biosci Biotechnol Biochem* 73:502–507.

Zubik, L., and M. Meydani. 2003. Bioavailability of soybean isoflavones from aglycone and glucoside forms in American women. *Am J Clin Nutr* 77:1459–1465.

7

Biological Functions and Traditional Therapeutic Uses of Kochujang (Red Pepper Paste)

Dae Young Kwon and Soon-Hee Kim

CONTENTS

7.1 Introduction 165
7.2 History and Tradition 166
7.3 Production Methods 169
7.4 Nutritional and Functional Effects 172
     7.4.1 Medicinal Effects of Kochujang Written in Literature 172
     7.4.2 Biological Functions 172
          7.4.2.1 Nutritional and Functional Components 173
          7.4.2.2 Functionality of Red Pepper and Capsaicin 173
          7.4.2.3 Functionality of Kochujang 174
7.5 Conclusion 178
References 179

7.1 Introduction

Korean cuisine is characterized by a complete meal setting of rice, kuk, kimchi, banchan, and jang on the table, which is in contrast to the courses served in Western styles of food (Kim et al., 2016). Jang is an essential component of Korean food and is produced through fermentation. Although jang is frequently used as an ingredient, it is often served on its own. Doenjang, kochujang (or gochujang), kanjang and jeotgal are examples of jang that take a few months of fermentation to produce (Shin and Jeong, 2015; Koo et al., 2016). Most types of jang, except for jeotgal, are fermented bean products. Jang can be used as a major ingredient in kuk and chigae and as a condiment with fresh vegetables, sashimi, cooked fish, shellfish, and meat. In addition, jang is used as a seasoning to balance the salt concentration (kan) of food (Jang et al., 2016). The majority of Korean foods are seasoned with jang rather than salt, because jang is made from fermented beans and thus contains rich amino acids and volatile aromatic compounds that enhance the smell and flavors of food (Shin and Jeong, 2015). As jang is used in most kuk and banchan, many have stated that jang decides the flavor of a food.

Kochujang is a fermented and aged bean product made from soybean powder, red pepper powder, and rice flour (Shin and Jeong, 2015), and is used as a seasoning in kuk and banchan, or as a condiment itself. Kochujang is one of the most frequently consumed foods by Koreans. According to the 2015 National Nutrition Survey conducted by the Korea Health Industry Development Institute, kochujang was ranked as the 14th most frequently consumed food in Korea (KHIDI, 2015). The reported average daily intake of kochujang was 6.11 g; it was the second-most consumed seasoning after kanjang (KHIDI, 2015). The *Heobaekjeongjip*, a book written in the fifteenth century by Gwidal Hong (1438–1504), stated that "the quality of kochujang decides the farming success of that year." This statement demonstrates the importance of jang in Korean food beyond its nutritional value (Hur, fifteenth century). Although many regions have traditionally made kochujang, the most famous region is Sunchang. Generally, kochujang produced in Sunchang is the highest selling product in Korea. The outstanding flavor and functional effects of Sunchang kochujang are due to the geographical characteristics that provide a congenial climate for fermentation and a great environment for growing high-quality red peppers.

7.2 History and Tradition

Kochujang has more than thousand years long history (Kwon et al., 2017). The oldest written reference to kochujang is found in the *Hyangyak-jipsongbang*, a Korean medical book that listed medicinal herbs for doctors, published in 1433 during the 15th year of the reign of King Sejong in the Chosun dynasty (Figure 7.1). This book refers to kochujang or gochojang as chojang, and gochu as gocho or gochu (Kwon et al., 1433). However, the early references to kochujang are primarily focused on its medicinal properties rather than its role as a food additive. For example, kochujang was often used to promote digestive issues caused by weaknesses in the spleen and stomach (Cham, 850; Chun, 1460).

In the "Yangrobongchinseo" chapter of *Hyangyak-jipsongbang*, a porridge made with carp, rice, tangerine peels, green onions, and kochujang was recommended for elderly people who suffered from loss of appetite or dysentery (Kwon et al., 1433). Chojang and chosi (fermented soybean products used to make kochujang) were introduced in a Korean medical encyclopedia called the *Uibangyuchi* (1445, in the 27th year of King Sejong) (Han et al., 1445). The book recommended a dish made with kochujang and rice (hwangjagyegogi; similar to modern Korean spicy chicken stew) for elderly people with weak spleens and stomachs (Han et al., 1445). These records show that kochujang was used to improve appetites, recover strength, and promote digestion. According to the *Siknyochanyo* (1460; 4th year of King Sejo; Figure 7.2)

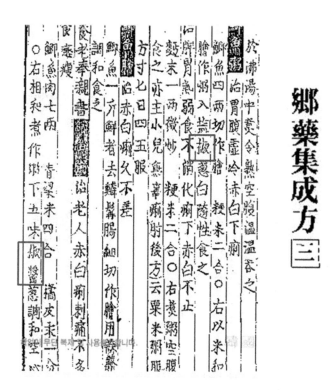

FIGURE 7.1
The first written reference to kochujang. *Hyangyak-jipsongbang* (1443), a medical book published in the 15th year of the reign of King Sejong, suggested kochujang carp stew to improve spleen and stomach functions for those suffering from loss of appetite or digestion dysfunction.

(Chun, 1460), written by royal physician Sunui Jun, and *Uirimchwalyo* (Yang, sixteenth century), written by Yesu Yang, spicy carp porridge and hwangja-gyetang made with kochujang and chicken were effective in improving cold symptoms, diarrhea, and weakness. The *Sauikyeongheombang*, a medical book written by four doctors, also detailed the efficacy of kochujang and red peppers based on their experiences (Lee et al., seventeenth century).

Although most of the old references only mentioned the medicinal usage of kochujang, it is believed that kochujang was also enjoyed as a food earlier than the first relevant record appeared because food records were generally made when a food had therapeutic effects or when it caused illness, which contrasts with the current tendency of having interest in food itself or for a recipe. *Siksanjip*, published by Manbu Lee (1664–1731) and written 200 years after the *Sauikyeongheombang*, stated, "We made fragrant alcohol and kochujang to pour over the hearse like a stream during the funeral" (Lee, eighteenth century). *Bukheonjip*, written by Chuntaek Kim (1670–1717), recorded that "he encouraged me to have a drink during the meal with kochujang, ginger, and kimchi" (Kim, eighteenth century). These are the first records

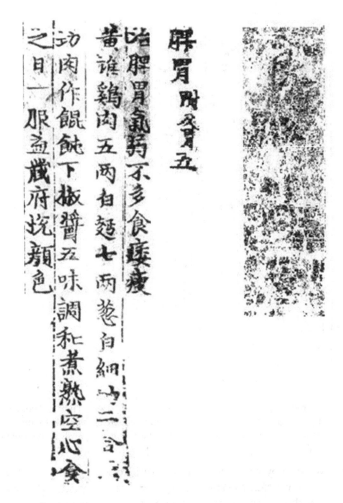

FIGURE 7.2
A written record of kochujang used for therapeutic purposes. *Siknyo-chanyo* said that kochujang helps to relieve the symptoms of nausea, lack of digestion, etc.

of kochujang as a food and demonstrate the consumption of kochujang in daily diets and on special occasions.

Kochujang was also widely enjoyed by the royal family. According to oral traditions, King Taejo Sungkye Lee tasted kochujang at the Manil temple in Sunchang with a Buddhist monk name Muhak before he founded Chosun. Not being able to forget the taste of kochujang, he asked for it to be sent as an offering to the royal palace. If this tradition is true, it may have been the reason why kochujang, especially Sunchang kochujang, was enjoyed by the Chosun royal family. The *Seungjeongwonilgi* (25th year of King Yeongjo, July 24, 27th year; May 18; and 33rd year May 7; records of the king's commands and his interactions with officials, written on a daily basis by Seungjeongwon, the royal secretariat during the Chosun dynasty) mentioned that kochujang was served to King Yeongjo and that he enjoyed it and that some officials had recommended kochujang to the king (Anonymous, 1799). The *Naegakilryeok* (a diary recorded on September 19, 1781) included in the *Kyujangkakilgi* (records of the king's commands and affairs of the royal palace, written on a daily basis by Kyujangkak) stated that "vegetables, fruits, and kochujang were prepared," which shows that kochujang was central banchan for Koreans at this time (Anonymous, 1781).

As it was with the royal family, kochujang was also a popular food product with ordinary citizens. A war diary titled *Yanghouseonbongilgi* (1894) from the Donghak Peasant Revolution, which began in 1894 and was initiated by citizens in response to corrupt officials and social turmoil, listed kochujang and kimchi as military supplies (Anonymous, 1894). The inclusion of kochujang on this list demonstrates its role and importance in being valued as highly as kimchi in the diets of citizens (Chung, 2016).

Kochujang was also cited as the most missed food by Koreans living abroad. In the *Byeolkeongon* (1928), Yugyeong stated that he missed kimchi and kochujang the most while in a foreign country (You, 1928). "The Shade of a Willow Tree," an essay on August by Kwanbin Ok published in *Dongkwang* (1931), a monthly magazine from the time of the Japanese occupation, also mentioned that "one spoon of kochujang brings the fragrance of the clear water in my hometown" (Ok, 1931). These records imply that kochujang had become an indispensable and representative item in Korean cuisine.

7.3 Production Methods

One of the major ingredients of kochujang is kochujang meju, which is made from cooked soybeans and nonglutinous rice with a 6:4 ratio. This mixture is then woven with straw and dried for 2–3 months. The manufacturing process of kochujang meju is shown in Figure 7.3. Kochujang is made from meju powder mixed with malt, salt, rice flour, and red pepper powder (Shin and Jeong, 2015). The typical recipe for kochujang is 25% red pepper powder, 22.2% glutinous rice, 5.5% meju powder, 12.8% salt, 5% malt, and 29% water.

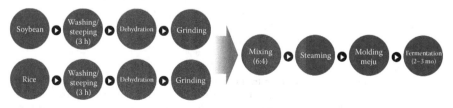

FIGURE 7.3
Manufacturing process of kochujang meju.

Once these ingredients are mixed and placed in a crock, it takes approximately 6 months to a year for fermentation to occur (Shin and Jeong, 2015). The manufacturing process of kochujang is shown in Figure 7.4. During the process, the microorganisms present in the mixture are simplified over time; they receive protein from the soybeans and carbohydrates from the rice (Shin et al., 2011). During fermentation, the microorganisms break down these proteins and starches. It has been reported that *Firmicutes* are most abundant in kochujang in bacteria phylum level, and as a family *Bacillaceae* make up the majority of the population (Figure 7.5) (Nam et al., 2012; MIFI, 2016). *Candida*

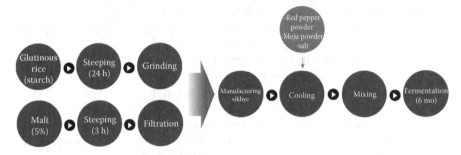

FIGURE 7.4
Typical manufacturing process of traditional kochujang.

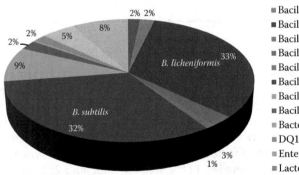

FIGURE 7.5
The distribution of microorganisms in traditional kochujang. The effects of the microorganisms found in kochujang produced in Jeonbuk areas were observed through pyrosequencing of the 16s rRNA gene (MIFI, 2016). As kochujang produced by traditional methods uses natural microorganisms present in ingredients and external environmental conditions, bacterial distribution of kochujang can vary.

and *Zygosaccharomyces* are rich in kochujang among yeasts (Lee et al., 1996; Jang, 2011). These are different from the dominant fungi and yeast found in meju in which *Aspergillus* spp. and *Rhizopus* spp. are most abundant. These findings demonstrate the change in microbial composition during fermentation.

According to historical references, the methods used to produce kochujang have not changed much over time. The first written description of how to produce kochujang is "Sunchang gochojangjobeop," found in the *Somunsaseol*, published by Sipil Lee (1700). It described a dried powdered mixture of boiled soybeans, baekseolgi (steamed white rice cake), red pepper powder, malt, and glutinous rice as the main ingredients of kochujang. This recipe is not much different from the modern recipe, except for the addition of abalone, large shrimp, and mussels. This difference is believed to have occurred because it was an offering to the king. The *Jeungbosallimkyeongje*, written by Jungrim Yu, explained not only the typical production methods but also the characteristics of the ingredients and useful tips (You, 1766). (In this book, Jungrim Yu did not refer to gocho as cho or gocho, but as mancho, a term used in China when describing red peppers from Taiwan and Indonesia.) When making kochujang meju, salt can be used as a seasoning, but high-quality cheongjang can also be used, because it improves the flavor of the kochujang; pan-fried sesame seeds can be added but can taste stale. Too much glutinous rice flour can cause sourness and red pepper powder should be added carefully. Strained tofu that is made from 1 mal (Korean unit of measurement) of soybeans can be added with other ingredients; dried kelp or fish, especially herring, can enhance the flavors of kochujang.

Although traditional methods have been used to produce kochujang, modified commercial methods for the mass industrial production of kochujang having uniform quality in a shortened processing time. The main difference between commercial and traditional methods is that the former uses koji instead of kochujang meju (Kwon et al., 2014). Koji is prepared by inoculating 0.1% *Aspergillus oryzae* in steamed and cooled wheat flour and then fermenting at 35°C for 40–48 h. In addition, commercially produced kochujang mainly has wheat flour or nonglutinous rice instead of glutinous rice as the grain ingredient and is sweetened using starch syrup rather than saccharified grain such as malt. The mixture of koji, steamed rice or wheat flour, red pepper powder, and starter culture is ripened by fermentation at room temperature for 16–60 days. Commercial production of kochujang is completed by adding starch syrup, sterilizing at 85°C for 10 min, and packaging.

Taken together, the main difference between traditional and modified commercially produced kochujang is the fermentation method—that is, the type of microorganisms used: natural diverse microorganisms in the former or a few selective seed microorganisms in the latter. Because of the combined fermentation by the different microorganisms used, the traditional kochujang not only has various flavors but also yields varying fermentation products with time. However, the modified commercially produced kochujang can maintain uniform quality and shows few changes in quality over time; fermentation products are also not relatively complicated. In recent years, traditional kochujang has been preferred because of its rich flavor and various functional ingredients produced by natural fermentation. Therefore, efforts have been made to improve the quality of commercial kochujang similar to that of traditional kochujang as well as to shorten the processing time.

7.4 Nutritional and Functional Effects

7.4.1 Medicinal Effects of Kochujang Written in Literature

As mentioned earlier, records about kochujang written in *Hyangyakjipsongbang* (1443), *Uibangyuchi* (1445), *Sikryochanyo* (1460), *Uirimchwalyo*, and *Sauikyeongheombang* explained the use of kochujang as a medicinal food because, at that time, food records were generally made when a food had an extraordinary functional effect (i.e., medicinal effects) and oriental medicine basically considered eating a healthy food as a kind of therapy (Chung, 2016). These records strongly suggest that kochujang has apparent efficacy to improve health. Specifically, they said that kochujang helps to promote digestive issues caused by weaknesses in the spleen and stomach. They mainly focused on physical movement of digestive organs because detailed molecular biology might not have been known at that time. The efficacy of kochujang can be agreed upon nowadays and the hot spiciness of kochujang is responsible for this. As well as appetite- and digestion-promoting effects, kochujang was used to relieve the symptoms of vomiting and diarrhea (Noh, 1826). Also, it was written that the tang boiled kochujang with carp porridge or chicken is effective in restoring strength from the overall sense of energy deprivation (Chun, 1460). It was even reported kochujang was pasted on the area of a boil after acupuncture treatment (Uihwi 1871; Byun et al., 1898). Furthermore, the book *Sujinkyungheomsinbang* (Lee, 1913) states that people will get better by taking kochujang tea when they are undergoing back pain. Korean people have eaten kochujang for a thousand years for its good taste and to maintain the body by improving dynamic behavior of the gut and intestine with development of fermentation technology in terms of food treatment. Inevitably, biotechnology-based sciences will be necessary to obtain evidence for these functions and to evaluate the written literature.

7.4.2 Biological Functions

In recent days many efforts have been conducted to study the biological functions of kochujang based on the old literature in terms of animal tests and human intervention tests. Meanwhile, the present lifestyle, food resources, and medical environment are different from those in the past. In the past, food resources were not abundant, and thus excessive calorie intake was not a problem. Further, eating well was important because medicines had not been developed. When diseases occurred, patients lost their appetite and could not eat well; hence, their immunity was lowered and the illness often worsened. Therefore, in the past, the functionality of kochujang was regarded as important for health, because it contributed remarkably to nutrition by promoting appetite and food intake and stimulating the digestive tract to help improve digestion.

However, in modern society, overnutrition has become a more serious problem than nutritional deficiency. Infectious diseases, which were a major health problem in the past, have been largely overcome by the development of therapeutic agents. Thus, the present situation has changed remarkably from the past, when an increase in the immunity of patients via the recovery of the general health condition was considered essential. Chronic diseases such as obesity, diabetes, and cardiovascular diseases caused by excessive nutrition are emerging as the major health problems. Recent studies on the effectiveness of kochujang have mainly focused on the prevention and treatment of metabolic diseases such as obesity and diabetes; they have revealed that kochujang has anticancer and analgesic effects. Therefore, this chapter focuses on the effects of kochujang on the improvement of obesity and metabolic diseases.

7.4.2.1 Nutritional and Functional Components

Kochujang consists of 44.6% water, 43.8% carbohydrates, 4.9% protein, and 1.1% fat. In every 100 g of kochujang, there are 178 kcal, 822 mg of potassium, and 408 mg of vitamin A (National Standard Nutritional database). Major bioactive compounds in chili pepper are carotenoids, capsaicinoids, and flavonoids. In addition, vitamin C is abundant in chili (1.2 mg/g) and all these compounds have the antioxidant property (Shaha et al., 2013). As for the quantity, carotenoids are more abundant than capsaicinoids such as capsaicin and dihydrocapsaicin (carotenoids, 1.1 mg/g; capsaicinoids, 550 μg/g of chili) (Al Othman et al., 2011; Shaha et al., 2013). However, capsaicin has been most intensively studied among the functional components in chili, perhaps because it is responsible for the pungency, the uniqueness of chili.

7.4.2.2 Functionality of Red Pepper and Capsaicin

As red pepper powder makes up 25% of kochujang, the health benefits of kochujang can be associated with capsaicin, the main component of red pepper powder. It has been reported that 100 g of kochujang contains 5 mg of capsaicin. (Ham et al., 2012). The representative biological function of capsaicin is related to metabolic syndrome, except for pain relief and anticancer activity.

Antiobesity effect of capsaicin: Capsaicin stimulates hormone-sensitive lipase (HSL) via its receptor—transient receptor potential cation channel subfamily V member 1 (TRPV1)—to increase lipolysis, which degrades triglycerides (TGs) stored in the adipocytes (Lee et al., 2011; Chen et al., 2015). Capsaicin also promotes thermogenesis by increasing the expression of uncoupling protein 2 (UCP2), which dissipates energy into heat and promotes the consumption of stored energy (Lee et al., 2011; McCarty et al., 2015). In addition, in muscle cells, capsaicin activates AMP-activated protein kinase (AMPK) to increase the expression of carnitine palmitoyltransferase 1α (CPT1α), which is a rate-limiting enzyme for the transfer of fatty acids to the mitochondria, thereby facilitating β-oxidation (Lee et al., 2011). These functions of capsaicin promote fatty acid oxidation in the muscle cells, thereby increasing energy expenditure. In conclusion, capsaicin decomposes the stored fat into fatty acids and promotes the consumption of the degraded fatty acid, thereby improving obesity.

Antidiabetic effect of capsaicin: On the other hand, capsaicin increases insulin sensitivity by decreasing blood glucose and insulin levels in both fed and fasted states (Ahuja et al., 2006; Chaiyasit et al., 2009). Several studies reported that capsaicin activates AMPK, which is a master regulator to facilitate glucose uptake and fatty acid oxidation (Joo et al., 2010; Kang et al., 2011). Indeed, capsaicin stimulated the glucose uptake through AMPK activation in muscle cell lines (Kim et al., 2013).

Functionality of red pepper: Although conducting *in vitro* and in animal studies to determine the efficacy of foods is considered adequate, investigating the effects directly in human subjects is more reasonable. A total of 487,000 adults aged 30 years or older from China were surveyed for 5 years to determine the relationship between the intake of red peppers and the risk of death. According to this study, people who ingested red pepper six to seven times a week had a significantly lower total mortality rate than those who consumed less pepper (hazard ratio [HR]: 0.82–0.86; HR values varied according to the conditions of the multivariate models) (Lv et al., 2015). In addition, those who consumed red peppers six to seven times a week had lower mortality from ischemic heart disease (HR: 0.73–0.78), diabetes mellitus (HR: 0.59–0.82), and respiratory illness (HR: 0.57–0.71). However, mortality from cancer, cerebrovascular diseases, and infectious diseases was not found to be associated with red pepper intake. Some studies have shown that consumption of excessively spicy foods such as red pepper increases the incidence of gastric cancer (Lopez-Carrillo et al., 1994). However, according to the large Chinese cohort study conducted by Lv et al. (2015), cancer mortality was 0.95 (95% CI, 0.88–1.03) in people who consumed spicy foods six to seven times a week. In other words, no difference was found in the incidence of cancer between people who consumed more red pepper and those who consumed less pepper.

7.4.2.3 Functionality of Kochujang

Among the ingredients of kochujang, red pepper powder is present in the largest portion, and its pungent taste provides a unique feature to kochuang different from other kinds of soybean-fermented jangs. Therefore, capsaicin, a bioactive component of red pepper powder, might likely be responsible for the functionality of kochujang. However, kochujang also has other ingredients,

Biological Functions and Traditional Therapeutic Uses of Kochujang

such as meju powder obtained from soybean, besides red pepper powder. Further, since the fermentation of microorganisms causes the enzymatic degradation of components and produces various fermentation products, there is a difference in composition of ingredients themselves and kochujang.

Therefore, here we introduce the results of evaluating the efficacy of kochujang itself. Thus far, kochujang has been shown to be associated with the improvement of metabolic diseases such as obesity, diabetes, and hyperlipidemia. This is similar to the functionality of capsaicin.

Antiobesity effect of kochujang: In a high-fat-diet-induced obese model, rats fed a diet containing 10% freeze-dried kochujang powder showed reduced body weight, epididymal adipose tissue, and liver weight by 14%, 17%, and 60%, respectively, compared with those of the control group, without toxicity and any change of dietary intake (Shin et al., 2016). The adipocyte size and serum leptin level also significantly decreased in the kochujang-fed rats. The activities of fatty acid synthase (FAS) or glucose-6-phosphate dehydrogenase (G6PDH) in the liver and adipose tissue, which are involved in lipid synthesis and accumulation, were reduced by the intake of kochujang. These results suggest that kochujang reduces obesity by inhibiting fat accumulation in the adipose tissue and liver (Shin et al., 2016).

In another study of pancreatectomized diabetic rats, rats that were provided a high-fat diet including 5% freeze-dried kochujang for 8 weeks showed 20% weight loss, decreased serum leptin levels, and reduced adipose fat tissue (Kwon et al., 2009). Similar results were obtained in an *in vitro* experiment in which 3T3-L1 adipocytes were treated with 1 mg/mL of kochujang extract; the expression of genes involved in fat accumulation such as peroxisome proliferator-activated receptor gamma (PPARγ), CCAAT/enhancer-binding protein alpha (C/EBPα), and sterol-regulatory element-binding protein 1c (SREBP-1c) was significantly suppressed. Intracellular lipid content also decreased after kochujang treatment (Ahn et al., 2006; Kong and Park, 2008). Therefore, the leptin secretion level, which is known to be proportional to the intracellular fat content, also decreased after treatment with kochujang. In addition, the activity of hormone-sensitive lipase (HSL), which contributes to TG breakdown, increased after treatment with kochujang, which might also contribute to weight loss (Ahn et al., 2006).

Preventive effect on metabolic diseases by kochujang: Excess energy is accumulated in the adipocytes as a form of TG, and if the capacity of the adipocytes is exceeded, fat overflows into the blood and accumulates in the nonadipose tissue such as the liver or muscle (Gregor and Hotamisligil, 2011). This interferes with insulin signal transduction, resulting in abnormal function and insulin resistance. Because this series of actions is mutually influential, disorders such as obesity, hyperlipidemia, fatty liver, and insulin resistance occur almost simultaneously. Therefore, when obesity is reduced, hyperlipidemia and insulin resistance are also often improved. Ingestion of kochujang not only reduced fat accumulation in the adipose tissue and liver, but also reduced the levels of TG and low-density lipoprotein cholesterol (LDL-C) in the blood by about 30% and 37%, respectively, in high-fat diet-induced obese rats (Shin et al., 2016). In another study on obese mice fed a high-fat diet, kochujang intake significantly decreased serum total cholesterol and LDL-C levels, along with a reduction of body and fat tissue weight and blood glucose level (Koo et al., 2008). This might be because kochujang lowered the expression of acetyl-CoA carboxylase, which is involved in lipid synthesis, and increased the expression of acyl-CoA synthase, CPT-1, and UCP1, which are related to lipid oxidation, thereby lowering fat synthesis and promoting energy consumption (Figure 7.6) (Koo et al., 2008).

Kochujang has been shown to improve hyperlipidemia in human as well as animal studies. Sixty overweight men and women with a BMI ≥ 23 kg/m^2 and a waist–hip ratio (WHR) ≥ 0.90 for men and ≥ 0.85 for women were provided with 32 g/day of kochujang for 12 weeks. This resulted in a 6% reduction of visceral fat as measured by CT scans, a 16% reduction of serum triglyceride, and a 20% reduction of ApoB (p < 0.05) (Figure 7.7), although subject weight and WHR remained unchanged (Cha et al., 2013). When 30 hyperlipidemic subjects (110–190 mg/dL LDL-C or 200–260 mg/dL total cholesterol) were given 34.5 g/day of kochujang for 12 weeks, their total cholesterol and LDL-C were reduced by 10% and 15%, respectively (p < 0.01) (Lim et al., 2015).

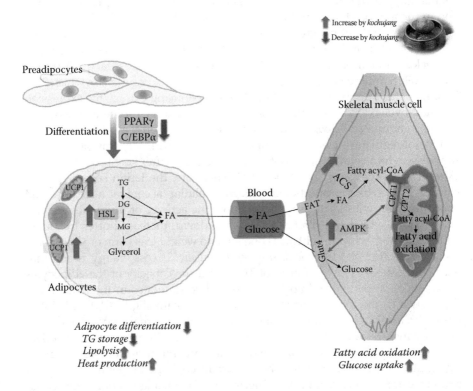

FIGURE 7.6
Functional mechanisms involved in anti-obesity effect of kochujang. Kochujang lowers gene expression involved in lipid synthesis and increases gene expression related to lipid oxidation, thereby lowering fat synthesis and promoting energy consumption.

Biological Functions and Traditional Therapeutic Uses of Kochujang

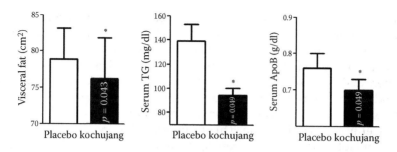

FIGURE 7.7
Improvement of visceral fat and blood lipid levels by kochujang intake. Sixty overweight men and women were provided with 32 g/day of kochujang for 12 weeks. Visceral fat areas were measured by CT scans. (From Cha, Y.S. et al. 2013, *Nutrition and Metabolism (London)* 10:24.)

Taken together, the experimental results for kochujang itself showed that it is mainly effective in metabolic diseases such as obesity, diabetes, and hyperlipidemia. Capsaicin is presumed to contribute to the efficacy of kochujang. In fact, when the effect of mixed raw materials of kochujang was compared with that of fermented aged kochujang, the mixed sample also induced adipose tissue weight loss and lowered serum LDL-C levels. However, feeding of kochujang was more effective in reducing body weight, blood leptin, and TG levels, and accumulated lipid content in the adipose and liver tissues compared with the mixed raw materials of kochujang (Figure 7.8) (Shin et al., 2016).

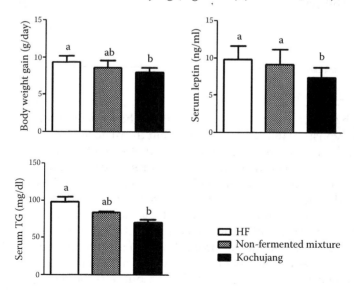

FIGURE 7.8
Comparison of efficacy between fermented kochujang and nonfermented kochujang. Sprague–Dawley rats were fed high-fat diets containing 10% nonfermented mixtures of raw materials or 10% fermented kochujang for 5 weeks. Values are expressed as mean ± SE of rats ($n = 8$ for each group). (From Shin, H.W. et al. 2016, *Journal of Food Science Technology* 53:1004–1013.)

In addition, leptin secretion levels decreased with increasing fermentation time of kochujang (Kong and Park, 2008). The inhibitory effect of kochujang on cancer cell proliferation was also found to increase with the fermentation period (data not shown; Kim et al., 2005). Meanwhile, meju powder, which makes up 5% of kochujang, is rich in isoflavonoids, such as daidzin and genistin from soybeans. During the fermentation process, microorganisms transform daidzin and genistin into daidzein and genistein by eliminating glucoside. This transformation increases the bioavailability of isoflavone and, as a result, the *in vivo* efficacy (Shin et al., 2016). Taken together, these results suggest that various fermented products by microorganisms, as well as capsaicin and meju powder, increase the functionality of kochujang, although capsaicin plays an important role in its functionality.

In recent years, efforts have been made continually to increase the taste and functionality of kochujang by evaluating its sensory, physicochemical, and functional properties depending on the changes in raw materials and fermenting microorganisms. For example, the addition of freeze-dried garlic powder to kochujang further decreased the production of PPARγ, C/EBPα, SREBP-1c, tumor necrosis factor-α, and leptin, implying that garlic-containing kochujang has greater inhibitory efficacy in adipocyte differentiation and lipogenesis (Kong and Park, 2008). Further studies on kochujang that have more scientific basis and improved functionality might improve its applicability.

7.5 Conclusion

Although direct references to kochujang have been found since the Chosun dynasty (1400s), it is assumed that the history of kochujang is longer than the written record, considering that a length of time is required for changes in food culture and that Koreans have used jang and red peppers for a long time. In Korean cuisine, kochujang is used as a seasoning in kuk and banchan and as a condiment for vegetables, fish, shellfish, and meat. Kochujang is an essential part of the Korean diet and has become one of the most frequently consumed foods. Kochujang is also known for its therapeutic effects, such as promoting appetite and the health of digestive organs. In addition, kochujang has been shown to reduce abdominal fat and blood lipid levels in animals and humans. Sunchang kochujang has been the most popular kochujang product since the Chosun dynasty, as mentioned in multiple historical sources. Sunchang kochujang is still widely enjoyed for its high-quality flavor, fragrance, and color.

References

Ahn, I.S., M.S. Do, S.O. Kim et al. 2006. Antiobesity effect of kochujang (Korean fermented red pepper paste) extract in 3T3-L1 adipocytes. *Journal of Medicine and Food* 9:15–21.

Ahuja, K.D., I.K. Robertson, D.P. Geraghty, and M.J. Ball. 2006. Effects of chili consumption on postprandial glucose, insulin, and energy metabolism. *American Journal of Clinical Nutrition* 84:63–69.

Al Othman, Z.A., Y.B. Ahmed, M.A. Habila, and A.A. Ghafar. 2011. Determination of capsaicin and dihydrocapsaicin in *Capsicum* fruit samples using high performance liquid chromatography. *Molecules* 16:8919–8929.

Anonymous. 1781. *Naegakilryeok*. Korea.

Anonymous. 1799. *Seungjungwon-ilki* (Diary of King Chosun Royal Secretariat). Korea.

Anonymous. 1894. *Yanghouseonbongilgi*. Korea.

Byun, S.C., M.K. Byun, and J.K. Byun. 1898. *Bongnam-ilg*. Korea.

Cha, Y.S., S.R. Kim, J.A. Yang et al. 2013. Kochujang, fermented soybean-based red pepper paste, decreases visceral fat and improves blood lipid profiles in overweight adults. *Nutrition and Metabolism (London)* 10:24.

Chaiyasit, K., W. Khovidhunkit, and S. Wittayalertpanya. 2009. Pharmacokinetics and the effect of capsaicin in *Capsicum frutescens* on decreasing plasma glucose level. *Journal of Medical Association of Thailand* 92:108–113.

Cham, E. 850. *Sikui-simgam*. Book for alimentotherapists. China.

Chen, J., L. Li, Y. Li et al. 2015. Activation of TRPV1 channel by dietary capsaicin improves visceral fat remodeling through connexin43-mediated Ca2+ influx. *Cardiovascular Diabetology* 14:22.

Chun, S.E. 1460. *Siknyo-chanyo*. Korea.

Chung, K.R. 2016. Effects of Kochujang in old Korean Documents. *Journal of Korean Contents Society* 9:55–622.

Gregor, M.F., and G.S. Hotamisligil. 2011. Inflammatory mechanisms in obesity. *Annual Review of Immunology* 29:415–445.

Ham, H., M. Sung, Y. Kim et al. 2012. Determination of capsaicinoids in selected commercial pepper powders and pepper-containing products using HPLC and method validation. *Journal of Korean Society of Food Science and Nutrition* 41:870–874.

Han, K.H., W.J. Yim, and C. Kwon. 1445. *Euibangyuchi*. Korea.

Hur, B.J., Heo, B.J. Fifteenth century. *Heobaekjeongjip*. Korea.

Jang, D., A. Lee, S. Kang, S. Lee, and D. Kwon. 2016. Does siwonhan-mat represent delicious in Korean foods? *Journal of Ethnic Foods* 3:159–162.

Jang, S.J., Y.J. Kim, J. M. Park, and Y.S. Park. 2011. Analysis of microflora in *Gochujang*, Korean traditional fermented food. *Food Science and Biotechnology* 20:1435–4140.

Joo, J.I., D.H. Kim, J.W. Choi, and J.W. Yun. 2010. Proteomic analysis for antiobesity potential of capsaicin on white adipose tissue in rats fed with a high-fat diet. *Journal of Proteome Research* 9:2977–2987.

Kang, J.H., G. Tsuyoshi, H. Le Ngoc et al. 2011. Dietary capsaicin attenuates metabolic dysregulation in genetically obese diabetic mice. *Journal of Medicine and Food* 14:310–315.

KHIDI. 2015. *2015 Korea National Health and Nutrition Examination Survey*. Korea: Korea Health Industry Development Institue

Kim, C.T. Eighteenth century. *Bukheonjip*. Korea.

Kim, S.H., J.T. Hwang, H.S. Park, D.Y. Kwon, and M.S. Kim. 2013. Capsaicin stimulates glucose uptake in C2C12 muscle cells via the reactive oxygen species (ROS)/AMPK/p38 MAPK pathway. *Biochemical and Biophysics Research Communications* 439:66–70.

Kim, S.H., M.S. Kim, M.S. Lee et al. 2016. Korean diet: Characteristics and historical background. *Journal of Ethnic Foods* 3:26–31.

Kim, S.O., C.S. Kong, J.H. Kim et al. 2005. Fermented wheat grain products and kochujang inhibit the growth of AGS human gastric adenocarcinoma cells. *Journal of Food Science and Nutrition* 10:349–352.

Kong, C.S., and K.Y. Park. 2008. Antiobesity effect of garlic-added kochujang in 3T3-L1 adipocytes *Journal of Food Science and Nutrition* 13:66–70.

Koo, B., S.H. Seong, D.Y. Kown, H.S. Sohn, and Y.S. Cha. 2008. Fermented kochujang supplement shows antiobesity effects by controlling lipid metabolism in C57BL/6J mice fed high fat diet. *Food Science and Biotechnology* 17:336–342.

Koo, O., S. Lee, K. Chung et al. 2016. Korean traditional fermented fish products: Jeotgal. *Journal of Ethnic Foods* 3:107–116.

Kwon, C., H.T. Yu, J. Roh, and Y. Park. 1433. *Hyangyak-jipsongbang*, (vol. 3). Korea.

Kwon, D.Y., K.R. Chung, and H.J. Yang. 2017. *The Truth of Birth and Propagation of Korean Red Pepper(Kochu)*. Seoul: FreeAcademy Press.

Kwon, D.Y., S.M. Hong, I.S. Ahn et al. 2009. Kochujang, a Korean fermented red pepper plus soybean paste, improves glucose homeostasis in 90% pancreatectomized diabetic rats. *Nutrition* 25:790–799.

Kwon, D.Y., D.J. Jang, H.J. Yang, and K.R. Chung. 2014. History of Korean gochu, gochujang, and kimchi. *Journal of Ethnic Foods* 1:3–7.

Lee, I.J. 1913. *Sujinkyungheomsinbang*. Korea.

Lee, J.M., J.J., Oh, N.S., and Han, M.S. 1996. Bacterial distribution of kochujang. *Korean Journal of Food Science and Technology* 28:260–266.

Lee, M.B. Eighteenth century. *Siksanjip*. Korea.

Lee, M.S., C.T. Kim, I.H. Kim, and Y. Kim. 2011. Effects of capsaicin on lipid catabolism in 3T3-L1 adipocytes. *Phytother Res* 25:935–939.

Lee, S.H., D.K. Chae, R. Park, and Y. Hur. Seventeenth century. *Sauikyeongheombang*. Korea.

Lee, S.P. 1700. *Somunsaseol*. Korea.

Lim, J.H., E.S. Jung, E.K. Choi et al. 2015. Supplementation with *Aspergillus oryzae*-fermented kochujang lowers serum cholesterol in subjects with hyperlipidemia. *Clinical Nutrition* 34:383–387.

Lopez-Carrillo, L., M. Hernandez Avila, and R. Dubrow. 1994. Chili pepper consumption and gastric cancer in Mexico: A case-control study. *American Journal of Epidemiology* 139:263–271.

Lv, J., L. Qi, C. Yu et al. 2015. Consumption of spicy foods and total and cause specific mortality: Population based cohort study. *British Medical Journal* 351:h3942.

McCarty, M.F., J.J. DiNicolantonio, and J.H. O'Keefe. 2015. Capsaicin may have important potential for promoting vascular and metabolic health. *Open Heart* 2:e000262.

MIFI. 2016. Annual report on the study of strategy for industrialization of K-GRAS. Seoul: Microbial Institute for Fermentation Industry.

Nam, Y.D., S.L. Park, and S.I. Lim. 2012. Microbial composition of the Korean traditional food "kochujang" analyzed by a massive sequencing technique. *Journal of Food Science* 77:M250–256.

National standard nutritional database. Agro-Food Integrated Information System. National Institute of Agricultural Sciences (http://koreanfood.rda.go.kr/kfi /fct/fctFoodSrch/list).

Noh, S.C. 1826. *Nohsangchu-ilgi*. King Sunjo 26th year, August Korea.

Ok, K.B. 1931. The shade of a willow tree. *Dongkwang* 24.

Shaha, R.K., S. Rahman, and A. Asrul. 2013. Bioactive compounds in chilli peppers (*Capsicum annuum* L.) at various ripening (green, yellow and red) stages. *Annals of Biological Research* 4:27–34.

Shin, D.H., and D. Jeong. 2015. Korean traditional fermented soybean products: Jang. *Journal of Ethnic Foods* 2:2–7.

Shin, D.H., D.Y. Kwon, Y.S. Kim, and D.Y. Jung. 2011. *Science and technology of Gochujang*. Seoul: Health Edu.

Shin, H.W., E.S. Jang, B.S. Moon et al. 2016. Anti-obesity effects of gochujang products prepared using rice koji and soybean meju in rats. *Journal of Food Science Technology* 53:1004–1013.

Uihwi. 1871. *Keumrisanin*. Korea.

Yang, Y.S. Sixteenth century. *Uirimchwalyo*. Korea.

You, J. 1766. *Jeungbosallimkyeongje*. Korea.

You, K. 1928. *Byeolkeongon*. 12:148–149.

8

Jeotgal (Fermented Fish): Secret of Korean Seasonings

Ok Kyung Koo and Young Myoung Kim

CONTENTS

8.1 Introduction 183
8.2 History 185
8.3 Classification 187
    8.3.1 Classification by Main Ingredients 188
    8.3.2 Classification by Seasoning 189
        8.3.2.1 Kimchi and Jeotgals 191
    8.3.3 Regional Jeotgals 192
        8.3.3.1 Regional Jeotgals by Main Ingredients 192
        8.3.3.2 Regional Jeotgal Recipes 194
8.4 Composition 195
    8.4.1 General Composition 195
        8.4.1.1 Amino Acids 196
        8.4.1.2 Nucleotides 197
        8.4.1.3 Fatty Acids 197
        8.4.1.4 Flavor Compounds 199
    8.4.2 Microbial Ecology 199
        8.4.2.1 Microflora 199
        8.4.2.2 Microbial Community during Fermentation 200
        8.4.2.3 Microorganisms 204
8.5 Health Benefits 205
8.6 Conclusion 208
References 209

8.1 Introduction

Food technology has been developed based on the strong demand for the consumption of safe, tasty, and healthy food (Kim et al., 2016). People have developed their own unique ways to preserve food products in good condition and the most prevalent method has been through fermentation, the addition of salt, and dehydration for reducing water activity to protect food against the growth of spoilage and pathogenic microorganisms. Fermented foods have been produced using beans, fish, and meat, which were referred to as jang, in the Orient (Choi, 2012). Jang made with beans is dujang (doenjang in Chapter 5), with fish, is eojang, and with meat is yukjang (Choi, 2012). Eojang, which is now commonly called jeotgal, is a traditional fermented fish food in Korea, produced from the whole meat and/or internal organs of fish and shellfish (Figure 8.1). Fish and shellfish are highly perishable due to the high moisture content and nutritive elements such as protein and fat for the growth of spoilage microorganisms (Park et al., 1997). Therefore, jeotgal has been produced using salt and fermentation to avoid deterioration from spoilage, autolysis, and microbial activities and to enhance the preservation. The process also enhances jeotgal with its own unique umami flavor from the production of free amino acids and the decomposition of adenosine triphosphate (ATP) to hypoxanthine (Lee et al., 1987). The salt concentration, fermentation, and curing conditions such as temperature and time can be the major extrinsic factors affecting the quality of jeotgal (Kim, 2014; Kim et al., 2016).

The development of jeotgal in Korean cuisine has been closely connected to grain-based main dishes, especially rice. Since traditional Korean food was based on vegetables and grains, animal protein sources were significantly limited (Jo, 2010). In addition, carbohydrates in rice need sodium ion for digestion and absorption in the small intestine, so salted food such as

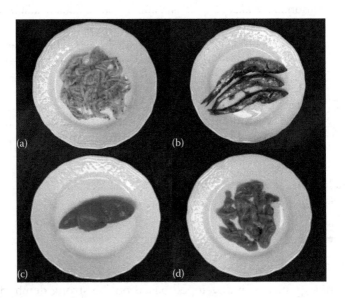

FIGURE 8.1
Jeotgals produced with whole fish: (a) Saeu-jeot (small shrimp) and (b) myeolchi-jeot (anchovy); jeotgals produced with the internal parts of fish: (c) myeongran-jeot (roe from pollack) and (d) changnan-jeot (intestine of pollack). (Modified from Koo, O.K. et al. 2016. *J Ethn Foods* 3(2):107–116. With permission.)

jeotgal has been a great source to support nutrition. Fermented jeotgal also provides rich flavor to enhance the taste of rice and to ease chewing and swallowing it (Jo, 2010). Jeotgal is also rich in proteases and lipases to assist the digestion of meat proteins so that saeu-jeot (small shrimp) has been used as dipping sauce for broiled pig's feet (jokbal), and blood/noodle sausages (sundae). Jeotgal has also been used as folk remedies for digestive problems by consuming persimmon, meat, and other foods. Jeotgal has been used as an important condiment for substituting salt or soy sauce in Korean style stews (chigae) (Kim et al., 2016), or improving flavor of kimchi or infants' food (Kim, 2014).

Fermented fish foods have been produced in various ways across Asia, Europe, South America, Africa, and other countries: fish, fish sauce, fish paste, and other types of food. Fermented fish products include anchovies from the Mediterranean countries and South America, bagoong from the Philippines, and guedj from Senegal (Tanasupawat and Visessanguan, 2014). Liquid types of fish sauces are aekjeot from Korea (Mheen, 1993), shotssuru from Japan (Itoh et al., 1993), nuoc-man from Vietnam (Kim, 2014), hakarl from northern Europe (Skåra et al., 2015), and Worcestershire sauce from England and others (Ricke et al., 2013). Fish pastes include prahok from Cambodia, shrimp paste from China, and padaek from Laos and others (Ricke et al., 2013). Since Asian countries mainly consume rice, these types of fermented fish foods are consumed as protein sources or condiments in Korea, while Europeans consume them as condiments (Thapa, 2016).

Jeotgal is an important part of Korean cuisine because of its nutritional value, healthful effects on digestion and appetite, and beneficial microorganisms. In this chapter, we introduce the historical and cultural background of jeotgal; classify jeotgal by main ingredients, types, and regions; discuss the microbiology of jeotgal and main composition of jeotgal for flavor; and show the high added nutritional value and beneficial effects of the Korean fermented fish food.

8.2 History

It is still unknown when jeotgal was first produced in Korea since no clear documentation has been found. The history of jeotgal was reviewed in detail by Koo et al. (2016), and it is summarized in this chapter.

The first document on jeotgal was discovered in historical Chinese literature—Sigyung (551–477 BCE) (Anonymous, 3000–2500 BCE) and Lyeki (Anonymous, 500 BCE–1 CE)—that were written in Han dynasty (202 BCE–CE 220). This literature is the bible of Confucianism, describing the courtesy observed during the Zhou dynasty (1046–256 BCE). In this document, jeotgal was written as "hae," while later it was written as "ja," as shown in Figure 8.2.

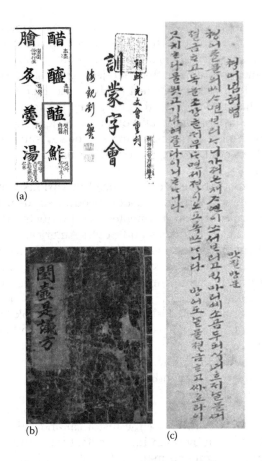

FIGURE 8.2
Ancient literature from the Orient that mentioned jeotgal: (a) jeot written in Chinese characters by Choi (1527); (b) book cover of food-dimibang; (c) the recipe of chongeo-jeot (herring) written inside the *Eumsik-dimibang* by Jang, 1670. (Modified from Koo, O.K. et al. 2016. *J Ethn Foods* 3(2):107–116. With permission.)

This was its first description as Korean food introduced by *Cheminyosul* (CE 532), the oldest Chinese agriculture technology handbook (Ka, 532). Ja was prepared by fish that was salted and wrapped in lotus leaves, influenced by the Kokuryu (37 BCE–CE 668) or Baekje (18 BCE–CE 660) dynasty (Ka, 532).

The first literature written in Korea was *Samkuksaki*, the history of the Kokuryu, Backje, and Shilla dynasties, which stated that jeotgal was served at the royal wedding for King Sinmun (CE 681–692) of the Shilla dynasty (Kim, 683). This record showed the apparent evidence of thousands of years of jeotgal history that was clearly described in historical Korean literature. Ever since, numbers of documents have introduced jeotgal in the Chosun

Jeotgal (Fermented Fish) 187

dynasty, which occurred after the three dynasties, and then the Koryo dynasty. In the literature, jeotgal was not only prepared with fish but also with other types of meat, such as pork, rabbit, or venison, and consumed with kimchi (Han, 2010).

Jeotgal was also used as one of the cruel execution methods used in the Koryo dynasty, described as "like making a person into jeotgal," which was introduced in the Koryosa (history of the Koryo dynasty) and the Koryosajeolyo (brief history of the Koryo dynasty) (Kim and Jung, 1451; Kim, 1452). The *Sallimkyongje*, an agriculture and life guidebook written by Mansun Hong in the eighteenth century, introduced the recipe of saeu-jeot (small shrimp) and recommended adding the saeu-jeot to soup with meat, fish, or tofu (Hong, 1700). Jeotgal was served on special occasions such as royal court ceremonies, ancestral rites, and parties. In these cases, fermented meat and fish were both served: rabbit-jeot, venison-jeot, pork-jeot, and fish-jeot (Lee, 1540; Anonymous, 1697).

The *Siuijonseo*, a cookbook written in the late 1890s, exclusively illustrated the recipes of the various types of fermented fish products that are mostly consumed today (Anonymous, 1890), although fermented meat products were not introduced in this cookbook. Based on the literature, fermented fish products were more popular with the common people, while fermented meat products were consumed on special occasions by the royal family. Meat such as livestock cattle (beef, beef tripe, beef heart), pork (pork meat, pork rind), deer, lamb, and rabbit, and birds, including sparrows, were used. Bamboo shoots, eggs, and duck eggs were also found in the literature to have been used as jeotgal (Lee and Lee, 1989). Jeotgal currently refers only to fermented fish products.

8.3 Classification

According to Suh and Yoon (1987), there are about 145 species reported as jeotgal and they can be classified by the main ingredients, processing methods, and processing regions in Korea. Any fresh fish, mollusks, and crustaceans can be used to make jeotgal, and it is generally named after the main ingredients. There are about 87 species of whole fish, 32 species of crustaceans, 14 species of Pelecypoda or Gastropoda, 10 species of cephalopods, and 2 species of sea cucumbers or sea urchins (Suh and Yoon, 1987). Table 8.1 summarizes some of the popular jeotgals in Korea; they are separated by the types of main ingredients. As shown in Table 8.1, specific parts of the fish, such as intestine, roe, and gills are also used to produce jeotgal and, depending on the parts of fish, there are 118 species of flesh or whole body, 15 species of intestine, and 12 species of roe (Suh and Yoon, 1987).

188　　　　　　　　　　　　　　　　　　　　　*Korean Functional Foods*

TABLE 8.1

Classification of Jeotgals Based on the Main Ingredients

Types of Main Ingredients	Jeotgal Name (Main Ingredients)
Fish	
Whole fish	Myeolchi-jeot (anchovy), baendaengi-jeot (herring), jeoneo-jeot (gizzard shad), junchi-jeot (Chinese herring), kalchi-jeot (cutlassfish), choki-jeot (croaker), whangseokeo-jeot (yellow corvina), godeungeo-jeot (mackerel), kanari-jeot (sand eel), mineo-jeot (croacker), domi-jeot (sea bream), byungeo-jeot (pomfret), kajami-jeot (flatfish), kongchi-jeot (saury), dongtae-jeot (frozen pollack), bangeo-jeot (icefish)
Intestine	Changnan-jeot (pollack), haesam-changja-jeot (sea cucumber), kodeungeo-changja-jeot (mackerel), kalchi-sok-jeot (cutlass), chuneobam-jeot (gizzard shad), jogi-sok-jeot (yellow corvina), jeoneobam-jeot (stomach of gizzard shad)
Roe	Myeong-ran-jeot (pollack), gea-jeot (crab), taegu-al-jeot (cod), saeu-al-jeot (small shrimp), sungeo-al-jeot (mullet), yuneo-al-jeot (salmon)
Gills	Taegu-agami-jeot (cod), mineo-agami-jeot (croaker), myeongtae-agami-jeot (pollack), jogi-agami-jeot (yellow corvina)
Mollusks	
Pelecypoda	Kul-jeot (oyster), eorikul-jeot (oyster with hot pepper), bajirak-jeot (clam), jogae-jeot (shellfish), dongjuk-jeot (surf clam), daehap-jeot (clam), mat-jeot (razor clam), moshijogae-jeot (short necked clam), baekhap-jeot (large clam), honghap-jeot (mussel), junbok-naejang-jeot (ear shell), garibi-jeot (scallop), kijogae-jeot (pen shell)
Gastropoda	Obunjaki-jeot (supertexta), kolbangi-jeot (sea snail), sora-jeot (conch)
Cephalopods	Ojingeo-jeot (squid), koltuki-jeot (small squid), mooneo-jeot (octopus), nakji-jeot (small octopus), hanchi-jeot (cuttlefish)
Crustaceans	
Shrimp	Saeu-jeot (small shrimp), gonjangii-jeot (mysidacea), daeha-jeot (jumbo shrimp), toha-jeot (freshwater shrimp), choon-jeot (spring shrimp), chu-jeot (fall shrimp), o-jeot (May shrimp), yuk-jeot (June shrimp), ja-jeot (July shrimp), baekha-jeot (winter)
Crab	Ge-jeot (crab), tulge-jeot (hairy crab), bangke-jeot (three-spined shore crab), kotge-jang (blue crab), dolge-jang (stone crab), chamge-jeot (Chinese mitten crab)
Others	
	Gaebul-jeot (spoon worm), meongge-jeot (sea squirt), haesam-changja-jeot (sea cucumber), sungge-jeot (sea urchin)

Source: This table is modified from Koo, O. K. et al. 2016. *J Ethn Foods* 3(2):107–116.

8.3.1 Classification by Main Ingredients

Myeolchi-jeot produced with anchovy and saeu-jeot made with small shrimp are the most popular jeotgals consumed in Korea. Myeolchi-jeot production starts with washing fresh anchovies, draining them, and then salting by alternately layering anchovy and salt. Qualified refined salt with

Jeotgal (Fermented Fish)

a concentration of 20% to 30% is used and fermented for 2 to 3 months depending on the salt concentration and temperature (Lee and Choe, 1974). There are number of different kinds of saeu-jeot depending on the harvest season. Shrimp harvested and produced during spring are called choon-jeot and those harvested in autumn are called chu-jeot. This nomenclature applies the same to myeolchi-jeot (Song and Ahn, 2009). It is also called o-jeot, yuk-jeot, or ja-jeot depending on whether the harvest takes place in May, June, or July, respectively. To produce jeotgal, a salt concentration that is higher by 35% to 40% in summer and about 30% in winter is required for saeu-jeot since the hardness of the shell makes it difficult for salt to infuse into the meat. After washing with sea water or 3% to 4% of salted water, fresh shrimp is mixed with salt and stored for 4 to 5 months at 13°C to 20°C (Park et al., 1997).

Gills are rich in calcium and about 15% to 20% of refined salt is mixed with washed gills and fermented for up to 3 months. Since it takes a relatively long time for salt infusion into gills, other ingredients such as red pepper are added to maximize the salt infusion (Kim and Kim, 2014). For jeotgal production using roe and intestine, the whole part should be taken in order to realize the quality and unique texture and flavor.

Other special types of jeotgals are hongeo and gulbi. Hongeo is fermented skate that has a very unique and strongly pungent odor and taste by the conversion of urea to ammonia in skate during fermentation. Hongeo is served as a main dish rather than condiment and it contains high concentrations of glutamic acid (14.7%), aspartic acid (9.59%), and essential fatty acids (22.8%) such as linoleic acid, linolenic acid, and arachidonic acid (Kim and Jang, 2015). This jeotgal is highly preserved due to the ammonia limiting growth of microorganisms (Kim and Jang, 2015).

8.3.2 Classification by Seasoning

The most popular and traditional jeotgal is produced by simply adding salt and fermenting for certain periods as summarized in Figure 8.3 (Ka, 532; Anonymous, 1890; Lee et al., 2004). However, other seasonings have also been added to jeotgal to enhance the flavor, to induce the salt infusion into the main ingredients, or even to inhibit the fishy flavor during the fermentation. There are two types of seasoned jeotgal: spices are added to the fermented fish product or the seasoned fish is fermented (Figure 8.3). Fermentation of the seasoned fish is more common. Seasonings added for fermentation include honey, red pepper powder, shredded red pepper, black pepper, oil, anchovy fish sauce, akane, and others. Other subingredients are also added before fermentation: grains such as millet, rice, glutinous rice, and flour; vegetables such as radish, pepper, red-pepper leaf, and cucumber; fruits and nuts such as chestnut, pear, dates, and pine nuts; and others including kelp, rice-rinsed water, and water (Lee and Lee, 1989). Spices that are added after the fermentation process include green onions, garlic, ginger, red pepper

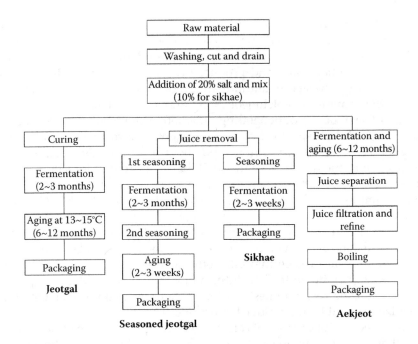

FIGURE 8.3
Production flow of jeotgal, seasoned jeotgal, sikhae, and aekjeot. (Modified from Lee, S.B. et al. 2004. *Fundamentals of food fermentation*. Hyoil. ISBN 89-8489-016-2.)

powder, shredded red peppers, sesame, green peppers, black pepper powder, vinegar, red chili-pepper paste with vinegar, oil, and others (Lee and Lee, 1989).

Eorikul-jeot (oyster) is one of the most popular seasoned jeotgals; red pepper, garlic, ginger, relish, scallion and others are added (Kwon et al., 2014). Kul-jeot is an oyster jeotgal without any seasonings but 20% of salt and is fermented for about 1 month (Kwon et al., 2014). The fermentation period is shorter for oyster than for other ingredients since oyster contains high levels of glycogen (Kwon et al., 2014).

Jeotgals that are produced with mollusks, including ojingeo-jeot (squid), nakji-jeot (small octopus), and others, also use seasonings such as red pepper, garlic, ginger, syrup, and others. They are prepared by removing the organs and bones (Jang, 1670; Lee, 1809; Anonymous, 1890). Other types of seasoned jeotgals are changnan-jeot (pollack) and myeongran-jeot (pollack). Changnan-jeot has a unique chewy texture since it is made with intestines of pollack. This jeotgal is seasoned with red pepper, ginger, sesame, scallion, and sesame oil. Myeongran-jeot is manufactured with the roe of pollack and the seasonings include red pepper, garlic, ginger, sesame, and sugar (Kim and Kim, 1991). In order to provide more clear and uniform color to the roe, natural coloring agents are incorporated in the jeotgal; some common

Jeotgal (Fermented Fish) 191

examples are red monad, annatto, ß-carotene, and red beet (Kim and Kim, 1991).

Sikhae is manufactured by fermentation of fish that is salted and mixed with cooked grains to produce lactic acid and reduce the pH to increase the preservability (Figure 8.3). A relatively low concentration of refined salt is added to fish—about 5% to 10%, which is incorporated with cooked grains including rice, glutinous rice, and flour, and seasonings such as red pepper and malt, and radish (Park et al., 1997). Depending on the region, about eight different combinations of cooked grains and seasoning produce sikhae (Rhee et al., 2011). The main ingredients are mostly low-fat and white plain fish such as flat fish, pollack, red tongue sole, rockfish, squid, and others. Due to the low sodium content, sikhae should be consumed within 2 weeks and kept under refrigerated conditions (Kim, 2008; Rhee et al., 2011). Kajami-sikhae is made with flat fish and it is the most popular sikhae. Five to ten percent of refined salt is added to flat fish and left for about 1 day. Then the seasonings are added with 20% to 50% w/w and the fish is cured for up to 2 weeks. Because of the low sodium concentration, it should be consumed within 1 to 2 weeks and only produced during fall and winter (Park et al., 1997).

Aekjeot is a fermented fish sauce in which the liquid is separated from jeotgal (Figure 8.3). It is produced by 25% salt and over a 1-year fermentation period, which is much longer than that for jeotgal. It is a popular seasoning or pickling to provide umami flavor for kimchi or salads. Any fish can be used to make aekjeot and sand lance and anchovy are commonly used.

8.3.2.1 Kimchi and Jeotgals

Jeotgals have been most frequently used as seasonings for kimchi; however, they are also used as seasonings in other cuisine, condiments, and side dishes for alcohol. Myeolchi-jeot (anchovy), saeu-jeot (shrimp), kalchi-jeot (cutlassfish), joki-jeot (yellow corvina), whangseokeo-jeot (young yellow corvina), and others (a total of 47 jeotgals) have been used in kimchi (Lee and Kong, 2004). People prefer kimchi made with jeotgal because it enhances the flavor, taste, and natural color of kimchi, helps preserve its quality, extends storage time, and improves its nutrition.

Saeu-jeot (shrimp) and myeolchi-jeot (anchovy) are the most popular jeotgals used in kimchi with fish sauces such as aekjeot and kkanari-aekjeot. Some of the unique jeotgals used for kimchi are kkoltugi-jeot on the east coast (Gangwon-do) and in the midwest area (Chungchungbuk-do), kul-jeot (oyster) in the southern and midwest areas (Chungchungnam-do and Jeollanam-do), and kalchisok-jeot in the southern area (Lee and Kong, 2004). A survey by Kim et al. (1998) showed that over 65.5% eat kimchi daily and about 96.3% used jeotgals for making kimchi. Among them, myeolchi-jeot (anchovy) and saeu-jeot (small shrimp) were the most popular to add to kimchi by 84.9% and 69.1%, respectively (Kim et al., 1998).

8.3.3 Regional Jeotgals

South Korea is a relatively small country with an area of 100,210 km² (Korea is 219,155 km² including North Korea); it has a variety of climate zones and topography and the nature to develop distinctive flavors of jeotgal by each region. The southern part of the peninsula has the most varieties of jeotgal: 99 jeotgals out of 145 made of whole fish and internal parts. Other areas produce 41 varieties in the central region, 34 in the northeastern part, and 32 in the northwest area (Suh and Yoon, 1987). Figure 8.4 summarizes the regional distribution of jeotgal by main ingredients.

8.3.3.1 Regional Jeotgals by Main Ingredients

Fish: Regional jeotgals have a close relationship with the fish produced in the region and are mostly related to seawater fish. Cold-water fish families mostly live off the east coast and the warm-water fish move along with the water temperature changes in the coastal area. When spring comes, warm-water fish such as mackerel, pike, anchovy, sardine, horse mackerel, and squid along the east coast move to the north when the water temperature rises. The southern part of the peninsula (Namhae area) is rich in fish since it is the junction area of the cold water and warm water. In particular, the sea near southern Dadohae has good environmental conditions for fish breeding and has many different kinds of fish. Warm-water fish families cannot stay along the west coast since the water is too shallow to have enough algae, and they can only be harvested during spring when the water temperature rises. In the southern provinces, many jeotgals are made up of intestines since the main parts of fish are mostly consumed and jeotgal is made with the by-products. In order to improve storage efficiency, fish intestines, which contain high concentrations of enzymes, are treated separately from the flesh (Suh and Yoon, 1987).

Pelecypoda and Gastropoda: The west coast has continental shelves and tideland along the coastline; Pelecypoda such as oysters, clams, Manila clams, moss clams, and surf clams undergo natural breeding and artificial reproduction. The southern sea has continental shelves deeper than those off the west coast; oysters, clams, Manila clams, and ark shells have undergone active propagation. In particular, crab is strongly productive in Jeolla-do (southwestern area) and Hwanghae-do (northwestern area). Mostly crab meat is used for jeotgal and the most widely distributed jeots are kul-jeot (oyster), jogae-jeot (shellfish), and bajirak-jeot (clam) (Suh and Yoon, 1987).

Cephalopods: Joetgal made by cephalopods is distributed all across the country; ojingeo-jeot (squid) is produced mostly in Gyeongsang-do (southeastern area), but also in Gyeonggi-do (province surrounding Seoul), Jeolla-do, and Pyongan-do (northwestern area). Mooneo-jeot (octopus) is made in Gyeongsang-do, Jeolla-do, Gangwon-do (mideastern area), and Hamgyong-do (far northeast area), while mooneo-sikhae is only in north Hamgyong-do (Suh and Yoon, 1987).

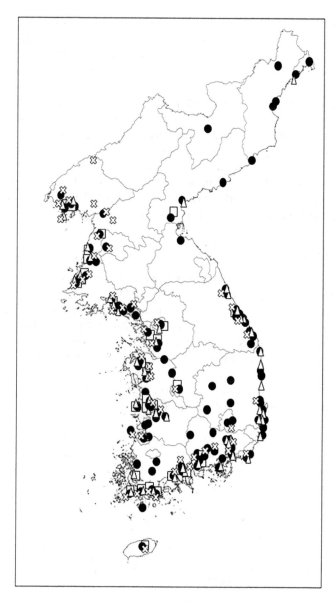

FIGURE 8.4
Distribution of jeotgals produced using fish in Korea (●), pelecypoda and gastropoda (□), cephalopods (Δ), crustaceans (✖). (Modified from Suh, H.K., and S.S. Yoon. 1987. *Korean J. Dietary Culture* 2(1):45–54.)

Crustaceans: Both marine crabs and freshwater crabs are used for jeotgal production in the western and southern parts of the peninsula. Jeotgal made by shrimp also uses freshwater and marine shrimp. Shrimp is distributed along the west coast and the central part of the east coast. Depending on harvest season, the common names refer to the months or seasons: o-jeot (May), yuk-jeot (June), ja-jeot (July), chu-jeot (fall), baekha-jeot (winter). Minmulsaeu-jeot (freshwater shrimp) are produced only in Jeolla-do, while busaeu-jeot (opossum shrimp) is produced in Gangneung (the east coast). Haesam-changja-jeot (sea cucumber intestines) along the south coast and sungge-jeot (sea urchins) are made with the gonads of sea urchins produced on Jeju Island. Inland, where mountain ranges block the coast area on the peninsula, jeotgal is not produced and there is limited access to it since travel to transport seafood is inconvenient (Suh and Yoon, 1987).

8.3.3.2 Regional Jeotgal Recipes

Jeotgal recipes are also different by region and they are varied in their production frequency, spices and other ingredients, or the type of jeotgal. The areas along the southern coast make myeolchi-jeot (anchovy) once a year during spring, while the east coast area produces it twice a year in spring and fall when they harvest anchovy is harvested. Anchovy is a warm-water fish and the warm water moves to the north in spring and fall along the east coast (Suh, 1987).

The Hamheung and Pukchong areas in North Korea add red pepper powder when making myeolchi-jeot (anchovy) to promote the fermentation process and to inhibit the fishy flavor by curing at low temperatures. Temperature can be the part of the main reason for different recipes by adding red pepper powder in jeotgal. For example, the annual average temperature of Hamheung and Pukchong is about 9.1°C~9.8°C and the annual average temperature of Gyeongju and Yeongdeok (southeast area), where red pepper powder is used, is about 13.3°C and 13.2°C, respectively. Northwest coastal areas make ge-jeot (crab) in brine, while the central and southern areas of the peninsula make it in soy sauce. Along the northwestern coast, blue crab and king crab are the main ingredients for ge-jeot and brine is used to increase the storage efficiency since fish cannot be caught during winter due to the frozen sea (Suh, 1987).

Sikhae is made only in the eastern part of the peninsula because the water along the western coast is too shallow to catch fish during winter and warm-water fish cannot stay. Therefore, jeotgal is developed on the west coast to store fishery products for long periods of time. However, the water along the east coast is too deep for the cold-water fish to be caught all year round. The total fermentation and storage period of sikhae is only about 1 month, which is too short a period in which to produce and store it on the west coast. In addition, the salt production of the east coast is very limited and sikhae requires less salt than other jeotgal (Suh, 1987).

8.4 Composition

8.4.1 General Composition

Proximate composition of major jeotgals, including myeolchi-jeot (anchovy), myeong-ran-jeot (pollack), and changnan-jeot (pollack), with the raw materials and after fermentation were compared and are demonstrated in Table 8.2 (Kim and Kim, 2014). The moisture content decreased during fermentation while the ash content increased in all jeotgals. Changnan-jeot showed a dramatic increase in carbohydrate content potentially due to addition of seasonings. Table 8.3 summarizes the composition of other major jeotgals,

TABLE 8.2

Proximate Composition of Myeolchi-Jeot (Anchovy), Myeong-Ran-Jeot (Pollack), and Changnan-Jeot (Pollack) Compared with the Raw Materials

		Moisture	Crude Protein	Crude Lipid	Carbohydrate	Ash
Myeolchi-jeot	Raw	74.3[a]	17	N/A[b]	1.4	4.3
	Jeotgal	61.1	13.1	N/A	0.2	24
Myeong-ran-jeot	Raw	73.5	22.4	1.5	1.5	1.1
	Jeotgal	66	20.5	3	2.7	7.8
Changnan-jeot	Raw	80.9	11.5	2.2	0.2	5.2
	Jeotgal	64.3	12.9	3.2	8.2	11.4

Source: Modified from Kim, Y.M. 2014b. In *Strategy for stimulation and development of fermented food sciences and related industry: The Korean Academy of Science and Technology.* 107–159. Songnam (Korea): KAST Research Report.
[a] Unit: Grams per 100 g of each material; the unit is applied to all components.
[b] N/A: Not available.

TABLE 8.3

Proximate Composition of Commercial Saeu-Jeot (Small Shrimp), Ojingeo-Jeot (Squid), and Myeolchi-Jeot (Anchovy)

	Moisture	Crude Protein	Salinity	pH	Nitrogen[a]
Saeu-jeot	63.2[b]	7.12	24.3	7.13	53.42 (VBN, mg%)
Ojingeo-jeot	69.9	13.1	5.92	5.36	46.33 (VBN, mg%)
Myeolchi-jeot	68.7	N/A[c]	22.0	5.69	1.43 (TN, %), 528.1 (NH_2-N, mg%)

Source: Modified from Kim, Y.M. 2014b. In *Strategy for stimulation and development of fermented food sciences and related industry: The Korean Academy of Science and Technology.* 107–159. Songnam (Korea): KAST Research Report.
[a] VBN: Volatile basic nitrogen; TN: total nitrogen; NH_2-N: ammonia nitrogen.
[b] Unit: Grams per 100 g of each material; the unit is applied to moisture, crude protein content, and salinity.
[c] N/A: Not available.

196   *Korean Functional Foods*

including saeu-jeot (small shrimp), ojingeo-jeot (squid), and myeolchi-jeot (anchovy) (Kim, 2014b). The salinity, pH, and nitrogen content are included in Table 8.3. Further compositional information is described in this section.

8.4.1.1 Amino Acids

Free amino acid production from the hydrolysis of meat protein from the main ingredients is the most distinctive compositional change of jeotgal during fermentation. Depending on the fish, compositional distribution of amino acid is different: Shrimp contains glycine, proline, alanine, and sesine; tuna, bonito, and mackerel contain histidine. Amino-nitrogen increased to twice its amount after 3 days of fermentation in ojingeo-jeot (squid) (Kaneko et al., 1992). Change in free amino acid content during the fermentation of saeu-jeot (small shrimp) with 30% salt is summarized in Table 8.4 (Chung and Lee, 1976). In raw shrimp, proline, arginine, alanine, glycine, lysine, and glutamic acids compose 68.4% of total amino acids; however, lysine, glutamic acid, methionine, alanine, aspartic acid and leucine were obtained after 72 days of fermentation. Total free amino acids increased to twice their amount up to 72 days of fermentation and declined after later stages of fermentation;

TABLE 8.4

Compositional Changes of Amino Acids during Fermentation of Saeu-Jeot (Small Shrimp) with 30% Salt at 20°C

Amino Acids	Raw Shrimp		Fermented for 72 Days	
	FAA Content (mg/100 g)	Percentage of Total Amino Acid	FAA Content (mg/100 g)	Percentage of Total Amino Acid
Lysine	969.8	8.14	3,586.5	13.10
Histidine	148.4	1.25	188.8	0.69
Arginine	1,738.2	14.59	Trace	–
Aspartic acid	323.2	2.71	2,516.8	9.20
Threonine	487.6	4.09	1,814.7	6.63
Serine	333.9	2.80	2,013.5	7.36
Glutamic acid	911.5	7.65	3,209	11.72
Proline	2,209.9	18.55	Trace	–
Glycine	1,038.7	8.72	1,950.6	7.13
Alanine	1,287.8	10.81	2,894.4	10.57
Valine	503.5	4.23	1,761.8	6.44
Methionine	333.9	2.80	3,146.1	11.49
Isoleucine	328.6	2.76	1,258.4	4.60
Leucine	699.5	5.87	2,453.9	8.97
Tyrosine	270.3	2.27	Trace	–
Phenylalanine	328.6	2.76	566.3	2.07
Total	11,913.4	100.00	27,370.8	100.00

Source: Data from Chung, S.Y., and E.H. Lee. 1976. *Bull Korean Fish Soc* 9:79.

Jeotgal (Fermented Fish) 197

the result was also applied in junbok-naejang-jeot (intestines of ear shell) (Li et al., 2014). Changes in the nitrogen compounds also peaked the concentration at 72 days and decreased afterwards. TMAO (trimethylamine N-oxide) decreased by microbial or enzymatic decomposition to TMA (trimethylamine), which showed increase during fermentation. Betaine also increased up to 72 days of fermentation and then decreased (Chung and Lee, 1976). Kul-jeot (oyster) showed increases in lysine, aspartic acid, cysteine, isoleucine, and tyrosine more than twice the original amounts (Kim et al., 1981). Kajami-sikhae (flat fish) contained amino nitrogen with 53.4% of total nitrogen and the free amino acids such as leucine, alanine, arginine, glutamine, isoleucine, and valine were over 7.0 mmol/CP 100 g (Jung et al., 1992).

8.4.1.2 Nucleotides

Adenosine triphosphate (ATP) is degraded to adenosine diphosphate (ADP), adenosine monophosphate (AMP), inosine monophosphate (IMP), hypoxanthine (Hx), and inosine (HxR) for additional flavor during fermentation (Oh et al., 1996). Among 19 jeotgal products, none contained IMP or GMP (Kaneko et al., 1992). The content of ATP-related compounds in myeolchi-jeot (anchovy) showed almost complete decrease of ATP, ADP, AMP, and IMP and significant increase of Hx and production of uric acid (Cho et al., 2000). Kajami-sikhae (flat fish) also showed significant decreases in ATP and ADP, while other nucleotides such as cytidine monophosphate (CMP) and cytidine triphosphate (CTP) were significantly increased (Jung et al., 1992).

8.4.1.3 Fatty Acids

Total lipids, nonpolar lipids, and phospholipids decreased during the fermentation process in myeolchi-jeot (anchovy) from the bacterial lipase activities (Kim et al., 1994). The total lipid content in jeotgals with whole fish such as myeolchi-jeot, jogi-jeot (yellow corvina), jeongeori-jeot (sardine), baendangi-jeot (large-eyed herring), and others was about 1.9% to 10.2% (myeolchi-jeot with 5.51% to 5.85%); jeotgals with intestine, gills, or roe in changnan-jeot (pollack); myeongran-jeot (pollack); kalchi-sok jeot (cutlass); jeoneobam-jeot (stomach of gizzard shad); and sunggeal-jeot (roe of sea urchin) were about 1.5% to 11.9%, and kalchi-sok jeot was the highest with 11.9%. Mollusks and crustaceans contained the lowest lipid content by 0.8% to 2.1% (Lee et al., 1986; Park and Park, 1993). The fatty acid compositional change of myeolchi-jeot with 20% salt during fermentation is summarized in Table 8.5. The major fatty acid ratios were 14:0, 16:0, 16:1, 18:1, 20:5, and 22:6; 16:0 contained the highest concentration during fermentation (Cha and Lee, 1985). The result was supported by other researchers and the jeotgals that contained highest ω-3 polyunsaturated fatty acid (PUFA) content was koltuki-jeot (small squid) by 39.1%. Eicosapentaenoic acid (EPA, 20:5) was observed especially in kul-jeot (oyster) by 17.7% and koltuki-jeot by 16.4%; docosahexaenoic acid (DHA, 22:6) was found in koltuki-jeot in 22.2% and

TABLE 8.5

Compositional Changes of Fatty Acids during Fermentation of Myeolchi-Jeot (Anchovy) with 20% Salt at 20°C

Saturated Fatty acids	Raw Anchovy (Area %)	Fermented 90 Days (Area %)	Monounsaturated Fatty Acids	Raw Anchovy (Area %)	Fermented 90 Days (Area %)	Polyunsaturated Fatty Acids	Raw Anchovy (Area %)	Fermented 90 Days (Area %)
12:00	0.2	0.5	14:01	0.4	0.7	18:02	1.1	1.8
14:00	6.4	9.3	15:01	0.2	0.5	18:03	2.1	1.1
15:00	0.8	1.2	16:01	8.6	10.6	20:04	1.9	1.4
16:00	20.7	26.8	17:01	0.8	0.8	20:05	15.5	6.7
17:00	1.1	2.5	18:01	11.6	12.4	22:03	1	0.7
18:00	3.3	4.8	20:01	1.9	2.8	22:04	0.4	0.3
20:00	0.8	2.2	22:01	3	3.8	22:05	1.5	0.7
22:00	0.5	1				22:06	16.3	7.6
Total	**33.8**	**48.3**		**26.5**	**31.6**		**39.8**	**20.3**

Source: Modified from Cha, Y.J., and E.H. Lee. 1985. *Bull Korean Fish Soc* 18(6):511–518.

Jeotgal (Fermented Fish) 199

saeu-jeot (small shrimp) in 15.1% to 21.5% (Lee et al., 1986; Park and Park, 1993; Kim et al., 1994). Overall, jeotgals did not show dramatic changes in fatty acid content during fermentation and preserved most PUFA due to the anaerobic condition to prevent oxidation of fatty acids by the juice formed from osmosis of fish with high salt content (Lee et al., 1986).

8.4.1.4 Flavor Compounds

Lipid components in fish and fishery products generate various unique flavors by varieties of volatile and nonvolatile fatty acids; the components can also be easily oxidized under aerobic conditions to cause lipid peroxidation resulting in offensive flavors. Other volatile organic compounds are also produced during the fermentation of jeotgal to bring its unique flavor. Volatile compounds in myeolchi-jeot (anchovy) were detected using simultaneous steam distillation solvent extraction/gas chromatography/mass spectrometry (Cha, 1993). The compounds that were identified include 17 aldehydes, 12 alcohols, 10 ketones, nitrogen- and sulfur-containing compounds, esters, furans, and others. Aldehydes were identified the most by oxidation of PUFA, and benzaldehyde with almond and peanut flavors was also detected in high ratios (Cha, 1993). Flavor compounds in saeu-jeot (small shrimp) were detected using vacuum simultaneous distillation-solvent extraction/gas chromatography/mass spectrometry/olfactometry and aroma extract dilution analysis. (Cha et al., 1999). The most significantly detected compounds were 2,3-butanedione (sour/buttery), 1-octen-3-one (earthy/mushroom), dimethyl trisulfide (cooked cabbage/soy sauce), and 2-acetylthiazole (grainy/nutty). Free amino acids identified as affecting the taste of saeu-jeot were aspartic acid, glutamic acid (sour/umami), arginine, methionine (bitter), and lysine (sweet/bitter) (Cha et al., 1999). During fermentation of ojingeo-jeot (squid), alcohols increased significantly; the major alcohol compounds were propanol, isoamyl alcohol, methionol, phenylethyl alcohol, and others (Choi et al., 1995). Isoamyl alcohol production was contributed by *Pseudomonas* and *Staphylococcus aureus* and was also observed in saeu-jeot. Methionol (3-methylthio-1-propanol) is a major flavor compound in soy sauce and phenylethyl alcohol was produced by the microbial oxidation, which is also a main rose flavor and frequently identified in foods (Choi et al., 1995). Action (3-hydroxy-2-butanone) was produced by *Pseudomonas*, which has a buttery flavor, and identified in saeu-jeot; phenylacetaldehyde, which has sweet flavor, was produced by *S. aureus* and identified also in myeolchi-jeot (Choi et al., 1995).

8.4.2 Microbial Ecology

8.4.2.1 Microflora

Jeotgal contains high sodium content, between 10 and 30% salt in general, that reduces or inhibits the growth of most microorganisms to cause spoilage or foodborne illness. However, halotolerant or halophilic microorganisms survive and promote the fermentation of jeotgal. Microorganisms present in jeotgal are from fish, shellfish, or other main ingredients, seasonings, or subingredients, and from the environment, including seawater, mud, processing plants, and food handlers (Roh et al., 2010). Marine bacteria are naturally halophilic with 3.5% salinity. Halotolerant or halophilic microorganisms such as *Staphylococcus aureus, Saccharomyces rouxii, Vibrio costicola, Paracoccus halodentrificase,* and others can survive and affect jeotgal fermentation. Some extremely halophilic bacteria, such as *Ectothiorhodospira halophile, Actinopolyspora halophilua, Halococcus,* and *Halobacterium* sp., have been isolated from the sea (Lee and Choe, 1974; Hur, 1996).

Indigenous microorganisms as well as the microbial community of the fermented product vary depending on the main ingredients. *Halobacterium* and *Halomonas,* which are halophilic and halotolerant bacteria, and other bacteria such as *Bacillus, Brevibacterium, Flavobacterium, Micrococcus, Pediococcus, Pseudomonas,* and *Staphylococcus* have been frequently isolated in jeotgal (Ahn et al., 1990; Jung and Park, 2004; Guan et al., 2011). Ham and Jin (2002) evaluated the bacterial distribution in 72 jeotgal products in Seoul markets, and the most bacterial isolates were coliforms by 35.5%, *Vibrio* spp. by 8.6%, and *Staphylococcus* spp. by 12.9%. Kim et al. (2009c) also analyzed the bacterial distribution in 17 jeotgal products and isolated 308 strains. The top five genera isolated from jeotgals were 70 *Bacillus,* 34 *Tetragenococcus,* 31 *Lactobacillus,* 19 *Leuconostoc,* and 5 *Weissella.* Lactic acid bacteria (LAB) such as *Lactobacillus, Leuconostoc, Lactococcus, Weissella, Tetragenococcus, Carnobacterium,* and *Marinilactibacillus* were occupied by 27.6% of all bacterial isolates. Halotolerant and halophilic bacteria including *Paracoccus, Psychrobacter, Salinicoccus, Halomonas, Cobetia,* and *Lentibacillus* were also isolated. Jeotgal that contained the most diverse bacterial community was gajami-sikhae, followed by garibi-jeot (scallop), gaebul-jeot (spoon worm), kijogae-jeot (pen shell), and jeoneo-bam-jeot (stomach of gizzard shad), which are mostly made by mollusks (Kim et al., 2009c). Most jeotgal showed that total aerobic/anaerobic count ranged from 10^3 to 10^5 colony-forming units (CFUs)/g (Kim et al., 2009c).

During the fermentation and ripening of jeotgal, autolytic enzymes from fish or the microorganisms present in jeotgal become involved in the protein degradation to amino acids. This process could be highly affected by the NaCl content and fermentation temperature to cause different flavors and preservatives. At 7.5% salt in changnan-jeot (pollack), the microbial activity for the protein degradation was observed during fermentation at 25°C; trimethylamine and total volatile basic nitrogen content were increased to 20.5 and 102.1 mg%, respectively. However, no microbial growth was observed in changnan-jeot (pollack) with 20% salt (Chae, 2011).

8.4.2.2 Microbial Community during Fermentation

The microbial community changes during fermentation and the major phylum changes from Proteobacteria to Firmicutes (Roh et al., 2010). Myeolchi-jeot

Jeotgal (Fermented Fish)

(anchovy) showed that total viable cell counts peaked between 30 and 60 days of fermentation and continuously decreased to less than the initial concentration. *Achromobacter, Brevibacterium, Pseudomonas, Bacillus,* and *Flavobacterium* were isolated during the early stage of fermentation. *Pediococcus, Halobacterium, Sarcina,* and *Micrococcus* were isolated during the intermediate stage. Yeasts such as *Saccharomyces* and *Torulopsis* were also observed in the intermediate and later stages of fermentation (Lee and Choe, 1974; Hur, 1996). Lee and Choe (1974) isolated *Halobacterium, Cutirubrum, Micrococcus morrhuae,* and *Sarcina litoralis* during the fermentation of myeolchi-jeot (Figure 8.5; Lee and Choe, 1974). *Bacillus, Rummeliibacillus, Sporosarcina,* and *Virgibacillus* were identified in myeolchi-jeot as well as *Halomonas, Kocuria,* and *Psychrobacter* (Guan et al., 2011).

Saeu-jeot (small shrimp) was studied to show the changes in microbial concentration by different salt levels and the result with that the optimal bacterial count was at 18% salt, while 3%, 8%, and 30% salt resulted in the complete reduction of total viable cell counts (Mok et al., 2000). The result was potentially because the halophile and halotolerant bacteria, such as *Halobacterium, Pediococcus, Sarcina,* and *Micrococcus morrhuae,* and yeast, such as *Saccharomyces* and *Torulopsis,* were dominant in 18% salt—the most optimal salt condition for fermentation also observed in other studies (Mok et al., 2000). Guan et al. (2011) have isolated other halophiles including *Halomonas, Salinicoccus, Salinimicrobium, Salinivibrio,* and *Staphylococcus* at similar salt concentrations; *Lactobacillus, Leuconostoc, Psychrobacter,* and *Weissella* were also isolated (Roh et al., 2010). *Staphylococcus* spp. was isolated dominantly in this study; it may have been involved in ripening of jeotgal and this bacterium may not actively be involved in proteolysis (Roh et al., 2010).

While culture-dependent methods have been mainly used to evaluate the microbial community in jeotgal, this method is time consuming and can only isolate and identify the microorganisms that are able to grow in the media. Therefore, amplicon sequencing methods have been recently applied to overcome the limitation of the culture-dependent method with the development of next-generation sequencing technology. These high-throughput microbial community analysis tools target 16S rRNA genes for sequencing, which makes it possible to investigate the microbial population including unculturable microorganisms as well as further investigate the targeted function for jeotgal fermentation.

Various types of jeotgals were analyzed using this tool and Roh et al. (2010) investigated the microbial communities of seven different jeotgals (Figure 8.6). Except for kapojingeo-jeot (cuttlefish), which was dominant in uncultured *Crenarchaeota,* most jeotgals primarily belonged to the family Halobacteriaceae (68.6% to 98.4%) (Roh et al., 2010). Saeu-jeot (small shrimp), jogae-jeot (shellfish), kul-jeot (oyster), and ge-jeot (crab) that were over 10% NaCl contained relatively higher numbers of Archea in the class Halobacteria of the family Halobacteriaceae. For bacterial sequences, most amplicons belonged to the order Lactobacillales (71.1% to 98.7%), except

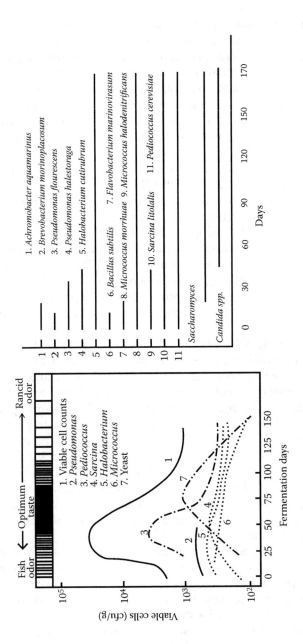

FIGURE 8.5
Microbial community changes of myeolchi-jeot (anchovy) during fermentation. (Modified figures from Lee, J.G., and W.K. Choe. 1974. *Korean J Fish Aquat Sci* 7(3):105–114; Hur, S.H. 1996. *Korean J Food Sci Technol* 25(5):885–891.)

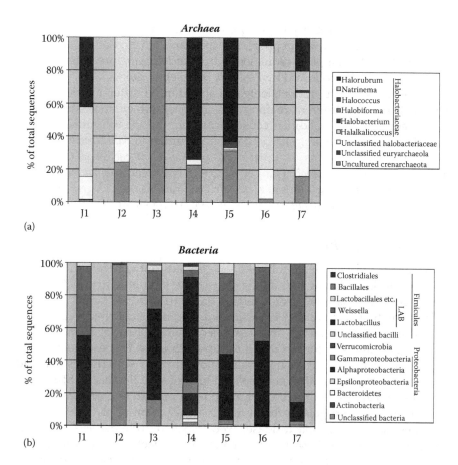

FIGURE 8.6
Microbial composition of seven different jeotgals from barcoded pyrosequencing analysis. (a) Archaeal and (b) bacterial composition of J1, shrimp; J2, shellfish; J3, cuttlefish; J4, oyster; J5, roe of pollack; J6, tripe of pollack; J7, crab. (Modified figures from Roh, S.W. et al. 2010. *Int J Syst Evol Microbiol* 4:1–16. With permission.)

jogae-jeot. Jogae-jeot showed Gammaproteobacteria composed of 98.8% of total sequences, which consisted mostly of the genus *Salinivibrio* of the order Vibrinoales (Rhee et al., 2011). Ojingeo-jeot (squid) contained genera *Leuconostoc* predominantly followed by *Bacillus*, *Staphylococcus*, *Psychrobacter*, *Paracoccus*, and others. While *Leuconostoc* does not have osmotic stress–related genes, these genes were identified in ojingeo jeot (Jung et al., 2013).

The microbial community in sikhae has been shown to be dominated by LAB. *Lb. sakei* was identified as the major bacteria in myeongtae-sikhae (pollack) by 74% at 10°C and 90% at 20°C, but was only 2% before fermentation. *Lb. sakei* was dominant also in kajami-sikhae, which contains over 90% of Leuconostocaceae and Lactobacillaceae families (Kim et al., 2014).

The difference in microbial composition of sikhae is mainly in subingredients such as cooked grains, red peppers, radishes, and others. Radish decreased Proteobacteria to complete reduction, while *Lactobacillus* presented 89% to 91% of total bacteria followed by *Weissella* (Jung et al., 2013).

As a fermented fish product, jeotgal is abundant in different microorganisms of fish from different regions and seasons, fermentation stages, and subingredients. This condition caused isolation and identification of novel bacteria such as genus *Jeotgalicoccus*, which is similar to *Salinicoccus* (Yoon et al., 2003b); *Proteus cibarius* (Hyun et al., 2016); *Weissella jogaejeotgali* (Lee et al., 2015); *Brevibacterium jeotgali* (Choi et al., 2013); *Halomonas cibimaris* (Jeong et al., 2013); *Kocuria atrinae* (Park et al., 2010); *Paenibacillus tyraminigenes* (Mah et al., 2008); *Salinicoccus jeotgali* (Aslam et al., 2007); and so on.

8.4.2.3 Microorganisms

Bacteria isolated from jeotgal have been studied to investigate the biological characteristics for further application in the food industry. *Bacillus* and its relatives were isolated from jeotgals on media with 15% NaCl and the isolates, such as *Virgibacillus halodentridicans* from myeolchi-jeot (anchovy) and *Staphylococcus equorum* from saeu-jeot (small shrimp), were able to grow under high salt concentration for up to 25% NaCl. These isolates and *Halobacillus treuperi* from saeu-jeot also showed protease activities (An and Lee, 2011). Kim et al. (2009b) also isolated halotolerant *Bacillus* sp. SJ-10 from ojingeo-jeot (squid) and the bacterium showed growth and protease activities on collagen and gelatin for up to 14% NaCl (Kim et al., 2009b). Other enzymes, such as β–galactosidase, were isolated from *Lactobacillus casei* no. 10 and no. 36 and *L. pentosus* no. 63 from saeu-jeot and myeolchi-jeot to show the activity on hydrolyzing lactose to glucose and galactose to combat lactose intolerance (Kim et al., 1996a).

The protease activities of the isolates can be used for their further application as starters in jeotgal and other food products. *Micrococcus, Pseudomonas,* and *Leuconostoc* isolated from changnan-jeot (pollack) with strong protease activities were able to shorten the fermentation period. These bacteria were inoculated in changnan-jeot (pollack) with 10^5 CFUs/g and the fermentation was shortened for up to 10 days at 0°C. Using the starter, the condition of the jeotgal's pH, volatile basic nitrogen (VBN), nitrogen basics (NH_2-N), free amino acid contents, and the sensory evaluation were performed to show the potential food application (Yoon et al., 2003a). *Bacillus subtilis* p-4 and *B. licheniformis* p-5 with strong proteolytic activities were also used in the large-scale production to accelerate the fermentation process (Cha and Lee, 1989). These isolates can be applied in other food products such as dairy products. *Lactobacillus casei* no. 10 and no. 36, and *L. pentosus* no. 63 isolated from saeu-jeot and myeolchi-jeot, were tested in yogurt and their physicochemical characteristics such as pH, titratable acidity, viscosity, and viable cell counts were evaluated (Kim et al. 1997).

Fermented jeotgal inhibits the growth of spoilage and pathogenic bacteria. Enterobacteriaceae were observed to be about 10^1 to 10^4 CFUs/g in saeu-jeot (small shrimp) and Gram-positive cocci were about 10^1 to 10^3 CFUs/g. *Salmonella* was not detected in these products while other bacteria such as *Staphylococcus xylosus, S. sciuri,* and nonvirulent *Vibrio* were isolated. When foodborne pathogens were inoculated in commercial saeu-jeot with 21.9% salt, LD50 during storage at 20°C for *Salmonella, E. coli* O26, and *S. aureus* was 10, 12, and 12 days, respectively (Oh et al., 2004). The bacterial reduction in jeotgal was due to the high salt concentration causing low water activity and antimicrobial activity by the chlorine ion from NaCl inhibiting the growth of bacteria. Also, bacteria grown during fermentation, such as *Lactococcus lactis* NK24, produced bacteriocin and other antimicrobial substances to reduce the growth of pathogenic bacteria (Kim et al., 1999b). *B. siamensis* RM502 isolated from ojingeo-jeot (squid) showed protease activities and antimicrobial activities against *S. aureus* and *V. parahaemolyticus* (Kim et al., 2013). Growth inhibition of *Listeria monocytogenes* by LAB isolated from various jeotgals was also observed (Kim et al., 2005). Antifungal activities of *B. atrophaeus, Virgibacillus pantothenticus,* and *B. subtilis* isolated from jeotgals were observed against plant pathogens such as *Fusarium oxysporum* and *Collectotrichum acutatum* (Kim et al., 2010).

8.5 Health Benefits

Jeotgal has been widely accepted as an important part of Korean fermented food for a nutritious and healthy diet—as a source of protein, minerals, and vitamins; probiotics; increased appetite by its umami flavor; and a good digestant (Kim et al., 1996b; Kim and Kim, 2014).

Proteins in fish, mollusks, crustaceans, and other marine by-products have also been studied for potential health benefits by bioactive peptides obtained during the fermentation process. Bioactive peptides are composed of 3~40 amino acid residues and have biological functions including antioxidant, antimicrobial, antiviral, antihypertensive, anticoagulant, antithrombotic, and other characteristics depending on their compositions and sequences (Lordan et al., 2011). These peptides can be obtained by enzymatic hydrolysis of proteins during fermentation, gastrointestinal digestion, and food processing (Daliri et al., 2017).

Antioxidant activities were observed in the peptides from jumbo squids and oysters. Tryptic hydrolysates of jumbo squid skin gelatin exhibited strong lipid peroxidation inhibition activities that were stronger than a natural antioxidant, α-tocoperol (Mendis et al., 2005). Hydrolysate of oyster obtained from an *in vitro* gastrointestinal digestion model also exhibited antioxidative activity against polyunsaturated fatty acid peroxidation without any cytotoxicity to a human embryonic lung fibroblast cell line (MRC-5) (Qian et al., 2008). The antioxidative activity of oyster hydrolysates was more effective than α-tocopherol. These activities were found to be caused by the presence of hydrophobic amino acids such as glycine, proline, aromatic amino acids, and histidine that were rich in gelatin peptides (Choi et al., 2015).

High blood pressure has been recognized as one of the most significant risk factors for cardiovascular disease and research on controlling angiotensin-I-converting enzyme (ACE) had been intensively performed since it has a critical role in regulation of blood pressure. ACE converts angiotensin-I to angiotensin-II, which is a potent vasoconstrictor. Synthetic drugs directly attack ACE and block the action of ACE with side effects including cough, skin rash, and angioneurotic edema. However, natural peptides, including cod frame, pollack skin, clam, mussel, oyster, shrimp, squid, and others, react with ACE to inhibit the action (Hartmann and Meisel, 2007; Alemán et al., 2011; Ngo et al., 2012). Nonapeptide isolated from oyster protein hydrolysate exhibited antihypertensive activity by inhibiting ACE activity on spontaneously hypertensive rats (Wang et al., 2008). Peptides extracted from myeolchi-aekjeot induced apoptosis in cancer cells (U937), and squid gelatin hydrolysates in human breast carcinoma (MCF-7) and glioma (U87) cell lines (Lee et al., 2003; Alemán et al., 2011). Natural anticoagulants were detected from yellowfin sole and their activities serve as a platelet aggregation inhibitor (Rajapakse et al., 2005). Low molecular weight peptides of pepsinolytic hydrolysates of Alaska pollack backbone demonstrated calcium-binding activities that can be further applied to the use of Ca supplements as alternatives to dairy products (Jung et al., 2006).

As the fermentation proceeds, jeotgal shows the increase in health benefits by increases in functional by-products including free amino acids, phytochemicals, and other metabolites from fermentation. Saeu-jeot (small shrimp) showed an increase of twice the total free amino acid content after 72 days of fermentation, and essential amino acids including lysine, glutamic acid, methionine, alanine, aspartic acid, and leucine increased 1.27- to 5.79-fold during the fermentation (Chung and Lee, 1976). Fermented myeolchi-jeot (anchovy) has anticancer activity and prevention of somatic mutation, while salted fresh anchovy causes comutation in *Drosophila*. Lee et al. (2000) tested the methanol extract of 0-, 6-, and 12-month fermented myeolchi-jeot with a *Drosophila* wing spot test system and the result showed 26.6% and 43.3% anticancer activities on 6- and 12-month fermented myeolchi-jeot while freshly produced myeolchi-jeot showed commutation effects (Lee et al., 2000). A similar result was observed by Jung (2000) in the SOS chromotest and, the longer the fermentation proceeded, the higher were the anticancer activities observed.

Cell cytotoxicity on liver hepatocellular carcinoma cell HepG2 showed the strongest inhibition activity on chuneobam-jeot (shad gizzard) by 77.6%, followed by kajami-sikhae (flat fish, 65.6%), ojingeojeot (squid, 57.6%), and koltugijeot (small squid, 57.5%). The result was dose dependent by polyunsaturated fatty acid (PUFA) such as eicosapentaenoic acid (EPA) and docosahexaenoic acid (DHA) content (Lim et al., 2001). Kajami-sikhae (flat fish) also showed stong HepG2 proliferation inhibition activity since sikhae contains highly bioactive grains and other subingredients such as garlic and hot pepper that enhance the anticancer activity (Park et al., 1991; Shoji et al., 1997).

Some of the protein hydrolysates by enzymes in jeotgal have been shown to have antioxidant properties (Kim, 2003). Myeolchi-aekjeot (anchovy sauce) that was fermented and cured for 5 years with 30% NaCl showed 3.3- and 2.1-fold higher contents of bioactive compounds than 1 and 3 years, respectively. The antioxidant activities were even higher than for doenjang and chongkukjang due to the glutamic acid and lysine contents (Kim, 2003). The ACE inhibitor activity was also observed in myeolchi-jeot, which contained threonine, glutamic acid, lysine, serine, and proline (Kim et al., 1993a). Whangseokeo-jeot (yellow corvina) that was fermented for 240 days at 25°C increased the radical scavenging activity and reducing power with the amino acids, reducing sugar and the carbonyl compounds formed by lipid peroxidation during the Maillard reaction (Kim et al., 2006).

Fermentation of jeotgal is performed by the combination of autolytic degradation and microbial activities where LAB and other bacteria are actively involved. *Lactobacillus paraplantarum, L. plantarum, L. pentosus,* and *Leuconostoc mesenteroides* isolated from ojingeo-jeot (squid), jokae-jeot (scallop), kul-jeot (oyster), changnan-jeot (pollock roe), and others have shown the production of conjugated linoleic acid (CLA) including *cis*-9, *trans*-11-CLA (Kim, 2014a). Probiotic potential by *L. plantarum* NK181 and *Pediococcus pentosaceus* isolated from commercial jeotgals was observed by the resistance to gastric juice and bile salts (Kim et al., 2005: Lee et al., 2006, 2014). *Lactobacillus* ML 36, Ml 128, and ML 178 and yeasts YK 33 and YK 61 were isolated from ojingeo-jeot, kalchisok-jeot (cutlass), koltuki-jeot (small squid), and myeolchi-jeot (anchovy) and were seen as potential probiotics by the resistance to artificial gastric and bile juice. They also showed resistance to rifamycin, streptomycin, tetracycline, and nisin (Kim et al., 2005). *L. plantarum* NK181 showed radical scavenging activity and cholesterol reduction activities to Caco-2 cells (Lee et al., 2006). *L. brevis* BH-21 from myeolchi-jeot was able to produce γ-aminobutyric acid (GABA) (Jeon et al., 2004). *Bacillus subtilis* W-1 induced apoptosis, a programmed cell death, and growth inhibition of lung cancer cell A549 and ovarian cancer cell SK-OV3 as antitumor agent (Park et al., 2004). Myulchikinase (MK) with a size of 28 kDa isolated from myeolchi-jeot showed cytotoxicity to tumor cell line and plasminogen activator type fibrinolytic enzyme activity in a plasminogen-rich fibrin plate but not in a plasminogen-free fibrin plate. This salt tolerance enzyme was able to maintain the activity up to 30% NaCl (Yang et al., 2005).

Anti-inflammatory effects to human mast cell line (HMC)-1 was observed in the supernatant of *B. subtilis* J80 and G147 isolates by the production of histamine release (28.5% by J80, 41.1% by G147). The proinflammatory cytokines such as tumor necrosis factor (TNF)-α (66.7% by J80) and interleukin (IL)-6 (38.5% by J80 and 41.1% by G147) were produced to activate HMC-1 (Ko et al., 2011). *Lactococcus lactis* NK34 induced the production of IL-1α and inhibition of the formation of preneoplastic lesions (Lee et al., 2007). Other bacteria such as *Alishewanella jeotgali* KCTC 22429, *Halomonas jeotgali* KCTC 22487, *Carnobacterium jeotgali* KCTC 13251, and *Marinilactibacillus psychrotolerans* NBRC 10002 isolated from jeotgal showed immunological effects. These bacteria modulated the function of dendritic cells by maturation and cytokine production such as inteleukin-12 in mouse bone marrow-derived dendritic cells. In addition, high lymphocyte stimulatory capability of these isolates suggested that not only LAB but also other bacteria in jeotgal had immunostimulating functions (Moon et al., 2014).

8.6 Conclusion

Jeotgal is a generally favorable food for Korean consumers, mostly due to its unique flavor and tastes to enhance the appetites (Oh, 2009; Seo, 2011). About 16.0% of Koreans consume jeotgal once or twice a week as side dishes (over 60%) or as seasonings (about 37.6%) for kimchi, soup, and other menus (Kim et al., 2009a). Over 65.5% of Koreans eat kimchi daily and about 96.3% of kimchi contains jeotgal (Kim et al., 1998). Among jeotgals, myeolchi-jeot (anchovy) and saeu-jeot (small shrimp) are most popular for adding to kimchi by 84.9% and 69.1%, respectively (Kim et al., 1998). For other purposes, saeu-jeot (69.6%), myeongran-jeot (pollack) (66.9%), myeolchi-jeot (65.5%), ojingeo-jeot (squid) (63.2%), and changnan-jeot (pollack) (49.3%) are the most popularly consumed jeotgals (Oh, 2009).

Jeotgal's unique flavor is formed during the fermentation process; the hydrolysis of meat protein by microbial fermentation and endogenous proteases is mainly involved. Appropriate salt concentration is an important factor to bring the best flavor and taste palatability as well as preservation by the inhibition of growth of spoilage and pathogenic bacteria. However, there has been increasing demand for the consumption of low-salt jeotgal by increasing health concerns about hypertension and diabetes from high sodium intake and the changes in appetite (Kim and Lee, 1991). In order to keep the storage period, nutrition, and palatability, scientists have been researching the development of effective manufacturing processes with low-salt jeotgal. Gamma-irradiation was applied to increase the preservability of ojingeo-jeot, and the intervention technology was able to lengthen the shelf-life by up to 30 days and to keep the flavor, general content, water activity, and pH of the jeotgal with 10% salt (Kim et al., 1999a). Plant extracts from bay leaf, green tea, and pine needles were also tested in low-salt ojingeo-jeot, and its quality and bioactivities were determined (Hong and Kim, 2013). Other

Jeotgal (Fermented Fish)

low-salt jeotgals such as myeolchi-jeot (anchovy), myeongran-jeot (pollack), and jogi-jeot (yellow corvina) were analyzed for their amino acid composition, volatile compounds, and fatty acid composition (Cha et al, 1986; Park et al., 2002; Han et al., 2005).

For more than a thousand years of history, jeotgal has been the center of the secret of Korean seasonings. It comes in the form of varieties of fermented fish and shellfish-based condiments, and it has also been a good nutritional supplier, health supplement, and flavor and appetite enhancer, with a rich and savory taste. The health benefits of jeotgal were introduced in this chapter with the metabolites from the fermentation of microorganisms; the benefits include antioxidants and antidiabetics, reducing body fat, and boosting immune systems. With intensive research and development on low-sodium jeotgal, this high-value-added food will be able to keep its reputation as one of the important traditional Korean fermented foods globally.

References

Ahn, Y.S., C.J. Kim, and S.H. Choi. 1990. Production of protease by the extreme halophile, *Halobacterium* sp. *J Korean Agric Chem Soc* 33:247–251.

Alemán, A., E. Pérez-Santín, S. Bordenave-Juchereau, I. Arnaudin, M.C. Gómez-Guillén, and P. Montero. 2011. Squid gelatin hydrolysates with antihypertensive, anticancer and antioxidant activity. *Food Res Int* 44:1044–1051.

An, D.H., and J.H. Lee. 2011. Isolation of bacteria from jeotgal using high-salt-content media and their growths in high-salt condition. *Korean J Microbiol Biotechnol* 39(3):294–300.

Anonymous. 3000–2500 BCE. *Sigyung.* China.

Anonymous. 500 BCE–CE 1. *Lyeki.* China.

Anonymous. 1697. *Jongmyouikue:* Korea National Central Museum, Korea.

Anonymous. 1890. *Siuijonseo.* Korea.

Aslam, Z., J.H. Lim, W.T. Im, M. Yasir, Y.R. Chung, and S.T. Lee. 2007. *Salinicoccus jeotgali* sp. nov., isolated from jeotgal, a traditional Korean fermented seafood. *Int J Syst Evol Microbiol* 57:633–638.

Cha, Y.J. 1993. Volatile flavor components in Korean salt—Fermented anchovy. *J Korean Soc Food Nutr* 21(6):719–724.

Cha, Y.J., and E.H. Lee. 1985. Studies on the processing of low salt fermented sea foods 7. Changes in volatile compounds and fatty acid composition during the fermentation of anchovy prepared with low sodium contents. *Bull Korean Fish Soc* 18(6):511–518.

Cha, Y.J., H. Kim, S.M. Jang, and J.Y. Park. 1999. Identification of aroma-active compounds in Korean salt-fermented fishes by aroma extract dilution analysis—2. Aroma-active components in salt-fermented shrimp on the market. *J Korean Soc Food Nutr* 28(2):319–325.

Cha, Y.J., and E.H. Lee. 1989. Studies on the processing of rapid fermented anchovy prepared with low salt contents by adapted microorganism 1. Biochemical characterization of proteolytic bacteria and their extracellular protease isolated from fermented fish paste. *Kor J Soc Fish Aquat Sci* 22(5):363–369.

Cha, Y.J., D.C. Park, and E.H. Lee. 1986. Studies on the processing of low salt fermented sea foods 10. Changes in volatile compounds and fatty acid composition during the fermentation of yellow corvenia prepared with low sodium contents. *Bull Korean Fish Soc* 19(6):529–536.

Chae, S.K. 2011. Studies on microbial and enzymatic actions during the ripening process of salted Alaska pollack tripe. *Korean J Food & Nutr* 24(3):340–349.

Cho, Y.J., Y.S. Im, D.H. Seo, T.J. Kim, J.G. Min, and Y.J. Choi. 2000. Enzymatic method for measuring ATP related compounds in jeotkals. *J Korean Fish Soc* 33(1):16–19.

Choi, D.K. 2012. The appearance of salted seafood in the east Asia and Vietnam's nuoc mam. *Asian Comp Folklore* 48:102–146.

Choi, E.J., S.H. Lee, J.Y. Jung, and C.O. Jeon. 2013. *Brevibacterium jeotgali* sp. nov., isolated from jeotgal, a traditional Korean fermented seafood. *Int J Syst Evol Microbiol* 63:3430–3436.

Choi, J.H., K.T. Kim, and S.M. Kim. 2015. Biofunctional properties of enzymatic squid meat hydrolysate. *Prev Nutr Food Sci* 20(1):67–72.

Choi, S.H., S.I. Im, S.H. Hur, and Y.M. Kim. 1995. Processing conditions of low salt fermented squid and its flavor components—1. Volatile flavor components of low salt fermented squid. *J Korean Soc Food Nutr* 24(2):261–267.

Choi, S.J. 1527. *Hunmongjahoe*. Korea.

Chung, S.Y., and E.H. Lee. 1976. The taste compounds of fermented *Acetes chinensis*. *Bull Korean Fish Soc* 9:79.

Daliri, E.B.M., D.H. Oh, and B.H. Lee. 2017. Bioactive peptides. *Foods* 6(32):1–21.

Guan, L., K.H. Cho, and J.H. Lee. 2011. Analysis of the cultivable bacterial community in jeotgal, a Korean salted and fermented seafood, and identification of its dominant bacteria. *Food Microbiol* 28:101–113.

Ham, H.J., and Y.H. Jin. 2002. Bacterial distribution of salt-fermented fishery products in Seoul Garak wholesale market. *J Fd Hyg Safety* 17(4):173–177.

Han, J.S., H.R. Cho, and H.S. Cho. 2005. Study for the establishment of the quality index of low-salted myungran-jeot. *Korean J Food Cookery Sci* 21(6):440–446.

Han, Y.Y. 2010. A documentary analysis on hae (salted fermented sea foods) of kind, cooking method munmyoseokjeon. *J Korean Classics* 34:395–415.

Hartmann, R., and H. Meisel. 2007. Food-derived peptides with biological activity: From research to food applications. *Curr Opin Biotechnol* 18:163–169.

Hong, M.S. 1700. *Sallimkyongje*. Korea.

Hong, W.J., and S.M. Kim. 2013. Quality characteristics, shelf-life, and bioactivities of the low salt squid jeot-gal with natural plant extracts. *J Korean Soc Food Sci Nutr* 42(5):721–729.

Hur, S.H. 1996. Critical review on the microbiological standardization of salt-fermented fish product. *Korean J Food Sci Technol* 25(5):885–891.

Hyun, D.W., M.J. Jung, M.S. Kim et al. 2016. *Proteus cibarius* sp. nov., a swarming bacterium from jeotgal, a traditional Korean fermented seafood, and emended description of the genus *Proteus*. *Int J Syst Evol Microbiol* 66(6):2158–2164.

Itoh, H., H. Tachi, and S. Kikuchi. 1993. Fish fermentation technology in Japan. In: *Fish fermentation technology*. ed. C.H. Lee, K.H. Steinkraus, and P.J. Alan Reilly, 181–185. Tokyo: United Nation University Press.

Jang, K.H. 1670. *Eumsik-dimibang*. Korea.

Jeon, J.H., Kim. H.D., Lee, H.S., and B.H. Ryu. 2004. Isolation and identification of *Lactobacillus* sp. produced γ-aminobutyric acid (GABA) from traditional salt fermented anchovy. *Korean J. Food & Nutr* 17(1):72–79.

Jeong, S.H., J.H. Lee, J.Y. Jung, S.H. Lee, M.S. Park, and C.O. Jeon. 2013. *Halomonas cibimaris* sp. nov., isolated from jeotgal, a traditional Korean fermented seafood. *A Van Leeuw J Microb* 103:503–512.

Jo, S.J. 2010. Terms and categories of commercialized Gomso jeotgal: A case study of a salted seafood market in Gomso bay. *Korean Cultural Anthropol* 43(2):3–44.

Jung, H.S., S.H. Lee, and K.L. Woo. 1992. Effect of salting levels on the changes of taste constituents of domestic fermented flounder sikhae of Hamkyeng-Do. *Korean J Food Sci Technol* 24(1):59–64.

Jung, J.J., S.J. Choi, C.O., Jeon, and W.J. Park. 2013. Pyrosequencing-based analysis of the bacterial community in Korean traditional seafood, ojingeo jeotgal. *J Microbiol Biotechnol* 10:1428–1433.

Jung, K.O. 2000. Studies on enhancing cancer chemo-preventive effects of kimchi and safety of salts and fermented anchovy. PhD dissertation, Pusan National University, Korea.

Jung, W.K., R. Karawita, S.J. Heo, B.J. Lee, S.K. Kim, and Y.J. Jeon. 2006. Recovery of a novel Ca-binding peptide from Alaska pollack (*Theragra chalcogramma*) backbone by pepsinolytic hydrolysis. *Proc Biochem* 41:2097–2100.

Jung, Y.J., and D.H. Park. 2004. Physiology and growth properties of halophilic bacteria isolated from jeotgal (salted seafood). *Kor J Microbiol* 40:263–268.

Ka, S.H. 532. *Cheminyosul, Pokja method, Woo-ujang method*. China.

Kaneko, K, C.H. Kim, and T. Kaneda. 1992. Comparative study on content and composition of oligopeptide, free amino acids, 5′-ribonucleotides, and free sugars in salted preserves produced at Korea and Japan. *Korean J Dietary Culture* 7(3):253–58.

Kim, B.S. 683. *Samkuksaki (History of Three Korean Kingdoms)*, vol. 8, Korea.

Kim, C.Y., J.H. Pyeun, and T.J. Nam. 1981. Decomposition of glycogen and protein in pickled oyster during fermentation with salt. *Bull Korean Fish Soc* 14(2):66–71.

Kim, D.S., C. Koizumi, B.Y. Jeong, and K.S. Jo. 1994. Studies on the lipid content and fatty acid composition of anchovy sauce prepared by heating fermentation. *Bull Korean Fish Soc* 27(5):469–475.

Kim, E.M., Y.M. Kim, J.H. Jo, and S.J. Woo. 1998. A study on the housewives' recognition and preference of seafoods and fermented seafoods add kimchi. *Korean J Dietary Culture* 13(1):19–26.

Kim, E.Y., D.G. Kim, Y.R. Kim, S.Y. Choi, and I.S. Kong. 2009b. Isolation and identification of halotolerant *Bacillus* sp. SJ-10 and characterization of its extracellular protease. *Korean J Microbiol* 45(2):193–199.

Kim, H.R., S.H. Han, B. Lee, D.W. Jeong, and J.H. Lee. 2013. Analysis of the bacterial community in ojingeo-jeotgal and selection of *Bacillus* species inhibiting the growth of food pathogens. *Korean J Microbiol Biotechnol* 41(4):462–468.

Kim, H.J., M.J. Kim, T.L. Turner et al. 2014. Pyrosequencing analysis of microbiota reveals that lactic acid bacteria are dominant in Korean flat fish fermented food, gajami-sikhae. *Biosci Biotechnol Biochem* 78:1611–1618.

Kim, H.J., N.K. Lee, S.M. Cho, K.T. Kim, and H.D. Park. 1999b. Inhibition of spoilage and pathogenic bacteria NK24, a bacteriocin produced by *Lactococcus lactis* NK24 from fermented fish food. *Korean J Food Sci Technol* 31:1035–1043.

Kim, J.E., J.H. Kim, and I.K. Jeong. 2009a. Perception and utilization of salted seafood in Korean women. *Fam Environ Res* 47(6):11–20.

Kim, J.H., K.H. Lee, H.J. Ahn, B.S. Cha, and M.W. Byun. 1999a. Effects of gamma irradiation on microbiological and sensory qualities in processing of low salted and fermented squid. *Korean J Food Sci Technol* 31(4):1050–1056.

Kim, J.H., Y.H. Rhee, H.J. Na, Y.K. Lee, and S.Y. Shin. 1997. Physico-chemical characteristics of yogurt by *Lactobacillus* spp. from pickle. *Agric Chem Biotechnol* 40(1):12–17.

Kim, J.H., Y.H. Rhee, M.K. Oh, Y.K. Lee, and S.Y. Shin. 1996a. Microbiology fermenation biotechnology: β-galactosidase activity of *Lactobacillus* spp. from pickles. *Agric Chem Biotechnol.* 39(6):437–442.

Kim, J.S. 1452. *Koryosajeolyo.* Korea.

Kim, J.S., and I.J. Jung. 1451. *Koryosa; era of Seongjong.* Korea.

Kim, J.S., and K.H. Kim. 2014. Processing and characterization of salt-fermented fish (jeotgal) using seafood by-products in Korea. In *Seafood processing byproducts.* New York: Springer, 63–99.

Kim, J.S., G.S. Moon, K.H. Lee, and Y.S. Lee. 2006. Studies on quality changes and antioxidant activity during the fermentation of the salt fermented whangseoke. *J Korean Soc Food Sci Nutr* 35:171–176.

Kim, M.S., E.J. Park, M.J. Jeong, S.W. No, and J.W. Bae. 2009c. Analysis of prokaryote communities in Korean traditional fermented food, jeotgal, using culture-dependent method and isolation of a novel strain. *Korean J Microbiol* 45(1):26–31.

Kim, N.J. 2014a. Novel lactic acid bacteria producing high conjugated linoleic acids from Korean traditional fermented fish, jeot-gals, and their potential probiotic properties. MS thesis, Chonbuk National Univ.

Kim, S.H., and D.J. Jang. 2015. Fabulous Korean ethnic foods; namdo. In *Korea Food Research Institute,* 155. Seoul, Korea: Elsevier.

Kim, S.H., M.S. Kim, M.S. Lee et al. 2016. Korean diet: Characteristics and historical background. *J Ethn Foods* 3:26–31.

Kim, S.J., S.J. Ma, and H.L. Kim. 2005. Probiotic properties of lactic acid bacteria and yeasts isolated from Korean traditional food, jeot-gal. *Korean J Food Presev* 12(2):184–189.

Kim, S.M. 2003. The functionality of anchovy sauce. *Food Indust Nutr* 8:9–17.

Kim, S.M., and G.T. Lee. 1991. The shelf-life extension of low salted myungran-jeot. 1. The effects of pH control on the shelf-life of low-salted myungran-jeot. *J Korean Fish Soc* 30:459–465.

Kim, S.M., T.G. Lee, Y.B. Park et al. 1993. Characteristics of angiotensin-I converting enzyme inhibitors derived from fermented fish product. *Bull Korean Fish Soc* 26:321–329.

Kim, T.S., G.H. Lee, G.J. Kim, S.W. Lee, K.S. Park, and J.W. Park. 2010. Antifungal activity of bacterial strains isolated from tidal mudflat and salted seafood (traditional jeotgal) against six major plant pathogens. *Korean J Pestic Sci* 14(4):421–426.

Kim, Y.J., K.S. Sung, C.K. Han, J.H. Jeong, and T.S. Kang. 1996b. Effects of proteolytic enzymes on the production of fermented beef or pork with addition of fermented shrimp. *Korean J Anim Sci* 38:275–282.

Kim, Y.M. 2008. Present status and prospect of fermented seafood industry in Korea. *Food Sci Indust* 41(4):16–33.

Kim, Y.M. 2014b. Jeotgal. In *Strategy for stimulation and development of fermented food sciences and related industry: The Korean Academy of Science and Technology.* 107–159. Songnam (Korea): KAST Research Report.

Kim, Y.M., and D.S. Kim. 1991. Korean jeotgal—The raw materials and the products. Changjo, Korea.

Ko, Y.J., H.H. Kim, E.J. Kim et al. 2011. Anti-allergic inflammatory effect of bacteria isolated from fermented soybean and jeotgal on human mast cell line (HMC-1). *J Life Sci* 21(3):393–399.

Koo, O.K., S.J. Lee, K.R. Chung, D.J. Jang, H.J. Yang,. and D.Y. Kwon. 2016. Korean traditional fermented fish products: Jeotgal. *J Ethn Foods* 3(2):107–116.

Kwon, D.Y., D.J. Jang, H.J. Yang, and K.R. Chung. 2014. History of Korean gochu, gochujang, and kimchi. *J Ethn Foods* 1:3–7.

Lee, B. 1809. *Kyuhapchonso.* Korea.

Lee, E.H., C.B. Ahn, K.S. Oh, J.S. Kim, S.K. Jee, and J.G. Kim. 1987. The taste compounds of damchi-jeotguk-concentrated sea mussel extract. *Korean J. Food Culture* 2(1):25–31.

Lee, E.H., K.S. Oh, T.H. Lee, C.B. Ahn, and Y.J. Cha. 1986. Fatty acid composition of salted and fermented sea foods on the market. *Korean J Food Sci Technol* 18(1):42–47.

Lee, H. 1540. Toekyejip, Eonhaengnok, Yupyun. Korea.

Lee, H.J., K.O. Jung, S.H. Jeon, K.Y. Park, and W.H. Lee. 2000. Effects of salt and fermented anchovy extract on the somatic mutagenicity in *Drosophila* wing spot test system. *J Korean Soc Food Sci Nutr* 29:1139–1144.

Lee, J.G., and W.K. Choe. 1974. Studies on the variation of microflora during the fermentation of anchovy, *Engraulis Japonica. Korean J Fish Aquat Sci* 7(3):105–114.

Lee, K.W., J.Y. Park, H.D. Sa et al. 2014. Probiotic properties of *Pediococcus* strains isolated from jeotgals, salted and fermented Korean sea-food. *Anaerobe* 8:199–206.

Lee, M.H., and Y.J. Kong. 2004. Salted fish. In *Gimmyoungsa.* ISBN 406-2003-036

Lee, M.Y., and H.G. Lee. 1989. A bibliographical study on the shikke. *Korean J Dietary Culture* 4(1):39–51.

Lee, N.K., H.W. Kim, H.I. Chang et al. 2006. Probiotic properties of *Lactobacillus plantarum* NK181 isolated from jeotgal, a Korean fermented food. *Food Sci Biotechnol* 15:227–231.

Lee, N.K., J.E. Noh, G.H. Choi et al. 2007. Potential probiotic properties of *Lactococcus lactis* NK34 isolated from jeotgal. *Food Sci Biotechnol* 16:843–7.

Lee, S.B., K.H. Ko, J.Y. Yang, S.H. Oh, and J.K. Kim. 2004. *Fundamentals of food fermentation.* Hyoil. ISBN 89-8489-016-2.

Lee, S.H., H.J. Ku, M.J. Ahn et al. 2015. *Weissella jogaejeotgali* sp. nov., isolated from jogae jeotgal, a traditional Korean fermented seafood. *Int J Syst Evol Microbiol* 65:4674–4681.

Lee, Y.G., J.Y. Kim, K.W. Lee, K.H. Kim, and H.J. Lee. 2003. Peptides from anchovy sauce induce apoptosis in a human lymphoma cell (U937) through the increase of caspase-3 and -8 activities. *Ann N Y Acad Sci* 1010:399–404.

Li, J.L., B.S. Kim, and S.G. Kang. 2014. Preparation and characteristics of *Haliotis Discus Hannai Ino* (abalone) viscera jeotgal, a Korean fermented seafood. *Korean J Food Preserv* 21(1):1–8.

Lim, H.S., S.H. Kim, E.J. Yoo, D.S. Kang, M.R. Choi, and S.H. Song. 2001. Anticancer effect of extracts from the marine and salted fish products. *Korean J Life Sci* 11:48–53.

Lordan, S., R.P. Ross, and Stanton, C. 2011. Marine bioactives as functional food ingredients: Potential to reduce the incidence of chronic diseases. *Mar Drugs* 9(6):1056–1100.

Mah, J.H., Y.H. Chang, and H.J. Hwang. 2008. *Paenibacillus tyraminigenes* sp. nov. isolated from myeolchi-jeotgal, a traditional Korean salted and fermented anchovy. *Int J Food Microbiol* 127:209–214.

Mendis, E., N. Rajapakse, H.G. Byun, and S.K. Kim. 2005. Investigation of jumbo squid (*Dosidicus gigas*) skin gelatin peptides for their *in vitro* antioxidant effects. *Life Sci* 77:2166–2178.

Mheen, T. 1993. Microbiology of salted-fermented fishery products in Korea. In *Fish fermentation technology*. ed. C.H. Lee, K.H. Steinkraus, and P.J. Alan Reilly, 231–247, Tokyo: United Nation University Press.

Mok, C.K., J.Y. Lee, and J.H. Park. 2000. Microbial changes in salted and fermented shrimp at different salt level during fermentation. *Korean J Food Sci Technol* 32(2):444–447.

Moon, S.Y., E.J. Park, and H.G. Joo. 2014. Bacterial strains isolated from jeotgal (salted seafood) induce maturation and cytokine production in mouse bone marrow-derived dendritic cells. *J Vet Sci* 54(3):139–146.

Ngo, D.H., T.S. Vo, D.N. Ngo, I. Wijesekara, and S.K. Kim. 2012. Biological activities and potential health benefits of bioactive peptides derived from marine organisms. *Int J Biol Macromol* 51:378–383.

Oh, B.H. 2009. A study of utilization of Korean jeot-kals of housewives in Seoul area. *Korea Hotel Resort Casino Association* 8(2):155–169.

Oh, O.H., M.S. Kim, B.S. Suh, M.H. Kim, and J.S. Han. 1996. A study on taste and storage in kimchi with different kinds of jeotkal. *J Resource Development* 15(1):123–129.

Oh, S.H., O.S. Heo, O.K. Bang, H.C. Chang, H.S. Shin, and M.R. Kim. 2004. Microbiological safety of commercial salt-fermented shrimp during storage. *Korean J Food Sci Technol* 36(3):507–513.

Park, B.H., and Y.H. Park. 1993. Fatty acid composition of salt—Fermented seafoods in Chonnam area. *J Korean Soc Food Nutr* 22(4):465–469.

Park, C.K., T.J. Kang, and K.O. Cho. 2002. Studies on the processing of rapid- and low salt-fermented liquefaction of anchovy (*Engrulis japonica*) (II). Changes in the amino acids from oligopeptides during fermentation. *Korean J Dietary Culture* 17(4):363–376.

Park, E.J., M.S. Kim, S.W. Roh, M.J. Jung, and J.W. Bae. 2010. *Kocuria atrinae* sp. nov., isolated from traditional Korean fermented seafood. *Int J Syst Evol Microbiol* 60:914–918.

Park, J.K., Y.U. Cho, Y.J. Choi, Y.K. Jeong, and S.W. Gal. 2004. Antitumor activity of *Bacillus subtilis* SW-1 isolated from jeotgal. *J Life Sci* 14(5):815–820.

Park, K.Y., S.H. Kim, M.J. Suh, and H.Y. Chung. 1991. Inhibitory effects of garlic on the mutagenicity in *Salmonella* assay system and on the growth of HT-29 human colon carcinoma cells. *Kor J Food Sci Technol* 23:370–374.

Park, Y.H., D.S. Jang, and S.B. Kim. 1997. *Utilization of fishery products*. Seoul, Korea: Hyungseol.

Qian, Z.J., W.K. Jung, H.G. Byun, and S.K. Kim. 2008. Protective effect of an antioxidative peptide purified from gastrointestinal digests of oyster, *Crassostrea gigas*, against free radical induced DNA damage. *Biores Technol* 99:3365–3371.

Rajapakse, N., W.K. Jung, E. Mendis, S.H. Moon, and S.K. Kim. 2005. *Life Sci* 76:2607–2619.

Rhee, S.J., J.E. Lee, and C.H. Lee. 2011. Importance of lactic acid bacteria in Asian fermented foods. *Microb Cell Fact* 10:S5.

Ricke, S.C., O.K. Koo, and J.T. Keeton. 2013. Fermented meat, poultry and fish products. In *Food microbiology: Fundamentals and frontiers*. 4th ed. ed., M.P. Doyle and R.L. Buchanan, 857–80. Washington, DC: ASM Press.

Roh, S.W., K.H. Kim, Y.D. Nam, H.W. Chang, E.J. Park, and J.W. Bae. 2010. Investigation of archaeal and bacterial diversity in fermented seafood using barcoded pyrosequencing. *Int J Syst Evol Microbiol* 4:1–16.

Seo, J.W. 2011. Analyses of consumption patterns and buying defined factors on salted seafood-based on housewives' survey in Gwang-ju. *Korean Food Marketing Association* 28(4):55–76.

Shoji, F., T. Nobuyasu, H. Takaki, and W. Hideki. 1997. Cancer prevention by organosulfur compounds from garlic and onion. *J Cellular Biochem* 27:100–107.

Skåra, T., L. Axelsson, G. Stefansson, B. Ekstrand, and H. Hagen. 2015. Fermented and ripened fish products in the northern European countries. *J Ethn Foods* 2:18–24.

Song, K.E., and J.Y. Ahn. 2009. Change in spatial characteristics of jeotgal production. *Korea Soc Local His Cul* 6:158–171.

Suh, H.K. 1987. A study on the regional characteristics of Korean chotkal—The ways of preservation of chotkal. *Korean J Dietary Culture* 2(2):149–161.

Suh, H.K., and S.S. Yoon. 1987. A study on the regional characteristics of Korean chotkal—The kinds and materials of chotkal. *Korean J. Dietary Culture* 2(1):45–54.

Tanasupawat, S., and W. Visessanguan. 2014. Fish fermentation In *Seafood processing technology, quality and safety*, ed. I. S. Bosiaris, 177–207. West Sussex, UK: Wiley Blackwell.

Thapa, N. 2016. Ethnic fermented and preserved fish products of India and Nepal. *J Ethn Foods* 3:69–77.

Wang, J., J. Hu, J. Cui et al. 2008. Purification and identification of a ACE inhibitory peptide from oyster proteins hydrolysate and the antihypertensive effect of hydrolysate in spontaneously hypertensive rats. *Food Chem* 111:302–308.

Yang, W.S., H.S. Lim, K.T. Chung et al. 2005. Characterization of a fibrinolytic enzyme from pickled anchovy. *J Life Sci* 15(3):434–438.

Yoon, J.H., J.H. Kang, M.J. Park, Y.J. Kim, and M.S. Lee. 2003a. Shortening of fermentation period of *changran-jeotgal* using microorganism. *J Kor Fish Soc* 36(4):327–332.

Yoon, J.H., K.C. Lee, N. Weiss, K.H. Kang, and Y.H. Park. 2003b. *Jeotgalicoccus halotolerans* gen. nov., sp. nov. and *Jeotgalicoccus psychrophilus* sp. nov., isolated from the traditional Korean fermented seafood jeotgal. *Int J Syst Evol Microbiol* 53:595–602.

9

Sikcho (Korean Vinegar)

Kwang-Soon Shin and Hoon Kim

CONTENTS

9.1 History of Vinegar Fermentation 217
9.2 Production 219
9.3 Acetic Acid Bacteria 221
9.4 Varieties 222
9.5 Major Constituents 224
9.6 Physiological Functions 226
9.7 Conclusion 229
References 229

9.1 History of Vinegar Fermentation

Recent consumer interest in the relationship between diet and health has increased the demand for naturally fermented foods, such as vinegar. Vinegar, one of the most typical fermented foods, is a flavored liquid essentially containing 4%–20% acetic acid. According to the Korean Food Code, vinegars can be classified into two main categories: namely, fermented vinegar and synthetic vinegar. Fermented vinegar, perhaps better known as common vinegar, is prepared by acetic acid fermentation from raw materials, such as grains, fruits, and wines, among others, or their ripening mixtures with saccharified liquors from cereals or squeezed juices from fruits. In contrast, synthetic vinegar is prepared by the dilution of glacial acetic acid with water.

Vinegar is one of the oldest cooking ingredients and has been widely used in both the East and the West over thousands of years as a flavoring agent and a preservative (Lee et al., 2015). Indeed, according to the Vinegar Institute, the use of vinegar can be traced back over 10,000 years in history, with the manufacture and sale of flavored vinegars dating back almost 5,000 years. More specifically, in the sixth century BC, such flavored vinegars were sold to gourmets in Babylonia. In addition, the use of vinegar for medicinal purposes was recorded in the Old Testament and by Hippocrates (Conner and Allgeier, 1976).

The word *vinegar* has been in use in the English language since the fourteenth century, when the fermented liquid first arrived in the British Isles. The word itself originates from the French *vinaigre*, a word that simply means "sour wine" and comes from the Latin *vinum acre*, "sour wine," or, more commonly, *vinum acetum*, "wine vinegar." In addition, the word *aceum*, meaning "vinegar" in the most proper sense, is derived from the verb *acere*, meaning "to become pungent, go sour," and is similar to the ancient Greek ἀκμή [akmé], "spike," while the Greek word for vinegar is ὄξοσ [óxos] (i.e., sharing and pungent). Looking to another ancient culture, the Hebrew word for vinegar used in the Old Testament is *koe-metz* (also transliterated as *chomets, homets*), meaning "pungent" or "fermented."

In Korea, the origins of vinegar production and use are generally unclear. However, there is an old saying in Korean that "wine becomes vinegar when it is changed." We therefore expect that vinegar production and use began together with the development of wine. In addition, "The Record of the Three Kingdoms" in China states that "the people of Goguryeo enjoyed brewing themselves," suggesting that wine and vinegar were produced and used prior to the period of the Three Kingdoms in Korea. Furthermore, the *Jibongyuseol*, which was the first Korean encyclopedia and was written in 1614 by Yi Su-Kwang, states that "another name for vinegar is a liquor made from nonglutinous rice." This traditional vinegar has been used for centuries as an ingredient for cooking, such as a flavoring agent and a preservative. Moreover, a number of pieces of literature, such as the *Kosachoalyu* (sixteenth century), the *Sanlimkyungje* (seventeenth and eighteenth centuries), and the *Dongkuksesiki* (nineteenth century), mentioned ingredients and formulae for vinegar production, and were published during the Chosun dynasty (1392–1910).

In terms of additional uses for vinegar besides cooking, the medical use of vinegar for the treatment of various diseases, such as furuncle and palsy, was described in the *Hyangyakgugeupbang*, a Korean book of medicine written in the tenth century. Additionally, the *Donguibogam* Korean traditional medical encyclopedia, published in 1610 by oriental medical practitioner Heo Jun, states that "vinegar is innoxious, tastes sour, makes our body warm, removes a furunculus, and remedies the vertigo" (Figure 9.1). The English version of *Donguibogam* is now available in many overseas libraries; a study regarding the history of Korean traditional vinegars based on systematic research of old literature can be found in a review by Lim and Cha (2010). In their research, types and characteristics of the vinegars produced in the Chosun dynasty were well characterized with reference to representative old literature published from the fifteenth to the nineteenth centuries— for example, *Sangayorok* (ca. 1459), *Sikryochanyo* (1460), *Sooeunjabbang* (1540s), *Gosachalyo* (1554), *Dongeuibogam* (1613), *Sasichanyocho* (1655), *Jubangmoon* (end of the 1600s), *Shinganguwhang* (1660), *Eumsikdimibang* (1670s), *Yorok* (1680s), *Chisengyoram* (1691), *Sanrimkyoungje* (1715), *Eumsikbo* (1700s), *Onjubeop*

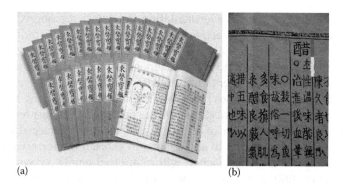

FIGURE 9.1
(a) The original *Donguibogam*, a Korean traditional medical encyclopedia published in 1610 by Heo Jun and (b) the vinegar item stated in the chapter "Tangaek-pheon" of *Donguibogam*.

(late 1700s), *Sulmandeununbeop* (end of the 1700s), *Kyuhapchongseo* (1809), *Imwonsipyukji* (1827), *Jungildangjabji* (1856), *Sulbitneunbeop* (end of the 1800s), *Siuijeonseo* (end of the 1800s), and *Buinpilji* (1915).

9.2 Production

In the case of fermented vinegar, the vinegar is produced via a two-step fermentation process carried out by several microorganisms, including molds, yeasts, and bacteria (Rainieri and Zambonelli, 2009). As vinegar production can be associated with different microorganisms, this suggests that vinegar contains not only acetic acid, but also various other metabolic compounds that modify the flavor and taste of the resulting final product (Lee et al., 2015). The first step in the production process is ethanol fermentation, where simple sugars present in the raw material are converted into ethanol by yeast, such as *Saccharomyces cerevisiae*. The resulting ethanol is further oxidized to acetic acid by acetic acid bacteria during the second step, which ultimately results in the preparation of acetic acid from various sugary and starchy materials by these sequential fermentation steps (Gullo et al., 2014).

In the context of the fermentation system employed, vinegar production can be separated into two different classes: namely, an independent two-step fermentation and a simultaneous two-step fermentation. Of these two systems, traditional Korean fermented vinegars have generally been prepared by the latter, where alcoholic fermentation by yeast and acetic acid fermentation by acetic acid bacteria occur simultaneously. However, vinegar production via fermentation can be split into a further two main methods—that is, a slow process involving static surface fermentation, and a fast submerged fermentation process. Generally, static fermentation is employed in the traditional production of vinegar (Nanda et al., 2001). This process proceeds slowly over the course of months or a year, and as such, vinegar is primarily produced by the more rapid submerged fermentation process on an industrial scale. Indeed, the latter of these two processes has several advantages, including high yields and process speeds (Gullo et al., 2014). More specifically, the fast fermentation process involves the addition of a "mother of vinegar" bacterial culture to the ethanol-containing liquid to accelerate and shorten the fermentation process, with completion being reached within approximately 3 days. However, although the traditional method is not costly because longer time is needed than industrial production to complete the fermentation period, the traditional method is advantageous in terms of its superior product quality (e.g., flavor and taste) and the abundance of functional ingredients (e.g., organic acids, minerals, and polyphenols) in the final product. A schematic outline of the methods employed in vinegar production is provided in Figure 9.2.

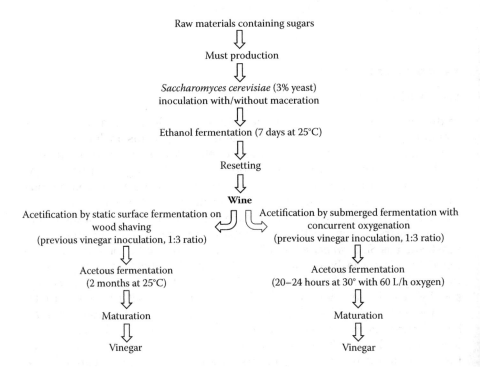

FIGURE 9.2
Schematic outline showing the methods employed in vinegar production. (Adapted from Budak N.H. et al. 2014. *J Food Sci* 79:R757–764.)

9.3 Acetic Acid Bacteria

Acetic acid bacteria are a group of bacteria that belong to the Acetobacteriaceae family. In addition to their application in vinegar production, they play important roles in plant-associated nitrogen-fixing bacteria and in the symbiosis of insects and human pathogens (Pedraza, 2008; Kim et al., 2012). They belong to the group of obligate aerobes (i.e., they require oxygen to grow) and are Gram-negative bacteria (Budak et al., 2014). In addition, these bacteria do not form spores and take the form of ellipsoidal or rod-shaped cells (Sengun and Karapinar, 2004). More specifically, *Acetobacter* and *Gluconobacter* are the two main genera employed in vinegar production, where the choice of culture dictates the specific production method. It is well known that the genus *Acetobacter* oxidizes alcohol preferentially over glucose, whereas the genus *Gluconobacter* preferentially oxidizes glucose over ethanol (Swings and De Ley, 1981; Yamada, 2000; Giudici et al., 2009). Indeed, the various acetic acid bacteria species isolated from different kinds of vinegar have been characterized in a recent article by Budak et al. (2014). During the acetic acid fermentation step, the oxidation of a carbon source (i.e., ethanol) into a corresponding organic acid (i.e., acetic acid) takes place (Adachi et al., 2003; Gullo et al., 2014). This biotransformation to yield acetic acid under the action of acetic acid bacteria is therefore the key step in this process (Solieri and Giudici, 2009):

$$2C_2H_5OH + O_2 \rightarrow 2CH_3CHO + H_2O \rightarrow 2CH_3COOH$$
$$+ H_2O(\Delta H = -493\,kJ/mol)$$

As stated previously, acetic acid bacteria belong to the group of obligate aerobic bacteria, which means that they carry out oxidative reactions and channel the released electrons to molecular oxygen (Mamlouk and Gullo, 2013). For this reason, the acetic acid fermentation process is otherwise known as oxidative fermentation. Acetic acid bacteria have also been associated with the production of several other foods, including nonfermented foods. During vinegar production, acetic acid bacteria partially oxidize ethanol via two successive catalytic reactions involving alcohol dehydrogenase (ADH) and a membrane-bound aldehyde dehydrogenase (ALDH). The complete oxidation of ethanol is achieved at the cytoplasmic level by nicotinamide adenine dinucleotide (NAD)-ADH and NAD-ALDH. The produced acetic acid can then be further utilized by acetyl CoA synthase and via the tricarboxylic acid (TCA) or Krebs cycle (Mamlouk and Gullo, 2013). The membrane-bound ADH and ALDH complexes are tightly linked to the respiratory chain, which transfers electrons via ubiquinone and a terminal ubiquinol oxidase to oxygen as the final electron acceptor (Matsushita et al., 2004).

Thus, ADH oxidizes ethanol to acetaldehyde, which is further oxidized to acetic acid by ALDH as follows:

Alcohol dehydrogenase (ADH):

$$CH_3CH_2OH + \text{pyrroloquinoline quinone (PQQ)} \rightarrow CH_3CHO + PQQH_2$$

Aldehyde dehydrogenase (ALDH):

$$CH_3CHO + PQQ + H_2O \rightarrow CH_3COOH + PQQH_2$$

9.4 Varieties

As vinegar is generally an inexpensive product, its production requires low-cost raw materials, such as substandard fruits, seasonal agricultural surpluses, by-products from food processing, and fruit waste (Solieri and Giudici, 2009). Indeed, vinegar can be produced from a range of starch- or sugar-containing food sources for its ultimate use in a variety of food applications. As outlined in Table 9.1, many types of vinegars exist worldwide, including apple cider vinegar, wine vinegar, sake lees vinegar, spirit vinegar, balsamic vinegar, beer vinegar, cane vinegar, champagne vinegar, coconut vinegar, malt vinegar, persimmon vinegar, potato vinegar, and rice vinegar.

In Korea, grains were the most preferred raw ingredient in traditional vinegar production. Grain vinegars were produced primarily from rice, wheat, barley, and millet. Depending on the raw material of grain vinegars, traditional Korean grain vinegars were called micho (nonglutinous rice vinegar), sajeolcho (glutinous rice vinegar), jinmaekcho (wheat vinegar), daemaekcho (barley vinegar), and changpocho (millet vinegar) (Lim and Cha, 2010). The most popular vinegar in Korea was brown rice vinegar prepared from bran-containing unpolished brown rice mixed with nuruk, a Korean fermentation starter that induces static surface fermentation (Kim et al., 2016b). In addition, Korean brown rice vinegar is similar to Chinese and Japanese black vinegar (*heicu* in Chinese and *kurosu* in Japanese) (Murooka et al., 2009). Fermentation methods for rice vinegar include the traditional static method and the recently developed continuous-culture and batch-culture methods (Nanda et al., 2001). While a number of companies manufacture brown rice vinegar via a modern submerged fermentation process, it is mainly produced using the traditional technique based on a simultaneous two-step fermentation process.

Sikcho (Korean Vinegar) 223

TABLE 9.1

Overview of Vinegars Found Worldwide

Category	Raw Material	Vinegar Name	Geographical Distribution
Vegetable[a]	Rice	Rice vinegar	East and Southeast Asia
	Bamboo sap	Bamboo vinegar[b]	Japan, Korea
	Malt	Malt vinegar	Northern Europe, USA
	Palm spa	Palm vinegar, toddy vinegar	Southeast Asia, Africa
	Barley	Beer vinegar	Germany, Austria, Netherlands
	Millet	Black vinegar	China, East Asia
	Wheat	Black vinegar	China, East Asia
	Sorghum	Black vinegar	China, East Asia
	Tea and sugar	Kombucha vinegar	Russia, Asia
	Onion	Onion vinegar	East and Southeast Asia
	Tomato	Tomato vinegar	Japan, East Asia
	Sugarcane	Cane vinegar	France, United States, Philippines, Japan
Fruit	Apple	Cider vinegar	United States, Canada
	Grape	Raisin (grape) vinegar	Turkey, Middle East
		Wine vinegar	Widespread
		Sherry (jerez) vinegar	Spain
		Balsamic vinegar	Italy
	Coconut	Coconut water vinegar	Philippines, Sri Lanka
	Date	Date vinegar	Middle East
	Mango	Mango vinegar	East and Southeast Asia
	Red date	Jujube vinegar	China
	Raspberry	Raspberry vinegar	East and Southeast Asia
	Blackcurrant	Blackcurrant vinegar	East and Southeast Asia
	Blackberry	Blackberry vinegar	East and Southeast Asia
	Mulberry	Mulberry vinegar	East and Southeast Asia
	Plum	Ume-su	Japan
	Cranberry	Cranberry vinegar	East and Southeast Asia
	Persimmon	Persimmon vinegar	South Korea, Japan
Animal	Whey	Whey vinegar	Europe
	Honey	Honey vinegar	Europe, America, Africa

Source: Solieri L., and P. Giudici. 2009. In *Vinegars of the world*, ed. L. Solieri, and P. Giudici, 1–16. Springer, Milan, Italy.

Note: Some content of this table is slightly modified.

[a] "Vegetable" is not a botanical term and it is used to refer to an edible plant part; some botanical fruits, such as tomatoes, are also generally considered to be vegetables.

[b] Obtained by bamboo sap fermentation.

On the other hand, traditional fruit vinegars in Korea were produced mainly from jujube (daechucho) in addition to plum (maejacho), persimmon (gamcho), peach (dochobang), and akebia berry (moktongcho) (Lim and Cha, 2010). Recently, diverse fruit vinegars, such as apple and persimmon vinegars, have been available in the Korean market. Such fruit vinegars exhibit unique aromas and flavors, as the flavors of the original fruits remain in the final product. In addition, fruit vinegars contain high concentrations of various polyphenolic compounds (Conner and Allgeier, 1976; Matsuo and Ito, 1978), which originate from the raw materials, the added nutrients, and even from the water used for dilution. Furthermore, although the majority of fruit vinegars are produced in Europe, where there is a growing market for high-price vinegars made solely from specific fruits, a number of varieties are produced in Asia. For example, persimmon and apple vinegars have recently become popular in South Korea.

9.5 Major Constituents

As a number of organic acids and amino acids are naturally found in a variety of cereals and fruits, vinegars prepared via the fermentation of such raw materials contain a variety of organic acids (e.g., acetic, lactic, ascorbic, citric, malic, propionic, succinic, and tartaric acids) and amino acids (e.g., essential amino acids and gamma-aminobutyric acid [GABA]) (Jeong, 2009; Budak et al., 2014). Indeed, Na et al. (2013) recently reported various properties (i.e., pH, total acids, free amino acids, total polyphenolics, and total flavonoids) of commercial Korean fermented vinegars prepared from different raw materials, and the results are presented in Table 9.2. According to their study, the total acid and free amino acid contents of brewing vinegar were the highest among the seven commercial vinegars examined, while persimmon vinegar contained the highest GABA content. These commercial vinegars also contained a variety of polyphenolic compounds, including gallic, caffeic, syringic, and coumaric acids, which are well known to play an important role in the antioxidant activity of vinegar (Lee et al., 2009; Cejudo-Bastante et al., 2010; Qiu et al., 2010). In addition, Jeong et al. (2011) reported a comparative study of volatile compounds in four commercial vinegar-based beverages manufactured in Korea, Italy, and Japan. Using a solid-phase microextraction–gas chromatography/mass selective detector (SPME-GC/MSD) method, they analyzed a total of 179 volatile flavor compounds: namely, 12 acids, 27 esters, 20 alcohols, 13 aldehydes, 72 terpenes, 14 aromatic hydrocarbons, 11 ketones, and 10 miscellaneous compounds. They found that Italian and Japanese vinegar-based beverages contained similar flavor compositions (i.e., acids, ketones, and esters), while the major components in Japanese yuzu-ponz and Korean vinegar beverages were terpenes (79.6%) and acids (81.0%), respectively.

To date, the majority of compositional studies on vinegar have focused on the low molecular weight components outlined before. However, the chemical properties and biological activities of polysaccharide-based

TABLE 9.2

Chemical Characteristics of Various Korean Commercial Vinegars Fermented from Different Ingredients

Sample	pH	Total Acid (% as Acetic Acid)	Total Amino Acid (mg/100 g)	Total Polyphenol (mg/kg)	Total Flavonoid (mg/kg)
Fig vinegar	3.37 ± 0.08^b	5.48 ± 0.10^b	358.89	320.94 ± 20.74^b	91.75 ± 3.55^b
Brown rice vinegar	2.53 ± 0.06^c	6.57 ± 0.12^a	10.92	21.34 ± 2.08^c	5.86 ± 0.39^f
Apple vinegar	2.54 ± 0.07^c	6.33 ± 0.13^a	56.85	41.97 ± 4.60^d	9.41 ± 0.75^e
Persimmon vinegar	3.60 ± 0.09^a	4.38 ± 0.08^c	353.02	485.13 ± 27.16^a	194.85 ± 6.18^a
Brewing vinegar	3.37 ± 0.10^b	4.54 ± 0.06^c	521.05	284.10 ± 21.43^b	86.05 ± 3.24^c
Rice vinegar	2.62 ± 0.05^c	5.28 ± 0.11^b	122.31	83.86 ± 10.19^c	17.41 ± 0.92^d
Plum vinegar	2.39 ± 0.04^d	6.51 ± 0.09^a	103.52	44.41 ± 3.24^d	8.61 ± 0.43^e

Source: Na H.S. et al. 2013. *Korean J Food Preserv* 20:482–487.

Notes: Some content of this table is slightly modified. Results were expressed as means ± standard deviations.

[a-e] Different superscript letters indicate significant difference ($p < 0.05$) considered by Duncan's multiple range test.

macromolecules in vinegar have not yet been investigated in detail. This is due to the presence of small amounts of alcohol in some vinegars precipitating the high molecular weight materials, which results in the filtered vinegar product containing only small amounts of the macromolecules. However, a number of recent studies have reported that a low alcohol content may permit solubilization of specific macromolecules, such as polysaccharides. More specifically, some groups have focused on the study of carbohydrates as minor constituents of various traditionally fermented Korean vinegars (Matsuo and Ito, 1978; Kim et al., 2003; Qiu et al., 2010; Jeong and Cha, 2016).

9.6 Physiological Functions

Several physiological studies into the presence of bioactive substances in vinegar have proposed that the beneficial health effects of vinegar could be attributed to compounds such as polyphenols and organic acids. For example, the presence of such low molecular weight substances could account for the antioxidant (Lee et al., 2009; Chung et al., 2010; Hong et al., 2012; Park et al., 2012; Jo et al., 2013; Kim et al., 2013; Shin et al., 2014; Jeong and Cha, 2016; Yim et al., 2016), antimicrobial (Kim et al., 2003; Jeong and Cha, 2016), anticancer (Chung et al., 2010), antidiabetic (Lee et al., 2012), and antiobesity (Oh et al., 2014; Park et al., 2014) effects of Korean vinegars (Table 9.3). Based on these observations, a number of studies have suggested that the daily consumption of vinegar may promote human health and metabolism. Further details regarding the potential health benefits of vinegars can be found in a review by Budak et al. (2014).

In addition, the immunostimulatory activity of vinegar was recently investigated through the analysis of polysaccharides isolated from vinegar. For example, Kim et al. (2015) recently isolated six crude polysaccharides from commercially fermented vinegars manufactured from a range of raw materials, and evaluated their immunostimulatory activity using murine peritoneal macrophage cells. They reported that the polysaccharide isolated from fermented Korean vinegars, and in particular persimmon vinegar and brown rice vinegar, may confer immunostimulatory effects that are beneficial to human health. They also proposed the chemical structure of the immunostimulatory polysaccharide isolated from persimmon vinegar, assuming that it was likely produced during the fermentation process (Figure 9.3). Based on these results, the authors recently investigated the effects of the oral administration of vinegar polysaccharides (i.e., KPV-0 isolated from Korean persimmon vinegar, and KBV-CP isolated from Korean brown rice vinegar) on the intestinal

TABLE 9.3

Biological Activities of Various Korean Commercial Vinegars Fermented from a Range of Raw Materials

Vinegar	Additives[a]	Biological Activity	Ref.
Pear vinegar	–	Antioxidant	Yim et al. (2016)
Brown rice vinegar	Monascus-fermented soybean	Tyrosinase and elastase inhibition	Hwang et al. (2016)
Wheat vinegar	Mugwort	Antioxidant	Shin et al. (2014)
Black raspberry vinegar	–	Antioxidant	Park et al. (2012)
Cucumber vinegar	–	Antioxidant and hepatic aldehyde dehydrogenase activity	Hong et al. (2012)
Dropwort vinegar	Fermented dropwort extract	Inhibition of adipocyte differentiation and inflammation	Park et al. (2014)
Dropwort vinegar	Fermented dropwort extract	Protective effect on oxidative damage	Kim et al. (2013)
Ginseng vinegar	–	Lipid metabolism	Oh et al. (2014)
Mushroom vinegar	Three kinds of mushroom extract	Antioxidant and anticancer	Chung et al. (2010)
Onion vinegar	Yuza and apple extract	Antibiotic and antioxidant	Jeong and Cha (2016)
Onion vinegar	–	Stabilizes cerebral blood flow	Choi et al. (2012)
Yacon vinegar	–	Antidiabetic	Lee et al. (2012)
19 vinegars	–	Antioxidant	Lee et al. (2009)
6 vinegars	–	Immunostimulation	Kim et al. (2015)
3 vinegars	–	Immunostimulation	Kim and Shin (2014)
6 vinegars	–	Antioxidant	Jo et al. (2013)
5 vinegars		Antibiotic	Kim et al. (2003)

Source: Budak N. H. et al. 2014. *J Food Sci* 79:R757–764.
[a] "Additives" employed during preparation of the vinegar.

immune system using experimental mice. The results of this study led us to conclude that both KPV-0 and KBV-CP may stimulate the complete intestinal immune system (i.e., both the mucosal immune system and the systemic immune system) when taken orally (Lee et al., 2015; Kim et al., 2016b). We therefore concluded that, together with the low molecular weight compounds such as amino acids and polyphenols, the presence of high molecular weight polysaccharides in some vinegars appears to stimulate the intestinal immune system via oral consumption and could therefore be beneficial to human health.

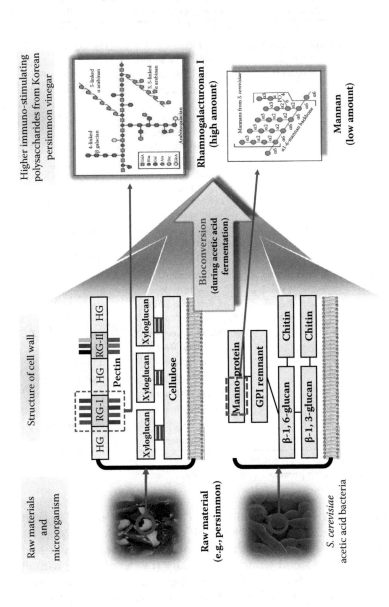

FIGURE 9.3
Proposed origin of the immunostimulatory polysaccharide. This polysaccharide likely originates from cell wall polysaccharides of the fermentative microbes and from the raw materials employed in vinegar production. HG, RG-I, and RG-II represent the homogalacturonan, and rhamnogalacturonan I and II regions, respectively, of the pectic polysaccharide in plant cell walls. (Based on Kim H. et al. 2016a. *Int J Biol Macromol* 89:319–327.)

9.7 Conclusion

Vinegar has been traditionally produced in Korea from cereals such as rice, barley, and corn over a number of centuries. In the 1970s, the development of synthetic vinegar resulted in a rapid increase in vinegar consumption, with this low-cost vinegar being produced and consumed until quite recently (Jeong, 2009). By the 1990s, the fermented vinegar market reached an industrial scale following the preparation of persimmon vinegar via fermentation from the pure raw material in the absence of additives. By the 2010s, Korea was exporting fermented vinegars to 42 countries due to a surplus, with the products of vinegar-based beverages accounting for the largest market share in Japan. Consequently, various major food companies in Korea, such as Daesang, Sampyo, CJ Cheiljedang, Woongjin, and Lottechilsung, launched a range of vinegar products manufactured on a large scale via the fast fermentation process. Meanwhile, medium- and small-sized enterprises joined the market race by launching traditionally fermented vinegars from functional raw materials, such as pomegranates, blueberries, mulberries, dropwort fruits, melons, peaches, potatoes, and jujubes.

As such, the competition to develop novel attractive vinegar products has recently intensified, with their development and application attracting growing attention. Based on our survey into vinegar research since 2010, we found that research trends tended to focus on the use of vegetables (i.e., edible plants such as black garlic, cucumber, dropwort, jujube, mulberry, onion, ginseng, wasabi, and yacon) in the development of novel vinegar products and their applications. Furthermore, current research tends to focus on the development of new vinegar products supplemented with biologically active additives (e.g., garlic, ginseng, jujube, and mushroom extracts) and the subsequent evaluation of their biological activities—in particular, their potential antioxidant effects. However, further studies related to the health effects of vinegar consumption by humans are necessary.

References

Adachi O., D. Moonmangmee, H. Toyama, M. Yamada, E. Shinagawa, and K. Matsushita. 2003. New developments in oxidative fermentation. *Appl Microbiol Biotechnol* 60:643–653.

Budak N.H., E. Aykin, A.C. Seydim, A.K. Greene, and Z.B. Guzel-Seydim. 2014. Functional properties of vinegar. *J Food Sci* 79:R757–764.

Cejudo Bastante M.J., E. Duran Guerrero, R. Castro Mejias, R. Natera Marin, M.C. Rodriguez Dodero, and C.G. Barroso. 2010. Study of the polyphenolic composition and antioxidant activity of new sherry vinegar-derived products by maceration with fruits. *J Agric Food Chem* 58:11814–11820.

Choi C.H., K.Y. Kim, W.S. Jeong et al. 2012. Effects of onion vinegar on the cerebral blood flow and the safety examination. *Korean J Orient Physiol Pathol* 26:657–664.

Chung B. H., H.S. Seo, H.S. Kim, S.H. Woo, and Y.G. Cho. 2010. Antioxidant and anticancer effects of fermentation vinegars with *Phellinus linteus, Inonotus obliquus,* and *Pleurotus ostreatus. Korean J Medicinal Crop Sci* 18:113–117.

Conner H. A., and R.J. Allgeier. 1976. Vinegar: Its history and development. *Adv Appl Microbiol* 20:81–133.

Giudici P., M. Gullo, and L. Solieri. 2009. Traditional balsamic vinegar. In *Vinegars of the world,* ed. L. Solieri, P. Giudici. 157–177. Springer, Milan, Italy.

Gullo M., E. Verzelloni, and M. Canonico. 2014. Aerobic submerged fermentation by acetic acid bacteria for vinegar production: Process and biotechnological aspects. *Process Biochem* 49:1571–1579.

Hong S.M., J.H. Lee, H.I. Lee, J.H. Jeong, and K.I. Seo. 2012. Development of functional vinegar by using cucumbers. *J Korean Soc Food Sci Nutr* 41:927–935.

Hwang J.Y., H.Y. Cho, and Y.H. Pyo. 2016. Effect of unpolished rice vinegar containing Monascus-fermented soybean on inhibitory activities of tyrosinase and elastase. *J Korean Soc Food Sci Nutr* 45:149–154.

Jeong E.J., and Y.J. Cha. 2016. Development of an onion vinegar beverage containing yuza (*Citrus junos Sieb* ex Tanaka) and its biological activity. *J Life Sci* 26:563–570.

Jeong E.J., S.Y. Jeon, J.H. Baek, and Y.J Cha. 2011. Volatile flavor compounds in commercial vinegar beverages derived from fruits. *J Life Sci* 21:292–299.

Jeong Y.J. 2009. Current trends and future prospects in the Korean vinegar industry. *Food Sci Ind* 42:52–59.

Jo D.J., E.J. Park, S.H. Yeo, Y.J. Jeong, and J.H. Kwon. 2013. Physicochemical and antioxidant properties of commercial vinegars with high acidity. *J Korean Soc Food Sci Nutr* 42:1204–1210.

Kim D.S., B.S. Hurh, and K.S. Shin. 2015. Chemical characteristics and immunostimulatory activity of polysaccharides from fermented vinegars manufactured with different raw materials. *J Korean Soc Food Sci Nutr* 44:191–199.

Kim D.S., and K.S. Shin. 2014. Chemical property and macrophage stimulating activity of polysaccharides isolated from brown rice and persimmon vinegars. *Korean J Food Nutr* 27:1033–1042.

Kim E.K., S.H. Kim, H.J. Nam et al. 2012. Draft genome sequence of *Gluconobacter morbifer* G707T, a pathogenic gut bacterium isolated from *Drosophila melanogaster* intestine. *J Bacteriol* 194:1245.

Kim H., H.D. Hong, H.J. Suh, and K.S. Shin. 2016a. Structural and immunological feature of rhamnogalacturonan I-rich polysaccharide from Korean persimmon vinegar. *Int J Biol Macromol* 89:319–327.

Kim H., H. Lee, and K.S. Shin. 2016b. Intestinal immunostimulatory activity of neutral polysaccharide isolated from traditionally fermented Korean brown rice vinegar. *Biosci Biotechnol Biochem:*1–8.

Kim M.J., J.H. Choi, S.H. Kwon, H.D. Kim, M.H. Bang, and S.A. Yang. 2013. Characteristics of fermented dropwort extract and vinegar using fermented dropwort extract and its protective effects on oxidative damage in rat glioma C6 cells. *Korean J Food Sci Technol* 45:350–355.

Kim O.M., D.J. Ha, and Y.J. Jeong. 2003. Antibacterial activity of vinegars on *Streptococcus mutans* caused dental caries. *Korean J Food Preserv* 10:565–568.

Lee M.K., S.R. Choi, J. Lee et al. 2012. Quality characteristics and anti-diabetic effect of yacon vinegar. *J Korean Soc Food Sci Nutr* 41:79–86.

Lee M.Y., H. Kim, and K.S. Shin. 2015. *In vitro* and *in vivo* effects of polysaccharides isolated from Korean persimmon vinegar on intestinal immunity. *J Korean Soc Appl Biol Chem* 58:867–876.

Lee S.M., Y.M. Choi, Y.W. Kim, D.J. Kim, and J.S. Lee. 2009. Antioxidant activity of vinegars commercially available in Korean markets. *Food Eng Prog* 13:221–225.

Lim E.J., and G.H. Cha. 2010. Study on manufacturing of vinegar through literatures of the Joseon dynasty. *J Korean Soc Food Cult* 25:680–707.

Mamlouk D., and M. Gullo. 2013. Acetic acid bacteria: Physiology and carbon sources oxidation. *Indian J Microbiol* 53:377–384.

Matsuo T., and S. Ito. 1978. The chemical structure of kaki-tannin from immature fruit of the persimmon (*Diospyros kaki L.*). *Agric Biol Chem* 42:1637–1643.

Matsushita K., H. Toyama, and O. Adachi. 2004. Respiratory chains in acetic acid bacteria: Membrane-bound periplasmic sugar and alcohol respirations. In *Respiration in archaea and bacteria: Diversity of prokaryotic respiratory systems*, ed. D. Zannoni, 81–99. Springer Netherlands, Dordrecht.

Murooka Y., K. Nanda, and M. Yamashita. 2009. Rice vinegars. In *Vinegars of the world*, ed. L. Solieri, P. Giudici, 121–33. Springer, Milan, Italy.

Na H.S., G.C. Choi, S.I. Yang et al. 2013. Comparison of characteristics in commercial fermented vinegars made with different ingredients. *Korean J Food Preserv* 20:482–487.

Nanda K., M. Taniguchi, S. Ujike et al. 2001. Characterization of acetic acid bacteria in traditional acetic acid fermentation of rice vinegar (komesu) and unpolished rice vinegar (kurosu) produced in Japan. *Appl Environ Microbiol* 67:986–990.

Oh Y.J., S.H. Kwon, K.B. Choi, T.S. Kim, and I.H. Yeo. 2014. Effect of vinegar made with hydroponic-cultured *Panax ginseng* C. A. Meyer on body weight and lipid metabolism in high-fat diet-fed mice. *Korean J Food Sci Technol* 46:743–749.

Park S., Chae K. S., Son R. H., Jung J. H., Im Y. R., and Kwon J. W. 2012. Quality characteristics and antioxidant activity of bokbunja (Black raspberry) vinegars. *Food Eng Prog* 16:340–346.

Park Y.H., J.H. Chioi, K. Whang, S.O. Lee, S.A. Yang, and M.H. Yu. 2014. Inhibitory effects of lyophilized dropwort vinegar powder on adipocyte differentiation and inflammation. *J Life Sci* 24:476–484.

Pedraza R.O. 2008. Recent advances in nitrogen-fixing acetic acid bacteria. *Int J Food Microbiol* 125:25–35.

Qiu J., C. Ren, J. Fan, and Z. Li. 2010. Antioxidant activities of aged oat vinegar in vitro and in mouse serum and liver. *J Sci Food Agric* 90:1951–1958.

Rainieri S., and C. Zambonelli. 2009. Organisms associated with acetic acid bacteria in vinegar production. In *Vinegars of the world*, ed. L. Solieri, and P. Giudici, 73–95. Springer-Verlag, Milan, Italy.

Sengun I.Y., and M. Karapinar. 2004. Effectiveness of lemon juice, vinegar and their mixture in the elimination of *Salmonella typhimurium* on carrots (*Daucus carota* L.). *Int J Food Microbiol* 96:301–305.

Shin J.H., K.M. Cho, and W.T. Seo. 2014. Enhanced antioxidant effect of domestic wheat vinegar using mugwort. *J Agric Life Sci* 48:95–104.

Solieri L., and P. Giudici. 2009. Vinegars of the world. In *Vinegars of the world*, ed. L. Solieri, and P. Giudici, 1–16. Springer, Milan, Italy.

Swings J., and J. De Ley. 1981. The genera *Gluconobacter* and *Acetobacter*. In *The prokaryotes: A handbook on habitats, isolation, and identification of bacteria*, ed. M.P. Starr, H. Stolp, H.G. Trüper, A. Balows, and H.G. Schlegel, 771–778. Springer, Berlin Heidelberg.

Yamada Y. 2000. Transfer of Acetobacter oboediens Sokollek et al. 1998 and Acetobacter intermedius Boesch et al. 1998 to the genus Gluconacetobacter as Gluconacetobacter oboediens comb. nov. and Gluconacetobacter intermedius comb. nov. Int J Syst Evol Microbiol 50 Pt 6:2225–2227.

Yim S.H., K.S. Cho, J.H. Choi et al. 2016. Physicochemical characteristics and antioxidant activity of pear vinegars using "Wonhwang," "Niitaka," "Chuhwangbae" fruits. *Korean J Food Preserv* 23:174–179.

10

Korean Ginseng: Composition, Processing, and Health Benefits

Boo-Yong Lee

CONTENTS

10.1 History 234
    10.1.1 Category 234
    10.1.2 Naming 235
10.2 Cultivation 235
    10.2.1 Cultivation History 235
    10.2.2 Cultivation Technology and Shape 236
10.3 Functional Ingredients 237
    10.3.1 Ginsenosides 237
    10.3.2 Other Functional Ingredients 239
    10.3.3 Comparison of Ginsenosides of Korean Ginseng
           and Foreign Ginsengs 240
    10.3.4 Production and Ginsenosides of Korean Red Ginseng 241
           10.3.4.1 Manufacturing Method... 241
           10.3.4.2 Conversion of Ginsenosides in Processing........... 241
    10.3.5 Manufacturing Method, Ginsenosides, and
           Functionality of Korean Black Ginseng 243
10.4 Excellence of Korean Ginseng 243
10.5 Korean Ginseng in Traditional Herbal Prescriptions 244
10.6 Processed Products 246
10.7 Functional Effects Proved by Modern Science 247
    10.7.1 Enhancement of Immune Function 247
    10.7.2 Antifatigue and Antistress Effects 248
    10.7.3 Antioxidative Stress Effect 248
    10.7.4 Antiaging Effect 248
    10.7.5 Antidiabetic Effect 250
    10.7.6 Antiobesity and Antihyperlipidemia Effects 250
    10.7.7 Effects of Blood Circulation Improvement and Lowered
           Blood Pressure 250
    10.7.8 Enhancement of Cognitive Performance 251
    10.7.9 Enhancement of Sexual Performance....................................... 251

234   *Korean Functional Foods*

      10.7.10 Hangover Reduction Effect..252
      10.7.11 Anticarcinogenic and Cancer-Preventive Effects..................252
      10.7.12 Antiviral and Anti-AIDS Effects..252
10.8   Conclusion..252
References..253

10.1 History

10.1.1 Category

Korean ginseng has been widely known as a mysterious "wonder drug," which has come down from thousands of years of existence in Asia. American ginseng (hwagi-sam), sanchi-sam, and even Siberian ginseng have been commercialized. However, there are plants with species different from *Panax ginseng* C. A. Meyer—Korean ginseng's scientific name—that belong to Araliaceae. They show difference in shape, components, and medicinal properties from Korean ginseng (Lee, 2008a).

More specifically, scientific names of American ginseng and sanchi-sam are *Panax quinquefolium* L. and *Panax notoginseng* Burkill, respectively; thus, they belong to the *Panax* genus, but are different species from Korean ginseng (Table 10.1). Siberian ginseng refers to a woody plant named *Eleutherococcus senticosus* Maxim, which does not belong to the *Panax* genus.

Panax ginseng C. A. Meyer is Korean ginseng's scientific name (1843). The word "panax" is of Greek origin; "pan" (meaning "all") is combined with "axos" (meaning "medicine"). Thus, it means that Korean ginseng is a "panacea" for all diseases.

The first scientific name for ginseng was *Panax schinseng* Nees (Lee, 1980). In 1833, Nees von Esenbeck of Germany described Korean ginseng as *Panax schinseng* var. *coraiensis* Nees in his book, *Icones Plantarum Medicinalium*. Therefore, this was the first, genuinely scientific name for Korean ginseng.

TABLE 10.1

Panax Genus Plants Used as Functional Foods and Medicines

Scientific Name	Leaf Shape	No. of Leaflets per Leaf	Root Shape	Place of Origin
Korean ginseng (Panax ginseng C. A. Meyer)	Long, oval shaped	5	Man shaped	Korea, Manchuria, Littoral Province of Siberia
American ginseng (hwagi-sam, *Panax quinquefolius* L)	Egg shaped	5	Cylinder shaped	United States, Canada
Sanchi-sam (*Panax notoginseng* Burkill)	Oval shaped	7	Small, carrot shaped	Yunnan Province, China

Korean Ginseng 235

However, *Panax ginseng* C. A. Meyer, identified 10 years later, became more widely known and was widely used as a scientific name for Korean ginseng.

10.1.2 Naming

The etymology of "Korea" has its roots in Goguryeo of the Three Kingdoms period. In China, there are as many as 92 records that Goguryeo frequently exchanged ginseng with the Wei dynasty of China, dispatching envoys and exchanging gifts. It can thus be easily speculated that ginseng may has been used as a tribute. Such records show that, from that time, Chinese ginseng and ginseng on the Korean Peninsula were differentiated, and the latter was called "Korean ginseng." There is no doubt that such frequent records on Korean ginseng were attributable to its excellence.

"Korean ginseng" once referred only to ginseng produced in Goguryeo; it was used as a common name indicating ginseng produced in the Three Kingdoms on the Korean Peninsula. The name "Korean ginseng" has a very long history. The same name had been long used through the Unified Silla period, Goryeo dynasty, and Joseon dynasty. Today, Korean ginseng refers to ginseng made in Korea and is used as a synonym for ginseng (Lee, 2008b).

10.2 Cultivation

10.2.1 Cultivation History

The exact period when Korean ginseng first started to be used for medicinal purposes in Korea is not known, yet it is considered to have been quite a long time ago. During the Three Kingdoms period, the medicinal efficacies of ginseng were widely known. It was recorded in *Myeonguibyeollok* (ancient medical literature) that Baekje and Goguryeo sent ginseng (wild ginseng) to China in AD 513 and AD 435–546, respectively. In addition, there is a record in *Chaebuwongu,* a Chinese historical literary work, that Silla sent ginseng to China in AD 627. As such, wild ginseng at that time was developed by private doctors through experience and used for medicinal purposes; it became gradually depleted, which naturally led to its cultivation (Compilation Committee, 1980).

Records on ginseng cultivation do not specify exact periods and mostly take the form of folklore. Although modality differs by regions, in most cases people prayed to the mountain god to cure diseases, have a child, or become rich. Under such guidance, they obtained ginseng seeds and planted them or relocated natural ginseng to other places, thus triggering ginseng cultivation.

When ginseng cultivation was still in initial stages, ginseng mainly referred to wild ginseng. The government ginseng diggers were called *chaesamgun* (ginseng digging man). There were a considerable number of wild ginseng diggers among the general public, other than the state diggers. Therefore, natural ginseng became depleted due to the prevalence of wild ginseng digging, so shortages became severe during the reign of King Seonjo (1567–1608) of the Joseon dynasty.

Afterwards, during the reign of King Sukjong and King Yeongjo of the Joseon dynasty, the forest area was reduced due to deforestation, so the amount of digging for natural ginseng rapidly decreased. However, demand for ginseng further increased, prompting cultivation of gasam (farmed ginseng) and jangnoisam (cultivated wild ginseng). There are records on gasam in *Jeongjongsillok* and other historical documents and there are records on how to cultivate gasam in *Imwonsipyukji* by Seo Yu-Gu. As such, cultivation methods for ginseng on flat land were gradually developed.

In the 1900s cultivation in forests was replaced by cultivation in fields, and large-scale artificial cultivation methods were developed mainly in the Kaesong area in Korea.

10.2.2 Cultivation Technology and Shape

Ginseng seeds are harvested around the end of July and, after the flesh is removed, the ginseng seeds remain. The seeds undergo pregermination treatment for seed germination in which seeds are mixed with sand for 100 days at 20°C and 10%–15% moisture. The seeds are sown in November when the length of the embryo bud grows to more than 5 mm and its testa is wide open. The wide-open testa of ginseng is sown on the bed soil created by mixing clean organic fertilizer and leaves of broad-leaved trees with clean soil without pathogenic bacteria. Only high-quality seeds of more than 4 mm are sown. After they are cultivated for 18 months, ginseng seedlings, which are 16 cm long and weigh 0.7 g, are produced (Compilation Committee, 1980; Choi, 1996).

Before planting ginseng, proper preparation of the soil in which it will be cultivated is conducted. Excessive fertilizers in the soil are absorbed and eliminated by growing rye, Sudan grass, and corn for 1–2 years. The cultivated green crops are supplied again to the soil (4.5 tons per 10 a) to increase organic content and the soil is plowed more than 15 times a year to improve physical properties of the soil and destroy pathogenic bacteria.

In order to control damage caused by harmful insects, new crop protective agents, which have less residue and are effective, are selected for use. In order to produce clean ginseng, pest control by natural substances has been adopted for practical use. To control root rot, which is one of the major causes of impairment from repeated cultivation, a combination of soil sterilization, use of microbial agents, and crop rotation cultivation is adopted in some regions (Choi, 1996).

The shapes of ginseng plants vary, depending on age, varieties, and the cultivation environment. In a 4-year-old ginseng plant, the aboveground

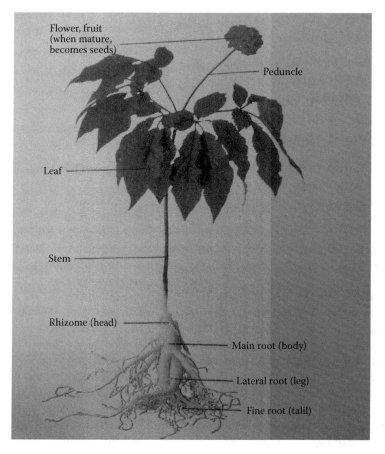

FIGURE 10.1
Name of each part of ginseng.

part has a flower, fruit, peduncle, leaves, and stem, while the underground part (root) has the latent bud, rhizome, fibrous root, main root, rootlets, and fine root (Figure 10.1).

10.3 Functional Ingredients

10.3.1 Ginsenosides

Carbohydrate, including free sugar and starch, comprises 60%–70% of Korean ginseng—the largest part. Korean ginseng contains medicinal ingredients that include ginsenosides; polysaccharide with immunostimulating activity; polyacetylene with anticarcinogenic effects; phenols with antioxidant effects;

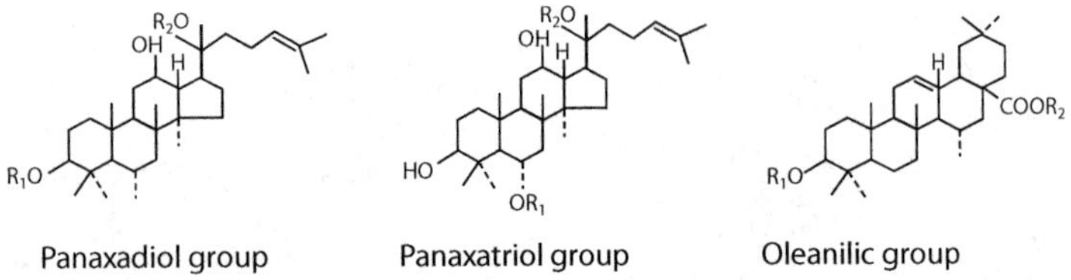

Panaxadiol group   Panaxatriol group   Oleanilic group

FIGURE 10.2
Chemical structure of the aglycone part of ginseng saponins.

gomisin, which protects the liver; and acidic peptide, which acts similarly to insulin (Park, 1996).

Ginseng saponins are called "ginsenosides," which means that glucosides are contained in ginseng. If the sugar part is eliminated from ginseng saponins, three types of aglycones remain: protopanaxadiol (PPD) (Shibata et al., 1965), protopanaxatriol (PPT) (Shibata et al., 1966), and oleanolic acid (Figure 10.2) (Horhammer et al., 1961). The etymological origin of "saponin" is sapo (meaning "soap") in Greek. When saponins are dissolved and shaken in water, they have foaming characteristics. It is reported that there are approximately 750 species of natural saponins and they are widely distributed in the plant kingdom. In general, saponins in plants normally show hemolysis action (dissolving blood corpuscles), but ginsenosides show almost no hemolysis even if taken in large quantities. It has been known since ancient times that long-term consumption of ginseng has no harmful effects on the body.

In terms of the chemical structure, saponins are glucosides that consist of sugar and aglycones. Depending on the frame structure of aglycones, saponins are classified into triterpenoid and steroid saponins. Triterpenoid saponins are again subclassified into lanostane, dammarane, ursane, and oleanane saponins.

Types of ginsenosides that have been discovered to date amount to a total of 38 types, of which the PPD type is 22 ginsenosides, the PPT type is 14 ginsenosides, and the oleanolic acid type is 2 ginsenosides.

PPD-type ginsenosides have glycosidic bonds at hydroxyl groups C-3 and C-20 of protopanaxadiol (see Figure 10.2). Major PPD-type ginsenosides include Ra_1, Ra_2, Rb_1, Rb_2, Rc, Rd, and Rg_3 (Sanada et al., 1974a). PPT-type ginsenosides have glycosidic bonds in the hydroxyl groups C-6 and C-20 of protopanaxadiol, and major PPT-type ginsenosides include Re, Rf, 20gluco Rf, Rg_1, Rg_2, and Rh_1 (Sanada et al., 1974b). Oleanolic acid-type ginsenosides include Ro and polyactyleneginsenoside Ro, discovered by the University of Illinois in 2002 (Zhang et al., 2002).

There are ginsenosides that are commonly contained in both red ginseng and white ginseng, but there are also ginsenosides that are uniquely found only in either red or white ginseng. A total of 24 ginsenosides have been found to exist in white ginseng and a total of 32 ginsenosides in red ginseng (Table 10.2). Ginsenosides Rg_3, Rg_2, and Rh_2, which are common in red

Korean Ginseng

TABLE 10.2

Types of Ginsenosides in Korean Ginseng

Type	Ginsenosides	Total (38 Types)
PPD	Ginsenosides Ra_1, Ra_2, Ra_3, Rb_1, Rb_2, Rb_3, Rc, Rd, Rg_3; quinquenoside R_1; malonyl ginsenosides[b] Rb_1, Rb_2, Rc, Rd; koryoginsenoside[b] R_1, R_2; ginsenosides Rh_2[a], Rs_1[a], RS_2[a], RS_3[a]; 20S ginsenoside Rg_3; notoginsenoside R_4[a]; ginsenoside Rg_5	22
PPT	Ginsenosides Re, Rf, Rg1, Rg2, Rg6a, Rh1; notoginsenoside R1; 20 glucoginsenoside Rf; koryoginsenoside R1; ginsenoside Rf2; 20R ginsenoside Rg2a, Rh1a; ginsenoside Rh4a; 20E ginsenoside F4	14
Oleanolic acid	Ginsenoside R_o, polyactyleneginsenoside R_o[b]	2

[a] Saponins unique to red ginseng (13 kinds).
[b] Saponins unique to white ginseng (seven kinds).

ginseng, do not exist in white ginseng. On the other hand, malonyl ginsenoside, Rb_1, Rb_2, Rc, and Rd exist only in white ginseng (Kitagawa et al., 1983). In particular, ginsenoside Rh_2, which is a unique constituent existing only in red ginseng, has been reported to exert strong inhibitory action on various cancer cells.

10.3.2 Other Functional Ingredients

In addition to saponins, ginseng contains a wide range of ingredients: polysaccharide, polyacetylene, phenolic compounds, essential oil components, peptide, alkaloid, and vitamins. These nonsaponin components also have many medicinal benefits, and important nonsaponin components with antioxidant activity are maltol and Arg-Fru-Glc (arginine-fructose-glucose) (Sanada et al., 1974a), which are generated during the red ginseng manufacturing process.

In the mid-1980s, about 20 kinds of polysaccharides: namely, panaxan A, B, C, D,...U, were isolated from Korean ginseng. Among them, there were neutral polysaccharides, including glucose, galactose, rhamnose, arabinose, and mannose, while acidic polysaccharides included acidic sugars such as uronic acid and galacturonic acid (Konno et al., 1984). Since 2000, acidic polysaccharide with strong immune activity has been isolated from Korean red ginseng and named red ginseng acidic polysaccharide (RGAP) (Park et al., 2001). The RGAP consists of 56.9% acidic sugar and 28.3% neutral sugar; most of the acidic sugar is glucuronic acid, which is assumed to play an important role in immunopotentiating activities.

Korean ginseng contains many kinds of polyacetylenes; major polyacetylenes include panaxynol, panaxydol, and panaxytriol. In particular, panaxydol, which exists only in ginseng, has outstanding inhibitory effects on the proliferation of cancer cells (Hwang, 1992). Panaxytriol is a polyacetylene

240   Korean Functional Foods

unique to red ginseng that is produced when the epoxy ring located at C-9 of panaxydol is hydrolyzed during the red ginseng manufacturing process.

Maltol, a kind of antioxidant phenolic compound, was first discovered in Korean red ginseng (Han et al., 1979). This is a substance produced by the pyrolysis of hexose when steamed at high temperatures during the manufacturing process of red ginseng.

Besides maltol, red ginseng contains antioxidant components, including salicylic acid, ferullic acid (Han et al., 1981), gentisic acid (Wee et al., 1989), caffeic acid, and vanillic acid. Such phenolic compounds show antioxidant effects in tissues of animals with extreme oxidative injury. Comparing the phenolic compounds found in Korean ginseng and American ginseng indicates that there are polyphenol components that exist only in Korean ginseng (Wee et al., 1998).

During the manufacturing process of red ginseng, Arg-Fru-Glc (AFG) and Arg-Fru are produced in large quantities, in addition to maltol. Relatively high proportions of AFG and Arg-Fru exist in red ginseng in 5.37% and 0.2%, respectively.

Korean ginseng contains essential oil compounds and nitrogen compounds that include water-soluble protein, peptide, pyroglutamic acid, and adenosine.

10.3.3 Comparison of Ginsenosides of Korean Ginseng and Foreign Ginsengs

Other varieties of ginseng currently are available in the global market along with Korean ginseng, American ginseng (hwagi-sam), and Chinese ginseng (sanchi-sam). However, Korean ginseng has more kinds of saponins than American or Chinese ginseng (Table 10.3) (Lee, 2007).

Korean ginseng, American ginseng (*Panax quinquefolium*), and Chinese ginseng (*Panax notoginseng*) show great differences in total saponin content and content ratio of each ginsenoside. American ginseng's main ingredients are protopanaxadiol (PPD)-type ginsenosides, including Rb_1, and it has less protopanaxatriol (PPT)-type ginsenosides. Compared to American ginseng, Korean ginseng has a balanced content of these ginsenosides (Han and Woo,

TABLE 10.3

Comparison of Kinds of Ginsenosides of Korean Ginseng and Foreign Ginsengs

Type	Korean Ginseng[a] (*Panax ginseng*)	American Ginseng (Hwagi-Sam) (*Panax quinquefolius*)	Chinese Ginseng (Sanchi-Sam) (*Panax notoginseng*)
PPD	21	13	14
PPT	15	5	15
Oleanolic acid	2	1	–
Total	38	19	29

[a] Figures combine the numbers of ginsenosides in red ginseng and white ginseng.

1974). In particular, ginsenoside Rf, which alleviates pain, does not exist in American ginseng.

10.3.4 Production and Ginsenosides of Korean Red Ginseng

10.3.4.1 Manufacturing Method

The basic process of red ginseng production from fresh ginseng simply consists of three steps: washing, steaming, and drying. Most manufacturers of red ginseng in South Korea produce red ginseng by utilization of traditional production processes, which can be summarized as follows. The fresh ginseng, grown for 4–6 years, is selected by size and shape; the dirt is shaken off; and then the root is washed with clean water. Subsequently, washed fresh ginseng is steamed for 1–3 h at 90°C–98°C (Figure 10.3). Then the steamed ginseng is dried by hot air and laid in the sun until its moisture contents drop to 15%–18% (Lee et al., 2015).

10.3.4.2 Conversion of Ginsenosides in Processing

Dammarane ginsenosides are characteristic components of ginseng and are considered to be its primary pharmacologically effective components. So far, about 50 kinds of ginsenosides have been identified from the ginseng root, and they are defined as protopanaxadiol and protopanaxatriol according to the dammarane skeleton (Christensen, 2009). Large numbers of ginsenosides in fresh ginseng are converted into different saponins by heat treatment during the red ginseng production process. Ginsenosides Rg_2, Rg_6, F_4, 20(E)-F_4, Rh_1, Rh_4, Rk_3, Rg_3, Rg_5, Rz_1, Rk_1, Rg_9, and Rg_{10} have been found in red ginseng, and these are converted from the major ginsenosides Rb_1, Rb_2, Re, Rd, Rg_1, and Re in fresh ginseng (Lee et al., 2013).

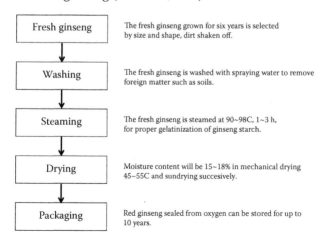

FIGURE 10.3
Process of manufacturing red ginseng from fresh ginseng.

Generally, ginsenosides are denatured by heat and acidic conditions. Red ginseng is treated with the heat process and the inner acidity is weakened by citric acid and other organic acids. Thus, in red ginseng production, ginsenosides must be denatured to the several converted ginsenosides. Conversions from each ginsenoside were estimated as follows: [$Rg_1 \rightarrow Rh_1 \rightarrow Rh_4$, Rk_3], [$Re \rightarrow Rg_2 \rightarrow F_4$, Rg_6], [$Rf \rightarrow Rg_9$, $20Z$-Rg_9, Rg_{10}], and [Rb_1, Rc, Rb_2, $Rd \rightarrow Rg_3 \rightarrow Rg_5$, Rk_1, Rz_1]. These results explain that the contents of the converted ginsenosides such as Rg_2, Rh_1, and Rg_3 progressively increase, and the contents of the natural ginsenosides such as Rg_1, Re, Rb_1, Re, and Rd progressively decrease in the red ginseng production process (Figure 10.4) (Lee, 2014).

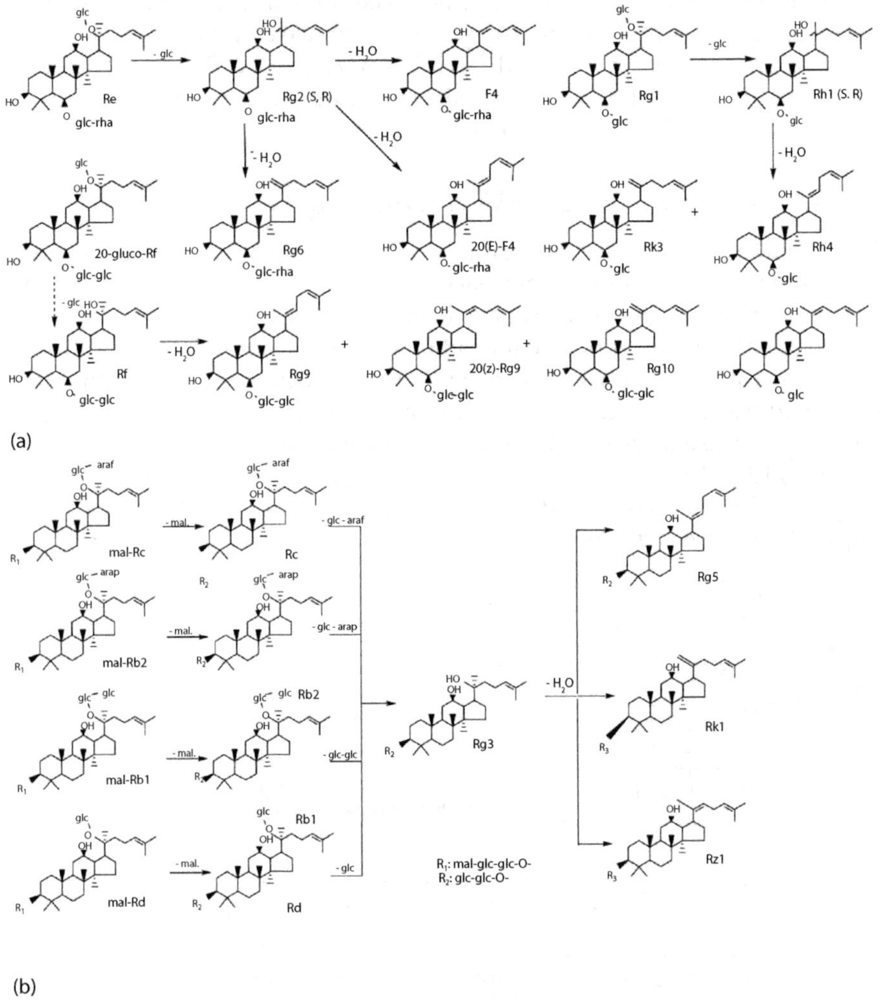

(a)

(b)

FIGURE 10.4
(a) The conversion mechanism of ginsenosides during the red ginseng process. (b) Protopanaxatriol ginsenosides.

10.3.5 Manufacturing Method, Ginsenosides, and Functionality of Korean Black Ginseng

Generally, Korean red ginseng is made by steaming fresh ginseng for 2–3 times. But Korean black ginseng (*Panax ginseng* C. A. Meyer) is steamed three to nine times and dried, and it shows strong black color through the Maillard browning reaction. It has been reported that some chemically deglycosylated and transformed saponins are obtained from black ginseng produced during intensive steaming. Ginsenosides Rg3, Rg4, Rg5, Rg6, Rh1, Rh2, Rh4, Rk1, and Rk3 have been known to be quite different from those of red ginseng, among which ginsenosides Rg3, Rg5, and Rk1 are considered to be major components (Nam et al., 2015).

Also, black ginseng has been recently found to demonstrate anticancer properties (Kim et al., 2008; Nam et al., 2014), to aid in recovery from learning and memory damages (Lee et al., 2010), and to show antihypotensive (Song et al., 2009), antidiabetic (Kim and Kang, 2009), antiobese (Song et al., 2006), tonic, and antiatopic activities (Shin et al., 2012), together with antioxidative (Lee et al., 2012) and exercise performance improving activities (Jo et al., 2010). These effects appear to be a little bit stronger than those of red ginseng. Such findings suggest that black ginseng might play an important role in the development of promising functional foods and drugs from the viewpoint of the chemical composition and biological activities of black ginseng as distinct from those of white and red ginsengs.

10.4 Excellence of Korean Ginseng

In oriental medicine, Korean ginseng has always been regarded as precious as distinguished from other ginsengs. Although there are no statistics available, the differentiation and excellence of Korean ginseng have long been recognized, both by those who are in engaged in oriental medicine and the general public. There are distinct differences in usages among ginsengs of different countries and although usages can be the same, Korean ginseng has been used in differentiation from other ginsengs, in terms of medicinal efficacies.

In terms of kinds of ginsenosides, Korean ginseng contains 38 ginsenosides and American ginseng has 19. Thus, the kinds of ginsenosides in American ginseng are much fewer than those in Korean ginseng. In particular, American ginseng contains less panaxatriol-type ginsenosides, which demonstrate antifatigue effects, antistress benefits, improvement of memory and learning functions, protection of tonic function, and defense effect radioactivity, compared to Korean ginseng. In terms of medicinal efficacy, it is considered that Korean ginseng, with more variety of ginsenosides, has strong and diverse physiological activities.

Korean ginseng contains many components other than saponins:

Polyacetylene compounds: More than 10 kinds of polyacetylene compounds have been isolated from Korean ginseng and it has been revealed that they have inhibitory action on the proliferation of cancer cells (Ames, 1985), antiplatelet activity (Park et al., 1990), and antioxidant activity (Kim et al., 1989).

Aromatic components: Since ancient times, it has been known that Korean red ginseng has an aroma different from that of red ginseng produced in other countries. According to sensory tests, Korean red ginseng has savory and sweet tastes, whereas Chinese red ginseng has aromas of dried tree roots and dried grass (Kim et al., 1993).

Acidic polysaccharides: Polysaccharides are compounds consisting of numerous monosaccharides and their molecular weight is approximately tens of thousands. Recently, they have been revealed to have various physiological activities, so active research on polysaccharides is under way. Among them, panaxan A-U (21 kinds) (Konno and Hikino, 1987), which lowers blood sugar, and polysaccharides with anticomplementary properties (Gao et al., 1989) have been isolated from Korean ginseng.

10.5 Korean Ginseng in Traditional Herbal Prescriptions

Ginseng is a medicinal plant that has been used in medical practices for more than 2,000 years (Park et al., 2012). The *Shennong Bencao Jing* (Shennong's herbal classic), one of the first books specializing in herbal medicine, was edited in the first century AD. In this text, ginseng was first recognized as a medicinal herb by medical practitioners. *Panax ginseng* is a traditional medicinal plant that has been used therapeutically for millennia in East Asia. In Korea, China, and Japan, ginseng is the most valuable of all medicinal herbs. The name *panax* means "all healing," which describes the traditional belief that ginseng can heal all aspects of the body. The most common ginsengs are Korean ginseng (*P. ginseng* C. A. Meyer), Chinese ginseng (*P. notoginseng* [Burk.] FH Chen), and American ginseng (*P. quinquefolium* L.).

Among the ginseng varieties, *P. ginseng* has been extensively researched and has received the most attention. *P. ginseng* is sensitive to the temperature and soil of the cultivated area. Therefore, it is cultivated in limited areas, including Korea, the Manchurian region of China (the region of Dongbei), and the maritime province of Siberia in Russia. Although it is not known whether historical documents described cultivated or wild ginseng, in the present review, we discuss historical accounts concerning *P. ginseng*, its role in traditional prescriptions, and experimental evidence from pharmacological and clinical studies of traditional prescriptions containing *P. ginseng* (Table 10.4).

TABLE 10.4

Summary of Pharmacological Activities of Ginseng-Containing Prescriptions Described in the *Shang-Han Lun* in either Animal or Human Studies

Name of Formula (in Korean)	Name of Formula (in Chinese)	Species	Pharmacological Evaluation
Banhasasim-tang	Ban-xia-xie-xin-tang	Human	Dyspepsia
		Human	Diarrhea
		Mice	Diarrhea
Sosiho-tang	Xiao-chia-hu-tang	Rat	Anaphylaxis
		Human	Hepatic injury
		Rat	Immune Modulation
Insam-tang	Ren-shen-tang	Mouse	Diabetes
Guibi-tang	Gu-pi-tang	Rat	Dementia
		Rat	Osteopenia
		Rat	Thrombocytopenic purpura
Sipjeondaebo-tang	Shi-quan-da-bu-tang	Mouse	Dementia
		Human	Atopic dermatitis
		Human	Anemia
		Human	Otitis
		Rat	Cancer
		Mouse	Immune modulation
Bojungikki-tang	Bu-zhong-yi-qi-tang	Human	Fatigue
		Rat	Diabetes
		Human	Immune modulation
		Hamster	Cancer
		Mouse	Lung injury
		Human	Inflammation
		Rat	Osteopenia
		Human	Atopic dermatitis
		Rat	Liver injury
		Mouse	Antibacterial
Insamyangyoung-tang	Ren-shen-yang-rong-tang	Mouse	Anemia
		Rat	Liver injury
		Mouse	Amnesia
		Rat	Immune modulation
Daegeonjung-tang	Da-jian-zhong-tang	Mouse	Colitis
		Rat	Liver injury
		Human	Gastrointestinal motility
		Human	Blood flow
Saengmaek-san	Sheng-mai-san	Rat	Diabetes
		Mouse	Amnesia
		Rat	Spinal cord injury
		Rat	Liver injury
		Rat	Cerebral ischemia
Siho-ga-yonggolmoryeu-tang	Chai-hu-jia-long-gu-muli-tang	Rabbit	Atherosclerosis

(Continued)

TABLE 10.4 (CONTINUED)

Summary of Pharmacological Activities of Ginseng-Containing Prescriptions Described in the *Shang-Han Lun* in either Animal or Human Studies

Name of Formula (in Korean)	Name of Formula (in Chinese)	Species	Pharmacological Evaluation
Sihokyeji-tang	Chai-hu-gui-zhi-tang	Rat	Gastric ulcer
		Rat	Liver injury
		Mouse	Hepatic drug-metabolizing
		Rat	enzyme activity
			Pancreatitis
Bekho-ga-insam-tang	Bai-hu-jia-ren-shen-tang	Rat	Water balance
		Rat	Salivary secretion
		Mouse	Atopic dermatitis
		Mouse	Antihyperglycemia
Ome-whan	Wu-mei-wan	Rat	Colitis

10.6 Processed Products

Historical records indicate that Korean ginseng was processed into a product by naturally drying fresh ginseng, which resembles the white ginseng of today. However, such white ginseng easily went stale during the rainy season, making it difficult to store it for more than a year. According to historical records, to store white ginseng for a long time, a ginseng processing method in which fresh ginseng was steamed and dried was developed during the reign of King Munjong of the Goryeo dynasty (Compilation Committee, 1980). Processing ginseng by steaming and drying is a manufacturing method that enables it to be stored longer. Thus, it can be regarded as the prototype of the red ginseng manufacturing method of today, which is one of the most representative Korean ginseng processing methods.

The manufacturing technology for red ginseng and white ginseng developed rapidly, and processed ginseng products were produced in large quantities during the late Joseon period under the reigns of King Yeongjo and King Jeongjo, respectively. In 1899, Naejangwon (the Office of Crown Property) under Gungmaebu (Ministry of the Royal Household) came to possess monopoly rights for red ginseng manufacturing. In Gaeseong, Samjeongguk was set up and equipped with red ginseng manufacturing facilities with which 6-year-old fresh ginseng was processed into red ginseng, red ginseng powder, red ginseng extract, red ginseng tablets, etc.

Korean ginseng is classified into four types of products, depending on the processing methods: white ginseng, red ginseng, taegeuk ginseng, and black ginseng. White ginseng is processed with mostly 4- to 5-year-old fresh ginseng, which is washed after removing unnecessary root hairs and either sun-dried or artificially dried to reduce the water content to 15% or less. Red ginseng is manufactured with 4- to 6-year-old fresh ginseng harvested from

September to November when ginseng's active ingredients are formed. Fresh ginseng is washed and steamed two or three times, and then either sun-dried or artificially dried to reduce the water content to 15% or less under strict sanitary control. Taegeuk ginseng is processed with fresh ginseng, which is washed and treated with heated water and dried to reduce its water content to 15% or less. Black ginseng is steamed three to nine times and dried to reduce its water content to 15% or less. Black ginseng shows a strong black color through the Maillard browning reaction.

Ginseng products are manufactured by processing of ginseng roots, which are produced primarily by processing fresh ginseng as their material. Major ginseng products are powder and extracts, which are also used as raw materials for a variety of Korean ginseng products. Ginseng powder products are produced by grinding primarily processed ginseng root into fine powder types of ginseng powder products including pure powder products and powder capsules and tablets that are easy to carry and convenient for taking consistent dosage amounts. Ginseng extract products are produced by extracting and condensing active components of ginseng, using primarily processed ginseng root with water as solvent. Korean ginseng (red ginseng) extract is one of the most representative Korean ginseng products and the most preferred by Korean and international consumers.

Moreover, ginseng extract is also used as a raw material for most processed ginseng products, including ginseng teas, beverages, candies, etc. Ginseng tea products are manufactured by using ginseng extract as the main material and mixing it with lactose and glucose, which is a binding agent, into granules or powder. Ginseng beverage products are manufactured by adding functional plant extracts or food additives.

10.7 Functional Effects Proved by Modern Science

10.7.1 Enhancement of Immune Function

Recently, research on red ginseng's immunoeffects has been receiving attention, and more interest has been directed at the immunity modulation action of polysaccharide rather than saponins. Saponins and polysaccharide promote cell proliferation of T-lymphocyte and, in particular, it has been reported that polysaccharide fractions increased Tc lymphocytes' power to destroy cancer cells three- to fourfold (Mizuno et al., 1994; Rivers et al., 2005). In particular, it has been reported that polysaccharide separated from extracts of tissue-cultured ginseng induced proliferation of B-cells and T-cells. In addition, studies indicate that ginseng saponins have an effect on recovery from inhibited immunity in cyclophosphamide-treated mice. It has been reported that Korean red ginseng increases activity of natural killer (NK) cells, which inhibits metastasis of cancer cells. There are numerous studies proving that Korean red ginseng increases the activity of NK cells (Yun et al.,1987).

In addition, numerous research results have been shown that Korean red ginseng intervenes in the generation and inhibition of cytokines (Kim et al., 1990).

10.7.2 Antifatigue and Antistress Effects

Dr. Brekhman, a pharmacologist in the then–Soviet Union, once explained ginseng's "effect of increasing nonspecific resistance" among its medicinal properties as a concept that illustrates ginseng's tonic effect. He said that ginseng boosted immunity under harmful conditions of a living body, thereby promoting immuno-ability in a nonspecific manner. He dubbed this the "adaptogen" effect (Brekhman and Dardymov, 1969).

In animal testing, restraint stress increased the concentration of polyamine in the brain, yet ginseng saponins inhibited polyamine production (Lee et al., 2006a). Restraint stress increases corticosteroid and interleukin (IL)-6 in blood, but Korean red ginseng inhibited them. Ginseng's recovery function was also proved to be effective in diminished motor function due to forced tightrope walking in mice. Moreover, Korean red ginseng enhances cardio-pulmonary function, thus speeding up recovery from fatigue, and research is being conducted on red ginseng's effects on various types of stress. Korean red ginseng also reduces anxiety symptoms (Han et al., 2005).

10.7.3 Antioxidative Stress Effect

Red ginseng and ginsenosides, the major bioactive constituents in red ginseng, have biological functions ameliorating various disease symptoms via antioxidant mechanisms in cells and animals (especially in rodents). Although there are limitations with respect to human studies on the effect of red ginseng, ingestion of red ginseng has also been shown to improve antioxidant activities in humans, determined by various biomarkers of oxidative stress. Taken together, results show that ingestion of red ginseng can be a preventive strategy against oxidative stress-associated chronic diseases (Table 10.5) (Lee et al., 2016).

10.7.4 Antiaging Effect

It has been reported that nonsaponin components of Korean red ginseng exhibit the scavenging effects of free radicals that are related to the ageing of cells. Moreover, phenolic compounds and maltol of ginseng are reported to play an important role in inhibiting ageing (Han et al., 1979). Recently, a variety of red ginseng products designed to prevent skin ageing have been under development (Chen et al., 1998).

Korean Ginseng

TABLE 10.5

Studies Showing Antioxidant Activity of Red Ginseng in Rodents

Disease Model	Inducer	Red Ginseng Type	Antioxidant Biomarker
Aging	12 months old	Red ginseng water extract	MDA ↓ SOD, CAT, GPx, GR, GST ↑ GSH, Vit C, Vit E ↑
Age-related male sexual dysfunction	12 months old	Red ginseng Water extract	MDA ↓ SOD, CAT, GPx, GR, GST ↑ GSH, Vit C, α-tocopherol ↑
Age-related renal injury	HFD, D-galactose	Red ginseng	8-OHdG ↓ AGE ↓
Hepatic disease	CCI4	Red ginseng essential oil	TBARS ↓ SOD, GPx, CAT ↑
Hepatic disease	Aflatoxin B1	Red ginseng extract	SOD, GPx, CAT ↑ MDA ↓
Alcoholic liver disease	Ethanol	Red ginseng water extract	4-HNE ↓ Nitrotyrosine ↓
Diabetes	Streptozotocin	Fermented red ginseng extract	GSH ↑ MDA ↓ SOD, CAT, GPx, GR ↑
Diabetes	Cyclosporine	Red ginseng water extract	8-OHdG ↓
Gastric ulcer	Hydrochloride/ ethanol indomethacin	Red ginseng powdered extract containing drug	TBARS ↓
High intensive exercise	Treadmill for 3 weeks	HRG	MDA ↓ SOD ↑
Arthritis	Murine type II collagen	Red ginseng Saponin extract	MDA ↓ Nitrotyrosine ↓ SOD, GSH, CAT ↑
Skin cancer	7,12-Dimethylbenz(a) anthracene Croton oil	Red ginseng hydroalcoholic extract	GSH, SOD, CAT, Vit C ↑, TBARS ↓

Notes: 4HNE = 4-hydroxy-2-nonenal; 8-OHdG = 8-hydroxydeoxyguanosine; AA = arachiodonic acid; AGE = advanced glycation end product; CAT = catalase; DCF = 2′,7′-dichroflurescein; GPx = glutathione peroxidase; GR = glutathione reductase; GSH = glutathione; HFD = high-fat diet; HRG = high pressure-treated red ginseng; HO-1 = heme oxygenase 1; MDA = malondialdehyde; NADPH = nicotinamide adenine dinucleotide phosphate; NMDA = N-methyl-D-aspartate; PCB126 = polychlorinated biphenyls; SOD = superoxide dismutase; TBARS = thiobarbituric acid-reacting substance; TRX = thioredoxin reductase; Vit = vitamin.

10.7.5 Antidiabetic Effect

After a single dose of ginseng administration, glucose tolerance tests showed that Korean red ginseng decreased blood glucose levels. When it is given to patients with diabetes, their blood sugar levels after meals are reduced because the ginseng increases insulin secretion (Lee et al., 2006b). In addition, it has been reported that ginsenosides increase insulin activity (Vuksan and Sievenppiper, 2005), although there is also a report that ginsenosides failed to lower blood sugar. Thus, more research is needed on this topic.

10.7.6 Antiobesity and Antihyperlipidemia Effects

Obesity is closely related to adult disease, and numerous study results on the effects of Korean red ginseng on lipid metabolism, hyperlipidemia, and hypercholesterinemia have been reported. In animal tests, ginseng saponins blocked the absorption of fat and cholesterol, thereby promoting metabolism (Kim and Park, 2003). In a human study, in which red ginseng products were administered for 4 weeks, body fat was decreased; a study conducted among obese women in their 20s also delivered a similar result. Korean red ginseng lowers total cholesterol, triglyceride, and low-density lipoprotein (LDL) in blood, expedites the breakdown of body fat, and is thus effective in preventing and treating hyperlipidemia (Yamamoto et al., 1983).

10.7.7 Effects of Blood Circulation Improvement and Lowered Blood Pressure

Ginsenosides relax blood vessels, thus increasing blood flow and improving blood circulation and cerebral blood flow. By relaxing the coronary arteries, ginsenosides protect against myocardial infarction, myocardial ischemia, and angina pectoris. Ginsenosides also inhibit platelet aggregation, showing antithrombotic and antiarrhythmic effects (Kim et al., 1994). It has been reported that platelet aggregation of coronary artery disease patients has been inhibited by ginsenosides; in particular, ginsenosides Rg1 and Rg3, which are the main saponin constituents, inhibit action and generation of thromboxane A2. Ginsenosides also prolong blood coagulation time by inhibiting platelet aggregation (Kim et al., 1999).

Nonsaponin constituents of red ginseng also have similar effects. Such effects work not only in coronary arteries, but also in the central nervous system, thus improving heart and cerebral ischemia (Park et al., 1995). Recently, the Korean Food and Drug Administration approved ginseng's functional effect of improving blood circulation by preventing blood clots.

Red ginseng had been traditionally known to raise blood pressure; hence hypertensive patients were advised not to consume it. However, there are now many reports that modern scientific evidence indicates that red ginseng actually lowers blood pressure. Clinical study shows that red ginseng lowers both diastolic and systolic pressure of hypertensive patients. In particular, ginsenosides, the major constituent of red ginseng, relax blood vessels by releasing NO (nitric oxide) from vascular endothelial cells (Sung et al., 2000; Kim et al., 2003).

10.7.8 Enhancement of Cognitive Performance

According to "A Clinical Study on Effects of Korean Ginseng on the Enhancement of Cognitive Performance and Anti-Dementia," a total of 30 Alzheimer's disease patients were given Korean ginseng in quantities of 4.5 or 9 g per day, starting in September 2006 (Lee et al., 2008). After 3 months, evaluation was conducted to determine whether their cognitive performance was enhanced. According to the results, the group given red ginseng showed improvement in MMSE (mini-mental state examination) and CDR (clinical dementia rating); such improvement of cognitive performance was more clearly observed in the 9 g/day group than the 4 g/day group. These results may be used as clinical data on Korean ginseng's effects on improving symptoms of dementia.

Korean ginseng is effective in treating memory disorders by improving learning and memory, and ginseng saponin enhances learning and memory in the maze test and passive avoidance test. In recent years, it has been frequently reported that Korean red ginseng is effective in preventing and treating Alzheimer's disease. It has been proven that Korean red ginseng inhibits the generation of the beta-amyloid protein and clinical studies also report that red ginseng enhances cognitive performance of dementia patients (Bao et al., 2005).

10.7.9 Enhancement of Sexual Performance

When 300 mg of Korean red ginseng was given to patients with psychogenic erectile dysfunction for 2 months in the form of nine capsules daily, the result showed that their sexual performance improved. All categories, including sexual desire, frequency of sexual intercourse, penile erection, and sexual satisfaction, showed improvement (Kim et al., 1998). In animal tests using mice and rats, Korean red ginseng not only reduced sexual behavior disorder caused by stress, but also enhanced sexual behavior. Moreover, it improved asthenespermia and oligospermia, which could be causes of male infertility (Murphy et al., 1998). The action mechanism for improving erectile dysfunction is as follows: Ginseng increases release of NO from slices of penile corpus cavernosum, thereby inducing the relaxation of the penile corpus cavernosum, which results in relaxation of blood vessels (Chen and Lee, 1995).

10.7.10 Hangover Reduction Effect

Korean red ginseng promotes alcohol metabolism and increases activity of alcohol dehydrogenase, thereby lowering blood alcohol concentration. It reduces lactate after alcohol drinking, reduces indexes related to liver toxicity that appear after alcohol intake is measured, and reduces liver cell toxicity (Lee and Kim, 2007).

10.7.11 Anticarcinogenic and Cancer-Preventive Effects

An epidemiologic study on anticarcinogenic and cancer-preventive effects of Korean ginseng showed that occurrence rate of cancer was significantly low in the group that took red ginseng. A 5-year study conducted to prove this also showed that cancer rates were lower in the group that took red ginseng and frequencies of various types of cancers were also low. Korean ginseng is known to have cancer-preventive effects through various mechanisms, such as antioxidant properties. In particular, Korean ginseng boosts immune functions and strengthens functions of NK cells and T-cells, while inhibiting cancer metastasis. However, there is some controversy regarding whether Korean red ginseng directly attacks cancer cells and whether its actions bring about changes in cell cycles. There are also some differences of view over its action on oncogene, its action to reduce resistance to multiple agents, the inhibition of angiogenesis, and inhibition of infiltration (Kenarova et al., 1990; Sonoda et al., 1998; Choi et al., 2002).

10.7.12 Antiviral and Anti-AIDS Effects

Korean red ginseng increased NK cell function in both AIDS patients and healthy persons. In particular, red ginseng was given to those infected with HIV (human immunodeficiency virus) in doses of 5.4 g daily and they survived more than 20 years without taking other AIDS medications (Sung et al., 2005, 2007). An increase in CD+4 cells after taking Korean red ginseng was confirmed and the red ginseng inhibited manifestation of resistance against ZDV (zidovudine, AIDS virus proliferation inhibitor). Thus, it was reported that a combination of red ginseng and AIDS drugs was more effective. Korean red ginseng is also effective in treating C-type hepatitis and inhibited inflammatory reactions caused by influenza virus infection.

10.8 Conclusion

Korean ginseng has a history of about 1500 years and has been regarded as the best medicinal plant cultivated by nature and people. Korea is the

Korean Ginseng 253

country from which this world-recognized ginseng originated. Generally, natural products that have medicinal effects have some toxicity as well. But Korean ginseng has almost no toxic properties. Thus, ginseng was regarded as a panacea from ancient times and it is continuously studied by scientific processes in the world. Its medical elements have been scientifically proven. There are magnificent medicinal effects and numerous stories of Korean ginseng. It is expected that this contribution will be an opportunity to understand its values and reputation.

References

Ames, B.N. 1985. Dietary carcinogens and anticarcinogens. Oxygen radicals and degenerative diseases. *Science* 221: 1256–1264.

Bao, H.Y., J. Zhang, S.J. Yeo et al. 2005. Memory enhancing and neuroprotective effects of selected ginsenosides. *Arch Pharm Res* 28: 335–342.

Brekhman, I.I., and I.V. Dardymov. 1969. New substances of plant origin which increase nonspecific resistance. *Annu Rev Pharmacol* 9: 419–430.

Chen, X., and T.J. Lee. 1995. Ginseniside-induced nitric oxide-mediated relaxation of the rabbit corpus cavernousm. *Br J Pharmacol* 115: 15–18.

Chen, Z.K., C.X. Fan, Y.H. Ye, L. Yang, Q. Jiang, and Q.Y. Xiang. 1998. Isolation and characterization of a group of oligopeptides related to oxidized glutathione from the root of *Panax ginseng. J Peptides Res* 52: 137–142.

Choi, K.T. 1996. Recent Korean ginseng cultivation. p. 1. Daejeon: Korea Ginseng & Tabaco Research Institute.

Choi, M.S., Y.H. Kim, and C.C. Jang. 2002. Effect of red ginseng extracts on the immune response in mouse. *J Basic & Life Res* 2(2): 47–50.

Christensen, L.P. 2009. Ginsenosides: Chemistry, biosynthesis, analysis, and potential health effects. *Adv Food Nutr Res* 55: 1–73.

Compilation Committee of the Korean Ginseng History. 1980. *Korean ginseng history,* 59. Kyunggi: Korean Ginseng Growers Association.

Gao, Q.P., H. Kiyohara, J.C. Cyong, and H. Yamada. 1989. Chemical properties and anticomplementary activities of polysaccharide fractions from roots and leaves of *Panax ginseng. Planta Medica* 55: 9–12.

Han, B.H., M.H. Park, Y.N. Han. 1981. Studies on the antioxidant components of Korean ginseng (I). Identification of phenolic acid. *Arch Pharm Res* 4(1): 53–58.

Han, B.H., M.H. Park, L.K. Woo, W.S. Woo, and Y.N. Han. 1979. Studies on the antioxidant components of Korea ginseng. *Korean Biochem J* 12(1): 33–40.

Han, B.H., and L.K. Woo. 1974. Dammarane glycosides of *Panax ginseng. Korean J Pharmacog* 5(1): 31–44.

Han, K., I.C. Shin, K.J. Choi, Y.P. Yun, J.T. Hong, and K.W. Oh. 2005. Korea red ginseng water extract increases nitric oxide concentrations in exhaled breath. *Nitric Oxide* 12(3): 159–162.

Horhammer, L., H. Wagner, and B. Loy. 1961. Contents of *Panax ginseng* root. *Preliminary report Pharm Ztg* 106: 1307–1311.

Hwang, W.I. 1992. Anti-cancer effect of Korean ginseng. *Korean J Ginseng Sci* 16: 170–171.

Jo, G.S., H.Y. Cha, H.J. Ji et al. 2010. Enhancement of exercise capacity by black ginseng extract in rats. *Lab Anim Res* 26: 279–286.

Kenarova, B., H. Neychev, C. Hadjiivanova, and V.D. Petkov. 1990. Immunomodulating activity of ginsenoside Rg1 from *Panax ginseng*. *Jpn J Pharmacol* 54(4): 447–454.

Kim, E.K., J.H. Lee, S.H. Cho et al. 2008. Preparation of black *Panax ginseng* by new methods and its antitumor activity. *Korean J Herbology* 23: 85–92.

Kim, H.J., D.S. Woo, G. Lee, and J.J. Kim. 1998. The relaxation effects of ginseng saponin in rabbit corporal smooth muscle: Is it a nitric oxide donor? *Br J Urol* 82: 744–748.

Kim, H.Y., Y.H. Lee, and S.I. Kim. 1989. Antihepatotoxic components of Korean ginseng. *Korean Biochem J* 22(1): 12–18.

Kim, J.Y., D.R. Germolec, and M.I. Luster. 1990. *Panax ginseng* as a potential immunomodulator: Studies in mice. *Immunopharmacol Immunotoxicol* 12(2): 257–276.

Kim, M.W., H.J. Sohn, K.J. Na, S.K. Kim, and J.N. Hur. 1993. Ginseng annual report (efficacy), 190. Daejeon: Korea Ginseng & Tabaco Research Institute.

Kim, N.D., S.Y. Kang, M.J. Kim, J.H. Park, and V.B. Schini. 1999. The ginsenoside Rg3 evokes endothelium-independent relaxation in rat aortic rings: Role of K+ channels. *Eur J Pharmacol* 367: 51–57.

Kim, N.D., S.Y. Kang, and V.B. Schini. 1994. Ginsenosides evoke endothelium-dependent vascular relaxation in rat aorta. *Gen Pharmacol* 25: 1071–1077.

Kim, N.D., E.M. Kim, K.W. Kang, M.K. Cho, S.Y. Choi, and S.G. Kim. 2003. Ginsenoside Rg3 inhibits phenylephrine-induced vascular contraction through induction of nitric oxide synthase. *Br J Pharmacol* 140(4): 661–670.

Kim, S.H., and K.S. Park. 2003. Effect of *Panax ginseng* extract on lipid metabolism in humans. *Pharmacol Res* 48(45): 511–513.

Kim, S.N., and S.J. Kang. 2009. Effects of black ginseng (9 times-steaming ginseng) on hypoglycemic action and changes in the composition of ginsenosides on the steaming process. *Korean J. Food Sci Technol* 41: 77–81.

Kitagawa, I., T. Taniyama, T. Hayashi, and M. Yoshikawa. 1983. Malonyl-ginsenosides Rb1, Rb2, Rc, and Rd, four new malonylated dammarane-type triterpene oligosaccharides from ginseng radix. *Chem Pharm Bull* 31: 3353–3356.

Konno, C., and H. Hikino. 1987. Isolation and hypoglycemic activity of panaxans M, N, O, and P, glycans of *Panax ginseng* roots. *Int J Crude Drug Res* 25: 53–56.

Konno, C., M. Sugiyama, M. Kano, M. Takahashi, and H. Hikino. 1984. Isolation and hypoglycemic activity of panaxans A, B, C, D and E, glycans of *Panax ginseng* roots. *Planta Medica* 50: 434–436.

Lee, C.B. 1980. *Korean graphic dictionary of plant*, 575. Seoul: Hyangmoonsa.

Lee, M.R., B.S. Yun, L. Liu et al. 2010. Effect of black ginseng on memory improvement in the amnesic mice induced by scopolamine. *J. Ginseng Res* 34: 51–58.

Lee, S.A., H.K. Jo, B.O. Im, S.G. Kim, W.K. Whang, and S.K. Ko. 2012. Changes in the contents of prosapogenin in the red ginseng (*Panax ginseng*) depending on steaming batches. *J. Ginseng Res* 36: 102–106.

Lee, S.D. 2007. Reviews in Ginseng research (I), 32–45. Seoul: The Korean Society of Ginseng.

Lee, S.D. 2008a. All about Korean ginseng, 67–107, Seoul: The Korean Society of Ginseng.

Lee, S.D. 2008b. All about Korean ginseng, 108–110, Seoul: The Korean Society of Ginseng.

Lee, S.H., B.H. Jung, S.Y. Kim, E.H. Lee, and B.C. Chung. 2006a. The antistress effect of ginseng total saponin and ginsenoside Rg3 and Rb1 evaluated by brain polyamine level under immobilization stress. *Pharmacol Res* 54: 46–49.

Lee, S.M. 2014. Thermal conversion pathways of ginsenoside in red ginseng processing. *Nat Prod Sci* 20: 119–25.

Lee, S.M., B.S. Bae, H.W. Park et al. 2015. Characterization of Korean red ginseng (*Panax ginseng* Meyer): History, preparation method, and chemical composition. *J Ginseng Res* 39: 384–391.

Lee, S.M., S.C. Kim, J.S. Oh, J.H. Kim, and M.K. Na. 2013. 20(R)-Ginsenoside Rf: A new ginsenoside from red ginseng extract. *Phytochem Lett* 6: 620–624.

Lee, S.S., and S.S. Kim. 2007. Reviews in ginseng research (l), 149–159. Seoul: The Korean Society of ginseng.

Lee, S.T., K. Chu, J.Y. Sim, J.H. Heo, and M. Kim. 2008. *Panax ginseng* enhances cognitive performance in Alzheimer disease. *Alzheimer Dis Assoc Disord* 22(3): 222–226.

Lee, W.K., S.T. Kao, I.M. Liu, and J.T. Cheng. 2006b. Mediation of beta-endorphin by ginsenoside Rh2 to lower plasma glucose in streptozotocin-induced diabetic rats. *Planta Medica* 72: 9–13.

Lee, Y.M., H.L. Yoon, H.M. Park, B.C. Song, and K.J. Yeum. 2016. Implications of red *Panax ginseng* in oxidative stress-associated chronic diseases. *J Ginseng Res* doi .org/10.1016/j.jgr.2016.03.003.

Mizuno, M., J. Yamada, H. Tarei, N. Kozukue, Y.S. Lee, and H. Tsuchida. 1994. Differences in immunomodulating effects between wild and cultured *Panax ginseng*. *Biochem Biophys Res Commun* 200: 1672–1678.

Murphy, L.L., R.S. Cadena, D. Chavez, and J.S. Ferraro. 1998. Effect of American ginseng (*Panax quinquefolium*) on male copulatory behavior in the rat. *Physiol Behav* 64: 445–450.

Nam, K.Y., J.E. Choi, S.C. Hong, M.K. Pyo, and J.D. Park. 2014. Recent progress in research on anticancer activities of ginsenoside-Rg3. *Korean J Pharmacogn* 45: 1–10.

Nam, K.Y., Y.S. Kim, M.Y. Shon, and J.D. Park. 2015. Recent advances in studies on chemical constituents and biological activities of Korean black ginseng (*Panax ginseng* C. A. Meyer). *Korean J Pharmacogn* 46(3): 173–188.

Park, J.D. 1996. Recent studies on the chemical constituents of Korean ginseng (*Panax ginseng* C.A. Meyer). *Korean J Ginseng Sci* 20: 389–415.

Park, H.J., D.H. Kim, S.J. Park, J.M. Kim, and J.H. Ryu. 2012. Ginseng in traditional herbal prescriptions. *J Ginseng Res* 36(3): 225–241.

Park, H.J., M.H. Lee, K.M. Park, K.Y. Nam, and K.H. Park. 1995. Effect of non-saponin fraction from *Panax ginseng* on cGMP and thromboxane A2 in human platelet aggregation. *J Ethnoparmacol* 49(3): 157–162.

Park, K.H., K.Y. Nam, K.J. Na et al. 1990. Ginseng annual report (efficacy), 85–122. Daejeon: Korea Ginseng & Tabaco Research Institute.

Park, K.M., Y.S. Kim, T.C. Jeong et al. 2001. Nitric oxide is involved in the immunomodulating activities of acidic polysaccharide from *Panax ginseng*. *Planta Medica* 67: 122–126.

Rivers, E., P.F. Ekholm, M. Inganils, S. Paulie, and K.O. Groenvik. 2005. The Rb1 fraction of ginseng elicits a balanced Th1 and Th2 immune response. *Vaccine* 23: 5411–5419.

Sanada, S., N. Kondo, J. Shoji, O. Tanaka, and S. Shibata. 1974a. Studies on the saponins of ginseng. I. Structures of ginsenoside-Ro, -Rb1, -Rb2, -Rc and -Rd. *Chem Pharm Bull* 22(2): 421–428.

Sanada, S., N. Kondo, J. Shoji, O. Tanaka, and S. Shibata. 1974b. Studies on the saponins of ginseng II. Structures of ginsenoside-Re, -Rf and -Rg2. *Chem Pharm Bull* 22(10): 2407–2412.

Shibata, S., O. Tanaka, T. Ando et al. 1966. Chemical studies on oriental plant drugs XIV. Protopanaxadiol. A genuine sapogenin of ginseng saponins. *Chem Pharm Bull* 14: 595–600.

Shibata, S., O. Tanaka, K. Soma, Y. Iida, T. Ando, and H. Nakamura. 1965. Studies on saponins and sapogenins of ginseng. The structure of panaxadiol. *Tetrahedron Lett* 3: 207–213.

Shin, Y.J., H.H. Jang, and G.Y. Song. 2012. Study on anti-atopic effects of black ginseng. *Korean J Aesthet Cosmetol* 10: 91–97.

Song, K.Y., H.J. Oh, S.S. Rho, Y.B. Seo, Y.J. Park, and C.S. Myung. 2006. Effect of black ginseng on body weight and lipid profiles in male rat fed normal diets. *Yakhak Hoeji* 50: 381–385.

Song, N.K., H.J. Choi, D.H. Kim, S.S. Roh, and Y.B. Seo. 2009. Effects of black ginseng on hypertension induced rats. *Korean J. Herbology* 24: 69–75.

Sonoda, Y., T. Kasahara, N. Mukaida, N. Shimizu, M. Tomota, and T. Takeda. 1998. Stimulation of interlukin-8 production by acidic polysaccharides from the root of *Panax ginseng*. *Immunopharmacol* 38: 287–294.

Sung, H., Y. Jung, M.W. Kang et al. 2007. High frequency of drug resistance mutations in human immunodeficiency virus type 1-infected Korean patients treated with HAART. *AIDS Res Human Retroviruses* 23: 1223–1229.

Sung, H., S.M. Kang, M.S. Lee, T.K. Kim, and Y.K. Cho. 2005. Korean red ginseng slows depletion of CD4 T cells in human immunodeficiency virus type 1-infected patients. *Clin Diagn Lab Immunol* 12: 497–501.

Sung, J., K.H. Han, J.H. Zo, H.J. Park, C.H. Kim, and B.H. Oh. 2000. Effects of red ginseng upon vascular endothelial function in patients with essential hypertension. *Am J Chinese Med* 28(2): 205–216.

Vuksan, V., and J.L. Sievenppiper. 2005. Herbal remedies in the management of diabetes: Lessons learned from the study of ginseng. *Nutr Metab Cardiovasc Dis* 15: 149–160.

Wee, J.J., J.D. Park, M.W. Kim, and H.J. Lee. 1989. Isolation of phenolic antioxidant components from *Panax ginseng*. *J Korean Agric Chem Soc* 32(1): 44–49.

Wee, J.J., J.Y. Shin, S.K. Kim, and M.W. Kim. 1998. The optimal steaming solvent for kujeungkupo (black ginseng) made using a content, radical scavenging of DPPH and ABTS, and COX-2 inhibition. *J Ginseng Res* 22(2): 91–95.

Yamamoto, M., A. Kunagai, and Y. Yamamura. 1983. Serum HDL-cholesterol-increasing and fatty liver-improving actions of *Panax ginseng* in high cholesterol diet-fed rats with clinical effect on hyperlipidemia in man. *Am J Chin Med* 11(1–4): 96–101.

Yun, Y.S., H.S. Moon, Y.R. Oh, S.K. Jo, Y.J. Kim, and T.K. Yun. 1987. Effect of red ginseng on natural killer cell activity in mice with lung adenoma induced by urethane and benzo(a)pyrene. *Cancer Detection Prevention* 26: 301–309.

Zhang, H., Z. Lu, G.T. Tan et al. 2002. Polyacetyleneginsenoside-Ro, a novel triterpene saponin from *Panax ginseng*. *Tetrahedron Lett* 43: 973–977.

11

Yangnyeom (Spices) and Health Benefits

Hye-Kyung Na and Young-Joon Surh

CONTENTS

11.1 Introduction and History...258
11.2 Nutritional Composition and Active Substances.............................258
    11.2.1 Nutritional Composition...258
    11.2.2 Active Substances..260
11.3 Disease Prevention and Other Beneficial Health Effects.................263
    11.3.1 Red Pepper..263
        11.3.1.1 Antioxidant Effects...263
        11.3.1.2 Anti-Inflammatory and Antiallergic Effects...........264
        11.3.1.3 Pain-Relieving Effects..264
        11.3.1.4 Antiobesity Effects...265
        11.3.1.5 Gastroprotective Effects.....................................266
        11.3.1.6 Neuroprotective Effects......................................266
        11.3.1.7 Cancer Chemopreventive and Therapeutic Effects...266
        11.3.1.8 Other Effects...268
    11.3.2 Ginger..269
        11.3.2.1 Antiemetic Effects...270
        11.3.2.2 Analgesic Effects...271
        11.3.2.3 Antioxidant Effects...271
        11.3.2.4 Chemopreventive and Anticarcinogenic Effects....272
    11.3.3 Garlic...273
        11.3.3.1 Cardioprotective Effect.......................................274
        11.3.3.2 Antihypertensive and Cholesterol-Lowering Effects...275
        11.3.3.3 Antidiabetic Effect..275
        11.3.3.4 Antioxidant Effects...276
        11.3.3.5 Immune Boosting Effects....................................276
        11.3.3.6 Protective Effects against Xenobiotic Toxicity........277
        11.3.3.7 Cancer Preventive and Anticancer Effects.............277
11.4 Other Spices...278
    11.4.1 Black Pepper..278
    11.4.2 Mustard..278
    11.4.3 Sesame Seed and Oil..279
11.5 Conclusion...280
References..281

11.1 Introduction and History

When making food, we use a variety of ingredients to create a distinctive flavor and color, while preserving the unique flavor of each food. For convenience, we call it as a yangnyeom. The Chinese characters 药 念 mean "to eat and to be like good medicine to the body." Yangnyeom includes some spices. Spices have also been widely used in folk medicine for thousands of years. The yangnyeom include soy sauce, green onion, sesame seed and oil, garlic, ginger, red pepper power, soybean paste, and pepper paste. Koreans used various spices for both culinary and medicinal purposes. The major spices most extensively used in Korea are red pepper (*Capsicum annum* L., Solanaceae), ginger (*Zingiber officinale* Roscoe, Zingiberaceae), and garlic (*Allium sativum*, Liliaceae).

Capsicum annuum (Solanaceae), commonly known as red pepper, is a major spice used in various Korean traditional cuisines. It is widely used as a seasoning in making kimchi, kochujang, and many ordinary foods in Korea. The consumption of red pepper per year in Korea is about 200,000 tons, which is equivalent to 2.5 kg per capita per year (about 7 g per person per day). For convenience, red pepper is often ground into a powder. Red pepper powder is the most heavily and most frequently consumed spice in Korea.

Ginger (*Zingiber officinale* Roscoe) belongs to the family Zingiberaceae. It originated in Southeast Asia and has been used in many countries as a spice and condiment to enhance flavor in cooking. Ginger is used as seasoning for making kimchi, bulgogi, and stew with fish. It masks the fishy smell of fish dishes.

Garlic (*Allium sativum*, Liliaceae) has been used not only as a spice but also as a medicinal product for over 3,000 years. Korea is the third largest producer of garlic in the world, and the majority of Korean foods contain garlic. Koreans mostly use garlic as a flavoring agent in diverse foods including soup, stew, and kimchi, and they also enjoy raw garlic and pickles.

11.2 Nutritional Composition and Active Substances

11.2.1 Nutritional Composition

The nutritional composition of red pepper, ginger, and garlic is shown in Table 11.1. Edible parts of red and green pepper are rich in vitamins A, B complex, and C. The vitamin C present in red pepper is not easily oxidized due to antioxidant properties of capsaicin, so its loss during cooking is less than that of vegetables. Fresh garlic, however, can cause indigestion, and its odor is a possible social deterrent. The garlic flavor is irritating, but when it is baked, the spicy flavor decreases and it tastes rather sweet.

Yangnyeom (Spices) and Health Benefits

TABLE 11.1

Nutritional Composition of Chili, Ginger, and Garlic

Item							Per 100 g Edible Portion									
	Energy (kcal)	Water (g)	Protein (g)	Fat (g)	Ash (g)	CHO (g)	Fiber (g)	Ca (mg)	P (mg)	Iron (mg)	Sodium (mg)	K (mg)	Vit. A (RE)	Vit. B1/2/6 (mg)	Vit. 6 (mg)	Vit. C (mg)
Dried red pepper	221	15.5	11	11	7.9	28.6	22	58	230	68	56	2930	4623	1.4	12.5	26
Green pepper	19	91.3	1.6	0.3	0.6	3.6	2.6	13	38	0.5	10	246	52	0.15	1.1	72
Ginger	53	83.3	1.5	0.2	1.1	13.9	1.6	13	28	0.8	5	344	–	0.07	1.0	5
Garlic	126	63.1	5.4	0	1.5	30.0	1.0	10	164	1.9	3	664	–	0.47	0.4	28

11.2.2 Active Substances

Capsaicin (Figure 11.1) is a major active compound from red peppers and is oil soluble. As illustrated in Figure 11.2, ginger constituents are grouped into two wide ranges of categories: volatiles and nonvolatiles (Jolad et al., 2004). Volatiles include sesquiterpene and monoterpenoid hydrocarbons providing the distinct aroma and taste of ginger. Nonvolatile pungent compounds include gingerols, shogaols, paradols, and zingerone that produce a "hot" sensation in the mouth. Gingerols, a series of chemical homologs differentiated by the length of their unbranched alkyl chains, were identified as the major active components in the fresh rhizome (Shukla and Singh, 2007). Gingerol analogs are thermally labile and easily undergo dehydration reactions to form the corresponding shogaols, which impart the characteristic pungent taste to dried ginger. Shogaols are important marker substances used for the quality control of many ginger-containing products, due to their diverse biological activities (Rahmani et al., 2014; Semwal et al., 2015). Paradol is similar to gingerol and is formed as a consequence of hydrogenation of shogaol.

On average, a garlic bulb contains about 1% alliin, a principal organosulfur compound in garlic (Amagase et al., 2001). Cutting or crushing garlic releases the vacuolar enzyme allinase, which rapidly converts alliin to allicin, a volatile organosulfur compound responsible for the characteristic pungent smell of garlic. Allicin has a strong antiseptic and antibacterial action, killing food poisoning bacteria as well as *Helicobacter pylori* causing gastric ulcers (Kockar et al., 2001). Allicin is relatively unstable and undergoes rapid decomposition to produce lipid-soluble organosulfur compounds, such as diallyl sulfide (DAS), diallyl disulfide (DADS), and diallyl trisulfide (DATS) (Figure 11.3). Besides oil-soluble organosulfur compounds, garlic contains water-soluble compounds. These include S-allyl cysteine (SAC), S-allyl mercaptocysteine (SAMC), and S-methyl cysteine, and γ-glutamyl cysteine derivatives (Amagase et al., 2001). While oil-soluble sulfur compounds are odorous, water-soluble compounds are odorless. Moreover, water-soluble compounds are more stable and safer than oil-soluble compounds.

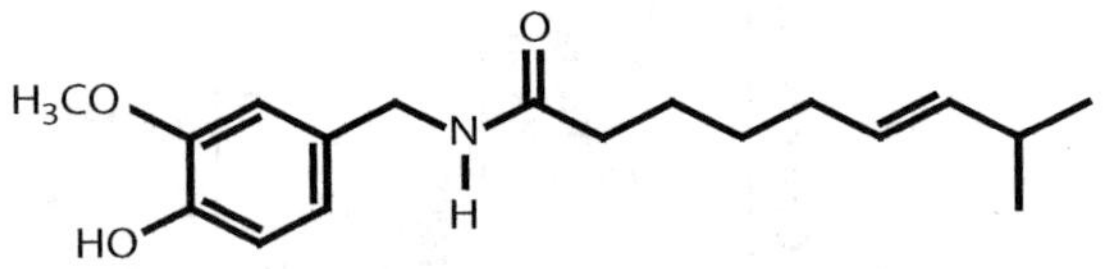

FIGURE 11.1
The chemical structure of capsaicin in red pepper.

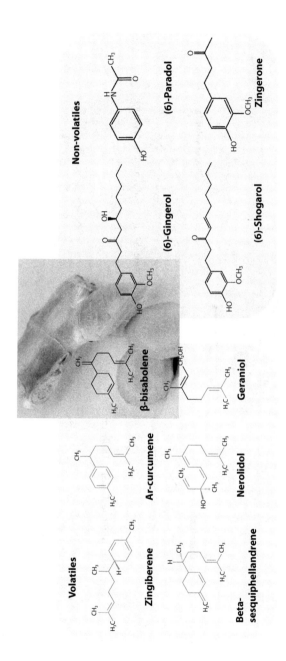

FIGURE 11.2
Chemical structures of volatile and nonvolatile compounds present in ginger.

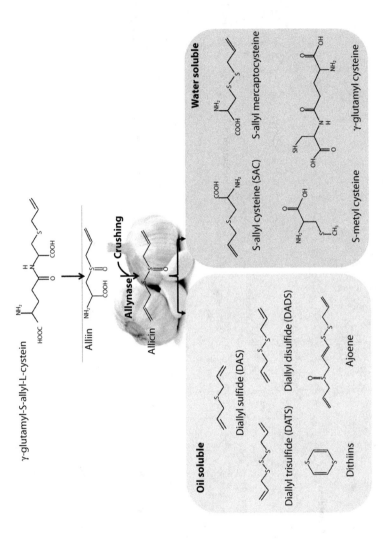

FIGURE 11.3
Chemical changes in garlic. Intact garlic bulbs contain large amounts of γ-glutamylcysteines. These compounds undergo hydrolysis and oxidation to produce alliin, which accumulates during storage of garlic bulbs. After processing, such as cutting, crushing, chewing, or dehydration, the vacuolar enzyme, alliinase, rapidly lyses alliin to form allicin. Allicin and other thiosulfinates instantly decompose to form other compounds, such as DAS, DADS, DATS, dithiins, and ajoene. Allicin also produces SAC and other water-soluble organosulfur compounds.

11.3 Disease Prevention and Other Beneficial Health Effects

Numerous studies have documented the antioxidant, anti-inflammatory, antimicrobial, and immunomodulatory effects of spices, which may account for their ability to prevent or treat several diseases. This is attributable to their biologically active components. We highlight the health benefits and disease-preventive effects of some spices and their bioactive substances.

11.3.1 Red Pepper

Capsaicin has been documented to be efficacious at doses comparable to usual human intake and has been clearly demonstrated to play numerous beneficial roles in health (Figure 11.4). These include cardioprotective, anti-lithogenic, anti-inflammatory, analgesic, thermogenic, antiobesity, antidiabetic, and gastroprotective effects (Srinivasan, 2016). The transient receptor potential cation channel subfamily V member 1 (TRPV1), also known as the capsaicin receptor or the vanilloid receptor 1, is known to mediate the majority of pharmacologic effects of capsaicin. This protein is a member of the TRPV group of the transient receptor potential family of ion channels (Clapham et al., 2005).

11.3.1.1 Antioxidant Effects

Like the majority of other spices, red pepper possesses pronounced antioxidant activity (Shobana and Naidu, 2000), which is attributable to the

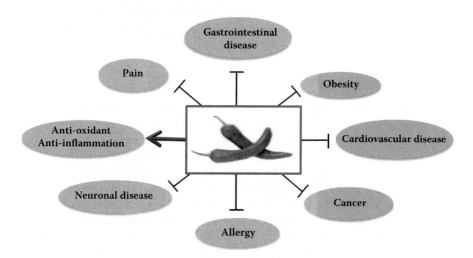

FIGURE 11.4
Beneficial health effects of capsaicin.

abundant presence of vitamin A, beta-carotene, and vitamin C. Besides these conventional antioxidant vitamins, capsaicin also has a capability to scavenge peroxy and hydroxyl radicals (Okada et al., 2002).

11.3.1.2 Anti-Inflammatory and Antiallergic Effects

Capsaicin has been shown to inhibit lipopolysaccharide (LPS)-induced production of proinflammatory cytokines, such as interleukin (IL)-1β, IL-6 and tumor necrosis factor (TNF)-α through activation of the peroxisome proliferator-activated receptor (PPAR) γ-liver X-receptor (LXR)-α axis. In addition, capsaicin suppressed the expression of p65, a functionally active subunit of the proinflammatory transcription factor NF-κB (Tang et al., 2015). *H. pylori* infection is one of causes of gastritis and stomach cancer. Capsaicin inhibited proliferation of *H. pylori* in cultured AGS gastric epithelial cells (Toyoda et al., 2016). Capsaicin also decreased the number of neutrophils in the antrum and corpus and mononuclear cell infiltration and heterotopic proliferative glands in the corpus of *H. pylori*-infected Mongolian gerbils. Further, mRNA expression of TNF-α and phosphorylation of IκB-α in the antrum were reduced by capsaicin (Toyoda et al., 2016).

Allergic rhinitis represents a global health problem believed to result from inflammation on the sensory nerves innervating the upper airway mucosa. Capsaicin blocks the axon reflex and may exert a curative effect on allergic rhinitis (Cheng et al., 2006). Allergic contact dermatitis is a common skin condition caused by a type-IV hypersensitivity reaction. This neuroimmune cross talk seems to be mediated by neuropeptides, such as substance P released from nerve fiber. Prolonged application of 8% topical capsaicin patches was found to be effective for temporary defunctionalization of peptidergic fibers implicated in allergic contact dermatitis (Andersen et al., 2017). Capsaicin inhibited ADP-induced platelet aggregation through TRPV1 (Almaghrabi et al., 2014).

11.3.1.3 Pain-Relieving Effects

Capsaicin has long been known to act selectively on a subpopulation of neurons to produce initial excitation, followed by a prolonged neuroinhibitory action commonly referred to as capsaicin desensitization (O'Neill, 1991). Neuropathic pain is difficult to treat, and the devastating condition can severely impact patients' quality of life. The 8% capsaicin patch can provide pain relief in patients with peripheral neuropathic pain (England et al., 2011; Kern et al., 2013). While releasing relatively large amounts of capsaicin, this patch rapidly defunctionalizes the cutaneous nociceptors (Derry et al., 2017). Painful diabetic neuropathy (PDN) is a debilitating consequence of diabetes. The treatment to provide total pain relief in PDN is difficult. Clinical guidelines recommend pain relief in PDN through topical application of capsaicin (Javed et al., 2015). A network meta-analysis suggests

Yangnyeom (Spices) and Health Benefits 265

that the capsaicin 8% patch is as effective as an oral centrally acting therapy in patients with PDN (van Nooten et al., 2017). An 8-week, double-blind, vehicle-controlled study indicated that topical capsaicin 0.075% cream was safe and effective in managing painful PDN (Scheffler et al., 1991). Topical application of either 0.01% or 0.025% oral capsaicin gel on the dorsal part of tongue was found to be an alternative for the short-term treatment of burning mouth syndrome (Jorgensen and Pedersen, 2017).

11.3.1.4 Antiobesity Effects

Obesity is caused by excessive accumulation of fat as the result of imbalance between energy intake and energy expenditure. Consumption of hot chili pepper, varying from a single meal to a continuous uptake for up to 12 weeks, facilitates weight loss through modulation of fat metabolism, energy expenditure, and thermogenesis. These antiobesity effects of chili pepper are attributable to activation of TRPV1 by its ingredient capsaicin (Varghese et al., 2017; Zheng et al., 2017). Stimulation of preadipocyte differentiation and proliferation as well as enhanced lipogenesis is a general mechanism underlying obesity. Capsaicin efficiently induces apoptosis and inhibits adipogenesis in 3T3-L1 preadipocytes and adipocytes (Hsu and Yen, 2007). Moreover, it significantly decreased the amount of intracellular triglycerides and glycerol-3-phosphate dehydrogenase activity and inhibited the expression of PPARγ, C/EBPα, and leptin (Hsu and Yen, 2007). Capsaicin not only suppresses the maturation of preadipocytes into adipocytes but also inhibits the differentiation of mesenchymal stem cells into adipocytes (Ibrahim et al., 2015). Fatty acids are degraded in the mitochondria via β-oxidation. The increase in fatty acid β-oxidation is negatively correlated with the body mass index. Capsaicin has been reported to increase lipolysis and induce fatty acid β-oxidation through modulation of hormone-sensitive lipase, acetyl-coA carboxylase, carnitine acyl transferase, and PPAR coactivator-1 (Rupasinghe et al., 2016).

Oral administration of capsaicin (2 mg/kg, p.o.) for 3 months modulates hypothalamic satiety-associated genotype, alters gut microbial composition, induces the "browning" genotype (brown adipose tissue-associated genes) in subcutaneous white adipose tissue and increases expression of thermogenesis and mitochondrial biogenesis genes in brown adipose tissue (Baboota et al., 2014). Obesity has a strong relationship to diabetes and insulin resistance. In obese individuals, the amount of nonesterified fatty acids, glycerol, hormones, cytokines, proinflammatory markers, and other substances involved in the development of insulin resistance is increased (Al-Goblan et al., 2014). Gestational diabetes mellitus may increase the future health risks of women and their offsprings. Capsaicin-containing chili supplementation improved postprandial hyperglycemia and hyperinsulinemia as well as fasting lipid metabolic disorders in women with gestational diabetes mellitus, and it decreased the incidence of newborns who were large for gestational age (Yuan et al., 2016).

11.3.1.5 Gastroprotective Effects

The therapeutic potential of chili and capsaicin has been well documented; however, they act as double-edged swords in many physiological circumstances (Maji and Banerji, 2016). In traditional medicine, chili has been used in the management of various gastrointestinal disorders such as dyspepsia, loss of appetite, gastroesophageal reflux disease, gastric ulcer, and so on (Maji and Banerji, 2016).

Intragastric application of capsaicin decreased the gastric acid secretion and basal acid output and enhanced the "nonparietal" component and gastric transmucosal potential difference in a randomized, prospective study of 84 healthy human subjects (Mozsik et al., 2005). Capsaicin at a low dose protected against gastric injuries induced by ethanol or indomethacin, which were attributed to stimulation of the sensory nerve endings (Mozsik et al., 2005). The capsaicin reactive receptor TRVP1 was detected in the gastrointestinal mucosa in patients with gastrointestinal disorders (Mozsik et al., 2007). Thus, application of capsaicin offers a new research tool for understanding the vanilloid-related events of human gastrointestinal functions (Mozsik et al., 2007).

11.3.1.6 Neuroprotective Effects

Stroke is a major cause of morbidity and mortality in the middle-aged and elderly. Global brain ischemia followed by reperfusion in rodents and humans usually results in delayed neuronal death in the CA1 region of hippocampus. Neuronal apoptosis is associated with brain damage elicited by ischemia–reperfusion. Pretreatment with capsaicin (3–30 µM) markedly attenuated hypoxia–reoxygenation (H/R)-induced apoptosis in hippocampal neurons (Guo et al., 2008). Intracellular accumulation of reactive oxygen species (ROS), which were greatly increased after H/R, was significantly inhibited by capsaicin. Capsaicin also markedly induced the phosphorylation of Akt in hippocampal neurons (Guo et al., 2008).

11.3.1.7 Cancer Chemopreventive and Therapeutic Effects

Considering the frequent consumption of capsaicin as a food additive and its current medicinal use, correct assessment of hazardous effects of this compound is important. Genotoxic and carcinogenic activities of capsaicin and chili extracts have been studied, but results are conflicting and discordant (Surh and Lee, 1996). Mammalian metabolism of capsaicin has been reported (Surh et al., 1995). Capsaicin appears to interact with xenobiotic metabolizing enzymes, particularly microsomal cytochrome P450-dependent monooxygenases, which are involved in activation as well as detoxification of various chemical carcinogens and mutagens. Hepatic cytochrome P450 2E1 (CYP2E1) catalyzes the conversion of capsaicin to reactive species such as the phenoxy radical intermediate capable of covalently binding to the active site of the

Yangnyeom (Spices) and Health Benefits

enzyme as well as tissue macromolecules. While covalent modification of protein and nucleic acids leads to toxicity, including necrosis, mutagenesis, and carcinogenesis, suicidal inhibition of microsomal cytochrome P450 may prohibit further activation of capsaicin and also of toxic xenobiotics. Capsaicin possesses the chemoprotective activity against some chemical carcinogens and mutagens (Surh et al., 1995).

The inhibition by capsaicin of microsomal monooxygenases involved in carcinogen activation implies its chemopreventive potential. Capsaicin attenuated the mutagenicity of vinyl carbamate (VC) and N-nitrosodimethylamine (NDMA) in *Salmonella typhimurium* TA100. Pretreatment of female ICR mice with a topical dose of capsaicin inhibited skin carcinogenesis. Capsaicin suppresses VC- and NDMA-induced mutagenesis or tumorigenesis, in part, through inhibition of the cytochrome P450 2E1 isoform responsible for activation of these carcinogens (Surh et al., 1995).

Lung cancer is a serious health problem in most developed countries and its incidence rate is increasing profusely. Hematological parameters and the histochemical analysis of mast cells showed abnormal changes, and the immunoblotting analysis revealed increased proinflammatory protein expression of TNF-α, IL-6, cyclooxygenase-2 (COX-2), and NF-κB in lung tumor formed in mice administered with benzo(a)pyrene (Anandakumar et al., 2012). Capsaicin (10 mg/kg body weight) administration to lung-cancer-bearing mice considerably attenuated all these abnormalities (Anandakumar et al., 2012). Capsaicin decreased the viability of CE 81T/VGH human esophagus epidermoid carcinoma cells via induction of G0-G1 phase cell cycle arrest and apoptosis. Capsaicin-induced apoptosis was associated with the elevation of intracellular ROS and Ca^{2+} production. BAPTA, an intracellular Ca^{2+} chelator, significantly inhibited capsaicin-induced apoptosis (Wu et al., 2006).

The expression of the TRPV1 gene and protein expression was inversely correlated with glioma grading, with marked loss of TRPV1 expression in the majority of grade IV glioblastoma multiforme. Capsaicin triggered apoptosis of U373 glioma cells. Capsaicin-induced apoptosis involved Ca^{2+} influx, mitochondrial permeability transmembrane pore opening and mitochondrial transmembrane potential dissipation, caspase 3 activation, and oligonucleosomal DNA fragmentation. These effects were markedly inhibited by the TRPV1 antagonist capsazepine (Amantini et al., 2007). Capsaicin inhibits complex-I and complex-III activity in pancreatic cancer cells, but not in normal HPDE-6 cells. This causes ROS generation and severe mitochondrial damage leading to apoptosis in pancreatic cancer cells. Furthermore, tumors from mice fed 2.5 mg/kg capsaicin show decreased superoxide dismutase (SOD) activity and an increase in intracellular glutathione (GSH) levels as compared to controls (Pramanik et al., 2011).

Aberrant activation of β-catenin/TCF signaling is related to the invasiveness of pancreatic cancer. Capsaicin treatment inhibits the activation of disheveled (Dsh) protein DvI-1 in several pancreatic cancer cell lines. Capsaicin treatment induced glycogen synthase kinase-3β, an enzyme involved in phosphorylation and subsequent proteasomal degradation of β-catenin and further activated the adenomatous polyposis coli and Axin multicomplex, thereby stimulating the proteasomal degradation of β-catenin (Pramanik et al., 2015). Expression of TCF-1 and β-catenin-responsive proteins, c-Myc and cyclin D1 also decreased in response to capsaicin treatment. Further, capsaicin reduced the interaction between β-catenin and TCF-1 in the nucleus. Capsaicin also inhibited orthotopic tumor growth, which was associated with inhibition of β-catenin/TCF-1 signaling (Pramanik et al., 2015). The anticarcinogenic potential of capsaicin was investigated using the transgenic adenocarcinoma of the mouse prostate (TRAMP) model, which mimics the progression of human prostate cancer. The capsaicin treatment resulted in a significant reduction in the metastatic burden compared to the controls. *In vitro* studies revealed a dose-dependent reduction in the invasion and migration capacity of prostate cancer PC3 cells upon capsaicin treatment (Venier et al., 2015).

Capsaicin sensitizes the cancer cells to radiotherapy. Oral administration of capsaicin with γ-irradiation reduced the tumor growth to a greater extent than capsaicin or γ-radiation treatment alone (Venier et al., 2015).

Association between capsaicin intake and gastric cancer development has been conflicting. The consumption of capsaicin has been speculated to increase the risk of gastric cancer. Analysis of 2,452 gastric cancer cases and 3,996 controls showed significant protection and susceptibility, with low and medium-high intake of capsaicin, respectively (Pabalan et al., 2014). In another study, the risk of gastric cancer was increased significantly among high-level consumers of capsaicin (90–250 mg of capsaicin per day— approximately 9–25 jalapeño peppers per day) as compared to low-level consumers (0–29.9 mg of capsaicin per day—approximately zero to less than three jalapeño peppers per day), and this effect was independent of *H. pylori* positivity (López-Carrillo et al., 2003). According to this study, no significant interaction was found between capsaicin intake and *H. pylori* infection on gastric cancer risk (López-Carrillo et al., 2003).

11.3.1.8 Other Effects

11.3.1.8.1 Cardioprotective Effects

Dietary capsaicin has favorably impacted endothelium-dependent vasodilation in rodents. TRPV1-mediated induction of LXRα in foam cells promotes cholesterol export, antagonizing plaque formation (McCarty et al., 2015). In rodent studies, capsaicin-rich diets have shown favorable effects on atherosclerosis, metabolic syndrome, diabetes, obesity, nonalcoholic fatty liver, cardiac hypertrophy, hypertension, and stroke risk. Application of capsaicin patch was found to increase exercise time to ischemic threshold in patients with angina. Significant increase in nitric oxide (NO) release was observed when human umbilical vein endothelial cells were incubated with capsaicin (25 μM), and this effect was inhibited by capsazepine. Capsaicin

(1 μM) decreased formation of apoptotic nuclei in human vascular endothelial cells treated with LPS and improved endothelial function and protected against LPS-induced apoptosis. Thus, regular consumption of chili pepper may promote endothelial health and reduce the cardiovascular disease risk (Chularojmontri et al., 2010).

11.3.1.8.2 Amelioration of Physical Fatigue and Improvement of Performance

Capsaicin has been shown to improve mitochondrial biogenesis and ATP production. Capsaicin supplementation dose dependently reduced serum lactate, ammonia, and levels of blood urea nitrogen and creatine kinase, and increased glucose concentration after a 15-min swimming test. In addition, capsaicin also increased hepatic glycogen content, an important energy source for exercise. These results suggest that capsaicin supplementation may have a wide spectrum of bioactivities for promoting health, performance improvement, and fatigue amelioration (Hsu et al., 2016).

11.3.2 Ginger

The pungent fractions of ginger—namely, gingerols, shogaols, paradols, and volatile constituents like sesquiterpenes and monoterpenes—are mainly attributed to the health-enhancing perspectives of ginger. The main pharmacological actions of ginger and its ingredients include immunomodulatory, antitumorigenic, anti-inflammatory, antiapoptotic, antihyperglycemic, antilipidemic, and antiemetic effects (Mohd Yusof, 2016) (Figure 11.5). According to a large cross-sectional study, ginger has a potential preventive property against some chronic diseases, especially hypertension and

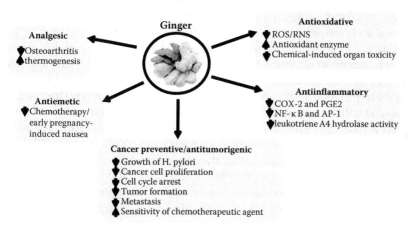

FIGURE 11.5
Beneficial health effects of ginger.

coronary heart disease (Wang et al., 2017). It also has anti-inflammatory and antioxidative properties for controlling the process of aging (Park et al., 2014). Furthermore, ginger has antimicrobial potential as well, which can help in treating infectious diseases (D'Souza et al., 2017). It is considered a safe herbal medicine with only a few insignificant adverse side effects (Ali et al., 2008). The National Center for Complementary and Alternative Medicine (NCCAM) has evaluated the results of the available studies, rating the reports from "suggestive" (for short-term use of ginger for safe relief from pregnancy-related nausea and vomiting) to "mixed" (when used for nausea caused by motion sickness, chemotherapy, or surgery) to "unclear" (for treating rheumatoid arthritis, osteoarthritis, or joint and muscle pain) (Hoffman, 2007). The role of ginger in reducing the extent of cardiovascular disorders, diabetes mellitus, and digestive problems has also been described in detail (Butt and Sultan, 2011).

11.3.2.1 Antiemetic Effects

Nausea and vomiting are physiological processes experienced by every human being at some stage of life. However, when these symptoms recur frequently, they can significantly reduce the quality of life and can also be detrimental to health. Existing antiemetic agents are ineffective against certain stimuli, are relatively expensive, and possess side effects. Various preclinical and clinical studies have shown ginger to exert antiemetic effects against different emetogenic stimuli (Palatty et al., 2013). Nausea and vomiting in early pregnancy (NVEP) are commonly encountered in family medicine. The use of ginger (~1 g daily) for at least 4 days is associated with a fivefold likelihood of improvement in NVEP according to the meta-analysis by Thomson et al. (2014). Ginger did not pose a significant risk for spontaneous abortion compared to placebo (Viljoen et al., 2014). Similarly, ginger did not pose a significant risk for the side effects of heartburn or drowsiness. According to the Norwegian Mother and Child Cohort Study, the use of ginger during pregnancy was not associated with any increased risk of congenital malformations (Heitmann et al., 2013). No increased risk for stillbirth/perinatal death, preterm birth, low birth weight, or low Apgar score was detected for women exposed to ginger during pregnancy compared to women who had not been exposed (Heitmann et al., 2013). Based on this evidence, ginger could be considered a harmless and possibly an effective alternative option for women suffering from nausea and vomiting in pregnancy (Viljoen et al., 2014).

Despite advances in antiemetic therapy, chemotherapy-induced nausea and vomiting still pose a significant burden to patients undergoing chemotherapy. Substantial research has revealed that ginger exerts multiple beneficial effects on nausea and vomiting in cancer patients undergoing chemotherapy (Marx et al., 2017).

11.3.2.2 Analgesic Effects

Osteoarthritis (OA) is a degenerative joint disease associated with increased pain and disability and a simultaneous decline in the quality of life of sufferers. While there is no cure for OA, management ideally combines nonpharmacological strategies, including complementary therapies and pain-relieving medication. Topical ginger treatment has the potential to relieve symptoms, improve overall health, and increase independence of people with chronic OA (Leach and Kumar, 2008; Therkleson, 2014). Ginger has been commonly prescribed by herbalists for sufferers of OA due to its unique qualities of heat circulatory stimulation, anti-inflammation, and analgesia (Therkleson, 2010, 2014).

The thermogenetic effect of ginger is attributed to [6]-gingerol and hexahydrocurcuminas through TRPV1-stimulating activity (Yoshitomi et al., 2017). Ginger has shown promising preliminary evidence for a chondroprotective effect in OA prevention and treatment (Leong et al., 2013).

11.3.2.3 Antioxidant Effects

Ginger shows antioxidant activity. The isolated antioxidants are divided into two groups: gingerol-related compounds and diarylheptanoids (Masuda et al., 2004). Antioxidant effects of ginger contribute to chemical- or chemotherapy-induced cytotoxicity. A daily supplement of ginger extract starting 3 days prior to chemotherapy has been shown to significantly elevate antioxidant activity and reduce oxidative stress in patients who received moderate to high emetogenic potential adjuvant chemotherapy compared to a placebo (Danwilai et al., 2017).

Oral dietary supplementation with ginger protects against cadmium-induced lipid peroxidation and liver toxicity. In addition, the ginger administration provoked an improvement in hematological indices (Onwuka et al., 2011). [6]-Shogaol may have more potent bioactivity than [6]-gingerol. [6]-Shogaol-rich extract derived from ginger induces the nuclear factor E2-related factor2 (Nrf2)/antioxidant response element (ARE) and heme oxygenase-1 expression *in vitro* and *in vivo* (Bak et al., 2012). Moreover, [6]-shogaol-rich extract decreased the diethylnitrosamine (DEN)-mediated elevations of serum aspartate transaminase and alanine transaminase as well as the DEN-induced hepatic lipid peroxidation (Bak et al., 2012). Administration of [6]-shogaol-rich extract to mice also restored the activity and protein expression of hepatic antioxidant enzymes such as superoxide dismutase, glutathione peroxidase, and catalase, which were repressed by DEN treatment (Bak et al., 2012). In addition, pretreatment with ginger prior to gentamycin administration significantly protected the kidney and attenuated oxidative stress by modulating renal damage and antioxidant indices

(Ademiluyi et al., 2012). Coadministration of the [6]-gingerol-rich fraction exhibited chemoprotection against hematotoxicity caused by the fungicide, carbendazim, augmented antioxidant status, and prevented oxidative damage in the kidneys and livers of rats (Salihu et al., 2016). Pretreatment of HepG2 cells with ginger extract significantly inhibited the production of ROS, DNA strand break, and cytotoxicity induced by aflatoxin B1 (Vipin et al., 2017). Ginger extract also showed a significant hepatoprotective effect, which was attributed to its inhibition of the lipid peroxidation and enhancement of Nrf2-mediated antioxidant enzyme activities (Vipin et al., 2017).

11.3.2.4 Chemopreventive and Anticarcinogenic Effects

Ginger has antitumorigenic effects in different cancer models. The anticancer properties of ginger are attributed to the presence of certain pungent vallinoids—namely, [6]-gingerol and [6]-paradol, as well as some other constituents like shogaols, zingerone, etc. *H. pylori* is the primary etiological agent associated with peptic ulcer disease and the development of gastric cancer. The methanol extract of ginger rhizome and gingerol inhibited the growth of CagA+ *H. pylori* strains *in vitro*. [6]-Gingerol appeared to be more effective than [6]-shogaol in terms of inhibiting *H. pylori* growth (Mahady et al., 2003). The anticarcinogenic effect of ginger and its components is mediated by modulation of a wide range of signaling molecules. [6]-Gingerol suppresses anchorage-independent growth of HCT116 colorectal cancer cells by inhibiting leukotriene A4 hydrolase activity (Jeong et al., 2009). [6]-Gingerol effectively suppressed tumor growth *in vivo* in nude mice, an effect that was mediated by inhibition of leukotriene A4 hydrolase activity. Moreover, mice fed [6]-gingerol survived significantly longer than vehicle-treated controls (Jeong et al., 2009). [6]-Gingerol inhibited both the vascular endothelial growth factor- and basic fibroblast growth factor-induced proliferation of human endothelial cells and caused cell cycle arrest in the G1 phase (Kim et al., 2005a). Moreover, intraperitoneal administration of [6]-gingerol to mice reduced the number of lung metastasis of B16F10 melanoma cells after tail-vein injection, with preservation of apparently healthy behavior (Kim et al., 2005a). In addition, mice subjected to free access to extract of ginger (0.125%) in drinking water exhibited significant reduction in the development of mammary tumors (Nagasawa et al., 2002).

[6]-Gingerol inhibited 12-O-etradecanoylphorbol-13-acetate (TPA)-induced TNF-α production, ornithine decarboxylase activity, and skin tumor promotion in female ICR mice (Park et al., 1998). Topically applied [6]-gingerol inhibited TPA-induced phosphorylation of p65 at Ser 536 and its interaction with the coactivator cAMP response element-binding protein-binding protein (CBP/p300) in mouse skin, thereby rendering NF-κB transcriptionally inactive (Kim et al., 2005b). In addition, [6]-gingerol has been shown to inhibit UVB-induced activation of NF-κB and COX-2 expression in hairless mouse skin as well as in an immortalized human keratinocytes cell line

Yangnyeom (Spices) and Health Benefits

(Kim et al., 2007a). [6]-Gingerol induced apoptosis in gastric cancer cells by blocking TRAIL-induced NF-κB activation (Ishiguro et al., 2007). It also inhibited the epidermal growth factor-induced cell transformation and activator protein-1 (AP-1) activation (Bode et al., 2001). In contrast, [6]-paradol had no effect on epidermal growth factor-induced AP-1 transactivation (Bode et al., 2001). [6]-Paradol exerts its primary inhibitory effect on cell transformation through induction of apoptosis. [10]-Gingerol was more potent than [6]-gingerol and at least as potent as [8]-gingerol for the inhibition of triple-negative human (MDA-MB-231, MDA-MB-468) and mouse (4T1, E0771) mammary carcinoma cell growth (Bernard et al., 2017). The inhibitory effect of [10]-gingerol on the growth of MDA-MB-231 cells was associated with a reduction in the number of rounds of cell division and S-phase cell cycle arrest, as well as induction of apoptosis (Bernard et al., 2017).

Ginger acts as an adjuvant to chemotherapeutic agents. Coadministration of ginger extract alongside doxorubicin (DOX) markedly increased the survival rate, decreased the tumor volume, and increased the level of phosphorylated AMPK. In addition, the histopathological results demonstrated enhanced apoptosis and absence of multinucleated cells in the tumor tissue of the ginger extract + DOX group (El-Ashmawy et al., 2017). Daily administration of ginger extract starting 3 days prior to chemotherapy has been shown to significantly elevate antioxidant activity and reduce oxidative marker levels in patients who received moderate to high-emetogenic-potential chemotherapy (Danwilai et al., 2017). Sonodynamic therapy involves the combined use of ultrasound-induced cavitation in the presence of a chemical agent known as a "sonosensitizer," with the resulting cellular damage and cytotoxicity being synergistically greater than the additive effects of each element alone. Sonodynamic therapy offers a less invasive but more targeted treatment than that achievable with conventional cancer therapies. Ginger extracts act as sonosensitizers and induce a synergistic increase in the observed cell death (Prescott et al., 2017).

11.3.3 Garlic

Garlic was selected as one of ten health foods by *Time* magazine in 2002; the National Cancer Institute first introduced garlic among 48 anticancer products. It is considered one of the best disease-preventive foods. Health benefits of garlic do not depend on freshness or pungency. Scientific studies show that aged garlic extract, which is odorless and richer in antioxidants than fresh or other forms of garlic preparations, is more effective for human health in boosting immunity and protecting against cardiovascular disease, cancer, aging, and drug toxicity (Lee et al., 2016).

Studies over the past few decades have extended the scope of beneficial effects associated with garlic use. These include antiseptic, antiviral, bactericidal, fungicidal, antidiabetic, antihypertensive, and cancer-preventive properties (*vide infra*). Among the water-soluble compounds, SAC has been extensively studied and shown to possess various biological activities, such as anticancer, antioxidant, cholesterol-lowering, antihepatotoxic, and neuroprotective effects (Colin-Gonzalez et al., 2012). S-1-propenyl-L-cysteine (S1PC) is a stereoisomer of SAC, an important sulfur-containing amino acid that accounts for the pharmacological effects of aged garlic extract. S1PC exists only in trace amounts in raw garlic, but its concentration increases almost up to a level similar to that of SAC in aged garlic extract (Kodera et al., 2017). S1PC showed immunomodulatory effects *in vitro* and *in vivo*, and it reduced blood pressure in a hypertensive animal model (Kodera et al., 2017). A pharmacokinetic study revealed that S1PC was readily absorbed after oral administration in rats and dogs with bioavailability of 88%–100% (Kodera et al., 2017).

11.3.3.1 Cardioprotective Effect

Preclinical and clinical evidence has shown that garlic reduces risks associated with cardiovascular disorders (CVDs) by reducing blood cholesterol, inhibiting platelet aggregation, and lowering blood pressure. Hydrogen sulfide (H_2S), much like NO, is an endogenously produced gaseous signaling molecule that plays a critical role in many physiologic processes and has been shown to exert cytoprotective actions in various models of CVD and cardiovascular injury (Elrod et al., 2007). Benavides et al. (2007) showed that garlic-derived polysulfides such as DATS and DADS are H_2S donors in the presence of thiols and thiol-containing compounds (i.e., GSH), independent of the H_2S-forming enzymes cystathionine γ-lyase, cystathionine β-synthase, and 3-mercatopyruvate sulfurtransferase. In CVD models, the administration of H_2S prevents myocardial injury and dysfunction. Intravenous or intraperitoneal administration of DATS at the time of reperfusion ameliorated myocardial injury, as observed by reduced areas of infarction and decreased circulating concentrations of cardiac troponin I, a marker of cardiac injury (Predmore et al., 2012). In mice genetically deficient in the H_2S-producing enzyme cystathionine γ-lyase, the administration of DATS at the time of reperfusion restored the H_2S concentrations and reduced an infarction size (King et al., 2014). It is speculated that H_2S-mediated cardioprotection may be mediated via cross talk with NO and is dependent on NO signaling (Altaany et al., 2013).

The NO donors, such as sodium nitroprusside, enhanced activity of cystathionine β-synthase (Eto and Kimura, 2002). Moreover, H_2S increased the endothelial cell proliferation, adhesion, and microvessel tube formation (Cai et al., 2007). H_2S enhanced endothelial NO synthase activity and significantly increased NO bioavailability (Bir et al., 2012), thereby improving the vascular function.

Yangnyeom (Spices) and Health Benefits

11.3.3.2 Antihypertensive and Cholesterol-Lowering Effects

Hypertension affects one in four adults and contributes to approximately 40% of cardiovascular-related deaths. In both clinical and preclinical models, dietary garlic intake has been shown to reduce blood pressure (Harauma and Moriguchi, 2006; Ried et al., 2008). A randomized, placebo-controlled, clinical trial was conducted on CAD patients, aged 25 to 75 years old. The patients were randomly divided into two groups: the garlic group, receiving garlic powder tablets (400 mg garlic) twice daily and the placebo group, receiving placebo for 3 months (Mahdavi-Roshan et al., 2016). After the 3 months, the effect of garlic on systolic blood pressure was significant, and this effect was more pronounced in hypertensive patients. The molecular mechanisms involved in reduction of blood pressure are associated with NO production. Takashima et al. (2017) reported that aged garlic extract induced the concentration-dependent vasorelaxation of isolated rat aortic rings through production of NO in the presence of L-arginine. In addition, the effect of aged garlic extract was inhibited by an NO synthase inhibitor and a NO scavenger. Moreover, treatment of the aorta with aged garlic extract significantly increased NO production (Takashima et al., 2017).

Garlic seems to decrease cholesterol synthesis by inhibiting hydroxymethyl-glutaryl-CoA reductase and its downstream enzyme, sterol 4α-methyl oxidase, in the cholesterol synthesis pathway (Singh and Porter, 2006; Ha et al., 2015). Several meta-analyses have shown that garlic intake was associated with markedly decreased levels of total cholesterol (Ried et al., 2013; Kwak et al., 2014). Although available data suggest that garlic is superior to placebo in reducing total cholesterol levels, the effects are largely modest. Therefore, the use of garlic for hypercholesterolemia is still questionable (Stevinson et al., 2000).

11.3.3.3 Antidiabetic Effect

The ingestion of garlic juice has been shown to facilitate the utilization of glucose in rabbits (Jain and Vyas, 1975). *S*-allyl cysteine sulfuxide (alliin), a sulfur-containing amino acid in garlic, attenuated diabetic conditions in rats almost to the same extent as did the antidiabetic drug glibenclamide and insulin (Augusti and Sheela, 1996). In streptozotocin-induced diabetic rats, elevated levels of glucose, cholesterol, and triglycerides, the increment of the activities of alanine aminotransferase and aspartate aminotransferase, and increased food and water consumption were observed (Masjedi et al., 2013). These abnormal alterations were significantly attenuated in the rats orally administered garlic juice. In addition, administration of garlic juice ameliorated the abnormal histological signs, such as scattered degeneration of the hepatocytes with lymphocytic infiltration in the portal areas, decrease in the number and the size of pancreatic islets, and atrophy of pancreatic islets.

11.3.3.4 Antioxidant Effects

Garlic bulb extracts successfully prevented human vascular endothelial cell death and significantly inhibited ROS formation in oxidative stress conditions (Chen et al., 2013). Aged garlic extract contains SAC as its most abundant compound. SAC readily prevents oxidation and nitration of lipids (Imai et al., 1994; Moriguchi et al., 1996; Ide and Lau, 1997; Numagami and Ohnishi, 2001) and proteins (Maldonado et al., 2003) (Kim et al., 2006). SAC is known to scavenge superoxide anion $\left(O_2^{\cdot-}\right)$, hydrogen peroxide ($H_2O_2$), hydroxyl radical ($\bullet OH$), and peroxynitrite anion ($ONOO^-$) (Colin-Gonzalez et al., 2012). SAC administration (100 mg/kg for 5 consecutive days) is able to activate Nrf2 in homogenates of cerebral cortex (Colin-Gonzalez et al., 2012).

DAS protected against gentamicin induced-nephrotoxicity in Wistar rats through potentiation of renal antioxidant capacity (Kalayarasan et al., 2009). The antioxidant effects of DAS were attributed to enhanced expression of Nrf2 in DAS-treated Wistar rats. Antioxidant properties of DAS were also found to play a protective role in the rat model of hepatic ischemia–reperfusion injury (Shaik et al., 2008). Ischemia–reperfusion resulted in elevated plasma levels of alanine aminotransferase, aspartate aminotransferase and lactate dehydrogenase, markers for liver injury. DAS pretreatment suppressed the enhancement of aforementioned enzymes and also lipid peroxidation markers (lipid hydroperoxides and 15-isoprostane-F2t) in plasma and liver from rats subjected to ischemia–reperfusion injury.

11.3.3.5 Immune Boosting Effects

Numerous studies have addressed the effect of garlic on the immune system. Garlic is considered to act as an immune booster by actively strengthening the host immune response (Schafer and Kaschula, 2014). Garlic stimulates the functions of certain immune cells, such as macrophages, lymphocytes, natural killer cells, dendritic cells, and eosinophils (Arreola et al., 2015). Administration of aged garlic extract resulted in improved immune responses against experimentally implanted fibrosarcoma tumors in BALB/c mice. Aged garlic extract significantly inhibited tumor growth and increased the survival rate (Fallah-Rostami et al., 2013). The CD4+/CD8+ ratio and *in vitro* interferone-γ production of splenocytes were significantly increased in the group treated with aged garlic extract. In a randomized, double-blind, placebo-controlled, parallel-group trial, the intake of black-vinegar-mash garlic-containing food enhanced the immune function as represented by stimulation of secretory immunoglobulin A release in the saliva (Nakasone et al., 2016).

11.3.3.6 Protective Effects against Xenobiotic Toxicity

DAS can be metabolized by CYP enzymes to diallyl sulfoxide and, subsequently, to diallyl sulfone (DASO2), which act as competitive inhibitors to CYP 2E1 (Brady et al., 1991). CYP2E1 is known to metabolize many xenobiotics, including alcohol, and the analgesic drug acetaminophen in the liver. DAS has the protective effects on cytotoxicity caused by alcohol, analgesic drugs, and other xenobiotics by targeting CYP2E1 (Rao et al., 2015). DAS and its reactive metabolite, DASO2, have been shown to reduce carbon tetrachloride-, N-nitrosodimethylamine-, and acetaminophen-induced toxicity in rodents (Yang et al., 2001). Genotoxic effects of acrylamide are supposed to result from oxidative biotransformation to glycidamide. Glycidamide formation was diminished in the presence of the DAS (Taubert et al., 2006). In addition, DATS and DADS at a 10-fold higher dose significantly increased the activities of glutathione S-transferase, quinone reductase, and glutathione peroxidase, whereas DAS did not (Fukao et al., 2004).

11.3.3.7 Cancer Preventive and Anticancer Effects

Several epidemiological studies have revealed that dietary consumption of garlic is associated with the reduced risk for certain types of cancers, especially stomach and colon cancer (Challier et al., 1998; Fleischauer et al., 2000; Hsing et al., 2002; Galeone et al., 2006). In a case-control study conducted between 2005 and 2007 in Taiyuan, China, raw garlic consumption was associated with reduced risk of lung cancer (Myneni et al., 2016). The major organosulfur compounds that contribute to the anticancer properties of garlic include allicin, allixin, DAS, DADS, DATS, SAC, allylmercaptan S-allylmethyldisulfide, S-allylmethyltrisulfide, and ajoene (Dorant et al., 1993; Milner, 2001; Shukla and Kalra, 2007). It has been reported that allylsulfides inhibit both initiation and promotion stages of experimentally induced tumorigenesis (Shukla and Kalra, 2007).

Garlic-derived organosulfur compounds have been known to inhibit carcinogen-induced cell damage. For example, SAMC, a water-soluble derivative of garlic, elevated SOD by approximately 100%. In this study, SAMC inhibited benzo(a)pyrene-induced DNA damage, cell proliferation, ROS formation, and NF-κB activation (Wang et al., 2016). Oral administration of DATS suppressed the colon inflammation induced by dextran sodium sulfate, phosphorylation at the Tyr 705 residue of signal transducer and activator of transcription 3 (STAT3), and expression of its major target protein cyclin D1 in mouse colonic mucosa (Lee et al., 2013). DATS treatment reduced the incidence and the multiplicity of papillomas formed in 7,12-dimethylbenz(a)anthracene-initiated and TPA-promoted mouse skin carcinogenesis via suppression of COX-2 expression through down-regulation of AP-1 and c-Jun NH_2-terminal kinase

(Shrotriya et al., 2010). Oral administration of DATS (1–2 mg/day, thrice/week for 13 weeks) by gavage significantly inhibited progression to poorly differentiated prostate carcinoma and pulmonary metastasis in the TRAMP model without any side effects (Singh et al., 2008).

Garlic-derived organosulfur compounds have been shown to modulate a number of key molecules linked to the apoptotic pathway in various human cancer cells. Molecular mechanisms underlying their induction of apoptosis frequently involve activation of proapoptotic proteins (e.g., Bax, Bak, and Bim) and down-regulation of antiapoptotic proteins, such as Bcl-2 and X-linked inhibitor of apoptosis protein, disruption of mitochondrial transmembrane potential and generation of ROS (Xiao et al., 2006; Kim et al., 2007b; Choi and Park, 2012). DATS induced apoptosis in MCF-7 cells through generation of ROS and significantly reduced the tumor volume in MCF-7 xenograft mice (Na et al., 2012). In addition, organosulfur compounds from garlic sensitized the cancer cells against chemotherapeutic agents. Allicin enhanced chemotherapeutic response by suppression of solid tumor growth, and ameliorated hepatic injury induced by tamoxifen, which was widely used for treatment of hormone-dependent breast cancer (Suddek, 2014). Oral administration of allicin enhanced the expression of SOD and the level of GSH, and suppressed production of TNF-α in the rat liver (Suddek, 2014).

11.4 Other Spices

11.4.1 Black Pepper

Black pepper (*Piper nigrum* L.), one of the most widely used spices, has been known to possess antioxidant, antimicrobial, and gastroprotective effects. This spice is frequently added to Korean dishes, especially beef-based soup. Piperine is an alkaloid present in black pepper that is responsible for its distinct biting quality. Piperine has diverse pharmacological effects and hence confers several health benefits, such as reduction of insulin resistance, amelioration of inflammation, and improvement of hepatic steatosis (Derosa et al., 2016). Piperine has been reported to exert chemopreventive effects through several mechanisms, including potentiation of antioxidant defense capacity, induction of detoxifying enzymes, and suppression of stem cell self-renewal (Manayi et al., 2017). Moreover, piperine has exhibited antimutagenic activity as well as inhibited activity and expression of multidrug resistance transporters such as P-gp and MRP-1 (Manayi et al., 2017).

11.4.2 Mustard

Mustard is another widely used condiment worldwide. In Korea, it is frequently used as a condiment for sausages and cold meats and also often as an ingredient of salad dressings. The tastes of mustard range from sweet to spicy, and the grade of pungency is largely determined by the seed types used for preparation. Mustards prepared from white mustard (*Sinapis alba* L.) seeds usually have a less pungent flavor than mustards made from brown or black mustard (*Brassica nigra* L.) seeds.

The typical pungent taste and flavor are primarily caused by isothiocyanates, also known as mustard oils. They are breakdown products of glucosinolates, natural ingredients of mustard seeds, and are formed in a reaction catalyzed by the enzyme myrosinase after tissue injury. The mustard species differ in glucosinolate composition: Black and brown mustards contain primarily sinigrin, which is converted to the allyl isothiocyanate responsible for the more pungent taste of these seeds compared with white mustard. The relatively mild white mustard contains glucosinalbin, which is mainly converted to 4-hydroxybenzyl isothiocyanate. These ingredients have a strong antiseptic and antioxidant activity.

11.4.3 Sesame Seed and Oil

Sesame (*Sesamum indicum* L.) is an important oilseed crop that possesses a wide spectrum of pharmacological activities. Sesame seeds have long been used as a spice. The bioactive components present in the seed include vital minerals, vitamins, phytosterols, polyunsaturated fatty acids (PUFAs), tocopherols, and a unique class of lignans such as sesamin and sesamolin (Pathak et al., 2014). Phenylpropanoid compounds such as lignans along with tocopherols and phytosterols have antioxidant activity and increase the keeping quality of oil by preventing oxidative rancidity (Pathak et al., 2014). Sesame seed supplementation decreased serum TC, LDL-C, and lipid peroxidation, and increased antioxidant status in hyperlipidemic patients (Alipoor et al., 2012). White sesame seed oil has been used in cooking and food preparation for centuries. In Korea, it is frequently used as an ingredient of all dishes including parboiling vegetables, meats, salad dressings with soy source, etc. Many studies have been conducted to investigate its health-promoting effects. Consumption of white sesame seed oil significantly improved glucose control and other biomarkers of hepatic stress, as well as cardiac and renal health (Aslam et al., 2017). White sesame seed oil may also be a viable functional food to help reduce the detrimental effects of diabetes. Compared to other plant oils, sesame seed oil is highly stable to oxidation and has been demonstrated to have protective effects against ischemia–reperfusion injury in the rat brain (Jamarkattel-Pandit et al., 2010). In addition, clinical trials showed that the intake of sesame resulted in an increase in enzymatic and nonenzymatic antioxidants, as well as in a reduction in oxidative stress markers (Gouveia Lde et al., 2016). Sesamol, a lignan isolated from sesame seed oil, inhibited production of NO, PGE_2, and proinflammatory cytokines (Wu et al., 2015). Sesamol markedly suppressed mRNA and protein expression of iNOS and COX-2. Sesamol enhanced the cellular antioxidant capacity regulated by Nrf2 and its target protein heme oxygenase-1. Moreover, sesamol suppressed nuclear translocation of NF-κB and decreased MAPK activation, but it promoted AMPK activation.

Perilla oil is characterized by relatively small content of both saturated fatty acids and monounsaturated fatty acids and much higher amounts of PUFAs. Koreans use perilla oil, which contains n-3 PUFA. n-3 PUFA consumption has been demonstrated in association with a reduced risk of chronic diseases, including insulin resistance, cancer, and cardiovascular disease. Perilla oil intake may significantly lower serum lipids, strengthen hepatic fatty acid oxidation, and inhibit hepatic fatty acid synthesis, but at the same time may also lead to insulin resistance (Zhang et al., 2014).

11.5 Conclusion

In addition to being used in flavoring, coloring, and preserving foods, spices have been important components of folk medicine as natural healing remedies. There has been substantial scientific evidence for the health benefit of various spices. Traditionally, Korean cuisine uses diverse spices. The most frequently and heavily used spices in Korea include hot chili pepper, ginger, and garlic. With increasing interest in alternative and complementary medicine in the management of chronic ailments, research is emerging on the use of spices. Many metabolic disorders and age-related degenerative diseases are closely associated with oxidative stress and inflammation, two major culprits in the body.

Spices contain powerful antioxidants and anti-inflammatory principles. The anti-inflammatory ingredients of chili pepper, ginger, and garlic, a trio spice set most frequently used in Korean cuisine, have been shown to inhibit the promotion and progression of cancer by targeting proinflammatory signal transducing molecules, such as NF-κB and AP-1 transcription factors (Figure 11.6). They also block the initiation of carcinogenesis by activating Nrf2, a transcription factor involved in inducing antioxidant and carcinogen detoxifying enzymes (Figure 11.6). More definitive research is needed to identify molecular targets of spices and their pharmacologically and physiologically active ingredients. This will work in parallel with clinical trials that are intended to assess their preventive/therapeutic potential.

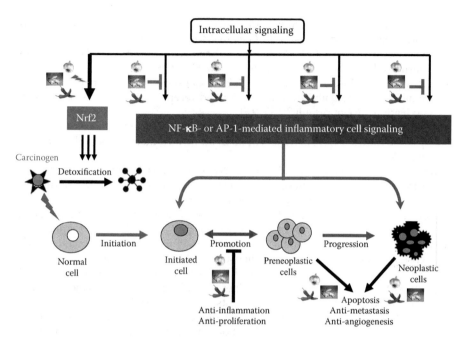

FIGURE 11.6
Modulation of multistage carcinogenesis by chili, ginger, and garlic.

References

Ademiluyi, A. O., G. Oboh, O. B. Ogunsuyi and A. J. Akinyemi. 2012. Attenuation of gentamycin-induced nephrotoxicity in rats by dietary inclusion of ginger (*Zingiber officinale*) and turmeric (*Curcuma longa*) rhizomes. *Nutr Health* 21: 209–218.

Al-Goblan, A. S., M. A. Al-Alfi and M. Z. Khan. 2014. Mechanism linking diabetes mellitus and obesity. *Diabetes Metab Syndr Obes* 7: 587–591.

Ali, B. H., G. Blunden, M. O. Tanira and A. Nemmar. 2008. Some phytochemical, pharmacological and toxicological properties of ginger (*Zingiber officinale* Roscoe): A review of recent research. *Food Chem Toxicol* 46: 409–420.

Alipoor, B., M. K. Haghighian, B. E. Sadat and M. Asghari. 2012. Effect of sesame seed on lipid profile and redox status in hyperlipidemic patients. *Int J Food Sci Nutr* 63: 674–678.

Almaghrabi, S. Y., D. P. Geraghty, K. D. Ahuja and M. J. Adams. 2014. Vanilloid-like agents inhibit aggregation of human platelets. *Thromb Res* 134: 412–417.

Altaany, Z., G. Yang and R. Wang. 2013. Crosstalk between hydrogen sulfide and nitric oxide in endothelial cells. *J Cell Mol Med* 17: 879–888.

Amagase, H., B. L. Petesch, H. Matsuura, S. Kasuga and Y. Itakura. 2001. Intake of garlic and its bioactive components. *J Nutr* 131: 955S–962S.

Amantini, C., M. Mosca, M. Nabissi et al. 2007. Capsaicin-induced apoptosis of glioma cells is mediated by TRPV1 vanilloid receptor and requires p38 MAPK activation. *J Neurochem* 102: 977–990.

Anandakumar, P., S. Kamaraj, S. Jagan et al. 2012. Capsaicin inhibits benzo(*a*) pyrene-induced lung carcinogenesis in an in vivo mouse model. *Inflamm Res* 61: 1169–1175.

Andersen, H. H., J. Elberling and L. Arendt-Nielsen. 2017. High-concentration topical capsaicin may abolish the clinical manifestations of allergic contact dermatitis by effects on induction and elicitation. *Med Hypotheses* 99: 53–56.

Arreola, R., S. Quintero-Fabian, R. I. Lopez-Roa et al. 2015. Immunomodulation and anti-inflammatory effects of garlic compounds. *J Immunol Res* 2015: 401630.

Aslam, F., S. Iqbal, M. Nasir et al. 2017. Evaluation of white sesame seed oil on glucose control and biomarkers of hepatic, cardiac, and renal functions in male Sprague–Dawley rats with chemically induced diabetes. *J Med Food* 20: 448–457.

Augusti, K. T. and C. G. Sheela. 1996. Antiperoxide effect of *S*-allyl cysteine sulfoxide, an insulin secretagogue, in diabetic rats. *Experientia* 52: 115–120.

Baboota, R. K., N. Murtaza, S. Jagtap et al. 2014. Capsaicin-induced transcriptional changes in hypothalamus and alterations in gut microbial count in high fat diet fed mice. *J Nutr Biochem* 25: 893–902.

Bak, M. J., S. Ok, M. Jun and W. S. Jeong. 2012. 6-Shogaol-rich extract from ginger up-regulates the antioxidant defense systems in cells and mice. *Molecules* 17: 8037–8055.

Benavides, G. A., G. L. Squadrito, R. W. Mills et al. 2007. Hydrogen sulfide mediates the vasoactivity of garlic. *Proc Natl Acad Sci U S A* 104: 17977–17982.

Bernard, M. M., J. R. McConnery and D. W. Hoskin. 2017. [10]-Gingerol, a major phenolic constituent of ginger root, induces cell cycle arrest and apoptosis in triple-negative breast cancer cells. *Exp Mol Pathol* 102: 370–376.

Bir, S. C., G. K. Kolluru, P. McCarthy et al. 2012. Hydrogen sulfide stimulates ischemic vascular remodeling through nitric oxide synthase and nitrite reduction activity regulating hypoxia-inducible factor-1alpha and vascular endothelial growth factor-dependent angiogenesis. *J Am Heart Assoc* 1: e004093.

Bode, A. M., W. Y. Ma, Y. J. Surh and Z. Dong. 2001. Inhibition of epidermal growth factor-induced cell transformation and activator protein 1 activation by [6]-gingerol. *Cancer Res* 61: 850–853.

Brady, J. F., H. Ishizaki, J. M. Fukuto et al. 1991. Inhibition of cytochrome P-450 2E1 by diallyl sulfide and its metabolites. *Chem Res Toxicol* 4: 642–647.

Butt, M. S. and M. T. Sultan. 2011. Ginger and its health claims: Molecular aspects. *Crit Rev Food Sci Nutr* 51: 383–393.

Cai, W. J., M. J. Wang, P. K. Moore et al. 2007. The novel proangiogenic effect of hydrogen sulfide is dependent on Akt phosphorylation. *Cardiovasc Res* 76: 29–40.

Challier, B., J. M. Perarnau and J. F. Viel. 1998. Garlic, onion and cereal fibre as protective factors for breast cancer: A French case-control study. *Eur J Epidemiol* 14: 737–747.

Chen, S., X. Shen, S. Cheng et al. 2013. Evaluation of garlic cultivars for polyphenolic content and antioxidant properties. *PLoS One* 8: e79730.

Cheng, J., X. N. Yang, X. Liu and S. P. Zhang. 2006. Capsaicin for allergic rhinitis in adults. *Cochrane Database Syst Rev*: CD004460.

Choi, Y. H. and H. S. Park. 2012. Apoptosis induction of U937 human leukemia cells by diallyl trisulfide induces through generation of reactive oxygen species. *J Biomed Sci* 19: 50.

Chularojmontri, L., M. Suwatronnakorn and S. K. Wattanapitayakul. 2010. Influence of capsicum extract and capsaicin on endothelial health. *J Med Assoc Thai* 93 Suppl 2: S92–101.

Clapham, D. E., D. Julius, C. Montell and G. Schultz. 2005. International Union of Pharmacology. XLIX. Nomenclature and structure–function relationships of transient receptor potential channels. *Pharmacol Rev* 57: 427–450.

Colin-Gonzalez, A. L., R. A. Santana, C. A. Silva-Islas et al. 2012. The antioxidant mechanisms underlying the aged garlic extract- and S-allylcysteine-induced protection. *Oxid Med Cell Longev* 2012: 907162.

D'Souza, S. P., S. V. Chavannavar, B. Kanchanashri and S. B. Niveditha. 2017. Pharmaceutical perspectives of spices and condiments as alternative antimicrobial remedy. *J Evid Based Complementary Altern Med*: 2156587217703214.

Danwilai, K., J. Konmun, B. Sripanidkulchai and S. Subongkot. 2017. Antioxidant activity of ginger extract as a daily supplement in cancer patients receiving adjuvant chemotherapy: A pilot study. *Cancer Manag Res* 9: 11–18.

Derosa, G., P. Maffioli and A. Sahebkar. 2016. Piperine and its role in chronic diseases. *Adv Exp Med Biol* 928: 173–184.

Derry, S., A. S. Rice, P. Cole, T. Tan and R. A. Moore. 2017. Topical capsaicin (high concentration) for chronic neuropathic pain in adults. *Cochrane Database Syst Rev* 1: CD007393.

Dorant, E., P. A. van den Brandt, R. A. Goldbohm, R. J. Hermus and F. Sturmans. 1993. Garlic and its significance for the prevention of cancer in humans: A critical view. *Br J Cancer* 67: 424–429.

El-Ashmawy, N. E., N. F. Khedr, H. A. El-Bahrawy and H. E. Abo Mansour. 2017. Ginger extract adjuvant to doxorubicin in mammary carcinoma: Study of some molecular mechanisms. *Eur J Nutr* Feb. 22.

Elrod, J. W., J. W. Calvert, J. Morrison et al. 2007. Hydrogen sulfide attenuates myocardial ischemia–reperfusion injury by preservation of mitochondrial function. *Proc Natl Acad Sci U S A* 104: 15560–15565.

England, J., T. Wagner, K. U. Kern, A. Roth-Daniek and A. Sell. 2011. The capsaicin 8% patch for peripheral neuropathic pain. *Br J Nurs* 20: 926–931.

Eto, K. and H. Kimura. 2002. A novel enhancing mechanism for hydrogen sulfide-producing activity of cystathionine beta-synthase. *J Biol Chem* 277: 42680–42685.

Fallah-Rostami, F., M. A. Tabari, B. Esfandiari, H. Aghajanzadeh and M. Y. Behzadi. 2013. Immunomodulatory activity of aged garlic extract against implanted fibrosarcoma tumor in mice. *N Am J Med Sci* 5: 207–212.

Fleischauer, A. T., C. Poole and L. Arab. 2000. Garlic consumption and cancer prevention: Meta-analyses of colorectal and stomach cancers. *Am J Clin Nutr* 72: 1047–1052.

Fukao, T., T. Hosono, S. Misawa, T. Seki and T. Ariga. 2004. The effects of allyl sulfides on the induction of phase II detoxification enzymes and liver injury by carbon tetrachloride. *Food Chem Toxicol* 42: 743–749.

Galeone, C., C. Pelucchi, F. Levi et al. 2006. Onion and garlic use and human cancer. *Am J Clin Nutr* 84: 1027–1032.

Gouveia Lde, A., C. A. Cardoso, G. M. de Oliveira, G. Rosa and A. S. Moreira. 2016. Effects of the intake of sesame seeds (*Sesamum indicum* L.) and derivatives on oxidative stress: A systematic review. *J Med Food* 19: 337–345.

Guo, S. Y., G. P. Yang, D. J. Jiang et al. 2008. Protection of capsaicin against hypoxia-reoxygenation-induced apoptosis of rat hippocampal neurons. *Can J Physiol Pharmacol* 86: 785–792.

Ha, A. W., T. Ying and W. K. Kim. 2015. The effects of black garlic (*Allium satvium*) extracts on lipid metabolism in rats fed a high fat diet. *Nutr Res Pract* 9: 30–36.

Harauma, A. and T. Moriguchi. 2006. Aged garlic extract improves blood pressure in spontaneously hypertensive rats more safely than raw garlic. *J Nutr* 136: 769S–773S.

Heitmann, K., H. Nordeng and L. Holst. 2013. Safety of ginger use in pregnancy: Results from a large population-based cohort study. *Eur J Clin Pharmacol* 69: 269–277.

Hoffman, T. 2007. Ginger: An ancient remedy and modern miracle drug. *Hawaii Med J* 66: 326–327.

Hsing, A. W., A. P. Chokkalingam, Y. T. Gao et al. 2002. Allium vegetables and risk of prostate cancer: A population-based study. *J Natl Cancer Inst* 94: 1648–1651.

Hsu, C. L. and G. C. Yen. 2007. Effects of capsaicin on induction of apoptosis and inhibition of adipogenesis in 3T3-L1 cells. *J Agric Food Chem* 55: 1730–1736.

Hsu, Y. J., W. C. Huang, C. C. Chiu et al. 2016. Capsaicin supplementation reduces physical fatigue and improves exercise performance in mice. *Nutrients* 8.

Ibrahim, M., M. Jang, M. Park et al. 2015. Capsaicin inhibits the adipogenic differentiation of bone marrow mesenchymal stem cells by regulating cell proliferation, apoptosis, oxidative and nitrosative stress. *Food Funct* 6: 2165–2178.

Ide, N. and B. H. Lau. 1997. Garlic compounds protect vascular endothelial cells from oxidized low density lipoprotein-induced injury. *J Pharm Pharmacol* 49: 908–911.

Imai, J., N. Ide, S. Nagae et al. 1994. Antioxidant and radical scavenging effects of aged garlic extract and its constituents. *Planta Med* 60: 417–420.

Ishiguro, K., T. Ando, O. Maeda et al. 2007. Ginger ingredients reduce viability of gastric cancer cells via distinct mechanisms. *Biochem Biophys Res Commun* 362: 218–223.

Jain, R. C. and C. R. Vyas. 1975. Garlic in alloxan-induced diabetic rabbits. *Am J Clin Nutr* 28: 684–685.

Jamarkattel-Pandit, N., N. R. Pandit, M. Y. Kim et al. 2010. Neuroprotective effect of defatted sesame seeds extract against in vitro and in vivo ischemic neuronal damage. *Planta Med* 76: 20–26.

Javed, S., I. N. Petropoulos, U. Alam and R. A. Malik. 2015. Treatment of painful diabetic neuropathy. *Ther Adv Chronic Dis* 6: 15–28.

Jeong, C. H., A. M. Bode, A. Pugliese et al. 2009. [6]-Gingerol suppresses colon cancer growth by targeting leukotriene A4 hydrolase. *Cancer Res* 69: 5584–5591.

Jolad, S. D., R. C. Lantz, A. M. Solyom et al. 2004. Fresh organically grown ginger (Zingiber officinale): Composition and effects on LPS-induced PGE2 production. *Phytochemistry* 65: 1937–1954.

Jorgensen, M. R. and A. M. Pedersen. 2017. Analgesic effect of topical oral capsaicin gel in burning mouth syndrome. *Acta Odontol Scand* 75: 130–136.

Kalayarasan, S., P. N. Prabhu, N. Sriram et al. 2009. Diallyl sulfide enhances antioxidants and inhibits inflammation through the activation of Nrf2 against gentamicin-induced nephrotoxicity in Wistar rats. *Eur J Pharmacol* 606: 162–171.

Kern, K. U., J. England, A. Roth-Daniek and T. Wagner. 2013. Is physician supervision of the capsaicin 8% patch administration procedure really necessary? An opinion from health care professionals. *J Pain Res* 6: 571–575.

Kim, E. C., J. K. Min, T. Y. Kim et al. 2005a. [6]-Gingerol, a pungent ingredient of ginger, inhibits angiogenesis in vitro and in vivo. *Biochem Biophys Res Commun* 335: 300–308.

Kim, J. K., Y. Kim, K. M. Na, Y. J. Surh and T. Y. Kim. 2007a. [6]-Gingerol prevents UVB-induced ROS production and COX-2 expression in vitro and in vivo. *Free Radic Res* 41: 603–614.

Kim, J. M., J. C. Lee, N. Chang, H. S. Chun and W. K. Kim. 2006. S-allyl-L-cysteine attenuates cerebral ischemic injury by scavenging peroxynitrite and inhibiting the activity of extracellular signal-regulated kinase. *Free Radic Res* 40: 827–835.

Kim, S. O., J. K. Kundu, Y. K. Shin et al. 2005b. [6]-Gingerol inhibits COX-2 expression by blocking the activation of p38 MAP kinase and NF-kappaB in phorbol ester-stimulated mouse skin. *Oncogene* 24: 2558–2567.

Kim, Y. A., D. Xiao, H. Xiao et al. 2007b. Mitochondria-mediated apoptosis by diallyl trisulfide in human prostate cancer cells is associated with generation of reactive oxygen species and regulated by Bax/Bak. *Mol Cancer Ther* 6: 1599–1609.

King, A. L., D. J. Polhemus, S. Bhushan et al. 2014. Hydrogen sulfide cytoprotective signaling is endothelial nitric oxide synthase-nitric oxide dependent. *Proc Natl Acad Sci U S A* 111: 3182–3187.

Kockar, C., M. Ozturk and N. Bavbek. 2001. *Helicobacter pylori* eradication with beta carotene, ascorbic acid and allicin. *Acta Medica (Hradec Kralove)* 44: 97–100.

Kodera, Y., M. Ushijima, H. Amano, J. I. Suzuki and T. Matsutomo. 2017. Chemical and biological properties of S-1-propenyl-l-cysteine in aged garlic extract. *Molecules* 22.

Kwak, J. S., J. Y. Kim, J. E. Paek et al. 2014. Garlic powder intake and cardiovascular risk factors: A meta-analysis of randomized controlled clinical trials. *Nutr Res Pract* 8: 644–654.

Leach, M. J. and S. Kumar. 2008. The clinical effectiveness of ginger (*Zingiber officinale*) in adults with osteoarthritis. *Int J Evid Based Healthc* 6: 311–320.

Lee, H. J., H. G. Lee, K. S. Choi, Y. J. Surh and H. K. Na. 2013. Diallyl trisulfide suppresses dextran sodium sulfate-induced mouse colitis: NF-kappaB and STAT3 as potential targets. *Biochem Biophys Res Commun* 437: 267–273.

Lee, H. S., W. C. Lim, S. J. Lee et al. 2016. Antiobesity effect of garlic extract fermented by *Lactobacillus plantarum* BL2 in diet-induced obese mice. *J Med Food* 19: 823–829.

Leong, D. J., M. Choudhury, D. M. Hirsh et al. 2013. Nutraceuticals: Potential for chondroprotection and molecular targeting of osteoarthritis. *Int J Mol Sci* 14: 23063–23085.

López-Carrillo, L., M. López-Cervantes, G. Robles-Díaz et al. 2003. Capsaicin consumption, Helicobacter pylori positivity and gastric cancer in Mexico. *Int J Cancer* 106: 277–282.

Mahady, G. B., S. L. Pendland, G. S. Yun, Z. Z. Lu and A. Stoia. 2003. Ginger (*Zingiber officinale* Roscoe) and the gingerols inhibit the growth of Cag A+ strains of *Helicobacter pylori*. *Anticancer Res* 23: 3699–3702.

Mahdavi-Roshan, M., J. Nasrollahzadeh, A. Mohammad Zadeh and A. Zahedmehr. 2016. Does garlic supplementation control blood pressure in patients with severe coronary artery disease? A clinical trial study. *Iran Red Crescent Med J* 18: e23871.

Maji, A. K. and P. Banerji. 2016. Phytochemistry and gastrointestinal benefits of the medicinal spice, *Capsicum annuum* L. (chilli): A review. *J Complement Integr Med* 13: 97–122.

Maldonado, P. D., D. Barrera, I. Rivero et al. 2003. Antioxidant S-allylcysteine prevents gentamicin-induced oxidative stress and renal damage. *Free Radic Biol Med* 35: 317–324.

Manayi, A., S. M. Nabavi, W. N. Setzer and S. Jafari. 2017. Piperine as a potential anticancer agent: A review on preclinical studies. *Curr Med Chem* May 23.

Marx, W., K. Ried, A. L. McCarthy et al. 2017. Ginger—Mechanism of action in chemotherapy-induced nausea and vomiting: A review. *Crit Rev Food Sci Nutr* 57: 141–146.

Masjedi, F., A. Gol and S. Dabiri. 2013. Preventive effect of garlic (*Allium sativum* L.) on serum biochemical factors and histopathology of pancreas and liver in streptozotocin-induced diabetic rats. *Iran J Pharm Res* 12: 325–338.

Masuda, Y., H. Kikuzaki, M. Hisamoto and N. Nakatani. 2004. Antioxidant properties of gingerol related compounds from ginger. *Biofactors* 21: 293–296.

McCarty, M. F., J. J. DiNicolantonio and J. H. O'Keefe. 2015. Capsaicin may have important potential for promoting vascular and metabolic health. *Open Heart* 2: e000262.

Milner, J. A. 2001. Mechanisms by which garlic and allyl sulfur compounds suppress carcinogen bioactivation. Garlic and carcinogenesis. *Adv Exp Med Biol* 492: 69–81.

Mohd Yusof, Y. A. 2016. Gingerol and its role in chronic diseases. *Adv Exp Med Biol* 929: 177–207.

Moriguchi, T., H. Saito and N. Nishiyama. 1996. Aged garlic extract prolongs longevity and improves spatial memory deficit in senescence-accelerated mouse. *Biol Pharm Bull* 19: 305–307.

Mozsik, G., J. Szolcsanyi and A. Domotor. 2007. Capsaicin research as a new tool to approach of the human gastrointestinal physiology, pathology and pharmacology. *Inflammopharmacology* 15: 232–245.

Mozsik, G., J. Szolcsanyi and I. Racz. 2005. Gastroprotection induced by capsaicin in healthy human subjects. *World J Gastroenterol* 11: 5180–5184.

Myneni, A. A., S. C. Chang, R. Niu et al. 2016. Raw garlic consumption and lung cancer in a Chinese population. *Cancer Epidemiol Biomarkers Prev* 25: 624–633.

Na, H. K., E. H. Kim, M. A. Choi et al. 2012. Diallyl trisulfide induces apoptosis in human breast cancer cells through ROS-mediated activation of JNK and AP-1. *Biochem Pharmacol* 84: 1241–1250.

Nagasawa, H., K. Watanabe and H. Inatomi. 2002. Effects of bitter melon (*Momordica charantia* L.) or ginger rhizome (*Zingiber offifinale* rosc) on spontaneous mammary tumorigenesis in SHN mice. *Am J Chin Med* 30: 195–205.

Nakasone, Y., N. Sato, T. Azuma and K. Hasumi. 2016. Intake of black-vinegar-mash-garlic enhances salivary release of secretory IgA: A randomized, double-blind, placebo-controlled, parallel-group study. *Biomed Rep* 5: 63–67.

Numagami, Y. and S. T. Ohnishi. 2001. S-allylcysteine inhibits free radical production, lipid peroxidation and neuronal damage in rat brain ischemia. *J Nutr* 131: 1100S–1105S.

O'Neill, T. P. 1991. Mechanism of capsaicin action: Recent learnings. *Respir Med* 85 Suppl A: 35–41.

Okada, Y., H. Okajima, Y. Shima and H. Ohta. 2002. Hydroxyl radical scavenging action of capsaicin. *Redox Rep* 7: 153–157.

Onwuka, F. C., O. Erhabor, M. U. Eteng and I. B. Umoh. 2011. Protective effects of ginger toward cadmium-induced testes and kidney lipid peroxidation and hematological impairment in albino rats. *J Med Food* 14: 817–821.

Pabalan, N., H. Jarjanazi and H. Ozcelik. 2014. The impact of capsaicin intake on risk of developing gastric cancers: A meta-analysis. *J Gastrointest Cancer* 45: 334–341.

Palatty, P. L., R. Haniadka, B. Valder, R. Arora and M. S. Baliga. 2013. Ginger in the prevention of nausea and vomiting: A review. *Crit Rev Food Sci Nutr* 53: 659–669.

Park, J. E., H. B. Pyun, S. W. Woo, J. H. Jeong and J. K. Hwang. 2014. The protective effect of *Kaempferia parviflora* extract on UVB-induced skin photoaging in hairless mice. *Photodermatol Photoimmunol Photomed* 30: 237–245.

Park, K. K., K. S. Chun, J. M. Lee, S. S. Lee and Y. J. Surh. 1998. Inhibitory effects of [6]-gingerol, a major pungent principle of ginger, on phorbol ester-induced inflammation, epidermal ornithine decarboxylase activity and skin tumor promotion in ICR mice. *Cancer Lett* 129: 139–144.

Pathak, N., A. K. Rai, R. Kumari and K. V. Bhat. 2014. Value addition in sesame: A perspective on bioactive components for enhancing utility and profitability. *Pharmacogn Rev* 8: 147–155.

Pramanik, K. C., S. R. Boreddy and S. K. Srivastava. 2011. Role of mitochondrial electron transport chain complexes in capsaicin mediated oxidative stress leading to apoptosis in pancreatic cancer cells. *PLoS One* 6: e20151.

Pramanik, K. C., N. M. Fofaria, P. Gupta et al. 2015. Inhibition of beta-catenin signaling suppresses pancreatic tumor growth by disrupting nuclear beta-catenin/TCF-1 complex: Critical role of STAT-3. *Oncotarget* 6: 11561–11574.

Predmore, B. L., K. Kondo, S. Bhushan et al. 2012. The polysulfide diallyl trisulfide protects the ischemic myocardium by preservation of endogenous hydrogen sulfide and increasing nitric oxide bioavailability. *Am J Physiol Heart Circ Physiol* 302: H2410–2418.

Prescott, M., J. Mitchell, S. Totti et al. 2017. Sonodynamic therapy combined with novel anti-cancer agents, sanguinarine and ginger root extract: Synergistic increase in toxicity in the presence of PANC-1 cells in vitro. *Ultrason Sonochem* May 13.

Rahmani, A. H., F. M. Shabrmi and S. M. Aly. 2014. Active ingredients of ginger as potential candidates in the prevention and treatment of diseases via modulation of biological activities. *Int J Physiol Pathophysiol Pharmacol* 6: 125–136.

Rao, P. S., N. M. Midde, D. D. Miller et al. 2015. Diallyl sulfide: Potential use in novel therapeutic interventions in alcohol, drugs, and disease mediated cellular toxicity by targeting cytochrome P450 2E1. *Curr Drug Metab* 16: 486–503.

Ried, K., O. R. Frank, N. P. Stocks, P. Fakler and T. Sullivan. 2008. Effect of garlic on blood pressure: A systematic review and meta-analysis. *BMC Cardiovasc Disord* 8: 13.

Ried, K., C. Toben and P. Fakler. 2013. Effect of garlic on serum lipids: An updated meta-analysis. *Nutr Rev* 71: 282–299.

Rupasinghe, H. P., S. Sekhon-Loodu, T. Mantso and M. I. Panayiotidis. 2016. Phytochemicals in regulating fatty acid beta-oxidation: Potential underlying mechanisms and their involvement in obesity and weight loss. *Pharmacol Ther* 165: 153–163.

Salihu, M., B. O. Ajayi, I. A. Adedara and E. O. Farombi. 2016. 6-Gingerol-rich fraction from *Zingiber officinale* prevents hematotoxicity and oxidative damage in kidney and liver of rats exposed to carbendazim. *J Diet Suppl* 13: 433–448.

Schafer, G. and C. H. Kaschula. 2014. The immunomodulation and anti-inflammatory effects of garlic organosulfur compounds in cancer chemoprevention. *Anticancer Agents Med Chem* 14: 233–240.

Scheffler, N. M., P. L. Sheitel and M. N. Lipton. 1991. Treatment of painful diabetic neuropathy with capsaicin 0.075%. *J Am Podiatr Med Assoc* 81: 288–293.

Semwal, R. B., D. K. Semwal, S. Combrinck and A. M. Viljoen. 2015. Gingerols and shogaols: Important nutraceutical principles from ginger. *Phytochemistry* 117: 554–568.

Shaik, I. H., J. M. George, T. J. Thekkumkara and R. Mehvar. 2008. Protective effects of diallyl sulfide, a garlic constituent, on the warm hepatic ischemia–reperfusion injury in a rat model. *Pharm Res* 25: 2231–2242.

Shobana, S. and K. A. Naidu. 2000. Antioxidant activity of selected Indian spices. *Prostaglandins Leukot Essent Fatty Acids* 62: 107–110.

Shrotriya, S., J. K. Kundu, H. K. Na and Y. J. Surh. 2010. Diallyl trisulfide inhibits phorbol ester-induced tumor promotion, activation of AP-1, and expression of COX-2 in mouse skin by blocking JNK and Akt signaling. *Cancer Res* 70: 1932–1940.

Shukla, Y. and N. Kalra. 2007. Cancer chemoprevention with garlic and its constituents. *Cancer Lett* 247: 167–181.

Shukla, Y. and M. Singh. 2007. Cancer preventive properties of ginger: A brief review. *Food Chem Toxicol* 45: 683–690.

Singh, D. K. and T. D. Porter. 2006. Inhibition of sterol 4alpha-methyl oxidase is the principal mechanism by which garlic decreases cholesterol synthesis. *J Nutr* 136: 759S–764S.

Singh, S. V., A. A. Powolny, S. D. Stan et al. 2008. Garlic constituent diallyl trisulfide prevents development of poorly differentiated prostate cancer and pulmonary metastasis multiplicity in TRAMP mice. *Cancer Res* 68: 9503–9511.

Srinivasan, K. 2016. Biological activities of red pepper (*Capsicum annuum*) and its pungent principle capsaicin: A review. *Crit Rev Food Sci Nutr* 56: 1488–1500.

Stevinson, C., M. H. Pittler and E. Ernst. 2000. Garlic for treating hypercholesterolemia. A meta-analysis of randomized clinical trials. *Ann Intern Med* 133: 420–429.

Suddek, G. M. 2014. Allicin enhances chemotherapeutic response and ameliorates tamoxifen-induced liver injury in experimental animals. *Pharm Biol* 52: 1009–1014.

Surh, Y. J., R. C. Lee, K. K. Park et al. 1995. Chemoprotective effects of capsaicin and diallyl sulfide against mutagenesis or tumorigenesis by vinyl carbamate and N-nitrosodimethylamine. *Carcinogenesis* 16: 2467–2471.

Surh, Y. J. and S. S. Lee. 1996. Capsaicin in hot chili pepper: Carcinogen, co-carcinogen or anticarcinogen? *Food Chem Toxicol* 34: 313–316.

Takashima, M., Y. Kanamori, Y. Kodera, N. Morihara and K. Tamura. 2017. Aged garlic extract exerts endothelium-dependent vasorelaxant effect on rat aorta by increasing nitric oxide production. *Phytomedicine* 24: 56–61.

Tang, J., K. Luo, Y. Li et al. 2015. Capsaicin attenuates LPS-induced inflammatory cytokine production by upregulation of LXR-alpha. *Int Immunopharmacol* 28: 264–269.

Taubert, D., R. Glockner, D. Muller and E. Schomig. 2006. The garlic ingredient diallyl sulfide inhibits cytochrome P450 2E1 dependent bioactivation of acrylamide to glycidamide. *Toxicol Lett* 164: 1–5.

Therkleson, T. 2010. Ginger compress therapy for adults with osteoarthritis. *J Adv Nurs* 66: 2225–2233.

Therkleson, T. 2014. Ginger therapy for osteoarthritis: A typical case. *J Holist Nurs* 32: 232–239.

Thomson, M., R. Corbin and L. Leung. 2014. Effects of ginger for nausea and vomiting in early pregnancy: A meta-analysis. *J Am Board Fam Med* 27: 115–122.

Toyoda, T., L. Shi, S. Takasu et al. 2016. Anti-inflammatory effects of capsaicin and piperine on *Helicobacter pylori*-induced chronic gastritis in Mongolian gerbils. *Helicobacter* 21: 131–142.

van Nooten, F., M. Treur, K. Pantiri, M. Stoker and M. Charokopou. 2017. Capsaicin 8% patch versus oral neuropathic pain medications for the treatment of painful diabetic peripheral neuropathy: A systematic literature review and network meta-analysis. *Clin Ther* 39: 787–803 e18.

Varghese, S. P. Kubatka, L. Rodrigo et al. 2017. Chili pepper as a body weight-loss food. *Int J Food Sci Nutr* 68: 392–401.

Venier, N. A., A. J. Colquhoun, H. Sasaki et al. 2015. Capsaicin: A novel radio-sensitizing agent for prostate cancer. *Prostate* 75: 113–125.

Viljoen, E., J. Visser, N. Koen and A. Musekiwa. 2014. A systematic review and meta-analysis of the effect and safety of ginger in the treatment of pregnancy-associated nausea and vomiting. *Nutr J* 13: 20.

Vipin, A., R. Rao, N. K. Kurrey, A. Appaiah and G. Venkateswaran. 2017. Protective effects of phenolics rich extract of ginger against aflatoxin B1-induced oxidative stress and hepatotoxicity. *Biomed Pharmacother* 91: 415–424.

Wang, K., Y. Wang, Q. Qi et al. 2016. Inhibitory effects of S-allylmercaptocysteine against benzo(a)pyrene-induced precancerous carcinogenesis in human lung cells. *Int Immunopharmacol* 34: 37–43.

Wang, Y., H. Yu, X. Zhang et al. 2017. Evaluation of daily ginger consumption for the prevention of chronic diseases in adults: A cross-sectional study. *Nutrition* 36: 79–84.

Wu, C. C. J. P. Lin, J. S. Yang et al. 2006. Capsaicin induced cell cycle arrest and apoptosis in human esophagus epidermoid carcinoma CE 81T/VGH cells through the elevation of intracellular reactive oxygen species and Ca2+ productions and caspase-3 activation. *Mutat Res* 601: 71–82.

Wu, X. L., C. J. Liou, Z. Y. Li et al. 2015. Sesamol suppresses the inflammatory response by inhibiting NF-kappaB/MAPK activation and upregulating AMP kinase signaling in RAW 264.7 macrophages. *Inflamm Res* 64: 577–588.

Xiao, D., K. L. Lew, Y. A. Kim et al. 2006. Diallyl trisulfide suppresses growth of PC-3 human prostate cancer xenograft in vivo in association with Bax and Bak induction. *Clin Cancer Res* 12: 6836–6843.

Yang, C. S., S. K. Chhabra, J. Y. Hong and T. J. Smith. 2001. Mechanisms of inhibition of chemical toxicity and carcinogenesis by diallyl sulfide (DAS) and related compounds from garlic. *J Nutr* 131: 1041S–1045S.

Yoshitomi, T., N. Oshima, Y. Goto et al. 2017. Construction of prediction models for the transient receptor potential vanilloid subtype 1 (TRPV1)-stimulating activity of ginger and processed ginger based on LC-HRMS data and PLS regression analyses. *J Agric Food Chem* 65: 3581–3588.

Yuan, L. J., Y. Qin, L. Wang et al. 2016. Capsaicin-containing chili improved post-prandial hyperglycemia, hyperinsulinemia, and fasting lipid disorders in women with gestational diabetes mellitus and lowered the incidence of large-for-gestational-age newborns. *Clin Nutr* 35: 388–393.

Zhang, T., S. Zhao, W. Li et al. 2014. High-fat diet from perilla oil induces insulin resistance despite lower serum lipids and increases hepatic fatty acid oxidation in rats. *Lipids Health Dis* 13: 15.

Zheng, J., S. Zheng, Q. Feng, Q. Zhang and X. Xiao. 2017. Dietary capsaicin and its anti-obesity potency: From mechanism to clinical implications. *Biosci Rep* 37.

12

Seed Oil (Sesame Seed, Perilla Seed)

JaeHwan Lee, Mi-Ja Kim,* and Mun Yhung Jung†

CONTENTS

12.1 Introduction 292
12.2 Sesame Seed and Sesame Seed Oil 292
    12.2.1 Importance 292
        12.2.1.1 History of Harvesting 292
        12.2.1.2 History as Food Ingredients 293
        12.2.1.3 Recipes 294
        12.2.1.4 Cultivation 296
    12.2.2 Chemical Composition 297
    12.2.3 Processing 297
    12.2.4 Beneficial Health Effects 301
        12.2.4.1 Effects on Lipid Metabolism 301
        12.2.4.2 Antioxidant Properties and Immunomodulating
                Effects 302
        12.2.4.3 Antihypertensive, Anticancer Effects,
                and Blood Sugar Regulation 302
12.3 Perilla Seeds and Perilla Seed Oil 303
    12.3.1 Leaves, Seed, and Seed Oil in Cuisine 303
    12.3.2 Fatty Acid Composition 305
    12.3.3 Health-Promoting Minor Components 306
    12.3.4 Nutty Flavors of Roasted Oil 309
    12.3.5 Oxidative Stability 309
    12.3.6 Health-Related Functionality 310
        12.3.6.1 Reduction of Risk for Coronary Heart Disease 310
        12.3.6.2 Improvement of Brain Health 311
        12.3.6.3 Reduction of Allergic Hypersensitivity 311
        12.3.6.4 Anticarcinogenic Activity 312
        12.3.6.5 Adverse Effects 312
12.4 Conclusion 313
References 313

---

* Dr. Lee and Dr. Kim contributed the sesame seed and sesame seed oil part of this chapter.
† Dr. Jung contributed the perilla seed and perilla seed oil part of the chapter.

12.1 Introduction

Sesame seeds (*Sesamum indicum*. L.), which originated from Africa (or some species from India), have been cultivated in North America, Africa, East Asia, India, and Turkey from 5,000 years ago as medicinal sources and food ingredients. Sesame seeds are important sources of dietary fat; amino acids, including arginine, phenylalanine, and glutamine; and many inorganic sources, including calcium, phosphorous, iron, and iodine. Also, beneficial health compounds like tocopherols, phytosterols, and lignans, including sesamolin, sesamin, and episesamin, are found in sesame seeds. Sesame seeds and sesame oils have been used as seasoning ingredients in Korean dishes due to their characteristic odor and taste.

Perilla (*Perilla frutescens*) is a plant of the mint family (Lamiaceae). Both perilla leaves and perilla seeds are used as ingredients in a range of Korean dishes. The fresh leaves (*deulkkae-nip* in Korean) are commonly used in salad dishes and as a veggie wrap (*ssam-chaeso* in Korean) for roasted meats. Roasted perilla seeds can also be used as an important ingredient in various Korean cuisines. Perilla seeds are, however, mainly used for the preparation of perilla seed oil (*deul-gireum* in Korean), which is an invaluable cooking and condiment oil in various cuisines in Korea. This chapter covers physicochemical properties, important major and minor components, and beneficial health functions of sesame seeds, sesame oils, perilla seeds, and perilla seed oil that are indispensable cooking ingredients in various Korean cuisines.

12.2 Sesame Seed and Sesame Seed Oil

12.2.1 Importance

In terms of cooking, sesame seeds can be classified into white-, black-, and yellow-colored seeds. Also, sesame oils from roasted sesame seeds, roasted whole sesame seeds, and a mixture of sesame seeds and salts have been used for preparation of traditional Korean cuisines including rice cake (called "tteok" in Korean) and snacks. Sesame oils are important condiments, providing a specific odor for foods like salad or cooked vegetables.

12.2.1.1 History of Harvesting

First, it is necessary to understand Korea's history briefly. Gojoseon was the first kingdom from 2333 BC and then three kingdoms, including Goguryeo, Baekje, and Silla, lasted from 57 BC to AD 668. The unification of the three kingdoms was done by Silla on the peninsula and then lasted from 676 to 935.

Seed Oil (Sesame Seed, Perilla Seed)

The Goryeo dynasty governed from 918 to 1392 and then the Joseon dynasty lasted about 500 years—from 1392 to 1897.

The usage of sesame seeds and sesame oils in Korea was first reported in the literature at the year of 683, which was the Shilla dynasty. A record on the sesame oil used for the lotus lantern for Buddha was written in *The Heritage of the Three States* (*Samguk Yusa*), which was published in 1281. However, sesame may have been cultivated on the Korean peninsula around 1000 BC, based on the carbonized sesame seeds found in China and Japan. The first sesame harvesting was recorded in 1123 in the Goryeo dynasty. Sesame harvesting methods were detailed 1429 (*Nongsa Jikseol*) or 1490 (*Sasichanyocho*) of the Joseon dynasty. Also, methods to produce sesame oils from sesame seeds were written in 1767 during this same dynasty (*Jeungbo Sallim Gyeongje*).

12.2.1.2 History as Food Ingredients

According to *The Chronicles of the Three States*, oil was part of Pyeback, which is a formal greeting ceremony from the newly wedded bride to her parents-in-law (AD 683). The oil was assumed to be sesame oil. In the Goryeo dynasty, tributes to China contained flavored oils, which were also presumed to be sesame oils (AD 945, 1072, 1080).

The purpose of using sesame oils was to provide characteristic and unique odor to foods. Generally, sesame oils are added to side dishes made of vegetables for salad purposes. Also, sesame oil is added to bibimbap, a Korean dish made of rice topped with vegetables. Sesame oil has been used in dough-making for noodles to prevent adhesion of noodles to each other and accelerate aging of noodles. Sesame seeds were used as coating materials outside of *han-gwa*, a general term for Korean traditional confectionery made of grain flower, honey, sugar, fruit, or edible root. A powdered form of sesame seeds was inserted inside a rice cake (called gyeongdan in Korean) or used as a soup ingredient. Powdered sesame seeds mixed with salts are popular condiments for many Korean dishes.

Historically, sesame seeds and sesame oils have been used since the Goryeo dynasty. Yumilgwa is a traditional Korean confectionary made by deep-fat frying a mixture of grain flower and honey and has two types of foods, including yakgwa and ganjeong. Yakgwa is a fried sweet dessert made from a pressed mixture of kneaded wheat flour, sesame oil, and honey. Gangjeong is dessert made from dried dough of rice flour. Yumilgwa has been supplied in national ceremonies. Records on the yumilgwa and sesame oil were first reported in the year 918 and several times in the Goryeo dynasty.

In the Joseon dynasty, yumilgwa was frequently used in big festivals and became popular among society's nobility. Sesame oil was also used for medicinal purposes for skin disease and other symptoms.

Korean rice cake (tteok in Korean) had sesame oil as an important ingredient. Among tteok, yakbab or yaksik is a cooked rice with sesame oil. Also,

294   *Korean Functional Foods*

hwajeon, a small sweet pancake with edible flower petals including azalea or chrysanthemum, needs sesame seeds and sesame oils.

12.2.1.3 Recipes

Some cookbooks have introduced recipes of traditional Korean dishes using sesame seeds or sesame oils. *Eumsik Dimibang*, *Jeungbo Sallim Gyeongje*, and *Gyuhap Chongseo* are some of representative books dealing with cooking recipes.

Eumsik Dimibang is a Koran cookbook written around 1670 by Lady Jang (1598~1680) during the Josen dynasty. *Jeungbo Sallim Gyeongje* is a Korean book on agriculture compiled by several authors in 1766. *Gyuhap Chongseo*, roughly translated as *Women's Encyclopedia*, is a compendium of advice for women, written by Lady Yi in 1809. *Siuijeonseo* is a Korean cookbook compiled in the late nineteenth century, the authors of which are not known. Tables 12.1 and 12.2 show representative cooking recipes using sesame seeds and sesame oils in old cookbooks (Choi 1998; Han 2005a,b; Hwang et al. 2010).

TABLE 12.1

Korean Cuisines Using Sesame Seeds and Oils in *Eumsik Dimibang*, *Jeungbo Sallim Gyeongje*, *Gyuhap Chongseo*, and *Siuijeonseo*

Cookbook	Ingredients	Cooking Methods	Number of Foods	Names of Foods
Eumsik Dimibang	Sesame seeds	Powder types	4	Mostly related to foods with meat
		Source types	3	Noodle-type foods
	Sesame oils	Frying	1	Gangjeong
		Mixing	13	Yakbab, dasik, etc.
		Spreading	1	Abalone preservation
Jeungbo Sallim Gyeongje	Sesame seeds	Raw seeds	12	Gochujang
		Roasted seeds	4	Yakkwa, dasik
	Sesame oils	Pan roasting	1	Roasted chicken
		Frying	3	Yakkwa
		Mixing	16	Yakbab
		Spreading	5	Platycodon, squid
Gyuhap Chongseo	Sesame seeds	Mixing	3	Pumpkin salad
		Spreading	6	Sliced meat
	Sesame oils	Powder	1	Yakbab
		Roasted seeds	9	Dumpling, steamed dish
Siuijeonseo	Sesame seeds	Mixing	44	Dumpling, bibimbab, sliced meat, noodle soup
	Sesame oils	Mixing	3	Bibimbab, pumpkin salad

Seed Oil (Sesame Seed, Perilla Seed)

TABLE 12.2

General Recipes of Korean Cuisine Using Sesame Seeds and Sesame Oils

Name of Cuisine	Representative Picture	Definition or Recipe
Bibimbap		Various marinated and/or cooked vegetables and stir-fried beef tossed thoroughly with cooked rice with the addition of gochu-jang as a seasoning condiment Sesame seed or sesame oil added/or served with bibimbap to provide unique flavor at the end of preparation
Namul (seasoned vegetables)		Side dish made by parboiling and seasoning vegetables Sesame seed and sesame oil added as seasoning at the final preparation to add flavor
Yaksik		Cooked glutinous rice mixed with honey, sugar, soy sauce, chestnut and jujube, etc., and steamed once more to make a dark, reddish, sweet rice cake Sesame oil added to season cooked glutinous rice
Gangjeong (variety of yugwa)		Traditional Korean sweet cookie made by puffed rice coated with various ingredients such as roasted sesame seed, black sesame seed, and crushed puffed rice with a syrup
Yeotgangjeong		Traditional Korean sweet cookie made by solidifying roasted grain or nuts with starch syrup Main ingredients (grain or nuts) are sesame seeds, beans, peanuts, etc.
Yakgwa		A cookie of deep-fried dough made of wheat flour, sesame oil, an alcoholic beverage, and honey

Note: Pictures and explanations of recipes were supervised by Prof. Chung LN at KyungHee Univ.

12.2.1.4 Cultivation

Sesame is the world's oldest oil crop; 37 species are found in the *Sesamum* genus, but only *Sesamum indicum* is cultivated widely. Other species are cultivated partly in Africa, India, or Sri Lanka (Hwang, 2005). Sesame seeds are an ovate shape 3–4 mm long and 1.5–2 mm wide and their color varies—white, black, gray, brown, red, and yellow. In Korea, white, black, and yellow sesame seeds are widely cultivated.

Major sesame-producing countries are China (about 30%), India (about 22%), Myanmar (about 8%), Sudan (about 4%), Uganda (about 4%), and others (about 32%). Production areas for sesame seeds in Korea have decreased gradually, even though consumption of sesame seeds has increased since 1990 (Table 12.3). Cultivation areas for sesame seeds in Korea changed from 31,077 ha in 2006 to 25,139 ha in 2015 (Table 12.3).

TABLE 12.3

Sesame Production, Cultivation Area, and Consumption in Korea Since 1990

	1990	1995	2000	2005	2010	2011
Consumption (1,000 tons)	57.8	88.9	101.6	100.6	94.0	96.3
Domestic production (1,000 tons)	38.1	31.9	31.7	23.5	12.8	12.7
Imported volume (1,000 tons)	15.0	42.0	70.0	66.6	75.6	76.6
Consumption per capita (kg)	1.3	1.9	2.0	1.9	2.0	1.8
Self-sufficiency rate (%)	67	32	26	23	15	13

Source: Rural Development Administration database, 2016.

Year	Cultivation Area (ha)	Increasing Rate (%)	Production per 10 h (kg)	Increasing Rate (%)	Domestic Production (ton)	Increasing Rate (%)
2006	31,077	−8.5	50	−27.5	15,489	−34.0
2007	31,321	0.8	56	12.0	17,506	13.0
2008	28,794	−8.1	68	21.4	19,472	11.2
2009	34,875	21.1	37	−45.6	12,780	−34.4
2010	27,154	−22.1	47	27.0	12,703	−0.6
2011	25,649	−5.5	37	−21.3	9,515	−25.1
2012	25,076	−2.2	39	5.4	9,690	1.8
2013	23,184	−7.5	53	35.9	12,392	27.9
2014	28,370	22.4	43	−18.9	12,158	−1.9
2015	25,139	−11.4	46	7.0	11,678	−3.9

Sources: Korean Statistical Information Service, 2016.

12.2.2 Chemical Composition

Sesame seed contains around 50% fat, 25% protein, 25% carbohydrates including fiber, and 5% ashes, although large variations have been observed depending on the variety, origin, color, and size of the seeds.

Sesame oil has less than 20% saturated fatty acid (mainly palmitic and stearic acids) and oleic and linoleic acids constitute almost all unsaturated fatty acid. The major form of sesame lipid is triacylglycerols and minor components are diacylglycerols, free fatty acids, polar lipids, and steryl esters. Unsaponifiable matter content is around 2% in sesame oils. Major unsaponifiable matters in sesame oils are sterols, triterpenes, triterpene alcohols, tocopherols, and sesame lignans. Sesamol may contain as high as 1.9% total sterols. Tocopherol content in sesame oil ranges from 330 to 1010 mg/kg oil. Generally, oils from black sesame seeds have a lower content of tocopherols than brown or white sesame seeds. γ-Tocopherol content is the highest and predominant in sesame oil, followed by δ- and α-tocopherols.

Sesame lignans are characteristic antioxidant compounds in sesame, and molecular structures of sesame lignans are shown in Figure 12.1. Lignans are formed by the oxidative coupling of p-hydroxyphenylpropane. Sesamin, episesamin, sesamolin, sesangolin, 2-episesalatin, sesamol, sesaminol, sesamol dimmer, samin, sesamolinol, pinoresiol, and P-1 are found in sesame (Figure 12.1). Sesame seeds have oil-soluble lignans, including sesamin and sesamolin, and water-soluble lignan glycosides, including pinoresinol glucosides and sesaminol glucosides. Sesamin has been found in other plants, but sesamolin is a characteristic lignan found only in sesame (Hwang, 2005). The content of sesamin is positively correlated with the oil content in seeds, whereas that of sesamolin does not show any correlation with the content of oils. The sesamin content (400–900 mg/100 g oil from white sesame; 100–500 mg/100 g oil from black sesame) is higher than that of sesamolin (100–400 mg/100 g oil from white sesame; 100–400 mg/100 g oil from black sesame) in sesame seeds, and the ratio of sesamolin to sasamin ranges from 0.2 to 1.0. Sesamol content in seeds is below 10 mg/100 g oil and usually increases during thermal treatment.

Lignan glycosides are the glycosylated forms of lignans including sesaminol, sesamolinol, and pinoresinol glucosides (Figure 12.1). Total contents of lignan glycosides are 100–170 mg/100 g white seed, with sesaminol triglucoside the most predominant compound (Hwang, 2005).

12.2.3 Processing

Sesame oil has been consumed worldwide. Depending on the region, different types of sesame oils are consumed, such as seed coat removal or roasting of the seeds. Major types of sesame oils are categorized into refined sesame oil from unroasted seeds, roasted sesame oil, and small mill sesame oil from roasted and dehulled seeds. Refined sesame oils are commonly used as salad

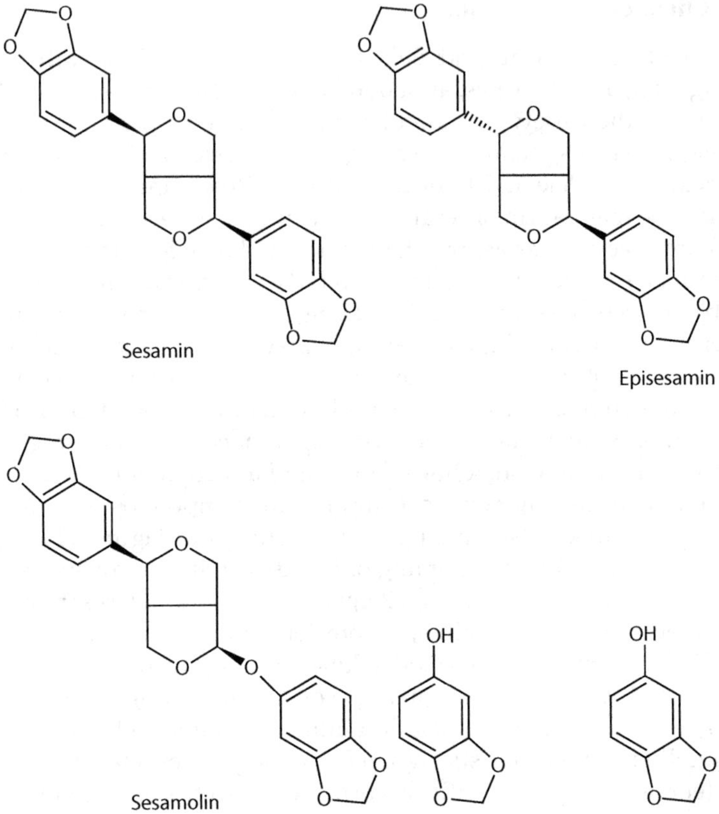

FIGURE 12.1
Molecular structures of sesamol, sesame lignans, and lignan glycosides in sesame seeds.
(*Continued*)

oil, and roasted sesame oil is popular in Asian countries including Korea, China, and Japan. Roasting is an important processing to develop desirable color, sensory attributes, and flavor for sesame oil through the Maillard reaction. Antioxidant properties, sesamol contents, and red color increased when sesame seeds were roasted at temperatures up to 220°C and then decreased, whereas flavor score proved to be optimal at 200°C. The recommended roasting conditions for sesame oils are 160°C for 25 min, 180°C for 25 min, 200°C for 15 min, or 220°C for 5 min (Yoshida and Takagi, 1997).

The roasting process significantly induces the changes of sesamin and sesamolin, which are major lignans in sesame seeds. These lignans have low antioxidant properties due to the lack of phenolic hydroxyl groups. Sesamol is the major antioxidant in sesame oils and is transformed from

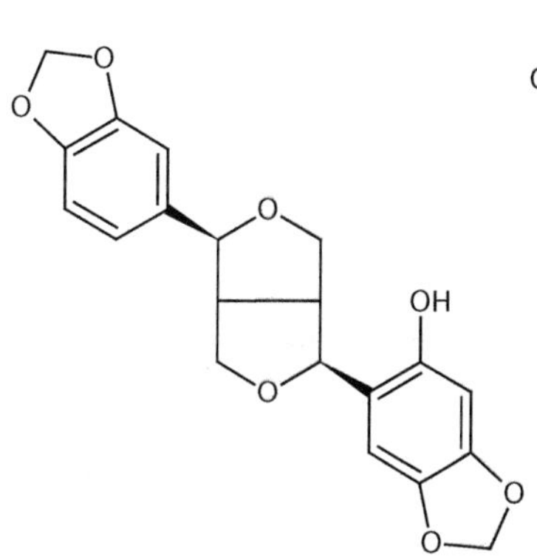

Seed Oil (Sesame Seed, Perilla Seed) 299

Sesaminol

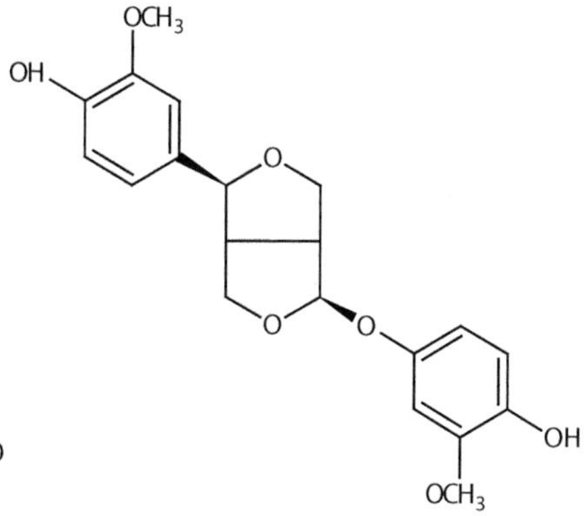

Pinoresinol

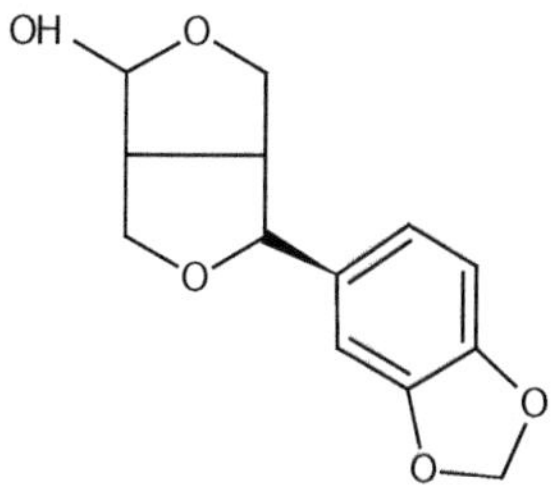

Samin

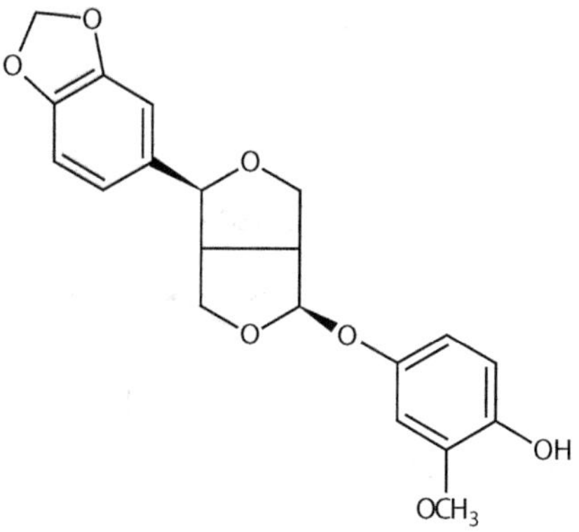

Sesamolinol

FIGURE 12.1 (CONTINUED)
Molecular structures of sesamol, sesame lignans, and lignan glycosides in sesame seeds.

(Continued)

the hydrolysis of sesamolin during heating. Sesame oil refining, especially the acidic anhydrous condition of bleaching, can increase the content of sesaminol from sesamolin. The heat stability of sesamol is relatively low and sesamol disappears at 180°C for 4 h, whereas sesaminol shows better heat stability. Sesamin undergoes epimerization upon heating with acid, and refining procedures like bleaching and deodorization cause significant changes in the contents of sesamin. Deodorization also destroys sesamol;

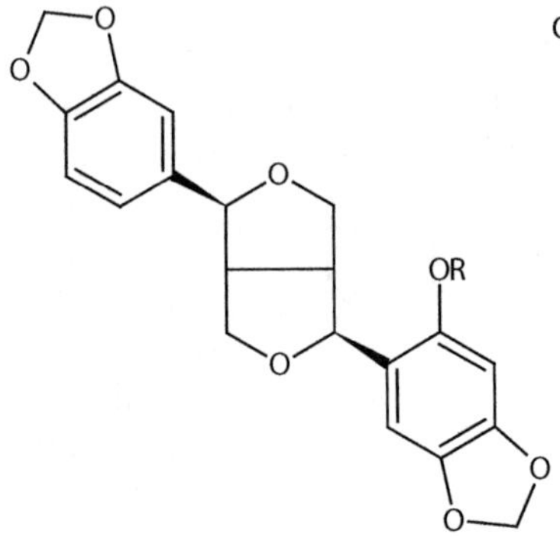

R = Glc

= Glc-Glc

= Glc-Glc-Glc

Sesaminol glucosides

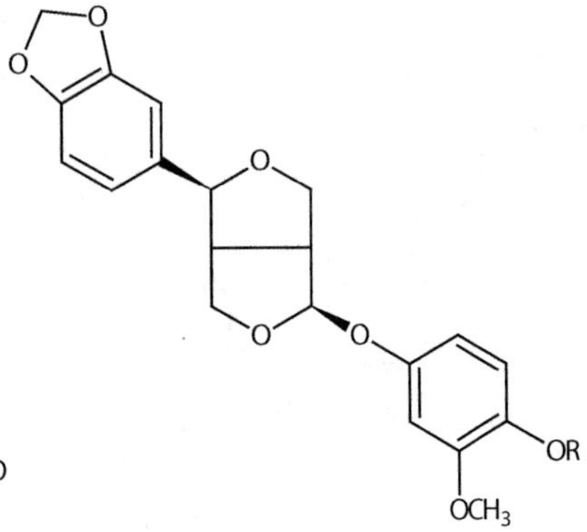

R = Glc

= Glc-Glc

Sesaminolinol glucosides

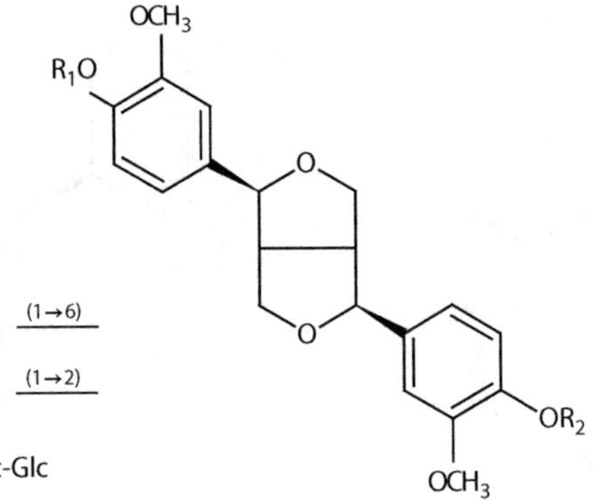

KP1: R_1 = H, R_2 = Glc Glc $\overset{(1 \to 6)}{\rule{1cm}{0.4pt}}$

KP2: R_1 = H, R_2 = Glc Glc $\overset{(1 \to 2)}{\rule{1cm}{0.4pt}}$

KP3: R_1 = H, R_2 = Glc-Glc-Glc

KP4: R_1 = Glc, R_2 = Glc

Pinoresinol glucosides

FIGURE 12.1 (CONTINUED)

Molecular structures of sesamol, sesame lignans, and lignan glycosides in sesame seeds.

commercial deodorized sesame oil contains trace amounts of sesamol (Hwang 2005).

Aroma characteristics of sesame oil have been reported by many researchers with different volatile analyzing methods. Major volatiles in sesame oils are pyrazines, furans, pyrroles, pyridines, and sulfur-containing compounds (Nakamura et al., 1989; Kim et al., 2000a; Park et al., 2011a). Kim et al. (2000a) reported 26 pyrazines, 11 pyridines, 9 thiazoles, 6 furans, 8 pyrroles, 5 phenols, 8 aldehydes, 8 hydrocarbons, 7 alcohols, 2 indoles, 3 ketones, 10 acids, 4 nitriles, 7 esters, and 5 other compounds from sesame oils prepared from sesame seeds roasted at 110°C to 230°C.

Odor-active volatiles, including 2-acetyl-1-pyrroline (roasty), 2-furfurylthiol (coffee like), 2-phenylethylthiol (rubbery), and 4-hydroxy-2,5-dimethyl-3(2H)-furanone (caramel-like), have been identified as important odor contributors for sesame oil by Schieberle (1996). As roasting temperature increased from 213°C to 247°C, total headspace volatiles and pyrazines increased significantly ($p < 0.05$). Also, the temperature of roasting was a more discriminating factor than time of roasting for the formation of volatiles in sesame oil. Volatiles with ion fragments of 52, 76, 53, and 51 amu, which are the major ion fragments from pyrazines, furans, and furfurals, played important roles in discriminating volatiles in sesame oils from roasted sesame seeds (Park et al., 2011a).

12.2.4 Beneficial Health Effects

Sesame and sesame oil have shown various health-promoting properties including cholesterol-modulating ability, antihypertensive properties, antioxidant activities, and regulation of blood sugar. Also, immune-modulating effects, antiaging effects, and bacteriocidal and fungicidal properties are reported in sesame and sesame oils.

12.2.4.1 Effects on Lipid Metabolism

Sesamin, one of the lignan compounds in sesame seeds, has been related to cholesterol-modulation effects, although other compounds, including sesamolin, sesaminol, and episesamin, have also demonstrated this activity. The cholesterol-modulating effects are associated with inhibition of δ-5-desaturase activity, enhance hepatic fatty acid β-oxidation, and decrease hepatic lipogenic activity (Jeng and Hou, 2005). δ-5-Desaturase is an enzyme in the conversion of dihomo-γ-linolenic acid to arachidonic acid. Sesame intake induced the increase in expression of mitochondrial and peroxisomal fatty acid oxidation enzymes (Ashakumary et al., 1999).

12.2.4.2 Antioxidant Properties and Immunomodulating Effects

Sesame oil has high oxidation resistance activity due to the presence of endogenous antioxidants including sesaminol, sesamolinol, pinoresinol, and sesamol. Sesaminol had a strong inhibitory effect on the peroxidation of low density lipoprotein (LDL) (Kang et al., 1998a, 2000) and is more effective in protecting LDL from oxidative stress than sesamolinol, pinoresinol, and even α-tocopherol, possibly because of the highly lipophilic characteristics of sesaminol. The lipophilicity may help sesaminol positioned within LDL particles.

Administration of sesamolin at 1% concentration in rats greatly reduced lipid peroxidation activity in liver and kidney (Kang et al., 1998a). However, sesamolin did not show appreciable antioxidant properties in *in vitro* assays. The metabolites of sesamolin—sesamol and sesamolinol—may be responsible for this antioxidant activity (Kang et al., 1998a). Sesame seeds or sesame oils, which are high in sesame lignans, could lower serum triacylglycerol levels through lowering activities of enzymes related to fatty acid synthesis (Sirato-Yasumoto et al., 2001).

Sesame oil has exceptionally high resistance against thermal oxidation. During heat treatment at a relatively high temperature like 180°C, sesamol was continuously generated with the decrease of sesamolin in sesame oil roasted at 230°C or 247°C, but not in sesame oil roasted at 213°C (Lee et al., 2010).

12.2.4.3 Antihypertensive, Anticancer Effects, and Blood Sugar Regulation

Sesame suppresses the development of hypertension in rats (Matsumura et al., 1998). Lowering blood pressure, as well as beneficial effects on lipid profiles and antioxidant properties, were also related to sesame administration (Sankar et al., 2011).

Sesame consumption is correlated with a significant reduction of blood glucose level and glycosylated hemoglobin level (Ramesh et al., 2005). Significant reduction in fasting blood sugar was dependent on the intake of sesame content (Mitra, 2007).

Sesame lignans, including sesamin and episesamin, could affect the metabolism of polyunsaturated fatty acids and prostaglandins. Prostaglandin is one of influential factors for mammary carcinogenesis. Sesamin at a 0.2% concentration reduced the cumulative number and mean number of mammary cancers (Hirose et al., 1992). Antitumor promotion activity of sesame components was also reported. Radical scavenging ability of sesame components was suggested as a major mechanism for the inhibition of tumorigenesis. When sesame components were consumed orally, the formation of skin papilloma was effectively limited, which implies that absorption of sesame components happened in digestive tracts and continued anticancer activity (Hwang, 2005). However, sesamol at 2.0% concentration showed forestomach carcinogenic activity in animal models (Akimoto et al., 1993). Notwithstanding this finding, human beings do not have a forestomach and their consumption of sesamol is much lower than the tested concentration.

12.3 Perilla Seeds and Perilla Seed Oil

12.3.1 Leaves, Seed, and Seed Oil in Cuisine

Perilla (*Perilla frutescens*) is a plant of the mint family (Lamiaceae). Perilla is classified into two main types—*Perilla frutescens* var. *frutescens* and *Perilla frutescens* var. *crispa*, which are cultivated mainly for the purpose of harvesting seeds and leaves, respectively. The fresh leaves (*deulkkae-nip* in Korean) have a characteristic mint-like aroma and are commonly used in salad dishes and as a veggie wrap (*ssam-chaeso* in Korean) for roasted meats. Perilla leaves (*deulkkae-nip*), which are typically used as a veggie wrap in Korean cuisine, are shown in Figure 12.2. Various types of perilla seeds cultivated in Korea are shown in Figure 12.3.

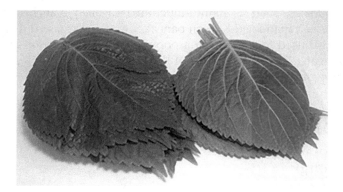

FIGURE 12.2
Perilla leaves used as a popular veggie-wrap for the roasted meats in Korean cuisine.

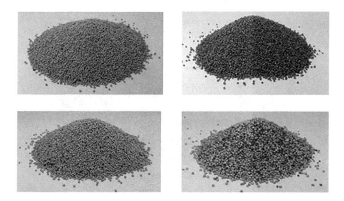

FIGURE 12.3
Different types of perilla seeds cultivated in Korea.

Perilla seeds contain approximately 40% oil and are mainly used for obtaining oil. In South Korea, 42,600 ha (59,000-ton seed production) were in production in 2015 (Statistics Korea, 2016). Perilla seed oil (deul-gireum in Korean) is used as a cooking and condiment oil in various different cuisine in Asia, mainly in Korea. The consumption of perilla seed oil as an edible oil is the highest in Korea, reaching almost 80% of total world consumption (Lee et al., 2014). Mechanical pressing following roasting the seeds is the most popular extraction method for obtaining perilla seed oil with its savory and nutty flavor. Perilla seed oils obtained by mechanical press extraction after different degrees of roasting are shown in Figure 12.4. Even though supercritical carbon dioxide (SC-CO_2) extraction technology has been recognized as a powerful tool for extracting oils from various oil-bearing sources, SC-CO_2 extraction technology is not yet commercially practiced for extracting oil from perilla seeds.

Perilla seed oil and sesame oil are the two main condiment oils used in Korean cuisine. Perilla seed oil is a common ingredient in a range of Korean traditional dishes, such as namul-muchim (seasoned blanched-vegetable side dishes), jeon (pan-fried Korean pancake), and gim (roasted dried laver). The oil is also used for preparing a popular dipping sauce for grilled and pan-fried meats. The typical recipe of the perilla seed oil dipping sauce for grilled and pan-fried meats is

Perilla seed oil (20 g)
Sugar (20 g)
Fermented soy sauce (20 g)
Vinegar (20 g)
Chopped garlic (5 g)

This dipping sauce is frequently used as a dressing source for preparing various vegetable salads in Korean cuisine. Perilla seed oil is also a popular

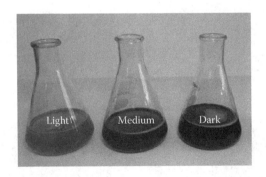

FIGURE 12.4
Perilla seed oils obtained by mechanical press extraction from the roasted perilla seeds with different degrees of roasting (light, medium, and dark roasted perilla seed oils).

ingredient as a condiment oil along with the sesame oil for the bibimbab (Korean traditional cuisine: cooked rice mixed with vegetables, beef, and red pepper paste). Perilla seed oil has been known to be the richest dietary source for omega-3 polyunsaturated fatty acid (PUFA). The quantity of α-linolenic acid (ALNA) is higher in perilla seed oil than in flaxseed oil, which is a well-known rich source of ALNA in Western countries.

12.3.2 Fatty Acid Composition

The oil content in a perilla seed is approximately 40% with a range of 33%–48% (Shin and Kim, 1994; Ding et al., 2012; Jung et al., 2012). The oil in perilla seeds consists of 91.2%–93.9% neutral lipids, 3.9%–5.8% glycolipids, and 2.0%–3.0% phospholipids (Shin and Kim, 1994). Perilla seed oil is an excellent source of plant-derived ω-3 fatty acid (ALNA) with an exceptionally low content of saturated fatty acids (less than 10% saturated fatty acids). The representative gas chromatogram of fatty acid methylesters from perilla seed oil is shown in Figure 12.5. The ALNA content in perilla seed oils was in the range of 53%–62% (Shin and Kim, 1994; Ding et al., 2012; Jung et al., 2012).

Perilla seed oil also contains significant amounts of other types of unsaturated fatty acids, including oleic acid (18:1) and linoleic acid (18:2). Wang et al. (2010) reported that perilla seed oil contained 7.38% palmitic acid, 1.93% stearic acid, 16.70% oleic acid, 14.91% linoleic acid, and 59.08% ALNA. Jung et al. (2012) reported that the fatty acid composition of press-extracted perilla seed oil was 5.85% palmitic acid, 1.92% stearic acid, 16.44% oleic acid, 14.10% linoleic acid, and 61.69% linolenic acid. The composition of the perilla seed oil is not dependent on the extraction method (mechanical pressing, solvent extraction, and SC-CO$_2$ extraction) (Jung et al., 2012). Lee et al. (2014) also reported that the fatty acid composition of perilla seed oil was 5.56% palmitic acid, 2.11% stearic acid, 16.78% oleic acid, 12.61% linoleic acid, and 62.29% linolenic acid.

The fatty acid composition in perilla seeds is associated with the cultivating climate, especially the growth temperature. Ding et al. (2012) reported

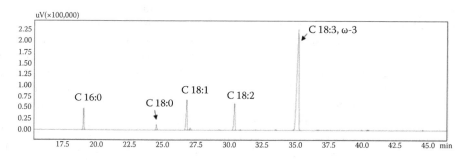

FIGURE 12.5
Representative gas chromatogram of fatty acid methylesters from perilla seed oil.

that the ratio of saturated over unsaturated fatty acids (SFA/UFA) in perilla seeds was positively associated with annual growth temperature. The fatty acid composition in the perilla seed oil might be different with country of origin of the seeds. Ding et al. (2012) reported that the relative ratios of monounsaturated over polyunsaturated fatty acids in Korea, China, and Thailand perilla seeds were 0.24, 0.20, and 0.15, respectively. ω-3 Fatty acids are well recognized as a health-promoting nutrient. Fish oils are a rich dietary source of ω-3 fatty acids such as eicosapentaenoic acid (EPA; 20:5) and docosahexaenoic acid (DHA; 22:6). ALNA can be transformed into the longer chain ω-3 fatty acids (EPA and DHA) in the human body (Ezaki et al., 1999; Burdge and Wotton, 2002; Burdge et al., 2002). Thus, ALNA is an alternative for fish-derived ω-3 fatty acid.

12.3.3 Health-Promoting Minor Components

Perilla seed oil is also a rich source of other beneficial health compounds including tocopherols, phytosterols, policosanols, and phospholipids. Total content of tocopherols in perilla oil is in the range of 400–780 mg/kg oil (Jung et al., 2012; Wang et al., 2010). The most abundant tocopherol in perilla oil is γ-tocopherol, followed by α-tocopherol and δ-tocopherol, in a decreasing order. Wang et al. (2010) reported that tocopherol content in perilla oil obtained from its raw seeds was 641.15 mg/kg oil. Jung et al. (2012) reported that tocopherol content in roasted perilla seed oil was 400.71 mg/kg oil. Lee et al. (2014) reported that roasted perilla seed oil contained 510.6 mg tocopherol per kilogram of oil with a composition of 37.2 mg α-tocopherol, 451.9 mg γ-tocopherol, and 14.9 mg δ-tocopherol/kg oil.

Perilla seed oil also contains high contents of phytosterols. β-Sitosterol is the most abundant phytosterol in perilla seed oil, followed by campesterol and stigmasterol in a decreasing order (Lee et al., 2014). β-Sitosterol consists of about 86% of the total phytosterol present in perilla seed oil. Lee et al. (2014) reported that phytosterol content in perilla seed oil was 2651.4 mg/kg oil with a composition of 236.7 mg campesterol, 138.5 mg stigmasterol, and 2276.1 mg β-sitosterol.

Perilla seed oil has been reported to be an exceptionally rich source of policosanols (Jung et al., 2011). The policosanol contents in 10 different commercial vegetable oils (soybean, corn, grapeseed, sesame, cottonseed, canola, ricebran, olive, perilla seed, and sunflower seed oils) were studied (Jung et al., 2011). Perilla seed oil contained the highest content of policosanols (427.8 mg/kg oil) among the 12 different vegetable oils tested. Octacosanol is the most predominant policosanol in perilla oil, representing 56% of the total policosanols (Jung et al., 2011). Figure 12.6 shows the representative gas chromatogram of policosanols in perilla seed oil as analyzed by gas chromatography-tandem mass spectrometry in multiple reaction monitoring mode. The press-extracted perilla seed oil contained high quantities of phospholipids (75.6 mg P/kg oil) (Jung et al., 2012).

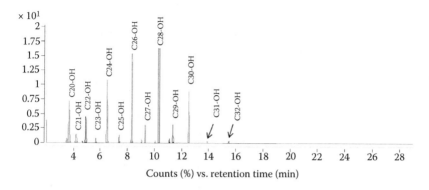

FIGURE 12.6
Representative gas chromatogram of policosanols in perilla seed oil as obtained by gas chromatography-tandem mass spectrometry in multiple reaction monitoring mode.

The quantities of tocopherols, sterols, policosanols and phospholipids in perilla oils obtained from roasted perilla seeds were greatly dependent on the extraction methods (supercritical carbon dioxide [SC-CO_2], mechanical press, and solvent extraction). Table 12.4 shows the fatty acid composition and contents of tocopherols, phytosterols, and policosanols in perilla seed oils obtained by different extraction methods (supercritical carbon dioxide extraction, mechanical extraction, and hexane extraction) (Jung et al., 2012). The SC-CO_2 extraction at 420 bar and 50°C and hexane extraction provided significantly higher oil yield than mechanical press extraction ($P < 0.05$). SC-CO_2 extraction performed at 420 bar and 50°C did not provide significantly different oil yield from hexane extraction ($P > 0.05$). Perilla oil obtained by SC-CO_2 extraction showed significantly higher tocopherol, phytosterol, and policosanol contents than the oils obtained by mechanical press and hexane extractions ($P < 0.05$) (Jung et al., 2012). The pressure during SC-CO_2 extraction greatly affected the tocopherol, phytosterol, and policosanol contents in the perilla oils. As the pressure increased, the contents of tocopherol, phytosterol, and policosanol in the perilla oil decreased. Jung et al. (2012) reported that tocopherol contents in perilla seed oil obtained by SC-CO_2 extraction under the pressures of 300, 360, and 420 bar at 50°C were 503.26, 444.83, and 420.16 mg/kg oil, respectively. These researchers also reported that the sterol contents in the perilla seed oils obtained by SC-CO_2 extraction under the pressures of 300, 360, and 420 bar at 50°C were 3664, 3717, and 3463 mg/kg oil, respectively. The authors also reported that policosanol contents in the oils obtained from perilla seeds under pressures of 300, 360, and 420 bar at 50°C were 655, 551, and 545 mg/kg oil, respectively (Jung et al., 2012). The hexane-extracted oil (131 mg P/kg oil) contains higher phospholipids than press-extracted oil (76 mg P/kg oil) and SC-CO_2-extracted perilla seed oil (0 mg P/kg). It is interesting to note that the SC-CO_2-extracted perilla seed oil did not contain detectable amounts of phospholipids. Kim et al. (1998) reported

TABLE 12.4

Fatty Acid Composition and Contents of Tocopherols, Phytosterols, and Policosanols in Perilla Seed Oils Obtained by Different Extraction Methods[a]

		Extraction Method		
	Components	SC-CO$_2$ Extraction	Mechanical Press (600 kgf/cm^2)	Solvent (Hexane)
Fatty acid composition (%)	Palmitic acid	5.9	5.9	6.0
	Stearic acid	1.9	1.9	1.9
	Oleic acid	16.4	16.4	16.4
	Linoleic acid	14.1	14.1	14.1
	Linolenic acid	61.7	61.7	61.6
Tocopherol contents (mg/kg oil)	α-Tocopherol	43.3	41.2	43.8
	β-Tocopherol	–	–	–
	γ-Tocopherol	363.5	346.6	344.6
	δ-Tocopherol	13.4	12.9	23.1
	Total	420.2	400.7	411.5
Sterol contents (mg/kg oil)	Campesterol	334.3	341.8	321.2
	Stigmasterol	198.5	176.6	177.5
	β-sitosterol	2930.0	2788.6	2773.9
	Total	3462.8	3280.0	3272.6
Policosanol contents (mg/kg oil)	C20-OH	8.5	4.6	4.5
	C21-OH	Trace	Trace	Trace
	C22-OH	15.4	7.5	7.8
	C23-OH	6.9	4.0	4.1
	C24-OH	56.3	21.3	24.6
	C25-OH	13.1	7.8	5.2
	C26-OH	78.7	44.2	48.5
	C27-OH	14.7	10.5	11.3
	C28-OH	250.7	129.9	148.5
	C29-OH	18.7	13.9	15.1
	C30-OH	53.4	30.4	32.8
	C31-OH	14.2	Trace	Trace
	C32-OH	14.4	Trace	Trace
	Total	544.9	274.1	302.4

Source: Jung, D. M. et al. 2011. *J Food Sci* 76:C891–899

[a] Supercritical carbon dioxide extraction, mechanical extraction, and hexane extraction.

that the phospholipid contents of perilla oil from unroasted raw perilla seeds obtained by SC-CO$_2$, mechanical press, and hexane extraction were <0.1, 0.9, and 30 mg P/kg oil, respectively. Phosphatidylethanolamine (50.4%–57.1%) and phosphatidylcholines (17.6%–20.6%) are the major phospholipid components with a small quantity of phosphatidic acid, lysophosphatidylcholine, phosphatidylserine, and phosphatidylinositol (Shin and Kim, 1994).

Seed Oil (Sesame Seed, Perilla Seed)

12.3.4 Nutty Flavors of Roasted Oil

Perilla seed oil is generally obtained by mechanical pressing after roasting the perilla seeds for the development of savory nutty flavor. The nutty flavor of perilla seed oil is believed to arise mainly from pyrazines formed during the roasting process. Pyrazines impart a nut-like flavor in various roasted, baked, and thermally processed foods via Maillard reactions between reducing sugars and amino groups (Guerra and Yaylayan, 2010; Lancker et al., 2010). Qualitative and quantitative information on pyrazines in roasted perilla seed oil has been available (Kim et al, 2000b; Park et al., 2011b; Kwon et al., 2013). Park et al. (2011b) identified four pyrazines (2-methylpyrazine, 2,5-dimethylpyrazine, trimethylpyrazine, and 2-ethyl-3,6-dimethylpyrazine) in perilla seed oil. Kim et al. (2000b) identified 12 pyrazines from perilla seed oils by dynamic headspace (HS) gas chromatography-mass spectrometry. Kwon et al. (2013) identified and quantitated 14 pyrazine compounds in perilla seed oils by (HS)-solid phase microextraction (SPME)-gas chromatography-tandem mass spectrometry.

Roasting considerably affects the quality and quantity of pyrazines in perilla seed oils. Kwon et al. (2013) reported that 2,5-dimethylpyrazine was the most predominant pyrazine found in lightly roasted perilla seed oil. However, 2-methylpyrazine was the most abundant pyrazine in the oil in dark roasted perilla seed oil. The total quantity of pyrazines in dark-roasted perilla seed oil was 17 times higher than that in lightly roasted perilla seed oil (Kwon et al., 2013). It was reported that total pyrazine contents in commercial perilla seed oils ($n = 7$) were in the range of 20.5–54.7 µg/g oil (Kwon et al., 2013). The result suggested that, for the extraction of commercial purposed perilla seed oils, roasting is generally practiced under the medium roasting condition. The total pyrazine contents in commercial perilla seed oil are similar to the previously reported values of total pyrazine contents in roasted soybean oil, red pepper seed oil, and peanut oils. Liu et al. (2011) reported that the total pyrazine content of unroasted peanut oil was 73.2 µg/g oil by HS-SPME-gas chromatography-mass spectrometry analysis. Jung et al. (1999) reported that the pyrazine contents in red pepper seed oil obtained from the roasted seeds were in the range of 26.3–131.0 µg/g oil.

12.3.5 Oxidative Stability

Perilla seed oil is highly susceptible to oxidation due to the high quantity of polyunsaturated fatty acid (ALNA) as compared to other vegetable oils such as soybean oil and corn oil. Lee et al. (2014) directly compared the oxidative stability of perilla seed oil with that of soybean oil under dark storage conditions in an oven at 60°C. The authors reported that the rate of peroxide formation in perilla seed oil was approximately three times higher than in soybean oil. Extraction method greatly influences the oxidative stability of perilla seed oil. Kim et al. (1998) reported that hexane-extracted oil obtained from raw perilla seeds showed the highest oxidative stability, followed by the mechanically pressed perilla oil and SC-CO$_2$-extracted oil in a decreasing order. Jung et al. (2012) reported that the press-extracted and hexane-extracted oils had much higher oxidative stability than SC-CO$_2$-extracted oil during storage in the oven under dark conditions at 60°C. However, the photooxidative stabilities of the oils were not considerably different with extraction methods.

12.3.6 Health-Related Functionality

Dietary lipids have been known to be concentrated energy sources and important functional and structural constituents in biological systems. Perilla oil from *P. frutescenes* seeds is a rich source of ALNA, which is a known precursor of EPA and DHA (Burdge and Wotton, 2002; Burdge et al., 2002). ALNA-rich perilla seed oil has been reported to have a range of beneficial activities, such as cardioprotective, antihypotensive, antiatherosclerotic, antiallergic, and anti-inflammatory activities; better brain function; and antitumor activity (Watanabe et al., 1989; de Lorgeril et al., 1994; Ezaki et al., 1999; Lanzmann-Petithory, 2001; de Wilde et al., 2003; Okuyama et al., 2007; Chung et al., 2013). Perilla leaf extract, which has perilla aldehyde as an effective component, has been shown to reduce body weight gain in obese experimental animals and to improve blood lipid profile by down-regulating adipogenic transcription factor and other specific target fat-accumulating genes (Kim and Kim, 2009).

12.3.6.1 Reduction of Risk for Coronary Heart Disease

Dietary ω-3 PUFA intake has been reported to reduce the risk for coronary heart disease by lowering heart rate and blood pressure, reducing platelet aggregation, and lowering triglyceride levels (Takeuchi et al., 2007; Harris et al., 2008). Chung et al. (2013) studied the effects of perilla seed oil supplement on the plasma level of cardioprotective polyunsaturated fatty acids in mice for a period of 8 weeks. The authors reported that perilla seed oil dietary supplements significantly increased EPA and DPA, known cardioprotective fatty acids, in the plasma of the mice. The EPA concentrations in mice plasma of the control group and the perilla seed oil supplemented group were 26.49 and 245.03 μM/L, respectively. The DPA concentrations in mice plasma of control and perilla seed oil supplemented groups were 12.20 and 44.71 μM/L, respectively.

Ezaki et al. (1999) studied the effects of long-term perilla seed oil intake on the fatty acid composition in serum and the risk factors of coronary heart disease in Japanese elderly subjects. The long-term (10-month) perilla oil intake (3 g ALNA/day) greatly increased serum EPA and DHA without any major adverse effects. Perilla oil has been reported to exert antiartheosclerosis activities in Japanese quail (Sadi et al., 1996). Dietary perilla oil exhibits a similar physiological activity to fish oil in modulating hepatic fatty acid

Seed Oil (Sesame Seed, Perilla Seed)

oxidation (Ide et al., 2000; Kim et al., 2004). Cha et al. (2016) reported that perilla oil reduced hypercholesterolemia, atheroma formation, fat accumulation, and lipid peroxidation in hepatic and renal tissues in rabbits fed a high-cholesterol diet, showing the preventive activity of perilla oil on diet-induced atherosclerosis. Jang et al. (2014) reported the inhibitory effects of perilla oil on the platelet aggregation *in vitro* and thrombosis *in vivo*. The authors concluded that perilla oil inhibited platelet aggregation by blocking thromboxane formation, thereby delaying thrombosis following oxidative arterial wall injury.

The hypotension activity of perilla seed oil has also been previously reported. Shimokawa et al. (1988) reported that the systolic blood pressure of stroke-prone spontaneously hypertensive rats (SHR-SP) was lower by about 10% in the perilla oil-fed group than in both the safflower oil-fed and conventional diet groups. Furthermore, the survival time of male and female SHR-SP rats fed the perilla diet was longer than those fed the safflower diet (Shimokawa et al., 1988). Thrombosis induced by embolic blood vessel occlusion is one of the primary known causes of cerebrovascular diseases, including angina and cerebral strokes. Platelet aggregation is a main known cause of the thrombus formation.

12.3.6.2 Improvement of Brain Health

Fish-derived ω-3 fatty acids (DHA and EPA) have long been known to exert beneficial brain health functions such as increased learning ability and prevention of Alzheimer's and Parkinson's diseases. Perilla seed oil with high α-linolenic acid has also been reported to have similarly beneficial brain health activities to the fish-derived ω-3 fatty acids. Lee et al. (2012) reported that perilla oil supplementation improved spatial learning and memory via differential expression of proteins in the hippocampus of rats. Dietary perilla oil supplementation induced changes in membrane fatty acid composition (especially DHA) as well as in the immunoreactivity in a neurogenesis region of the hippocampus (Lee et al., 2012). Kang et al. (2015) reported that perilla seed oil supplement significantly improved cognitive function, and significantly lowered acetylcholinesterase activity and malonaldehyde levels in brain tissue of the trimethyltin (TMT)-induced learning- and memory-impaired ICR mice. Furthermore, perilla oil significantly reduced oxidized glutathione level and increased superoxide dismutase (SOD) activity significantly in the mice study.

12.3.6.3 Reduction of Allergic Hypersensitivity

Perilla oil may be effective in reducing allergic hypersensitivity in humans. Numerous studies have shown that it is effective in suppressing a wide range of allergic mediators in experimental animals. Perilla seed oil may inhibit the generation of leukotrienes (LTs) by leucocytes in patients with asthma. Okamoto et al. (2000) studied the effects of the oil on the suppression of leukotriene C4 generation by leucocytes by comparing the clinical features of patients with asthma. The results showed that dietary perilla seed oil significantly decreased the generation of LTC4 in selected patients with asthma (Okamoto et al., 2000). Chang et al. (2009) reported that dietary perilla oil inhibits proinflammatory cytokine production in the bronchoalveolar lavage fluid of ovalbumin-challenged mice. Arya et al. (2013) reported that perilla seed oil significantly inhibited the gastric secretion, total acidity, and esophagitis index in albino rats. The research results of Arya et al. (2013) also showed clear evidence on the *in vitro* antihistaminic and anticholinergic activity of ALNA on isolated rat ileum preparation.

12.3.6.4 Anticarcinogenic Activity

Epidemiologic and experimental studies suggest that dietary fish oil and vegetable oil containing high ω-3 fatty acids decrease the risk of colon cancer (Narisawa et al., 1994; Onogi et al., 1996; Roynettea et al., 2004). Hirose et al. (1990) studied the effects of perilla oil supplement on 7,12-dimethylbenz[a] anthracene (DMIBA)- and 1,2-diinethylliydrazine (DMH)-induced mammary gland and colon carcinogenesis in female Sprague–Dawley (SD) rats as compared with soybean and safflower oil for 33 weeks. The results of histological examination showed that the numbers of mammary tumors per rat were significantly lower in the perilla oil diet group than in the soybean oil diet group. Furthermore, the perilla oil supplement group showed significantly lower colon tumor incidence (18.2%) than those on the safflower oil diet (47.4%). The numbers of colon tumors per rat were lowest in the perilla oil group, which also had significantly lower incidence of nephroblastomas (0%) than soybean oil diet group (23.8%). The results suggested that perilla oil may inhibit the development of mammary gland, colon, and kidney tumors. Narisawa et al. (1994) also reported that moderate amounts of dietary perilla oil supplementation significantly reduced the N-methyl-N-nitrosourea-induced colon cancer in female F344 rats.

12.3.6.5 Adverse Effects

High intakes (over 3 g per day) of ω-3 fatty acids including DHA, EPA, and α-linoleic acid may heighten the risk of increased bleeding of a patient who is also taking aspirin or warfarin. There is a potential risk of hemorrhagic stroke for those who take very large quantities of perilla oil over extended periods. Perilla ketones present in perilla leaves and seeds have been known to be potent pulmonary edemagenic agents for laboratory animals and livestock (Guerry-Force et al., 1988; Yu et al, 2016). There have been some reported cases of anaphylaxis caused by perilla seeds (Jeong et al., 2006; Min et al., 2006). A case on IgE-mediated occupational asthma induced by inhaling smoke from roasting perilla seeds has also been reported (Jung et al., 2013).

12.4 Conclusion

Overall, sesame seeds, sesame oils, perilla seeds, and perilla oils are irreplaceable food ingredients in Korean cuisine and Asian dishes due to their unique flavor quality and nutritional properties. Recent studies on elucidating the beneficial health properties of these seeds and oils can attract health-concerned consumers' attention. Sesame seeds have been regarded as healthy food ingredients (Cole et al., 2009) and their usage may extend to diverse areas in different forms. Based on the cumulative reported data, perilla seed and perilla seed oil also seem to benefit health at the normal dietary level without noticeable adverse effects. The intake of perilla seed oil containing high quantities of ω-3 fatty acids may reduce the risk of cardiovascular disease and heart attack by improving blood pressure and vascular resistance and lowering triacylglycerol levels. Furthermore, perilla seed oil may be responsible for anticancer, anti-inflammation, and improved brain function activities. Perilla seed oil is the rich source of α-linolenic acid, a plant-derived ω-3 fatty acid with the absence of mercury contamination risk.

References

Akimoto, K., Y. Kigawa, T. Akamatsu et al. 1993. Suppressive effect of sesamin against liver damage caused by alcohol or carbotetrachloride in rodents. *Ann Nutr Metab* 37:218–224.

Arya, E., S. Saha, S. A. Saraf, and G. Kaithwas. 2013. Effect of *Perilla frutescens* fixed oil on experimental esophagitis in albino Wistar rats. *BioMed Res Int* Article ID 981372, 1–6.

Ashakumary, L., I. Rouyer, Y. Takahashi, T. Ide, N. Fukuda, T. Aoyama, T. Hashimoto, M. Mizugaki, and M. Sugano. 1999. Sesamin, a sesame lignan, is a potent inducer of hepatic fatty acid oxidation in the rat. *Metabolism* 48:1303–1313.

Burdge, G. C., A. E. Jones, and S. Wootton. 2002. Eicosapentaenoic and docosapentaenoic acids are the principal products of alpha-linolenic acid metabolism in young men. *Br J Nutr* 88:355–363.

Burdge, G. C., and S. A. Wotton. 2002. Conversion of alpha-linolenic acid to eicosapentaenoic, docosapentaenoic and docosahexaenoic acids in young women. *Br J Nutr* 88:411–420.

Cha, Y., J. Y. Jang, Y. Ban et al. 2016. Anti-atherosclerotic effects of perilla oil in rabbits fed a high-cholesterol diet. *Lab Ani Res* 32(3):171–179.

Chang, H. H., C. S. Chen, and J. Y. Lin. 2009. Dietary perilla oil lowers serum lipids and ovalbumin-specific IgG1, but increases total IgE levels in ovalbumin-challenged mice. *Food Chem Toxicol* 47:848–854.

Choi, C. U. 1998. History and science of sesame oil and perilla oil. *P Korean Soc Food Cook Sci C* 14(4):443–452.

Chung, K. H., H. J. Hwang, K. O. Shin, W. M. Jeon, and K. S. Choi. 2013. Effects of perilla oil on plasma concentrations of cardioprotective (n-3) fatty acids and lipid profiles in mice. *Nutr Res Pract* 7(4):256–261.

Cole, C. F., J. Kotler, and S. Pai. 2009. Happy healthy muppets: A look at Sesame Workshop's Health Initiatives around the world. In *Igniting the power of community*, ed. P. A. Gaist, 227–295. New York: Springer.

de Lorgeril, M., S. Renaud, N. Mamelle et al. 1994. Mediterranean alpha-linolenic acid-rich diet in secondary prevention of coronary heart disease. *Lancet* 343(8911):1454–1459.

de Wilde, M. C., E. Hogyes, A. J. Kiliaan, T. Farkas, P. G. M. Luiten, and E. Farkas. 2003. Dietary fatty acids alter blood pressure, behavior and brain membrane composition of hypertensive rats. *Brain Res* 988:9–19.

Ding, Y., Y. Hu, L. Shi, M. A. Chao, and Y. J. Liu. 2012. Characterization of fatty acid composition from five perilla seed oils in China and its relationship to annual growth temperature. *J Med Plant Res* 6(9):1645–1651.

Ezaki, O., M. Takahashi, T. Shigematsu et al. 1999. Long-term effects of dietary a-linolenic acid from perilla oil on serum fatty acids composition and on the risk factors of coronary heart disease in Japanese elderly subjects. *J Nutr Sci Vitaminol* 45:759–772.

Guerra, P. V., and V. A. Yaylayan. 2010. Dimerization of azomethine ylides: An alternate route to pyrazine formation in the Maillard reaction. *J Agric Food Chem* 58:12523–12529.

Guerry-Force, M. L., J. Coggeshall, J. Snapper, and B. Meyrick. 1988. Morphology of noncardiogenic pulmonary edema induced by perilla ketone in sheep. *Am J Pathol* 133:285–297.

Han, B. J. 2005a. A study of use of sesame and sesame oil in traditional Korean cuisine. *J East Asian Soc Diet Life* 15(2):137–151.

Han, B. J. 2005b. *100 our cuisine (which we must know)*. Seoul, Korea: Hyunmoonsa.

Harris, W. S., M. Miller, A. P. Tighe, M. H. Davidson, and E. J. Schaefer. 2008. Omega-3 fatty acids and coronary heart disease risk: Clinical and mechanistic perspectives. *Atherosclerosis* 197:12–24.

Hirose, M., A. Masuda, N. Ito, K. Kamano, and H. Okuyama. 1990. Effects of dietary perilla oil, soybean oil and safflower oil on 7,12-dimethylbenz[a]anthracene (DMBA) and 1,2-dimethylhydrazine (DMH)-induced mammary gland and colon carcinogenesis in female SD rats. *Carcinogenesis* 11:731–735.

Hirose, N., F. Doi, T. Ueki et al. 1992. Suppressive effect of sesamin against 7,12-dimethylbenz[a]-anthracene induced rat mammary carcinogenesis. *Anticancer Res* 12:1259–1265.

Hwang, H. S., B. Y. Han, B. J. Han, and L. N. Chung. 2010. *Korean traditional cuisine by 3 generations*. Seoul, Korea: Kyomunsa.

Hwang, L. S. 2005. Sesame oil. In *Bailey's industrial oil & fat products*. 6th ed. F. Shahidi, ed., 537–576, vol. 2, New Jersey: Wiley.

Ide, T., H. Kobayashi, L. Ashakumary et al. 2000. Comparative effects of perilla and fish oils on the activity and gene expression of fatty acid oxidation enzymes in rat liver. *Biochim Biophys Acta* 1485:23–35.

Jang, J. Y., T. S. Kim, J. Cai et al. 2014. Perilla oil improves blood flow through inhibition of platelet aggregation and thrombus formation. *Lab Anim Res* 30(1):21–27.

Jeng, K. C. G., and R. C. W. Hou. 2005. Sesamin and sesamolin: Nature's therapeutic lignans. *Curr Enzym Inhib* 1:11–20.

Jeong, Y. Y., H. S. Park, J. H. Choi, S. H. Kim, and K. U. Min. 2006. Two cases of anaphylaxis caused by perilla seed. *J Allergy Clin Immu* 117:1505–1506.

Jung, D. M., M. J. Lee, S. H. Yoon, and M. Y. Jung. 2011. A gas chromatography-tandem quadrupole mass spectrometric analysis of policosanols in commercial vegetable oils. *J Food Sci* 76:C891–899.

Jung, D. M., S. H. Yoon, and M. Y. Jung. 2012. Chemical properties and oxidative stability of perilla oils obtained from roasted perilla seeds as affected by extraction methods. *J Food Sci* 77:C1249–1255.

Jung, M. Y., J. Y. Bock, S. O. Baik, J. H. Lee, and T. K. Lee. 1999. Effects of roasting on pyrazine contents and oxidative stability of red pepper seed oil prior to its extraction. *J Agric Food Chem* 47:1700–1704.

Jung, S., W. Y. Lee, S. J. Yong et al. 2013. Occupational asthma caused by inhaling smoke from roasting perilla seeds. *Allergy Asthma Resp Dis* 1:90–93.

Kang, J. Y., B. K. Park, T. W. Seung et al. 2015. Amelioration of trimethyltin-induced cognitive impairment in ICR mice by perilla oil. *Korean J Food Sci Technol* 47:373–379.

Kang, M. H., H. Katsuzak, and T. Osawa. 1998a. Inhibition of 2,2'-azobis(2,4-dimethylvaleronitrile)-induced lipid peroxidation by sesaminols. *Lipid* 33:1031–1036.

Kang, M. H., M. Naito, K. Sakak, K. Uchida, and T. Osawa. 2000. Mode of action of sesame lignans in protecting low-density lipoprotein against oxidative damage *in vitro*. *Life Sci* 66:161–171.

Kang, M. H., M. Naito, N. Tsujihara, and T. Osawa. 1998b. Sesamolin inhibits lipid peroxidation in rat liver and kidney. *J Nutr* 128:1018–1022.

Kim, H. K., S. Choi, and H. Choi. 2004. Suppression of hepatic fatty acid synthase by feeding alpha-linolenic acid rich perilla oil lowers plasma triacylglycerol level in rats. *J Nutr Biochem* 15(8):485–492.

Kim, I. H., M. H. Kim, Y. E. Kim, and C. Y. Lee. 1998. Oxidative stability and extraction of perilla seed oil with supercritical carbon dioxide. *Food Sci Biotech* 7:177–180.

Kim, H. W., K. M. Park, and C. U. Choi. 2000a. Studies on the volatile flavor compounds of sesame oils with roasting temperature. *Korean J Food Sci Technol* 32:238–245.

Kim, M. J., and H. K. Kim. 2009. Perilla leaf extract ameliorates obesity and dyslipidemia induced by high-fat diet. *Phytother Res* 23(12):1685–1690.

Kim, S. J., H. N. Yoon, and J. S. Rhee. 2000b. The effects of roasting temperatures on the formation of headspace volatile compounds in perilla seed oil. *J Am Oil Chem Soc* 77:451–456.

Kwon, T. Y., J. S. Park, and M. Y. Jung. 2013. Headspace–solid phase microextraction–gas chromatography–tandem mass spectrometry (HS-SPME-GC-MS) method for the determination of pyrazines in perilla seed oils: Impact of roasting on the pyrazines in perilla seed oils. *J Agric Food Chem* 61:8514–8523.

Lancker, F. V., A. Adams, and N. D. Kimpe. 2010. Formation of pyrazines in Maillard model systems of lysine-containing dipeptides. *J Agric Food Chem* 58:2470–2478.

Lanzmann-Petithory, D. 2001. Alpha-linolenic acid and cardiovascular diseases. *J Nutr Health Aging* 5(3):179–183.

Lee, J., S. Park, J. Y. Lee, Y. K. Yeo, J. S. Kim, and J. Lim. 2012. Improved spatial learning and memory by perilla diet is correlated with immunoreactivities to neurofilament and α-synuclein in hilus of dentate gyrus. *Proteome Sci* 10(1):72.

Lee, M. J., M. K. Cho, S. H. Oh et al. 2014. Fatty acid composition, contents of tocopherols and phytosterols, and oxidative stability of mixed edible oil of perilla seed and rice bran oil. *Korean J Food Nutr* 27:59–65.

Lee, S. W., M. K. Jeung, M. H. Park, S. Y. Lee, and J. H. Lee. 2010. Effects of roasting conditions of sesame seeds on the oxidative stability of pressed oil during thermal oxidation. *Food Chem* 118:681–685.

Liu, X., Q. Jin, Y. Liu et al. 2011. Changes in volatile compounds of peanut oil during the roasting process for production of aromatic roasted peanut oil. *J Food Sci* 76:C404–412.

Matsumura, Y., S. Kita, Y. Tanida et al. 1998. Antihypertensive effect of sesamin. III. Protection against development and maintenance of hypertension in stroke-prone spontaneously hypertensive rats. *Biol Pharm Bull* 21:469–473.

Min, S. Y., J. Y. Park, J. Y. Yoon et al. 2006. A case of perilla seeds-induced anaphylaxis. *Korean J Asthma Allergy Clin Imm* 26(1):94–97.

Mitra, A. 2007. Study on the benefits of sesame oil over coconut oil in patients of insulin resistance syndrome, notably type 2 diabetes and dyslipidaemia. *J Hum Ecol* 55:61–66.

Nakamura, S., O. Nishimura, H. Masuda, and S. Mihara. 1989. Identification of volatile flavor components of the oil from roasted sesame seeds. *Agric Biol Chem* 53:1891–1899.

Narisawa, T., Y. Fukaura, K. Yazawa, C. Ishikawa, Y. Isoda, and Y. Nishizawa, 1994. Colon cancer prevention with a small amount of dietary perilla oil high in alpha-linolenic acid in an animal model. *Cancer* 73:2069–2075.

Okamoto, M., F. Mitsunobu, K. Ashida et al. 2000. Effects of perilla seed oil supplementation on leukotriene generation by leucocytes in patients with asthma associated with lipometabolism. *Int Arch Allergy Imm* 122:137–142.

Okuyama, H., K. Yamada, D. Miyazawa, Y. Yasui, and N. Ohara. 2007. Dietary lipids' impacts on healthy ageing. *Lipids* 42(9):821–825.

Onogi, N., M. Okuno, C. Komaki et al. 1996. Suppressing effects of perilla oil on azoxymethane-induced foci of colonic aberrant crypts in rats. *Carcinogenesis* 17(6):1291–1296.

Park, M. H., M. K. Jeong, J. D. Yeo et al. 2011a. Application of solid phase-microextraction (SPME) and electronic nose techniques to differentiate volatiles of sesame oils prepared with diverse roasting conditions. *J Food Sci* 76:C80–88.

Park, M. H., N. G., Seol, P. S. Chang, S. H. Yoon, and J. H. Lee. 2011b. Effects of roasting conditions on the physicochemical properties and volatile distribution in perilla oils (*Perilla frutescens* var. *japonica*). *J Food Sci* 76:C808–815.

Ramesh, B., R. Saravanan, and K. V. Pugalendi. 2005. Influence of sesame oil on blood glucose, lipid peroxidation, and antioxidant status in streptozotocin diabetic rats. *J Med Food* 8:377–381.

Roynettea, C. E., P. C. Calderb, Y. M. Dupertuisa, and C. Pichard. 2004. n-3 Polyunsaturated fatty acids and colon cancer prevention. *Clin Nutr* 23:139–151.

Sadi, A. M., T. Toda, H. Oku, and S. Hokama. 1996. Dietary effects of corn oil, oleic acid, perilla oil, and evening primrose oil on plasma and hepatic lipid level and atherosclerosis in Japanese quail. *Exp Anim Tokyo* 45:55–62.

Sankar, D., A. Ali, G. Sambandam, and R. Rao. 2011. Sesame oil exhibits synergistic effect with anti-diabetic medication in patients with type 2 diabetes mellitus. *Clin Nutr* 30: 351–358.

Schieberle, P. 1996. Odour-active compounds in moderately roasted sesame. *Food Chem* 55:145–152.

Shimokawa, T., A. Moriuchi, T. Hori et al. 1988. Effect of dietary alpha-linolenate/linoleate balance on mean survival time, incidence of stroke and blood pressure of spontaneously hypertensive rats. *Life Sci* 43 (25):2067–2075.

Shin, H. S., and S. W. Kim. 1994. Lipid composition of perilla seed. *J Am Oil Chem Soc* 71:619–622.

Sirato-Yasumoto, S., M. Katsuta, Y. Okuyam, Y. Takahash, and T. Ide. 2001. Effect of sesame seeds rich in sesamin and sesamolin on fatty acid oxidation in rat liver. *J Agric Food Chem* 49:2647–2651.

Statistics Korea, 2016. Statistics for Major Agricultural and Livestock Food Products, Ministry of Agriculture, Food and Rural Affairs (Registered Publication Number: 11-1543000-000128-10).

Takeuchi, H., C. Sakurai, R. Noda et al. 2007. Antihypertensive effect and safety of dietary a-linolenic acid in subjects with high-normal blood pressure and mild hypertension. *J Oleo Sci* 56:347–360.

Wang, S., H. Hwang, S. H. Yoon, and E. Choe. 2010. Temperature dependence of autoxidation of perilla oil and tocopherol degradation. *J Food Sci* 75:498–505.

Watanabe, S., E. Suzuki, N. Kojima, R. Kojima, Y. Suzuki, and H. Okyuyama. 1989. Effects of alpha-linolenate/linoleate balance on collagen induced platelet aggregation and serotonin release in rats. *Chem Pharm Bull* 37(6):1572–1575.

Yoshida, H., and S. Takagi. 1997. Effects of seed roasting temperature and time on the quality characteristics of sesame (*Sesamum indicum*) oil. *J Sci Food Agric* 75:19–26.

Yu, H., J. Qiu, L. Ma, Y. Hu, P. Li, and J. Wan. 2016. Phytochemical and phytopharmacological review of *Perilla frutescens* L. (Labiatae), a traditional edible-medicinal herb in China. *Food Chem Toxicol* 108:1–17.

13

Health Benefit Effects of Jukyeom (Bamboo Salt)

Hyung-Min Kim, Jaehyun Ju, Phil-Dong Moon, Na-Ra Han,
Hyun-Ja Jeong, and Kun-Young Park

CONTENTS

13.1 Introduction: History...319
13.2 Processing 320
13.3 Composition..322
13.4 Functionality...323
    13.4.1 Antioxidative Activity 323
    13.4.2 Anticancer Activity...325
        13.4.2.1 *In Vitro* Anticancer Effects 325
        13.4.2.2 *In Vivo* Anticancer Effects..327
        13.4.2.3 Antimetastatic Activity of Bamboo Salt 327
    13.4.3 Obesity..329
    13.4.4 Immunity..332
    13.4.5 Allergy..333
    13.4.6 Allergic Rhinitis 334
    13.4.7 Atopy..334
    13.4.8 Hypertension 334
    13.4.9 Prevention of Cisplatin Ototoxicity 334
    13.4.10 Inflammation 336
    13.4.11 Antimicrobial Activity 336
    13.4.12 Prevention of Hepatic Damage 336
    13.4.13 Enamel Remineralization by Dentifrice 336
13.5 Conclusions...336
Acknowledgment...337
References..337

13.1 Introduction: History

Bamboo salt was first produced by Jin-pyo Yul-sa (famous Buddhist priest) during his meditation period at the famous Busa-Uibang (Buddhist retreat located atop Mt. Byun-san) in Korea about 1,300 years ago, and passed on mainly by Buddhist priests through generations as a folk medicine

319

(Zhao et al., 2013a). In the history of oriental medicine, many kinds of excellent traditional medical treatments have been developed among Koreans. Many natural ingredients have been utilized and transformed into traditional medicine that can help relieve illnesses. Bamboo was used by Koreans as an important medical material, containing different medicinal efficacies varying from its stub, roots, and leaves. About 1,000 years ago, some Korean medicine doctors and monks started to make medical salts by inserting sea salt in a thick bamboo cylinder (called Juk-Tong) and baking them together with pine tree firewood.

The ancient bamboo salt was baked only two or three times. It was used for special medicinal treatments. Eventually, it became clear that bamboo salt could only attain its full medical efficacy if it was baked nine times. Also, if the salt was completely molten, the toxic characteristic disappeared. Now bamboo salt is well known as one of the most famous traditional medical treatments, not only in Korea but also in many Asian countries. Many pharmaceutical scientists all around the world are researching bamboo salt's special therapeutic potential, such as its anticancer and antiviral effects (Zhao, 2011).

13.2 Processing

As shown in Figure 13.1, the manufacture of bamboo salt consists of a strict choice of raw materials, and repeated and detailed baking processes. Solar salt, which is manufactured by the natural evaporation process of sea water resulting in crystallization, must be rated "top tier" by a strict evaluation, based upon the mineral composition and hazardous material composition. Bamboo trees also need to have their quality evaluated before being cut and used as bamboo cylinders; they should be fresh and 3–5 years old. Then, the chosen solar salt is compressed into the bamboo cylinder, with the open side of the cylinder sealed with yellow clay. The sealed bamboo cylinder is put into a kiln fueled by pine tree wood for at least 8 hours at a temperature above 800°C. Baked bamboo salt is crushed into powder to be put into a new bamboo cylinder; there is one cycle of baking to be repeated eight times to form a gray-colored pigment. When the eighth cycle is complete, the salt bulk is put into a specialized melting pot fueled by pine tree and powdered pine resin to raise its temperature to 1500°C. Fully liquefied bamboo salt is then cooled and solidified into bulky purple bamboo salt, which is called ja-juk-yeom in Korean and also called nine-times-baked bamboo salt. The salt is crushed into a powder or tablet to be commercially available.

Health Benefit Effects of Jukyeom (Bamboo Salt)   321

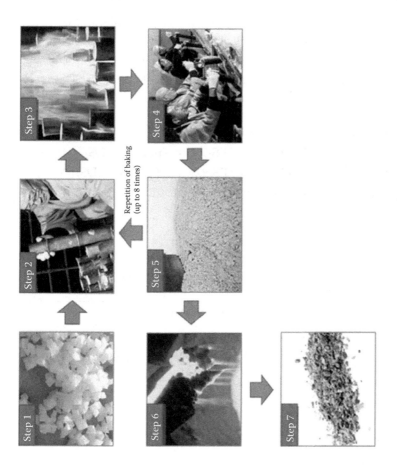

FIGURE 13.1
The craft of manufacturing bamboo salt. Step 1: choosing solar salt; step 2: choosing bamboo cylinders suitable for salt baking; step 3: loading bamboo cylinders with solar salt or prebaked bamboo salt at 800°C for 8 hours; step 4: powdering bulk bamboo salt to be poured into bamboo cylinders for repetition of the baking cycle; step 5: repeating baking cycle from step 2 through step 4 eight times; step 6: baking the ninth (final) time at 1500°C, followed by cooling.

13.3 Composition

Salt samples and devices related to the manufacture of bamboo salt underwent ICP-OES and/or ICP-MS analyses for evaluation of mineral composition. The detailed results are shown in Table 13.1 (Hwang et al., 2007).

Our observation showed that BS-1×—bamboo salt baked once (1×)—and BS-9×—bamboo salt baked nine times (9×)—contained lower levels of

Mg (3512 ppm for BS-1× and 1810 ppm for BS-9× vs. 4068 ppm for SDS (sun-dried salt = solar salt)

Ca (951 ppm for BS-1× and 1015 ppm for BS-9× vs. 1408 ppm for SDS)

S (1808 ppm for BS-1× and 488 ppm for BS-9× vs. 2813 ppm for SDS)

than SDS, but higher levels of

K (1936 ppm for BS-1× and 7976 ppm for BS-9× vs. 1542 ppm for SDS)

P (21 ppm for BS-1× and 404 ppm for BS-9× vs. 3 ppm for SDS)

Mn (3 ppm for BS-1× and 10 ppm for BS-9× vs. 2.8 ppm for SDS)

Zn (0.4 ppm for BS-1× and 3.1 ppm for BS-9× vs. 0.2 ppm for SDS)

than SDS.

TABLE 13.1

Mineral Contents of Various Salts and Raw Material for Bamboo Salt Manufacture Analyzed with ICP-OES and ICP-MS

	Salt Sample					Raw Yellow Mud
			BS			
Mineral	PS	SDS	BS1	BS9	Bamboo	
Pb	0.05	0.28	0.3	0.09	0.15	11
Mn	0.2	2.8	3	10	16	868
Zn	<0.1	0.2	0.4	3.1	11.2	57.7
Ge	<0.5	<0.5	<0.5	<0.5	<0.5	0.2
As	<0.25	<0.25	<0.25	<0.25	<0.25	4.4
Mg	22	4,068	3,512	1,810	252	3,801
Si	7	9	10	46	45	–
P	<3	<3	21	404	563	99
S	65	2,813	1,808	488	224	256
K	563	1,542	1,936	7,976	3,413	5,321
Ca	121	1,408	951	1,015	3,442	394
Fe	<1	13	12	189	39	50,376

Source: Hwang, K. M. et al. 2008. *J Med Food* 11:717–722.

Note: Data are in units of parts per million. PS: purified salt; SDS: sun-dried salt; BS1: bamboo salt baked once (same as BS-1×); BS9: bamboo salt baked nine times (same as BS-9×).

In particular, K contents of BS-9× were fivefold higher than those of SDS (Hwang et al., 2007). Also, bamboo itself was found to contain high amounts of K (3413 ppm) and P (563 ppm); raw yellow mud, which is used for sealing the bamboo cylinder, was found to contain high concentrations of Fe (50,376 ppm), K (5321 ppm), and Mn (868 ppm).

Potassium (K, kalium) functions as a catalyst in cellular physiological reaction and is involved in generation of energy and synthesis of glycogen and protein; however, the catalytic effect of potassium declines in high concentrations of sodium. Potassium plays an important role in transmission of nerve impulses and softens muscle. Symptoms of potassium deficiency may include weakness of muscles, impaired digestion, weakening of cardiac muscles and respiratory organs, paralysis, vomiting, diarrhea, irritability, and headache.

Iron (Fe, ferrum) is a component of heme that transports oxygen and electrons around the body. When iron is deficient, there is an inadequate supply of nutrients and oxygen. In iron deficiency, anemia, malaise, fatigue, stomatitis, anorexia, and aphylaxis against bacteria can occur.

Manganese (Mn) affects skeletogeny and functions of reproduction and the central nervous system. Deficiency of manganese occurs along with deficiency of vitamin K and can result in shortening of bone length, bowed legs, sexual dysfunction, infertility, and testicular involution.

Phosphorus (P) plays a critical role in the formation and maintenance of bone, because it is deeply involved with calcium metabolism. Phosphorus regulates the parathyroid hormone, plays an important role in cell metabolism, and strengthens bones in combination with calcium.

Zinc (Zn) is known to affect development of skin and bony skeleton and maintenance of hair. It is involved in digestion, respiration, insulin secretion, taste sense, and reproduction. Zinc helps to treat burns and wounds and to metabolize protein. In addition, zinc strengthens bones. In zinc deficiency, anorexia, growth retardation, body weight loss, dermatosis, dysgenesis of reproductive organs, pregnancy disorder, nonrestorative wound healing, and aphylaxis against various diseases can occur.

Based upon these facts, the unique manufacturing process of bamboo salt promotes accumulation of mineral compounds into salt bulk as the baking cycles are repeated (Kim, 2012a, 2012b).

13.4 Functionality

13.4.1 Antioxidative Activity

Normal human blood is slightly alkaline, with a pH value of 7.4 (Park et al., 2002). Most alkaline meals are known to have antioxidative properties sufficient to adjust blood pH (Choi et al., 2006). Antioxidative meals are found to scavenge reactive oxygen species, which are not just by-products of energy metabolism but also well known to cause cellular and genetic damage and eventually promote aging and serious diseases including cancer (Lee et al., 2005a).

The radical scavenging effects of salt samples on the DPPH radical were tested (Figure 13.2). Purified salt, solar salt, and bamboo salt (1×, 3×, and 9×) showed scavenging activity of the DPPH radical at concentrations ranging from 5% to 25%, respectively. At concentrations of 10%, the radical scavenging activities of purified salt, solar salt, bamboo salt (1×, 3×, and 9×) were 0.8%, 1.2%, 7.6%, 11.4%, and 18.4%, respectively. At concentrations of 20%, their activities showed results (0.8%, 2.1%, 16.5%, 21.2%, and 28.5%) similar to those at concentrations of 10%. The radical scavenging activity of bamboo salt (9×) was more potent than that of bamboo salt (3×) and bamboo salt (1×); the three kinds of bamboo salt samples showed much better radical scavenging activity than solar salt and purified salt. This indicates that the radical scavenging activity of bamboo salt was more potent than that of purified salt and solar salt—enough to eventually reduce the possibility of cancer.

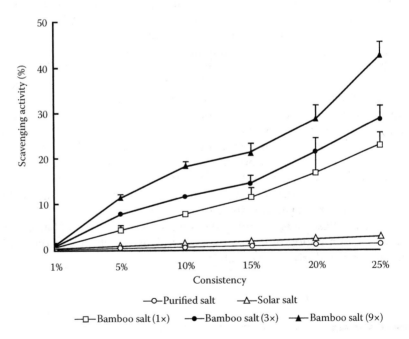

FIGURE 13.2
DPPH radical scavenging activity of salt samples. (From Zhao, X. 2011. Anticancer and antiinflammatory effects of bamboo salt and *Rubus coreanus* Miquel bamboo salt. PhD diss., Pusan National University, Busan, Korea.)

Health Benefit Effects of Jukyeom (Bamboo Salt) 325

13.4.2 Anticancer Activity

One clinical investigation referred to sodium as a dietary carcinogenic agent, whereas potassium was considered a dietary anticarcinogenic agent (Jansson, 1996). Fortunately, processing solar salt into bamboo salt reduces the Na/K ratio of salt and thus may partially account for the anticancer activity.

13.4.2.1 In Vitro *Anticancer Effects*

Buccal mucosa cancer: TCA8113 human tongue carcinoma cells, widely used for investigation of buccal mucosa cancer, were used to observe the anticancer effect of bamboo salt. By treatment of TCA8113 cells with a 1% concentration of salt, the growth inhibitory rate of purple bamboo salt was 61% higher than that of sea salt (27%) (Zhao et al., 2013b).

Gastric cancer cells: To evaluate the effects of bamboo salt on cell proliferation of AGS human gastric adenocarcinoma cells, the cells were cultured in the absence or presence of salt samples. After treatment for 48 hours, MTT assays were performed. Bamboo salt had a marked dose-dependent inhibitory effect on AGS cell growth. The growth of AGS cells following treatment with 0.5% concentration of purified salt, solar salt, BS-1×, BS-3×, and BS-9× was inhibited by 5%, 8%, 14%, 20%, and 25%, respectively. In addition, at 1% of the concentration, the growth inhibitory rates were 15%, 20%, 36%, 41%, and 51%, respectively ($p < 0.05$). The expression levels of members of the Bcl-2 family, such as Bax and Bcl-2, were characterized using RT-PCR and Western blotting analysis. Bamboo salt, solar salt, and purified salt induced down-regulation of antiapoptotic Bcl-2 protein levels as well as up-regulation of proapoptotic Bax protein levels. Bamboo salt (9×), bamboo salt (3×), and bamboo salt (1×) were more effective for the down-regulation of Bcl-2 and upregulation of Bax than the solar salt and purified salt. These results indicated that a portion of the antiproliferative activity of the bamboo salt was related to apoptosis mediated by up-regulation of Bax and down-regulation of Bcl-2 pathways; in particular, 9× baked bamboo salt showed the most noticeable effect (Park et al., 2013).

Liver cancer cells: Zhao et al. (2013a) investigated whether the anticancer actions of the bamboo salts were associated with inhibited expression of the inflammation-related genes NF-κB-P65, IκB-α, iNOS, and COX-2, as shown in Figure 13.3a. After a 48-hour incubation with 1% salt solutions, 9× bamboo salt showed anti-inflammatory activity in the HepG2 cells, as indicated by decreased protein expression of NF-κB along with increased IκB-α expression compared to cells

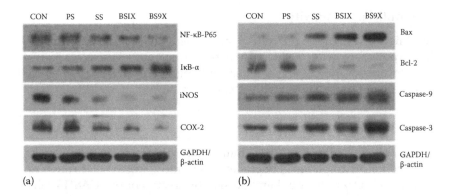

FIGURE 13.3
Changes in protein expression of (a) inflammation-related factors (NF-κB-P65, IκB, iNOS, and COX-2) and (b) apoptosis-related factors (Bax, Bcl-2, caspase-9, and caspase-3) in HepG2 cells. (From Zhao, X. et al., 2013, *J Environ Pathol Toxicol Oncol* 32:9–20.)

treated with the other types of salt. The levels of protein expression of COX-2 and iNOS were high in the untreated control HepG2 cells; however, these indicators were nearly undetectable in the presence of 9× bamboo salt. After incubation with 9× bamboo salt, the protein levels of COX-2 and iNOS were significantly decreased ($p < 0.05$). The mRNA levels of the related factors showed the same trend (data not shown).

Expression of Bax, Bcl-2, and caspase-9 and -3 in HepG2 cancer cells was also analyzed by RT-PCR and Western blotting. As shown in Figure 13.3b, treatment with 9× bamboo salt markedly promoted protein expression of proapoptotic Bax, while suppressing protein expression of antiapoptotic Bcl-2 ($p < 0.05$). These results suggest that 9× bamboo salt strongly induced apoptosis in the HepG2 cells via a Bcl-2-dependent pathway compared to the 1× bamboo, solar, and purified salts. Modest protein expression of caspase-9 and -3 was detected in the untreated control HepG2 cells, but higher expression levels were detected after the cells were treated with the salt samples. Protein expression of caspase-9 and -3 significantly increased in the presence of the bamboo salts with increasing salt-baking times. The mRNA levels of the related factors showed the same trend (data not shown). Overall, *in vitro* treatments with bamboo salt led to better anticancer efficacy than with PS and SS, and the efficacy of bamboo salt grew with increasing numbers of baking cycles.

Colon cancer cells: To elucidate the mechanisms underlying the inhibition of cancer cell growth by the bamboo salt samples, expressions of Bax and Bcl-2 in HCT-116 human colon carcinoma cells were measured by Western blot analysis after a 48-hour incubation with

1% salt solutions. Expression of proapoptotic Bax and antiapoptotic Bcl-2 showed significant changes ($p < 0.05$) in the presence of 9× bamboo salt. These results suggest that the salt induced apoptosis in the HCT-116 cells via a Bax and Bcl-2-dependent pathway. Apoptosis induction and expressions of COX-2 and iNOS also showed significant changes ($p < 0.05$) in the presence of 9× bamboo salt, accounting for the fact that the salt suppressed inflammatory reactions in the HCT-116 cells. The effects of this salt were greater than those of the 1× and 3× bamboo salt samples and even greater compared to the solar- and purified-salt samples (Zhao et al., 2013c).

13.4.2.2 In Vivo *Anticancer Effects*

Colon cancer models using AOM and DSS: Effects of bamboo salts on colon carcinogenesis were investigated by using an azoxymethane (AOM)/dextran sodium sulfate (DSS)-induced mouse model. The average colon length of the control group was 5.6 ± 0.6 cm, which was markedly shorter than that in the normal group (6.2 ± 0.5 cm), due to AOM/DSS-driven ulcerative colon cancer. The average colon length of the BS-9×-treated mice was 6.8 ± 0.2 cm, which was longer or close to that of the normal group, followed by BS3× (5.8 ± 0.2 cm), SS-Yb (5.5 ± 0.3 cm), and PS (5.0 ± 1.4 cm; $p < 0.05$; Figure 13.4a). The average colon tumor count of the control mice was 23.0 ± 3.3, whereas no tumors were found in the normal group. The average colon tumor count from the BS-9×-treated mice was 2.2 ± 1.7, which was significantly lower than that of the AOM/DSS-treated groups (90% inhibition) and close to that of the normal group ($p < 0.05$). In addition, the average colon tumor counts of the other groups were as follows: BS-3× (10.0 ± 0.8), SS-Yb (16.7 ± 1.5), and PS (18.2 ± 3.3; Figure 13.4b). Also, BS-treated mice exhibited suppressed expression of Bcl-2; increased expression of Bax, p53, and p21; and suppressed expression of inflammatory factors including COX-2 and iNOS, accounting for the lessened amount of tumor count in colon cancer (Ju et al., 2016).

13.4.2.3 *Antimetastatic Activity of Bamboo Salt*

To observe antimetastatic action of bamboo salt, we subcutaneously injected different salt solutions (400 and 800 mg/kg) into 6-week-old female BALB/c mice, followed by induction of experimental lung metastasis by injecting colon 26-M3.1 cells into the lateral tail vein (2.5×10^4 cells/mouse) after 2 days. The mice were sacrificed after 2 weeks. All bamboo-salt-treated mice had significantly fewer lung metastatic colonies than those treated with solar salt, purified salt, or control mice. The 9× bamboo salt was the most effective for inhibiting lung metastasis at a concentration of 400 mg/kg. This bamboo salt (inhibitory rate = 16%) inhibited tumor formation and lung metastasis to a greater degree than the 3× (inhibitory rate = 8%) and 1× (inhibitory rate = 4%) bamboo salts. Adversely, however, solar (inhibitory rate= –2%) and purified

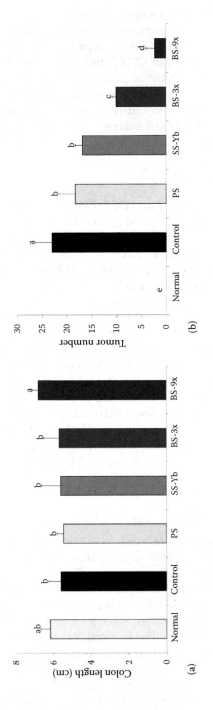

FIGURE 13.4
Changes in (a) colon length and (b) colon tumor counts by administration of salt samples to C57BL/6 mice with AOM/DSS-induced colon cancer. (From Ju, J. et al. 2016, *J Med Food* 19:1015–1022.)

(inhibitory rate = −4%) salts promoted metastasis. At 800 mg/kg, the inhibition rates associated with 9×, 3×, and 1× bamboo salts along with solar salt (SS) and purified salts (PS) were 20%, 16%, 6%, −10%, and −14%, respectively. Thus, the antimetastasis effect of bamboo salt was greater than that of SS and PS; the efficacy of bamboo salt was increased as the baking cycle was repeated (Zhao et al., 2013c).

Overall, bamboo salt exhibited *in vitro* anticancer effects on gastrointestinal cancer models such as buccal mucosa cancer, stomach cancer, liver cancer, and colorectal cancer, as well as *in vivo* anticancer effects on a colorectal cancer model. Many cancer patients benefit from the efficacy of bamboo salt itself and/or doenjang products made of bamboo salt for cancer treatment.

13.4.3 Obesity

Antiobesity effects of bamboo salt: Obesity is defined as accumulation of energy as adipose tissues for maintenance of metabolic balance, caused by energy intake beyond an individual's energy expenditure (Akoh, 1995; Hedley et al., 2004). Obesity is a significant public health problem and also leads to chronic diseases, such as diabetes, hypertension, stroke, cardiac myoinfarction, and cancer (Xavier and Sunyer, 2002; Lee et al., 2005b; Giri et al., 2006).

Thus, we used the high-fat diet (HFD) C57BL/6 mouse model by orally administering the salt samples at a concentration of 2,727 mg/kg per day (corresponding to a daily dose of 10 g for a 60 kg human) for 8 weeks (Ju et al., 2015). Addition of a salt sample significantly reduced the span of weight change compared with the HFD group ($p < 0.05$). Especially, the body weight change in the BS-9× group was smallest in the salt-administered groups, and it was similar to that of the normal diet group (Figure 13.5a). Mice food efficiency ratio (FER), which represents the changes in body weight divided by the consumed feed in a certain period, was also suppressed. Among the salt-administered groups, the BS-9× group showed the lowest FER (4.65%), which was significant compared with that of the HFD group ($p < 0.05$) (Figure 13.5b). Among all experimental groups, average weight of epididymal adipose tissue (EAT) in the BS-administered group was significantly lower compared with that of the HFD group ($p < 0.05$). Especially, the BS-9× group showed the lowest EAT weight among all salt-administered groups. BS-administered groups showed suppressed expression of PPARγ and C/EBPα compared with the HFD group. Especially, the hepatic expression of PPARγ was profoundly diminished in the BS-9× group. Taken together, bamboo salt, especially BS-9×, suppressed body weight increase by decreasing fat deposition in liver and adipose tissue without inducing anorectic activity (Ju et al., 2015).

Effects of bamboo salt on amelioration of diet-induced obesity and nonalcoholic fatty liver disease (NAFLD)/nonalcoholic steatohepatitis (NASH): Ju (2016) studied amelioiration of obesity itself and its hepatic complications (NAFLD and NASH) by administration of bamboo salt, using a C57BL/6

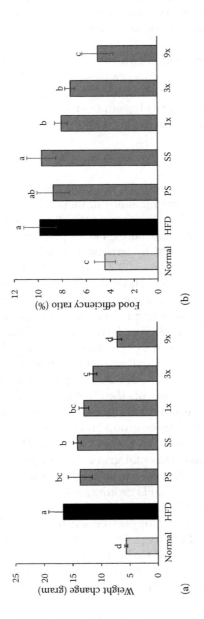

FIGURE 13.5
Changes in (a) body weight and (b) food efficiency ratio (body weight/total feed consumption) upon administration of salt. [a-d]Mean values with different superscript letters over the bars are significantly different ($p < 0.05$) according to Duncan's multiple range test. (From Ju, J. et al. 2015, *J Med Food* 18:706–710.)

mouse-based, diet-induced obesity (DIO) model. Obesity was induced by feeding 6-week-old C57BL/6 mice a high-fat diet (45% calories from fat) for 8 weeks. Then the mice were fed a high-fat diet mixed with 0.47% and 4% of salt sample (corresponding to daily administration of 5 and 42.5 g for a 60 kg human, respectively) for another 8 weeks. Induction of obesity by HFD led to significant increase in body weight, liver weight, and EAT weight during the entire 16 weeks. Administration of the bamboo salt to the mice by mixing it into a diet, however–even if applied in the midst of obesity induction– suppressed the progression of the DIO; the 9× BS group, especially, showed the strongest suppression of DIO of all the salt-administered groups.

Hepatic expression of PPARγ was promoted in the HFD group in comparison with that of the normal group, but its expression levels in BS groups were lower than that in the normal group. Expression of C/EBPα in the HFD group was similar with that in the normal one, but its expression levels in BS groups were lower than that in the normal group. Hepatic expression of FAS and SREBP-1c in the HFD group was promoted in comparison with those in the normal group, but their expression levels in BS groups were lower than those in the normal group (Ju, 2016). Also, administration of bamboo salt was found to promote hepatic β-oxidation. Expressions of PPARα, CPT-1, and ACO in the HFD group were lower than those in the normal one, BS groups showed promoted expression levels of the factors in comparison of normal group (Figure 13.6a).

Hepatic lipid accumulation is known to occur if the ratios of fatty acid synthesis and accumulation exceed the ratios of fatty acid degradation (Koteish and Diehl, 2001; Bradbury and Berk, 2004). Occurrence of NAFLD, which results from hepatic lipid accumulation, is found to have a strong relationship with insulin resistance and obesity (Day, 2002). Apolipoprotein B (apoB) is a major liver-derived, very low-density lipoprotein (VLDL); excretion of

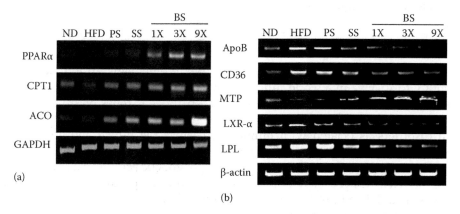

FIGURE 13.6
Changes in mRNA expression of (a) β-oxidation-related factors (PPAR-α, CPT-1, and ACO) and (b) NASH-related factors (ApoB, CD36, MTP, LXR-α, LPL) in livers from a DIO mouse model. (From Ju, J. 2016. Inhibitory effects on obesity and colon cancer by solar salt and bamboo salt in C57BL/6J mice. PhD diss., Pusan National University, Busan, Korea.)

VLDL containing apoB is thus well known to raise serum concentration of triglyceride (TG) and LDL. Also, microsomal triglyceride transfer protein (MTP) is expressed in endoplasmic reticulum of hepatocytes; thus, it is regarded as an important factor accounting for apoB-lipoprotein secretion (Tietge et al., 1999).

CD36 is also called fatty acid translocase; CD36-null mice have been found to be prone to NASH resulting from higher serum TG concentration and stronger hepatic insulin resistance than the wild-type mice (Anstee and Goldin, 2006). LXR-α is well known to activate lipogenic factors including fatty acid synthase (FAS) to eventually result in hepatic steatosis (Jin et al., 2013). Also, lipoprotein lipase (LPL) is inactive in a liver of nonobese status, but its expression is promoted resulting from progress of obesity (Pardina et al., 2009). Thus, our observation reached the NAFLD- and NASH-related factors including ApoB, CD36, MTP, LXR-α, and LPL, using liver samples from a C57BL/6 mice-based DIO model (Figure 13.6b). Hepatic expression of ApoB, CD36, LXR-α, and LPL in the HFD group was promoted in comparison with that in the normal group, but the expression levels in BS groups were lower than those in the normal group. Also, expression of MTP in the HFD group was lower than that in the normal group; BS groups showed promoted expression levels of the factors in comparison to the normal group. Such efficacies from bamboo salt groups were found to improve as baking cycles of bamboo salt accumulated.

Taking the preceding results together, bamboo salt suppressed the progression of obesity in a mouse model over 8 weeks postinduction. Also, bamboo salt reversed preexisting obesity in a DIO mouse model, while suppressing hepatic lipid accumulation by modulating mRNA expressions of related factors. Such efficacies were found to be promoted as baking times of bamboo salt accumulated.

13.4.4 Immunity

The immune system plays an important role in enhancing an individual's ability to survive in a world inhabited by pathogens and parasites (Greives et al., 2016). Immune response to microbial pathogens relies on innate and adaptive components (Hoffmann et al., 1999; Aderem and Ulevitch, 2000). In disorders associated with immunodeficiency, the innate and adaptive immune responses are reduced (Bonilla et al., 2005; Younger et al., 2015). Attenuation of immune functions, such as phagocytic activity, natural killer cell activity, delayed type hypersensitivity, antigen-specific antibody production, and T-cell proliferation, has resulted from deficiencies in minerals and vitamins (Kaminogawa and Nanno, 2004).

Immune cells are activated to improve the immune response against pathogens by immunomodulatory agents (Park et al., 2015). In general, immune cells, such as neutrophils and macrophages, regulate the innate immune response. Macrophages (major cells of the host defense system) suppress

Health Benefit Effects of Jukyeom (Bamboo Salt) 333

the invasion of microorganisms and foreign materials through phagocytic activities and lead to additional adaptive immune responses by synthesizing various inflammatory factors, including nitric oxide (NO) and tumor necrosis factor (TNF)-α (Adams and Hamilton, 1992; Aderem and Ulevitch, 2000; Park et al., 2015). Inducible NO synthase (iNOS) mediates the release of NO (Nathan, 1992). Expressions of TNF-α and iNOS are elevated by the translocation of nuclear factor-κB (NF-κB) to the nucleus and the degradation of inhibitors of NF-κB (IκB) (Jeong et al., 2014). In addition, T-cells play a critical role in immune functions. Th1 cytokines, such as interferon (IFN)-γ, interleukin (IL)-2, and TNF-α, regulate cell-mediated immune response and are produced by Th1 cells. Th2 cytokines, such as IL-4, IL-5, and IL-13, regulate humoral immune response and are produced by Th2 cells (Carter and Dutton, 1996). Acquired immune deficiency is induced by insufficient T-cell numbers (Linder, 1987).

The immune-enhancing effect of bamboo salt was evaluated in RAW264.7 macrophages and a forced swimming test (FST) animal model. Bamboo salt (BS) elevated the level of TNF-α through the activation of nuclear factor-κB in the RAW 264.7 cells. Immobility times in the FST were significantly reduced in the BS-fed group. Bamboo salt administration also resulted in increases in the levels of IFN-γ, IL-2, and TNF-α (Kim et al., 2016).

13.4.5 Allergy

Allergy is defined as an immune-mediated inflammatory response to common environmental allergens that are otherwise harmless (Douglass and O'Hehir, 2006). A variety of chemical mediators released from mast cells control immediate-type hypersensitivity reactions, such as urticaria, allergic rhinitis, and asthma (Miescher and Vogel, 2002). Among various substances released upon mast cell degranulation, histamine is one of the most characterized and potent vasoactive mediators implicated in the acute type of hypersensitivity reactions (Petersen et al., 1996). Histamine is released by compound 48/80 (Kim et al., 2003).

The secretory responses of mast cells can be induced by aggregation of their cell surface-specific receptors for immunoglobulin E (IgE) by the corresponding antigen (Metzger et al., 1986; Alber et al., 1991; Hong et al., 2003). It has been established that passive cutaneous anaphylaxis (PCA) resulted from the anti-IgE antibody as a typical *in vivo* animal model for immediate-type allergic reaction in anaphylactic reactions. Mouse skin is a useful site for studying PCA (Na et al., 2002).

Antiallergic effects of BS were measured on mast cell-mediated immediate-type allergic reactions. Bamboo salt suppressed an ear-swelling response induced by intradermal injection of compound 48/80 in mice. It also reduced histamine release from the rat peritoneal mast cells by compound 48/80. Furthermore, bamboo salt decreased passive cutaneous anaphylaxis (Shin et al., 2004).

13.4.6 Allergic Rhinitis

The preventive effect of bamboo salt was assessed in the ovalbumin (OVA)-induced allergic rhinitis (AR) animal model. Bamboo salt inhibited the number of rubs and levels of IgE, histamine, and IL-1β in serum. The level of IFN-γ was up-regulated, whereas the level of IL-4 was down-regulated in the spleen tissue of BS-treated mice. Numbers of eosinophils and mast cell infiltration increased by OVA sensitization were reduced by bamboo salt. The levels of inflammatory cytokines and caspase-1 activation were decreased by bamboo salt in the nasal mucosa of the AR mice. In activated human mast cells, bamboo salt suppressed the productions of IL-1β and thymic stromal lymphopoietin and activation of caspase-1 (Kim et al., 2012).

13.4.7 Atopy

Bambusae caulis in Liquamen (BCL; JukRyeok) is a nutritious liquid extracted from heat-treated fresh bamboo stems. The effect of *Bambusae caulis* in Liquamen was tested on 2,4-dinitrochlorobenzene-induced atopic dermatitis-like skin lesions in hairless mice. *Bambusae caulis* in Liquamen inhibited transepidermal water loss, melanin production, and erythema of skin. Serum level of IgE, number of leukocytes, and mRNA expressions of IL-4, IL-13, and TNF-α were reduced by application of *Bambusae caulis* in Liquamen (Qi et al., 2009).

13.4.8 Hypertension

Sodium is known as a major factor in the etiology of many cases of type I hypertension. Na^+-Cl^- cotransporter (NCC) plays a crucial role in sodium retention in renal distal convoluted tubes. Increases in NCC increase sodium retention, and it is critical in blood pressure increase. Comparison analysis of effects of various salts on hypertension was assessed in a hypertensive rat model. Purple bamboo salt, sun-dried salt, NaCl, or distilled water (DW, vehicle control) was administered orally for 8 weeks. Blood pressure of the purple bamboo salt-administered group was similar to that of the DW group, whereas the sun-dried salt (solar salt) and NaCl groups showed significantly increased blood pressure levels (Figure 13.7). Purple bamboo salt also suppressed NCC mRNA expression, unlike sun-dried salt or NaCl (Figure 13.8) (Kim et al., 2013).

13.4.9 Prevention of Cisplatin Ototoxicity

1. Bamboo salt oral administration. Cisplatin is an excellent therapeutic agent with ototoxic side effects. The preventive effect of bamboo salt was analyzed on cisplatin-induced apoptosis. Activations of caspase-3, -8, and -9 were inhibited by bamboo salt in cisplatin-treated HEI-OC1 cells. Bamboo salt reduced release of cytochrome c, translocation of

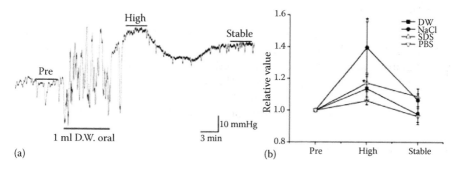

FIGURE 13.7
Effect of purple bamboo salt on blood pressure. (a) Scheme of blood pressure. (b) Relative blood pressure graph compared to the pre-stage. Pre: prestabilized stage before DW administration; high: 1 mL of DW administration after peaked and prolonged stage; stable: restabilized stage 20 min after high stage; DW, distilled water; SDS, sun-dried salt; PBS, purple bamboo salt (baked 9 times); *p < 0.05, significantly different from pre-stage.

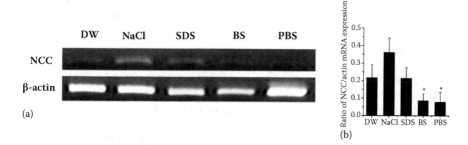

FIGURE 13.8
Effect of purple bamboo salt on NCC mRNA expression. (a) NCC mRNA expression levels in the kidney cortex tissue were analyzed by RT-PCR. (b) The levels of NCC mRNA expression were quantified by densitometry. DW: distilled water; SDS: sun-dried salt; BS: bamboo salt (baked three times); PBS: purple bamboo salt (baked nine times); *p < 0.05 significantly different from NaCl group.

apoptosis-inducing factor, and production of reactive oxygen species in cisplatin-treated HEI-OC1 cells. In addition, bamboo salt inhibited cisplatin-induced caspase-1 activation (Jeong et al., 2011).

2. Bamboo salt-pharmaceutical acupuncture. the preventive effect of bamboo salt pharmaceutical acupuncture was examined in cisplatin-treated mice and in the auditory cell line, HEI-OC1. Bamboo salt pharmaceutical acupuncture inhibited IL-6 production and caspase-3 activation induced by cisplatin in the cochlea. Bamboo salt decreased cisplatin-induced apoptosis and IL-6 production in HEI-OC1 cells. In addition, it reduced release of cytochrome c, activation of caspase-3, phosphorylation of extracellular signal-related kinase, and activation of nuclear factor-κB in HEI-OC1 cells (Myung et al., 2011).

13.4.10 Inflammation

Anti-inflammatory effects of bamboo salt were evaluated in human mast cell line (HMC-1 cells). Bamboo salt inhibited phorbol 12-myristate 13-acetate plus calcium ionophore A23187-induced productions of TNF-α, IL-1β, and IL-6. It reduced mRNA expression of TNF-α in HMC-1 cells. When NaCl was used to treat HMC-1 cells, the productions of TNF-α and IL-6 decreased, but the effect was notably less than that of BS-treated cells (Shin et al., 2003).

13.4.11 Antimicrobial Activity

The antimicrobial effect of bamboo salt was assessed using *Salmonella enteritidis*. Oxidation-reduction potential and pH values of the bamboo salt group stayed in the reduced (–105.7 to 52.5 mV) and alkaline (pH 8.4–9.3) states, while other salt groups (refined, baked, processed, and sea salts) became oxidized (182.6–248.0 mV) and changed acidic or neutral states (pH 5.5–7.8). Minimum inhibitory concentration values of 5.0% against *Salmonella enteritidis* were obtained for bamboo salt. On the other hand, minimum inhibitory concentration values of 5.0% were not observed for other salts (Moon et al., 2009).

13.4.12 Prevention of Hepatic Damage

The hepatoprotective effect of bamboo salt was evaluated for hepatic damage induced by carbon tetrachloride in Sprague–Dawley rats. Bamboo salt suppressed serum levels of aspartate aminotransferase, alanine aminotransferase, and lactate dehydrogenase. It also decreased the levels of proinflammatory cytokines, such as IL-6, IFN-γ, and TNF-α. The protective effect of BS was shown in histopathological sections of liver tissue. Bamboo salt reduced the mRNA levels and protein expressions of COX-2, iNOS, TNF-α, and IL-1β (Zhao et al., 2013d).

13.4.13 Enamel Remineralization by Dentifrice

The remineralization effect of a dentifrice with bamboo salt and NaF was examined on artificial caries-like enamel lesions, at both the surface and deep areas. Dentifrice containing bamboo salt and the positive control group up-regulated the surface hardness and down-regulated mineral loss of the artificial caries-like enamel lesions. Dentifrice containing bamboo salt reduced lesion depth compared to positive and negative control groups (Choi et al., 2012).

13.5 Conclusions

As referred to previously, bamboo salt has been found to have various health functionalities, owing to its special processing methods: repetition of a baking cycle with the salt stuffed into a bamboo cylinder and then baked at 800°C or above. Also, because of the unique mineral composition of bamboo salt, due to its special processing method, it has been found to reinforce health functionality in comparison with other types of salt, such as solar salt and/or purified salt. More detailed studies, however, are required to elucidate exactly which compound of bamboo salt can have such efficacies as have been described here, as well as the mineral composition of bamboo salt and structural changes during the baking process in the bamboo cylinder.

Acknowledgment

This work was supported by a grant 20130290 from Ministry of Oceans and Fisheries of Korea.

References

Adams, O. D., and T. A. Hamilton. 1992. *Molecular basis of macrophage activation and its origins*, 75–114, New York: Oxford University Press.

Aderem, A., and R. J. Ulevitch. 2000. Toll-like receptors in the induction of the innate immune response. *Nature* 406:782–787.

Akoh, C. C. 1995. Lipid-based fat substitutes. *Crit Rev Food Sci Nutr* 35:405–430.

Alber, G., L. Miller, C. Jelsema et al. Structure–function relationships in the mast cell high affinity receptor for IgE. Role of the cytoplasmic domains and of the beta subunit. *J Biol Chem* 266:22613–22620.

Anstee, Q. M., and R. D. Goldin. 2006. Mouse models in non-alcoholic fatty liver disease and steatohepatitis research. *Int J Exp Pathol* 87:1–16.

Bonilla, F. A., I. L. Bernstein, D. A. Khan et al. 2005. Practice parameter for the diagnosis and management of primary immunodeficiency. *J Allergy Clin Immunol* 94:S1–63.

Bradbury, M. W., and P. D. Berk. 2004. Lipid metabolism in hepatic steatosis. *Clin Liver Dis* 8:639–671.

Carter, L. L., and R. W. Dutton. 1996. Type 1 and type 2: A fundamental dichotomy for all T-cell subsets. *Curr Opin Immunol* 8:336–342.

Choi, C. H., M. O. Ha, H. J. Youn et al. 2012. Effect of bamboo salt-NaF dentifrice on enamel remineralization. *Am J Dent* 25:9–12.

Choi, S. Y., H. S. Cho, and N. J. Sung, 2006. The antioxidative and nitrite scavenging ability of solvent extracts from wild grape (*Vitis coignetiea*) skin. *J Korean Soc Food Sci Nutr* 35:961–966.

Day, C. P. 2002. Pathogenesis of steatohepatitis. *Best Pract Res Clin Gastroenterol* 16:663–678.

Douglass, J. A., and R. E. O'Hehir. 2006. 1. Diagnosis, treatment and prevention of allergic disease: The basics. *Med J Aust* 185:228–233.

Giri, S., R. Rattan, E. Haq et al. 2006. AICAR inhibits adipocyte differentiation in 3T3-L1 and restores metabolic alterations in diet-induced obesity mice model. *Nutr Metab (Lond)* 3:31–50.

Greives, T. J., N. A. Dochtermann, and E. C. Stewart. 2016. Estimating heritable genetic contributions to innate immune and endocrine phenotypic correlations: A need to explore repeatability. *Horm Behav* doi: 10.1016/j.yhbeh.2016.11.015.

Hedley, A. A., C. L. Ogden, C. L. Johnson et al. 2004. Prevalence of overweight and obesity among US children, adolescents, and adults, 1999–2002. *J Am Med Assoc* 291:2847–2850.

Hoffmann, J. A., F. C. Kafatos, C. A. Janeway et al. 1999. Phylogenetic perspectives in innate immunity. *Science* 284:1313–1318.

Hong, S. H., H. J. Jeong, and H. M. Kim. 2003. Inhibitory effects of *Xanthii fructus* extract on mast cell-mediated allergic reaction in murine model. *J Ethnopharmacol* 88:229–234.

Hwang, K. M., K. O. Jung, C. H. Song et al. 2008. Increased antimutagenic and anti-clastogenic effects of doenjang (Korean fermented soybean paste) prepared with bamboo salt. *J Med Food* 11:717–722.

Hwang, K. M., S. H. Oh, and K. Y. Park. 2007. Increased antimutagenic and *in vitro* anticancer effects by adding green tea extract and bamboo salt during doen-jang fermentation. *J Korean Soc Food Sci Nutr* 36:1–7

Jansson, B. 1996. Potassium, sodium, and cancer: A review. *J Environ Pathol Toxicol Oncol* 15:65–73.

Jeong, H. J., N. R. Han, K. Y. Kim et al. 2014. Gomisin A decreases the LPS-induced expression of iNOS and COX-2 and activation of RIP2/NF-κB in mouse perito-neal macrophages. *Immunopharmacol Immunotoxicol* 36:195–201.

Jeong, H. J., J. J. Kim, M. H. Kim et al. 2011. Specific blockage of caspase-1 activation by purple bamboo-salt prevents apoptosis of auditory cell line, HEI-OC1. *J Med Food* 14:53–61.

Jin, S. H., J. H. Yang, B. Y. Shin et al. 2013. Resveratrol inhibits LXRα-dependent hepatic lipogenesis through novel antioxidant Sestrin2 gene induction. *Toxicol Appl Pharmacol* 271:95–105.

Ju, J. 2016. Inhibitory effects on obesity and colon cancer by solar salt and bamboo salt in C57BL/6J mice. PhD diss., Pusan National University, Busan, Korea.

Ju, J., G. Y. Lee, Y. S. Kim et al. 2016. Bamboo salt suppresses colon carcinogenesis in C57BL/6 mice with chemically induced colitis. *J Med Food* 19:1015–1022.

Ju, J., J. L. Song, and K. Y. Park. 2015. Antiobesity effects of bamboo salt in C57BL/6 mice. *J Med Food* 18:706–710.

Kaminogawa, S., and M. Nanno. 2004. Modulation of immune functions by foods. *Evid Based Complement Alternat Med* 1:241–250.

Kim, H. M. 2012a. *Science of bamboo salt (1)*. Korea Bamboo Salt Industry Cooperative. 1–3.

Kim, H. M. 2012b. *Science of bamboo salt (2)*. Korea Bamboo Salt Industry Cooperative. 1–2.

Kim, K. Y., S. Y. Nam, T. Y. Shin et al. 2012. Bamboo salt reduces allergic responses by modulating the caspase-1 activation in an OVA-induced allergic rhinitis mouse model. *Food Chem Toxicol* 50:3480–3488.

Kim, M. S., H. J. Na, S. W. Han et al. 2003. *Forsythia fructus* inhibits the mast-cell-mediated allergic inflammatory reactions. *Inflammation* 27:129–135.

Kim, N. R., S. Y. Nam, K. J. Ryu et al. 2016. Effects of bamboo salt and its component, hydrogen sulfide, on enhancing immunity. *Mol Med Rep* 14:1673–1680.

Kim, Y. S, E. H. Lee, and H. M. Kim. 2013. Surprisingly, traditional purple bamboo salt, unlike other salts does not induce hypertension in rats. *TANG* 3:e16.

Koteish, A., and Diehl, A. M. 2001. Animal models of steatosis. *Semin Liver Dis* 21: 89–104.

Lee, J. M., K. T. Hwang, M. S. Heo et al. 2005a. Resistance of *Lactobacillus plantarum* KCTC 3099 from kimchi to oxidative stress. *J Med Food* 8:299–304.

Lee, W. J., E. H. Koh, J. C. Won et al. 2005b. Obesity: The role of hypothalamic AMP-activated protein kinase in body weight regulation. *Int J Biochem Cell Biol* 37:2254–2259.

Linder, J. 1987. The thymus gland in secondary immunodeficiency. *Arch Pathol Lab Med* 111:1118–1122.

Metzger, H., G. Alcaraz, R. Gogman et al. 1986. The receptor with high affinity for immunoglobulin E. *Annu Rev Immunol* 4:419–470.

Miescher, S. M., and M. Vogel. 2002. Molecular aspects of allergy. *Mol Aspects Med* 23:413–462.

Moon, J. H., H. A. Shin, Y. A. Rha, and A. S. Om. 2009. The intrinsic antimicrobial activity of bamboo salt against *Salmonella enteritidis*. *Mol Cell Toxicol* 5:323–327.

Myung, N. Y., I. H. Choi, H. J. Jeong et al. 2011. Ameliorative effect of purple bamboo salt-pharmaceutical acupuncture on cisplatin-induced ototoxicity. *Acta Otolaryngol* 131:14–21.

Na, H. J., H. J. Jeong, H. Bae et al. 2002. Tongkyutang inhibits mast cell-dependent allergic reactions and inflammatory cytokine secretion. *Clinica Chimica Acta* 319:35–41.

Nathan, C. 1992. Nitric oxide as a secretory product of mammalian cells. *FASEB J* 6:3051–3064.

Pardina, E., J. A. Baena-Fustegueras, R. Llamas et al. 2009. Lipoprotein lipase expression in livers of morbidly obese patients could be responsible for liver steatosis. *Obes Surg* 19:608–616.

Park, H. J., H. J. Yang, K. H. Kim et al. 2015. Aqueous extract of *Orostachys japonicus* A. Berger exerts immunostimulatory activity in RAW 264.7 macrophages. *J Ethnopharmacol* 170:210–217.

Park, K. S., K. A. Lee, and H. J. Kim. 2002. The effects of electric potential treatment on serum total cholesterol and triglyceride, blood glucose and blood pressure. *Korean J Sport Sci* 11:515–524.

Park, K. Y., X. Zhao, and S. H. Mun. 2013. Anticancer effects of bamboo salt on human cancer cells and on buccal mucosa cancer in mice. *FASEB J* 27 Supplement 639:4.

Petersen, L. J., H. Mosbech, and P. S. Skov. 1996. Allergen-induced histamine release in intact human skin *in vivo* assessed by skin microdialysis technique: Characterization of factors influencing histamine releasability. *J Allergy Clin Immunol* 97:672–679.

Qi, X. F., D. H. Kim, Y. S. Yoon et al. 2009. Effects of *Bambusae caulis* in Liquamen on the development of atopic dermatitis-like skin lesions in hairless mice. *J Ethnopharmacol* 123:195–200.

Shin, H. Y., E. H. Lee, C. Y. Kim et al. 2003. Anti-inflammatory activity of Korean folk medicine purple bamboo salt. *Immunopharmacol Immunotoxicol* 25:377–384.

Shin, H. Y., H. J. Na, P. D. Moon et al. 2004. Inhibition of mast cell-dependent immediate-type hypersensitivity reactions by purple bamboo salt. *J Ethnopharmacol* 91:153–157.

Tietge, U. J., A. Bakillah, C. Maugeais et al. 1999. Hepatic overexpression of microsomal triglyceride transfer protein (MTP) results in increased *in vivo* secretion of VLDL triglycerides and apolipoprotein B. *J Lipid Res* 40:2134–2139.

Xavier, F., and P. I. Sunyer. 2002. The obesity epidemic: Pathophysiology and consequences of obesity. *Obes Res* 10:97–104.

Younger, E. M., K. Epland, A. Zampelli et al. 2015. Primary immunodeficiency diseases: A primer for PCPs. *Nurse Practitioner* 40:1–7.

Zhao, X. 2011. Anticancer and anti-inflammatory effects of bamboo salt and *Rubus coreanus* Miquel bamboo salt. PhD diss., Pusan National University, Busan, Korea.

Zhao, X., X. Deng, K. Y. Park et al. 2013b. Purple bamboo salt has anticancer activity in TCA8113 cells *in vitro* and preventive effects on buccal mucosa cancer in mice *in vivo*. *Exp Ther Med* 5:549–554.

Zhao, X., J. Ju, H. M. Kim et al. 2013a. Antimutagenic activity and *in vitro* anticancer effects of bamboo salt on HepG2 human hepatoma cells. *J Environ Pathol Toxicol Oncol* 32:9–20.

Zhao, X., S. Y. Kim, and K. Y. Park. 2013c. Bamboo salt has *in vitro* anticancer activity in HCT-116 cells and exerts anti-metastatic effects *in vivo*. *J Med Food* 16:9–19.

Zhao, X., J. L. Song, J. H. Kil et al. 2013d. Bamboo salt attenuates CCl_4-induced hepatic damage in Sprague–Dawley rats. *Nutr Res Pract* 7:273–280.

14

Beneficial Effects of Cheonilyeom (a Mineral-Rich Solar Sea Salt) on Health and Fermentation

Jeong-Yong Cho, Lily Jaiswal, and Kyung-Sik Ham*

CONTENTS

14.1 Introduction 342
14.2 Salt in New Physiological Roles 342
    14.2.1 Activation of Immune System 342
    14.2.2 Obesity Control..343
14.3 Recent Debate on Salt Restriction 343
14.4 Types of Salt 344
    14.4.1 Rock Salt 344
    14.4.2 Solar Sea Salt..345
    14.4.3 Purified Salt..345
    14.4.4 Recrystallized Salt...345
14.5 Mineral Composition...345
14.6 Different Health Effects 346
    14.6.1 Oxidative Stress...347
    14.6.2 Effect of Heat-Treated Mineral-Rich Salt on Oxidative Stress ... 347
    14.6.3 Other Health Effects 349
14.7 Different Effects on Fermented Foods 349
    14.7.1 Fermented Vegetables...350
    14.7.2 Fermented Soybeans..352
    14.7.3 Fermented Seafood (Jeotgal)..353
14.8 Concluding Remarks 353
Acknowledgment...353
References..354

---

* Jeong-Yong Cho, Lily Jaiswal, and Kyung-Sik Ham contributed equally to this work.

14.1 Introduction

Dietary salt plays a crucial role in maintaining homeostasis in the body through regulating membrane potential, fluid volume, acid–base balance, nervous system, etc. Therefore, salt is an essential nutrient in humans. Across the world, many governments have recommended their people to reduce salt consumption for good health. However, recently, there has been a controversy among researchers over salt reduction for various health concerns, because the reduction of salt consumption increases plasma cholesterol, triglycerides, and renin activity that are known to be important biomarkers for cardiovascular diseases; this in turn increases cardiovascular disease-related mortality (Stolarz-Skrzypek et al., 2011; Graudal et al., 2012; O'Donnell et al., 2014). Thus, it is important to find an optimum salt intake in the context of maintaining health (Heaney, 2013). Another approach is to discover or develop salt that is better for our health compared to regular salt.

Various salts are found in the world, such as rock, solar sea, purified, and processed salts. Most do not contain minerals. However, some solar sea salts (mineral-rich salt, MRS), contain various minerals, including potassium (K), magnesium (Mg), calcium (Ca), etc. (Tan et al., 2012; Lee et al., 2014; Park et al., 2015; Hwang et al., 2016). Most previous studies undertaken used general table salt that contains above 99% NaCl. Recently, several studies have reported that MRS and its processed salts produced in Korea are expected to serve as an excellent dietary salt that can reduce the several health risks induced by mineral-deficient salt (MDS; regular salt). In this chapter, recent studies on the different biological effects of MRS and MDS in health and fermented foods are reviewed.

14.2 Salt in New Physiological Roles

The previously mentioned roles of salt have been renowned for a long time, but the recently unearthed new physiological role of salt has opened a substantial ground for debate on salt reduction. The new roles of salt contradict the well-established old beliefs of low salt intake for good health and compel us to reconsider the optimum intake amount. The newly reported functions of salt are discussed next.

14.2.1 Activation of Immune System

Several scientists have found that Na^+ acts as a functional component in skin, although the Na^+ function is unclear (Titze et al., 2004). It has been reported recently that a high-salt diet encourages Na^+ ions to be accrued in skin to

Beneficial Effects of Cheonilyeom on Health and Fermentation   343

provide protection against bacterial infection in humans and mice (Jantsch et al., 2014). It has been shown that augmented Na^+ accumulation creates a hypertonic environment in the skin, which stimulates macrophages to produce nitric oxide (NO) to facilitate pathogen removal.

14.2.2 Obesity Control

Recent epidemiological studies have reported a positive relationship between high salt intake and obesity, but most of these claims came from results of indirect research (Ma et al., 2015; Grimes et al., 2016; Moosavian et al., 2017). An interesting work that studied the direct relationship between salt intake and obesity was published recently that highlighted the role of dietary sodium against weight gain in $C_{57}BL/6J$ mice fed a high-fat diet (Weidemann et al., 2015). It was reported that high dietary sodium plays a significant role in antiobesity by inhibition of digestive efficiency through suppressing the renin–angiotensin system. In particular, dietary sodium suppressed digestive efficiency in a dose-dependent manner.

14.3 Recent Debate on Salt Restriction

Several reports and statistics pointed out that high sodium intake causes several health problems in humans due to its implication in cardiovascular diseases (He and MacGregor, 2011), obesity (Ma et al., 2015), high blood pressure (Ma et al., 2015), inflammation, and autoimmune diseases (Yi et al., 2015). Recently, the Institute of Medicine (IOM, 2005) advocated a daily dietary sodium intake for a normal person to be <2300 mg/day. In addition, the American Heart Association has set a target by curtailing salt consumption to <1500 mg/day in people older than 51 and those of any age who have hypertension, diabetes, or chronic kidney disease. All the reports mentioned here and policies were in favor of low sodium diet intake for upholding good cardiovascular and renal health, but recent investigations contradict the incumbent notion of low salt intake.

Much evidence and many recent reports showed that low sodium intake might influence human health by augmenting insulin resistance, acuteness of cardiovascular diseases and its incidence, and levels of serum lipids as well as disturbing neurohormonal pathways (DiNicolantonio et al., 2013). In particular, the low sodium intake triggers renin–angiotensin–aldosterone and the sympathetic nervous system, which in turn favors insulin resistance.

For hypertensive and normotensive patients, the sodium reduction efficiently mitigated blood pressure by 3.5% and 1%, respectively, but it raised other parameters such as plasma, aldosterone, renin, epinephrine, and norepinephrine levels as well as serum lipids like cholesterol (2.5%) and triglyceride levels (7%) in the body (Graudal et al., 2012). Another significant finding against low salt consumption was reported at almost the same time (Stolarz-Skrzypek et al., 2011) on population-based cohort studies reflecting that the low sodium excretion raised cardiovascular disease-based mortality. O'Donnell et al. (2014) investigated the association of estimated sodium and potassium excretion with the risk of death and cardiovascular events using urine samples from 101,945 persons in 17 countries. They documented that sodium intake of 3~6 g (7.5~15 g salt) per day was associated with a lower risk of death and cardiovascular events than either a higher or lower sodium intake. This group also reported that low sodium intake (<3 g/day) increases the risk of cardiovascular events and death in both hypertensive and nonhypertensive people, as compared with moderate sodium intake (4~5 g/day) (Mente et al., 2016). However, high salt intake (≥7 g/day) caused the risk of cardiovascular events and death in hypertensive people, but not in nonhypertensive people.

However, the difference in opinion between high and low salt intake groups has provided substantial ground for debate, as the exact consequences of salt intake on health is ambiguous to date. Hence, to reduce salt-induced health problems and to establish the optimum daily dietary intake, in-depth study on salt intake should be warranted by keeping health perspective as a priority.

14.4 Types of Salt

Among the world's dietary salts, various types of salts are produced, predominantly from sea water and rock salts. Table salt is made chiefly from the various sea and rock salts; each kind of table salt differs widely in NaCl and mineral composition (Gao et al., 2014). The ratio of other minerals and NaCl remains virtually constant in all sea water across the world (Sverdrup et al., 1942). Indeed, the disparity in salt composition is attributed to its manufacturing process. Therefore, based on its manufacturing process, salt is chiefly categorized into four groups.

14.4.1 Rock Salt

The rock salt "halite" is mined from underground deposits that crystallize with sodium and chloride ions. This salt is formed by the evaporation of salty water, especially sea water for a long time after diastrophism. Large deposits of rock salt are found in the United States, Canada, South America, Europe, India, and China. Most rock salts do not contain minerals because they have been washed out for a long time. Rock salt is widely consumed as table salt.

14.4.2 Solar Sea Salt

Solar sea salt is produced by natural evaporation of sea water that contains about 3.5% NaCl. Climate is a very important factor in solar sea salt production. The sun and wind provide the energy to evaporate the sea water. The brine water is moved through a series of evaporating grounds to obtain concentrated sea water (Balarew, 1993). When the salt concentration of the brine water becomes about 25% NaCl, the water is introduced into the crystallizing ground to crystallize the salt. The salt concentration of brine water and crystallization time are important factors in increasing purity of solar sea salt. With the exception of a few sea salts, most solar sea salts do not contain minerals (Tan et al., 2012).

14.4.3 Purified Salt

Purified salt is made from sea water using an ion exchange membrane electrodialysis method. The ion exchange membrane electrodialysis separates and concentrates various electrically charged positive (Na^+, K^+, etc.) and negative (Cl^-, SO_4^{2-}, etc.) ions present in sea water. The salt concentrate contains about 15%~20% NaCl and this concentrate is boiled to crystallize the salt.

14.4.4 Recrystallized Salt

Recrystallized salt is made by recrystallization of solar sea salt dissolved in water. The brine is boiled, concentrated, and allowed to yield salt crystals. This method can produce finely textured, high-purity salt, although the production cost is high.

14.5 Mineral Composition

Most dietary salts consumed daily, including refined, purified, rock, and solar sea salts, are mainly composed of NaCl with a low amount of other minerals (Tan et al., 2012). Table salts consumed by many people are made from purified, solar sea, or rock salts that contain above 99% NaCl with a trace of other minerals (Tan et al., 2012; Lee et al., 2014; Park et al., 2015; Hwang et al., 2016). However, some solar sea salts produced in several countries, especially France and Korea, contain appreciable amounts of K, Mg, and Ca (Tan et al., 2012). Gao et al. (2014) compared the general composition and mineral contents in MRS (mineral-rich salt, Korean solar sea salt) and MDS (mineral-deficient salt, rock salt) (Table 14.1). The NaCl, moisture and sulfate SO_4^{2-} contents in MRS were $86.95 \pm 0.89\%$, $11.4 \pm 0.19\%$, and $2.7 \pm 0.01\%$, respectively. The Mg ($9{,}629.0 \pm 218.1$ ppm), K ($2{,}764.2 \pm 65.9$ ppm), and

TABLE 14.1

General Composition and Mineral Contents of Mineral-Rich
Solar Salt (MRS) and Mineral-Deficient Salt (MDS)

	MRS	MDS
NaCl (%)	86.95 ± 0.89	99.9 ± 0.06
Moisture (%)	11.4 ± 0.19	ND
TIS (%)	0.03 ± 0.01	0.01 ± 0.001
SO_4^{2-} (%)	2.7 ± 0.01	ND
K (mg/kg)	2764.2 ± 65.9	17.4 ± 1.1
Mg (mg/kg)	9629.0 ± 218.1	ND
Ca (mg/kg)	1365.4 ± 20.2	ND
Fe (mg/kg)	62.0 ± 0.8	1.0 ± 0.1
Sr (mg/kg)	4.9 ± 1.7	ND
Mn (mg/kg)	5.3 ± 0.6	0.01 ± 0.02
Zn (mg/kg)	0.5 ± 0.5	0.4 ± 0.2
Cu (mg/kg)	0.1 ± 0.0	ND

Source: Gao, T.C. et al. 2014. *Food Sci Biotechnol* 23: 951–956.
Note: Values are mean ± SD of three experiments. ND: not detected;
TIS: total insoluble solid.

Ca (1,365.4 ± 20.2 ppm) were major minerals in MRS; minor minerals such as Sr, Fe, Mn, etc. were also observed in MRS. The differences in the NaCl and other mineral contents in various salts could be due to the differences in marine environments and/or production methods.

14.6 Different Health Effects

Salt, an essential nutrient, is taken in the diet (high or low amounts) every day to maintain the electrolytic balance in the body. The previously mentioned kinds of salts have shown the remarkable variations in NaCl as well as other mineral content in different salts. It is believed that the minerals fortifying salt not only enhance its overall quality but also enable it to heal and prevent various diseases, unlike table salt. Therefore, the trend of incorporating minerals and other bioactive compounds in salts is in vogue. It has also been reported that the reduced Na intake in conjunction with increased K and/or Mg substantially affects the modulation of blood pressure and cardiovascular health (Karppanen et al., 1984; Geleijnse et al., 1994; Terukazu et al., 1998; Essiet et al., 2011).

However, mineral-fortified processed salts do not contain various minerals that are believed to be necessary for human health. It has also been considered that minerals in natural salts are not enough to be physiologically effective. Recently, *in vivo* health effects of MRS were investigated. Surprisingly, health effects of minerals in MRS were more significant than we thought previously. Part of the results will be summarized in the forthcoming sections.

14.6.1 Oxidative Stress

In the past two decades, due to unhealthy lifestyles, the level of oxidative stress has risen exponentially. The increased oxidative stress adversely affects human health by causing cancer, arthritis, inflammation, and heart disease (Brieger et al., 2012). Moreover, oxidative stress causes oxidation of DNA, lipids, proteins, and other biomolecules and triggers the activation of proinflammatory cytokines such as nuclear factor-kappaB (NF-κB). We evaluated the efficacy of MRS and MDS against oxidative stress (Gao et al., 2014) and found that MRS remarkably reduced plasma lipid oxidation, protein oxidation, and DNA damage in the liver, as well as protein expression of NF-κβ in adipose tissue (Figure 14.1). Since salt has a profound effect on body physiology and oxidative stress causes many diseases, MRS is worthy of further study as a candidate for good dietary salt.

14.6.2 Effect of Heat-Treated Mineral-Rich Salt on Oxidative Stress

MRS containing various minerals does not show *in vitro* antioxidant activity (Gao et al., 2014), although MRS caused less oxidative stress than MDS when the same amounts of NaCl were consumed by normal rats. Traditionally, many people in Korea have eaten MRS after it was roasted. Interestingly, we found that *in vitro* antioxidant activity is generated when MRS is roasted (RS) (Gao et al., 2015). RS scavenges superoxide radicals and inhibits DNA oxidation, as reflected in *in vitro* assays (Figure 14.2). Bamboo salt (BS), which is produced by roasting MRS with bamboo, is more effective in antioxidative

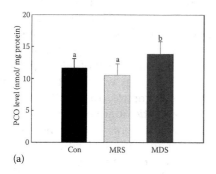 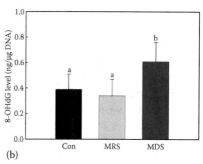

FIGURE 14.1
Protein oxidation (a) and DNA oxidation (b) in liver of rats orally administered with MRS and MDS for 7 weeks. (Based on Gao, T.C. et al. 2014. *Food Sci Biotechnol* 23: 951–956.) Con: control group; MRS: mineral-rich solar salt group; MDS: mineral-deficient salt group. Values are mean ± SD (n = 7 or 8). [a,b]Results with different letters on bars are significantly different ($p < 0.05$).

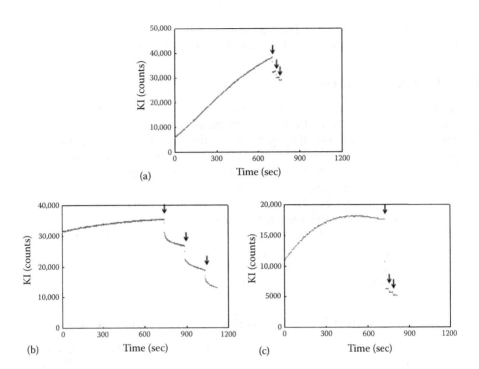

FIGURE 14.2
Superoxide radical-scavenging activities of MRS (a); RS (b); and BS (c). (Based on Gao, T.C. et al. 2015. *J Food Biochem* 39: 631–641.) The arrow indicates the addition of 5.0 mg salt solution in lucigenin/arginine/methylglyoxal-induced superoxide anion radical solution.

activity than RS. This result was consistent with the results of other studies on BS that demonstrated scavenging DPPH radical activity (Zhao et al., 2012) and inhibition of reactive oxygen species (ROS) formation in human astrocyte U373MG cells (Om and Jeong, 2007). We also investigated the effect of heat-treated MRS on oxidative stress in Sprague–Dawley (SD) rats orally administered various salts (1.8 g NaCl equivalent/kg) daily in SD rats for 7 weeks. The RS and BS groups had significantly lower levels of lipid peroxidation and protein oxidation and lower expression level of NF-κB p65, as well as higher total thiol contents than the MRS group, which indicated that RS and BS groups had reduced oxidative stress compared to the MRS group.

These results were correlated with *in vitro* antioxidative activity of the salts. Minerals contained in MRS might partially contribute to the reduction of oxidative stress induced by high salt intake, as discussed before. Although the mineral contents (Ca, Mg, K, etc.) in heat-treated MRS (especially, BS) are lower than MRS not treated with heat, heat-treated MRS has higher antioxidative activities *in vitro* and efficiently suppresses oxidative stress induced by a high-salt diet in an animal model compared with heat-treated MRS. This suggests that antioxidant is generated in MRS by heat treatment. These results warrant further study upon heat-treated MRS.

14.6.3 Other Health Effects

The generation of ROS has a direct nexus with mitochondrial dysfunction (MD) and endoplasmic reticulum (ER) stress. MD further causes the inactivation of several enzymes as well as insulin resistance. In recent investigation on the effect of MRS and BS on mitochondrial dysfunction, we found that a high-salt diet promoted insulin resistance by stimulating insulin receptor substrate 1 (IRS-1)ser307 expression and suppressing glucose transporter type 4 (GLUT4) expression in adipose and skeletal muscle tissues irrespective of types of salt used (Chanmuang, 2014). However, MRS and BS attenuated the progression of insulin resistance. In addition, MRS and BS raised mitochondrial membrane potential, ATP production, mitochondrial mass, cytochrome c, cytochrome c oxidase subunit III and GLUT4 expression, and, on the other hand, reduced ROS production when compared with MDS. The outcomes of MRS and BS on oxidative stress, mitochondrial dysfunction, and insulin resistance are promising.

As mentioned earlier, Weidemann et al. (2015) reported that dietary sodium prevents weight gain during a high-fat diet through suppressing digestive efficiency, with no effect on food intake, resting metabolic processes, or physical activity. Recently, it was reported that, compared to MDS, MRS caused less weight gain induced by a high-fat diet in C57BL/6J mice (Ju et al., 2016). MRS decreased levels of triacylglycerol, total cholesterol, leptin, and insulin in serum. In addition, MRS suppressed the expression of adipogenic- and lipogenic-related factors (peroxisome proliferator-activated receptor γ, CCAAT-enhancer-binding protein α, and fatty acid synthase), promoted the expression of β-oxidative factors (peroxisome proliferator-activated receptor α and carnitine palmitoyltransferase I), and reduced fat accumulation in the liver (Ju et al., 2016). The authors suggested that different antiobesity effects of MRS are due to mineral composition and other bioactive components resulting from the unique manufacturing processes.

14.7 Different Effects on Fermented Foods

Many Korean fermented foods, including vegetables (kimchi), seafoods (jeotgal), and beans (fermented soybeans) have been eaten for thousands of years (Park et al., 2014). Most of the fermented foods are generally made by adding high levels of salt to preserve them for a long time. Salting enables fermented foods to inhibit the growth of pathogenic and spoilage microorganisms during fermentation and preservation. Additionally, in the fermentation process, the presence of beneficial microbes under high salt concentrations affects the taste, rendering diverse flavor with beneficial health effects. Therefore, salt may play a crucial role in regulating the quality of fermented foods.

The fermented foods prepared with MRS taste better than those prepared with MDS containing only sodium chloride with a trace of minerals. Several scientists have also found that the useful microorganisms were more dominant in fermented foods prepared with MRS than the food with MDS. However, it seems practically challenging to find a significant difference in nutrients and beneficial health compounds among the fermented foods prepared with different salts. The reason might be due to the limitation of conventional analytical technologies used. Therefore, application of new technology such as metabolomics is required to find the differences among the fermented food made with different salts. New data obtained using metabolomics are introduced in the following sections.

14.7.1 Fermented Vegetables

Kimchi, a traditional Korean fermented food, is manufactured by fermenting vegetables with high salt concentration (2%–3% NaCl) (Cheigh and Park, 1994; Park et al., 2014). The major ingredients of kimchi are cruciferous vegetables, especially Chinese cabbage (baechu), and garlic, ginger, red pepper powder, etc. (Song, 2004). Many lactic acid bacteria (LAB), including *Leuconostoc* and *Lactobacillus*, and *Weissella* genera, are involved in kimchi fermentation (Ahn, 1988; Kim and Chun, 2005; Jung et al., 2011). The growth of microorganisms in kimchi fermentation is greatly influenced by starting ingredients. In particular, salt concentration and fermentation temperature significantly affect microbial communities during brining of Chinese cabbage and fermentation (Mheen and Kwon, 1984; Park and Kim, 1991; Park et al., 2003).

Salt inhibits the growth of the putrefactive microorganisms but promotes the growth of LAB during brining of Chinese cabbage and fermentation. It was reported that brined Chinese cabbage prepared with MRS had a lower number of total aerobic bacteria and a higher number of LAB than those of MDS (Choi et al., 2014). MRS stimulated more rapid growth of LAB during fermentation of kimchi compared to MDS (Han et al., 2009; Chang et al., 2010b, 2011). In contrast, several studies reported no difference in LAB count between kimchi prepared with MRS and MDS, which was fermented at above 20°C (Kim et al., 2005; Chang et al., 2010a). Chang et al. (2011) investigated the number of LAB during fermentation of kimchi at lower temperature (7°C), which was prepared with MRS and MDS and inoculated with *Leuconostoc citreum* G17. The LAB counts of the kimchi prepared with MRS increased to 9.26~9.42 log colony-forming units (CFUs)/mL at 12 days and then slightly decreased to 8.04~8.75 log CFUs/mL by 33 days of fermentation. In the case of the kimchi prepared with MDS, the LAB counts slowly increased to 8.99 log CFUs/mL at 27 days and then decreased to 7.92 log CFUs/mL at 33 days of fermentation.

These results suggest that MRS might stimulate the number of LAB in kimchi at low fermentation temperatures. In addition, minerals such as Mg and K contained in MRS promoted the growth of LAB during fermentation,

Beneficial Effects of Cheonilyeom on Health and Fermentation

suggesting that various minerals in MRS could be used as nutrient sources for LAB. However, the kimchi prepared with MRS aged for 4 years showed higher numbers of total microorganisms and LAB than that of 1-year-old MRS, although minerals in MRS aged for 4 years had lower mineral contents than those in 1-year-old MRS (Chang et al., 2011). Thus, it is important to discover optimum mineral contents in MRS that can stimulate the growth of LAB during kimchi fermentation.

There is no report available on chemical constituents and their composition in kimchi prepared with different types of salts. During kimchi fermentation, the types of salts could affect minor components rather than major components. Therefore, it would be very difficult to discern changes in chemical constituents and their composition by conventional methods such as liquid chromatography (LC) and gas chromatography (GC) analysis. Recently, studies have been conducted to identify the differences in chemical constituents and their composition in kimchi prepared by different types of salts through metabolomic analysis using GC–mass spectrometry (MS), LC-MS, and nuclear magnetic resonance (NMR) experiments. Jang et al. (2015) investigated volatile and nonvolatile metabolites in 40-day fermented radish water kimchi (dongchimi) prepared with MRS or MDS by using GC-MS and multivariate statistical analysis. Sulfur compound, free sugar, sugar alcohol, and lactic acid levels largely contributed to differences between MRS and MDS types. Sulfur compound levels were decreased by MRS, whereas it increased mannitol and lactic acid levels.

Several studies reported that kimchi prepared with MRS has a better crispy taste and flavor than kimchi prepared with MDS in sensory evaluation (Han et al., 2009; Chang et al., 2010b, 2011; Lee et al., 2012). Many scientists have suggested that kimchi prepared with MRS has more hardness than kimchi prepared with MDS, because various minerals (Mg and Ca) contained in MRS form a cross-linkage between the pectin of Chinese cabbage during brining and fermentation and suppress softness during fermentation (Mheen and Kwon, 1984; Lee et al., 1988). Jang et al. (2011) reported that kimchi prepared with MRS that aged for 4 years was more palatable than kimchi prepared with 1-year-old MRS. The contents of Ca, Mg, and SO_4^{2-}, bitter-taste-related compounds, decrease in MRS with aging (Kim et al., 1996). For long-term storage, kimchi prepared with MRS (aged for 4 years) was more suitable regarding fermentation characteristics and sensory evaluation than kimchi prepared with 1-year-old MRS (Chang et al., 2014). Therefore, it is important to find out optimum mineral contents in MRS that can enhance the taste and flavor of kimchi.

Kimchi has various beneficial health effects, including anticancer, antiobesity, anticonstipation, antioxidant, cholesterol reduction, fibrinolytic, antioxidative, and antiaging properties; brain health promotion; immunity-boosting properties, and skin health promotion (Cho et al., 1997; Lee et al., 2004; Islam and Choi 2009; Noh et al., 2009; Kim et al., 2011; Park et al., 2014). Information on different biological effects of MRS- and MDS-kimchi is limited. Based on *in vitro* inhibitory assays on cancer cells, several studies have reported that kimchi prepared with MRS had superior anticancer (cytotoxic) activity compared to that with MDS (Han et al., 2009; Yoon and Chang, 2011). In particular, kimchi prepared with MRS showed an excellent effect in inhibiting human gastric adenocarcinoma cells (AGS) and HT-29 human colon carcinoma cells compared to that prepared with MDS. Yoon and Chang (2011) also reported that kimchi prepared with MRS aged for 4 years was more effective in inhibiting the growth of gastric cancer cells (AGS) and intestinal cancer cells (HT-29) than that using 1-year-old MRS.

14.7.2 Fermented Soybeans

MRS has been widely used in fermented soybeans (doenjang and kanjang), traditional Korean fermented foods. As in kimchi, MRS enhances the quality and biological effects of fermented soybeans. Shim et al. (2016a) investigated microorganism properties of doenjang prepared with MRS aged for different periods (4 years and 1 year), and with MDS in starter and nonstarter fermentation for 13 weeks at 25°C. Doenjang prepared with MRS showed higher numbers of bacilli as well as much lower yeast counts during the fermentation than doenjang with MDS. In the case of nonstarter (rice straw) fermentation, *Debaryomyces hansenii* was the dominant yeast in doenjang prepared with MDS, whereas *Candida guilliermondii* and *Pichia sorbitophila* were found in doenjang prepared with MRS. The crude fat, protein levels, and sensory properties were higher in doenjang prepared with MRS than that prepared with MDS. The doenjang with MRS showed higher total phenolic contents than that with MDS (Shim et al., 2016b). These results are similar to the findings by Chang et al. (2010c). They also found that the browning reaction rate of doenjang prepared with MDS was faster than doenjang made with MRS.

Several *in vitro* studies have reported that deonjang prepared with MRS has superior anticancer and antioxidative activities compared to that prepared with MDS. However, as occurred with kimchi, studies on the differences in the biological effects of doenjang prepared with MRS or MDS are limited. Lee and Chang (2009) reported that deonjang prepared with MRS had an excellent growth inhibitory effect against human gastric adenocarcinoma cells (AGS) and HT-29 human colon carcinoma cells compared to that of doenjang made with MDS. Yoon et al. (2012) also reported that doenjang prepared with MRS aged for 4 years had strong inhibition activity against the growth of human gastric adenocarcinoma cells (AGS) and HT-29 human colon carcinoma cells than doenjang prepared with 1-year-old MRS. However, no difference in growth inhibition effect of doenjang prepared with MRS and MDS on BJ normal cells was noticed. Doenjang prepared with MRS showed higher *in vitro* antioxidative activities than that with MDS, as evaluated by ABTS, DPPH, and FRAP assays. These results suggest that MRS is far superior to MDS, especially regarding biological effect, and produces a doenjang with better quality.

14.7.3 Fermented Seafood (Jeotgal)

Jeotgal is a traditional Korean fermented food made by fermenting a mixture of fresh seafoods (fish, shellfish, shrimp, etc.) and salt (20%–25%) and is commonly used as a seasoning ingredient. Information on the fermentation characteristics of jeotgal prepared with different types of salts is much lower than that for kimchi and doenjang. Several studies (Chang and Rhee, 1986; Lee et al., 2008; Cho and Kim, 2010) have investigated the effects of various salts, including MRS, MDS, and others, on the physicochemical and sensory properties of fermented shrimp or anchovy. No significant differences in microorganisms or physicochemical and sensory properties among the samples were observed, although several factors appeared to be slightly different. Further systematic studies on various effects of different salts in microorganisms or physicochemical and sensory properties of jeotgal are required.

14.8 Concluding Remarks

Recently, the debate on salt restriction has been intensifying as more reports are coming out that low sodium intake increases health problems. We have to discover daily dietary salt intake that can minimize health problems. However, health problems induced by salt cannot be completely eliminated, even though the optimum daily dietary salt that can minimize health problems is taken. Recently, several studies reported that MRS containing minerals gave fewer health problems than those induced by MDS. Furthermore, MRS seems to be superior to MDS in the aspects of the quality and beneficial health effects of fermented foods prepared with salt. Current evidence suggests that minerals play a crucial role in reducing health problems induced by dietary salt as well as enhancing quality and biological effects of fermented foods. Korean solar sea salt and its processed salts (especially heat-treated salt) are considered to be good dietary salts that can reduce health problems induced by regular table salt. However, the biological advantages of minerals in mineral-rich salt for health and fermented foods are not fully understood. Further investigation on mineral function and mineral composition related to salt-induced health problems will enable us to develop a dietary salt that is better for our health.

Acknowledgment

This study was supported by a grant 20130290 from the Ministry of Oceans and Fisheries, Korea.

References

Ahn, S.J. 1988. The effect of salt and food preservation on the growth of lactic acid bacteria isolated from kimchi. *Korean J Soc Food Sci* 4: 39–50.

Balarew, C. 1993. Solubilities in seawater-type systems: Some technical and environmental friendly applications. *Pure Appl Chem* 65: 213–218.

Brieger, K., S. Schiavone, F.J. Miller, and K.H. Krause. 2012. Reactive oxygen species: From health to disease. *Swiss Med Weekly* 142: w13659.

Chang, J.Y., I.C. Kim, and H.C. Chang. 2011. Effect of solar salt on the fermentation characteristics of kimchi. *Korean J Food Preserv* 18: 256–265.

Chang, J.Y., I.C. Kim, and H.C. Chang. 2014. Effect of solar salt on kimchi fermentation during long-term storage. *Korean J Food Sci Technol* 46: 456–464.

Chang, M., I.C. Kim, and H.C. Chang. 2010c. Effect of solar salt on the quality characteristics of doenjang. *J Korean Soc Food Sci Nutr* 39: 116–124.

Chang, M.S., S.D. Cho, D.H. Bae, and G.H. Kim. 2010b. Safety and quality assessment of kimchi made using various salts. *Korean J Food Sci Technol* 42: 160–164.

Chang, M.S., S.D. Cho, and G.H. Kim. 2010a. Physiochemical and sensory properties of kimchi (Korean pickled cabbage) prepared with various salts. *Korean J Food Preserv* 17: 30–35.

Chang, P.K. and H.S. Rhee. 1986. Effects of the kind and concentration of salt on oxidation of lipids and on formation of flavor components in fermented anchovies. *Korean J Food Cookery Sci* 2: 38–44.

Chanmuang, S. 2014. Effects of various salts on insulin resistance, mitochondrial dysfunction, and blood pressure in rats. PhD diss., Mokpo Nat. Univ.

Cheigh, H.S. and K.Y. Park. 1994. Biochemical, microbiological and nutritional aspects of Kimchi (Korean fermented vegetable products). *Crit Rev Food Sci Nutr* 34: 175–203.

Cho, E.J., S.H. Rhee, S.M. Lee, and K.Y. Park. 1997. *In vitro* antimutagenic and anticancer effects of kimchi fractions. *J Korean Assoc Cancer Prevent* 2: 113–131.

Cho, S.D. and G.H. Kim. 2010. Changes of quality characteristics of salt-fermented shrimp prepared with various salts. *Korean J Food Nutr* 23: 291–298.

Choi, G.H., G.Y. Lee, Y.J. Bong et al. 2014. Comparison of quality properties of brined baechu cabbage manufactured by different salting methods and with different salts. *J Korean Soc Food Sci Nutr* 43: 1036–1041.

Dinicolantonio, J.J., A.K. Niazi, R. Sadaf et al. 2013. Dietary sodium restriction: Take it with a grain of salt. *Am J Med* 126: 951–955.

Essiet, S.S., J.K. Mika, H.N. Tarja et al. 2011. Feasibility and antihypertensive effect of replacing regular salt with mineral salt—Rich in magnesium and potassium—In subjects with mildly elevated blood pressure. *Nutr J* 10: 88–96.

Gao, T.C., J.Y. Cho, L.Y. Feng, S. Chanmuang, S.Y. Park et al. 2014. Mineral-rich solar sea salt generates less oxidative stress in rats than mineral-deficient salt. *Food Sci Biotechnol* 23: 951–956.

Gao, T.C., J.Y. Cho, Y. Feng, S. Chanmuang, S.Y. Park et al. 2015. Heat-treated solar sea salt has antioxidant activity *in vitro* and produces less oxidative stress in rats compared with untreated solar sea salt. *J Food Biochem* 39: 631–641.

Geleijnse, J.M., J.C.M. Witteman, A.A.A. Bak et al. 1994. Reduction in blood pressure with a low sodium, high potassium, high magnesium salt in older subjects with mild to moderate hypertension. *BMJ* 309: 436–440.

Graudal, N.A., T. Hubeck-Graudal, and G. Jürgens. 2012. Effects of low-sodium diet vs. high-sodium diet on blood pressure, renin, aldosterone, catecholamines, cholesterol, and triglyceride (Cochrane Review). *Am J Hypertens* 25: 1–15.

Grimes, C.A., D.P. Bolhuis, F.J. He, and C.A. Nowson. 2016. Dietary sodium intake and overweight and obesity in children and adults: A protocol for a systematic review and meta-analysis. *System Rev* 5: 7.

Han, G.J., A.R. Son, S.M. Lee et al. 2009. Improved quality and increased *in vitro* anticancer effect of kimchi by using natural sea salt without bittern and baked (guwun) salt. *J Korean Soc Food Sci Nutr* 38: 996–1002.

He, F.J. and G.A. MacGregor. 2011. Salt reduction lowers cardiovascular risk: Meta-analysis of outcome trials. *Lancet* 378: 380–382.

Heaney, R.P. 2013. Sodium: How and how not to set a nutrient intake recommendation. *Am J Hypertens* 26: 194–197.

Hwang, I.M., J.S. Yang, S.H. Kim et al. 2016. Elemental analysis of sea, rock, and bamboo salts by inductively coupled plasma-optical emission and mass spectrometry. *Anal Lett* 49: 2807–2821.

IOM (Institute of Medicine). 2005. Dietary reference intakes for water, potassium, sodium, chloride, and sulfate. Washington, DC: The National Academies Press.

Islam, M.S. and H. Choi. 2009. Antidiabetic effect of Korean traditional baechu (Chinese cabbage) kimchi in a type 2 diabetes model of rats. *J Med Food* 12: 292–297.

Jang, G.J., D.W. Kim, E.J. Gu et al. 2015. GC/MS-based metabolomic analysis of the radish water kimchi, donchimi, with different salt. *Food Sci Biotechnol* 24: 1967–1972.

Jantsch, J., V. Schatz, D. Friedrich et al. 2015. Cutaneous Na^+ storage strengthens the antimicroorganism barrier function of the skin and boost macrophage-driven host defense. *Cell Metabol* 21: 493–501.

Ju, J.H., J.L. Song, E.S. Park, M.S. Do, and K.Y. Park. 2016. Korean solar salts reduce obesity and alter its related markers in diet-induced obese mice. *Nutr Res Pract* 10: 629–634.

Jung, J.Y., S.H. Lee, J.M. Kim et al. 2011. Metagenomic analysis of kimchi, a traditional Korean fermented food. *Appl Environ Microbiol* 77: 2264–2274.

Karppanen, H., A. Tanskanen, J. Tuomilehto et al. 1984. Safety and effects of potassium- and magnesium-containing low sodium salt mixtures. *J Cardiovasc Pharmacol Ther* 6: S236–243.

Kim, B., K.Y. Park, H.Y. Kim et al. 2011. Anti-aging effects and mechanisms of kimchi during fermentation under stress-induced premature senescence cellular system. *Food Sci Biotechnol* 20: 643–649.

Kim, C.J., K.C. Kim, D.Y. Kim et al. 1996. *Fermentation engineering.* Seoul: Sunjin Munhoasa.

Kim, M. and J. Chun. 2005. Bacterial community structure in kimchi, a Korean fermented vegetable food, as revealed by 16S rRNA gene analysis. *Int J Food Microbiol* 103: 91–96.

Kim, S.J., H.L. Kim, and K.S. Ham. 2005. Characterization of kimchi fermentation prepared with various salts. *Korean J Food Preserv* 12: 395–401.

Lee, C.H., I.J. Hwang, and J.K. Kim. 1988. Macro- and micro-structure of Chinese cabbage leaves and their texture measurements. *Korean J Food Sci Technol* 16: 502–508.

Lee, I.S., H.S. Kim, and H.Y. Kim. 2012. Quality characteristic of baechu kimchi prepared with domestic and imported solar salts during storage. *Korean J Food Cookery Sci* 28: 363–364.

Lee, K.D., C.R. Choi, J.Y. Cho et al. 2008. Physicochemical and sensory properties of salt-fermented shrimp prepared with various salts. *J Korean Soc Food Sci Nutr* 37: 53–59.

Lee, S.M. and H.C. Chang. 2009. Growth-inhibitory effect of the solar salt-doenjang on cancer cells, AGS and HT-29. *J Korean Soc Food Sci Nutr* 38: 1664–1671.

Lee, Y.H., K.S. Ham, S.H. Han et al. 2014. Revealing discriminating power of the elements in edible sea salts: Line-intensity correlation analysis from laser-induced plasma emission spectra. *Spectrochim Acta Part B: Atom Spectro* 101: 57–67.

Lee, Y.M., M.J. Kwon, J.K. Kim et al. 2004. Isolation and identification of active principle in Chinese cabbage kimchi responsible for antioxidant activity. *Korean J Food Sci Technol* 36: 129–133.

Ma, Y., F.J. He, and G.A. MacGregor. 2015. High salt intake: Independent risk factor for obesity? *Hypertension* 66: 843–849.

Mente, A., M. O'Donnell, S. Rangarajan et al. 2016. Associations of urinary sodium excretion with cardiovascular events in individuals with and without hypertension: A pooled analysis of data from four studies. *Lancet* 388: 465–475.

Mheen, T.I. and T.W. Kwon. 1984. Effect of temperature and salt concentration on kimchi fermentation. *Korean J Food Sci Technol* 16: 443–450.

Moosavian, S.P., F. Haghighatdoost, P.J. Surkan, and L. Azadbakht. 2017. Salt and obesity: A systematic review and meta-analysis of observational studies. *Int J Food Sci Nutr* 68: 265–277.

Noh, J.S., H.J. Kim, M.J. Kwon, and Y.O. Song. 2009. Active principle of kimchi, 3-(4'-hydroxyl-3',5'-dimethoxyphenyl)propionic acid, retards fatty streak formation at aortic sinus of apolipoprotein E knockout mice. *J Med Food* 12: 1206–1212.

O'Donnell, M., A. Mente, S. Rangarajan et al. 2014. Urinary sodium and potassium excretion, mortality, and cardiovascular event. *New Engl J Med* 371: 612–623.

Om, A.S. and J.H. Jeong. 2007. Bamboo salts have antioxidant activity and inhibit ROS formation in human astrocyte U373MG cells. *Cancer Prevent Res* 12: 225–230.

Park, G., H. Yoo, Y. Gong et al. 2015. Feasibility of rapid classification of edible salts by a compact low-cost laser-induced breakdown spectroscopy device. *Bull Korean Chem Soc* 36: 189–197.

Park, J.A., G.Y. Heo, J.S. Lee et al. 2003. Change of microorganism communities in kimchi fermentation at low temperature. *Korean J Microbiol* 39: 45–50.

Park, K.Y., J.K. Jeong, Y.E. Lee, and J. Daily. 2014. Health benefits of kimchi (Korean fermented vegetables) as a probiotic food. *J Med Food* 17: 6–20.

Park, W.P. and Z.U. Kim. 1991. The effect of salt concentration on kimchi fermentation. *J Korean Chem Soc* 34: 295–297.

Shim, J.M., K.W. Lee, Z. Yao, H.J. Kim, and J.H. Kim. 2016a. Properties of doenjang (soybean paste) prepared with different types of salts. *J Microbiol Biotechnol* 26: 1533–1541.

Shim, J.M., K.W. Lee, Z. Yao, H.J. Kim, and J.H. Kim. 2016b. Proteases and antioxidant activities of doenjang, prepared with different types of salts, during fermentation. *Microbiol Biotechnol Lett* 44: 303–310

Song, Y.O. 2004. The functional properties of kimchi for the health benefits. *J Food Sci Nutr* 9: 27–33.

Stolarz-Skrzypek, K., T. Kuznetsova, L. Thijs et al. 2011. Fatal and nonfatal outcomes, incidence of hypertension, and blood pressure changes in relation to urinary sodium excretion. *JAMA* 305: 1777–1785.

Sverdrup, H.U., M.W. Johnson, and R.H. Fleming. 1942. Chemistry of sea water. In *The oceans their physics, chemistry, and general biology*. New York: University of California Press.

Tan, M.M., S. Cui, J.H. Yoo et al. 2012. Feasibility of laser-induced breakdown spectroscopy (LIBS) for classification of sea salts. *Appl Spectro* 66: 262–271.

Terukazu, K., I. Kazue, and K. Masumi. 1998. Reduction in blood pressure with a sodium-reduced, potassium and magnesium-enriched mineral salt in subjects with mild essential hypertension. *Hypertens Res* 21: 235–243.

Titze, J., M. Shakibaei, M. Schafflhuber et al. 2004. Glycosaminoglycan polymerization may enable osmotically inactive Na+ storage in the skin. *Am J Physiol Heart Circ Physiol* 287: H203–208.

Weidemann, B.J., S. Voong, F. Morales-Santiago et al. 2015. Dietary sodium suppresses digestive efficiency via the renin-angiotensin system. *Sci Rep* 5: article 11123.

Yi, B., J. Titze, M. Rykova et al. 2015. Effects of dietary salt levels on monocytic cells and immune responses in healthy human subjects: A longitudinal study. *Transl Res* 166: 103–110.

Yoon, H.H. and H.C. Chang. 2011. Growth inhibitory effect of kimchi prepared with four-year-old solar salt and topan solar salt on cancer cells. *J Korean Soc Food Sci Nutr* 40: 935–941.

Yoon, H.H., I.C. Kim, and H.C. Chang. 2012. Growth inhibitory effects of doenjang, prepared with various solar salts, on cancer cells. *Korean J Food Preserv* 19: 278–286.

Zhao, X., O.S. Jung, and K.Y. Park. 2012. Alkaline and antioxidant effects of bamboo salt. *J Korean Soc Food Sci Nutr* 41: 1301–1304.

15

Edible Korean Seaweed: A Source of Functional Compounds

Sanjeewa K. K. Asanka, Hyun-Soo Kim, and You-Jin Jeon

CONTENTS

15.1 Introduction 359
15.2 What Is Seaweed? 361
15.3 Traditional Korean Foods from Seaweed 363
    15.3.1 Edible Green Seaweed 364
    15.3.2 Edible Red Seaweed 365
    15.3.3 Edible Brown Seaweed 365
15.4 Bioactive Compounds 367
    15.4.1 Polysaccharides 367
        15.4.1.1 Fucoidans 367
        15.4.1.2 Laminarin 368
        15.4.1.3 Alginic Acid 368
        15.4.1.4 Carrageenans 369
        15.4.1.5 Ulvan 370
    15.4.2 Polyphenols 370
    15.4.3 Carotenoids 370
    15.4.4 Sterols 372
15.5 Potential Bioactive Properties as Functional Ingredients 372
    15.5.1 Antioxidant 372
    15.5.2 Anticancer 374
    15.5.3 Anti-Inflammation 375
    15.5.4 Antidiabetic and Antiobese 377
15.6 Conclusion 378
References 378

15.1 Introduction

Seaweed is a rich source of proteins, carbohydrates, lipids, vitamins, and other essential minerals for the body. In addition to the food value, seaweed contains diverse components with great pharmaceutical, cosmeceutical, and nutraceutical values. Within recent decades, the market for edible seaweed and functional foods produced from seaweed has increased with the discovery of long-term health benefits of seaweed consumption. South Korea is one of the larger consumers and producers of seaweed. Traditionally, Korean people consume seaweed as a vegetable or use it as a medicine. In this chapter, attention is given to discussing edible Korean seaweed and its potential bioactive properties.

Food is a vital part of life and it is more than merely the source of physical nourishment. Foods have been considered as a medium of emotional bonding, community building, social relations, and religious practices. Korean traditional cuisines are mainly based on rice, vegetables (bean curd, bean sprouts, bean paste, soy sauce, and seaweed), and meats. In general, Korean meals are served with one main dish and a number of side dishes together with soup. The contents of the main dish and side dishes are different among the provinces in Korea and even from family to family (Oum, 2005). Among the side dishes, kimchi is the most prominent in traditional Korean cuisine and is served with every meal. A typical adult Korean consumes an average of 50 ~ 200 g of kimchi per day and its market in Korea was more than 130 million USD in 2002 (Kim and Chun, 2005). In addition to kimchi, seaweed is also popular as a side dish and also as a soup ingredient, especially among older generations and lactating mothers (Kim, 1999). However, lack of collective information about edible Korean seaweed, food applications, nutrition value, and health promotion effects is minimizing the utilization of this invaluable natural resource as a functional food ingredient and nutraceutical. Herein we discuss the edible seaweed found in Korea, traditional food applications, and bioactive properties reported from edible seaweed.

Seaweed is one of the prominent primary producers in the marine food webs, rich in essential nutrients and bioactive compounds (Jibril et al., 2016). Seaweed is mainly categorized into three groups based on color: green (Chlorophyta), red (Rhodophyta), and brown (Laminariales). Compared to European countries, the use of seaweed as a food source and a medicine has a strong history in Asian countries including Korea, China, and Japan. In addition to its nutritious value, seaweed contains structurally diverse bioactive components including sulfated polysaccharides, phlorotannins, and pigments. Every year thousands of reports are published in reputable journals with bioactivities of crude and pure compounds isolated from edible seaweed. Therefore, the market value for seaweed-associated food products increases day by day. In contrast to Asian countries, most Western countries consume low amounts of seaweed and do not consider it as food source. However, during the last few decades, consumption of seaweed products has increased in many European countries (Yuan and Walsh, 2006; Mouritsen, 2009; Kasimala et al., 2015).

Korea is one of the highest consuming and producing countries of edible seaweed. Korean people traditionally consume seaweed as a raw product or after it has dried under sun. Within the Korean traditional diet, seaweed

Edible Korean Seaweed

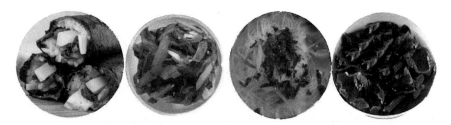

FIGURE 15.1
Popular seaweed foods in Korea. From left to right: gimpub prepared from dried laver seaweed; *Porphyra* spp., salad prepared from a brown seaweed; *Undaria pinnatifida*, soup prepared with dried laver seaweed; mi-yeok-guk soup prepared from dried miyeok.

commonly is consumed as a soup (mi-yeok-guk and mom-guk), snack (kimbugak), vegetable, pickle, or salad or is used to prepare gim-bap (a rolled mixture of gim and a steamed white rice, to which different land vegetables and meats are added) (Figure 15.1). Gim-bap is a popular food in Korea as a simple lunch or side dish. Dried and fresh gim is consumed by Koreans every day as a side dish. Mom-guk is a popular traditional soup on Jeju Island, and the soup is prepared from boiling *Sargassum* seaweed with pork bones (Kim, 2015; Fleurence and Levine, 2016). Harvesting from the wild and from cultivation (mariculture, land-based culture, and farming) are the major seaweed production methods. According to the FAO database, Chile is the highest seaweed collector from the wild in 2012 (436,035 tons) which accounts for 39% of total seaweed production from wild collection. However, in 2014 Korea alone commercially cultivated around 283,707 tons of sea mustard, 397,841 tons of lavar seaweed, 6,055 tons of green laver, and 16,563 tons of other brown seaweed species (FAO, 2014). The commercial seaweed farms in Korea are mainly concentrated on the west side of the southern coast, where almost 90% of the total production in Korea happens. Figure 15.2 illustrates the types of the edible seaweed and secondary metabolites responsible for the functional properties.

15.2 What Is Seaweed?

Terrestrial plants require a rigid structure to stand against gravity and most have well-developed root, leaf, and vascular systems. In contrast to terrestrial plants, seaweed requires a flexible structure to withstand the constant stress coming from the ocean currents and motion (Nautiyal, 2013). Generally, the term "seaweed" is used to define macroscopic, multicellular marine algal species (Lobban and Harrison, 1994). There are more than 10,000 known seaweed species, and many of them are edible and rich

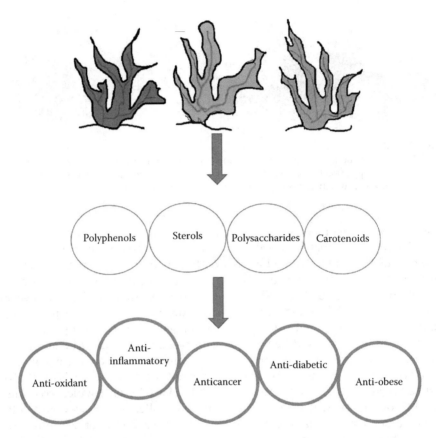

FIGURE 15.2
Some metabolites and their functional properties reported from Korean edible seaweed.

in essential nutrients (Mouritsen, 2009). The ecology of seaweed is dominated by two major environmental conditions: the presence of seawater and light sufficient to drive photosynthesis (Yoon et al., 2010). In addition to these major requirements, a firm attachment point is also essential for seaweed growth. Therefore, seaweed habitats are only in the intertidal and subtidal zones until the light is available for their photosynthesis (Gupta and Abu-Ghannam, 2011).

Seaweed can be classified into three major groups according to the seaweed's appearance: green seaweed (Chlorophyta), brown seaweed (Phaeophyta), and red seaweed (Rhodophyta) (Lobban et al., 1994; MacArtain et al., 2007). Green seaweed produces chlorophyll a and chlorophyll b in similar quantities like "higher" plants. Thus, due to the prominence of green color pigments, Chlorophyta seaweed has a green color appearance. In the case of Phaeophyta seaweed, it produces "fucoxanthin," a brown color xanthophyll pigment that masks other pigments such as chlorophylls a and c and other xanthophylls. Thus, Phaeophyta seaweed is brown in color. Rhodophyta seaweed produces a red color phycoerythrin, and phycocyanin masks the other green and yellow color pigments, including chlorophyll and beta-carotene (Gupta et al., 2011).

When considering the composition of seaweed, the fresh seaweed biomass contains a high amount of moisture and can account for up to 94% of the biomass. Like other plants, seaweed contains proteins, lipids, carbohydrates, vitamins (A, Bl, B12, C, D, E, folic acid, niacin, pantothenic acid, and riboflavin) and essential minerals (Ca, K, Na, and P). However, some studies have revealed that the nutrient composition of seaweed depends on the growth season and the area of production (Dhargalkar and Pereira, 2005; Holdt and Kraan, 2011). Traditionally, seaweed has been utilized as traditional cuisine and medicine in Asian countries such as Korea, China, and Japan (Sanjeewa et al., 2016). In addition to the nutritional value of seaweed, accumulated evidence has suggested that the metabolites (polysaccharides, polyphenols, sterols, and lipids) synthesized in seaweed possess numerous bioactive properties such as anticancer, anti-inflammation, and antioxidant properties (Lee et al., 2013). In contrast to Asians, Europeans consume less amounts of seaweed because of regulations and their food habits. However, because of the identification of invaluable health effects associated with seaweed, in order to increase seaweed consumption, European governments have started to adapt flexible rules on food products containing seaweed as an ingredient to increase seaweed consumption (Mabeau and Fleurence, 1993). Thus, food products containing seaweed as a functional ingredient appear to be continually growing in the market. Moreover, recent studies have demonstrated that polysaccharides, polyphenols, carotenoids, and sterols separated from brown seaweed have the potential to develop as functional materials due to the promising bioactivity.

15.3 Traditional Korean Foods from Seaweed

Seaweed has been used as human food since ancient times. This use has been traced back to the sixth century in China and fourth century in Japan. Especially, ancient Korean, Chinese, and Japanese people who lived near coastal areas highly preferred consuming seaweed as a main or side dish, or as a soup (Kılınç et al., 2013). Contemporary, seaweed-associated food products have been in high demand all around the world. Moreover, due to this high demand, several countries have already started commercial cultivation of edible seaweed species on a large scale (Hwang et al., 2007a). In the present section, attention is given to the literature about edible seaweed (green, red, and brown types) in Korea.

15.3.1 Edible Green Seaweed

Capsosiphon fulvescens (**mae-sang-i**) is an edible green seaweed. Mae-sang-i is predominant in regions of Korea such as GoHeung, GangJin in JeonNam, JangHeung, and WanDo. Moreover, mae-saeng-i has been traditionally used as a functional food for centuries in Korea (Park, 2005). Mae-sang-i's dried biomass contains polysaccharides (55%), proteins (30%), lipids (1%), and ash (13%). Moreover, mae-sang-i contains considerable amounts of Fe and Se compared to other seaweed it is also rich in Na, Mg, Ca, K, and P. Fructose, galactose, glucose, maltose, and sucrose are the major free sugar types present in mae-sang-i biomass (Yang et al., 2005), which is a popular dish in Korea due to its health-enhancing properties, such as addressing stomach disorders and hangovers (Hwang et al., 2008). Usually, Korean people consume this seaweed as a soup after boiling it with oysters or steaming mae-sang-i with rice to prepare gul-guk-bap. In addition, powdered mae-sang-i is popular because it can be added to diverse dishes such as juice, porridge, and soup.

Enteromorpha prolifera (**Ga-si-pa-rae**) is an abundant green seaweed in East Asian (Korea, China, and Japan) marine ecosystems (Cho et al., 2011b). This seaweed is consumed as a raw salad or boiled with hot water to consume as a soup or use as a sea vegetable. In addition, *E. prolifera* is used as an ingredient in cookies or meals or as a flavoring agent (Aguilera-Morales et al., 2005). The southern coast of Korea is popular for the cultivation of *Enteromorpha* species for traditional side dishes (Huh et al., 2004). The dried biomass contains 9%~14% proteins, 32%~36% ash, and n-3 and n-6 fatty acids (10.4 and 10.9 g/100 g of total fatty acids, respectively) (Aguilera-Morales et al., 2005). Thus, *E. prolifera* is a rich source of essential nutrients. Moreover, studies have revealed that the extracts and compounds collected from this seaweed have bioactive properties such as anticancer and anti-inflammation (Hiqashi-Okaj et al., 1999).

Caulerpa lentillifera (**Ba-da-po-do**), also known as seagrape/green caviar, is a green seaweed that is naturally distributed in tropical regions. *C. lentillifera* is usually consumed as a fresh salad or in a salt-preserved form. This seaweed contains around 10% protein, 16.76% polyunsaturated fatty acid (PUFA), and 30% dietary fibers from its dry weight. Moreover, *C. lentillifera* is rich in essential minerals (Na, K, Ca, and Mg) and omega-3 fatty acids (Matanjun et al., 2009). Moreover, some studies confirmed that the extracts separated from *C. lentillifera* have a potential to develop as anticancer, antioxidative, and antidiabetic agents (Nguyen et al., 2011; Sharma and Rhyu, 2014).

Enteromorpha linza, prefers to grow on rocky surfaces and rapidly colonizes bare surfaces (Cho et al., 2011a). Traditionally, *E. linza* has been consumed as a soup, seasoned cooked vegetables, or after mixing with vegetables and spices.

15.3.2 Edible Red Seaweed

Porphyra **spp. (Gim)** is one of the popular edible red seaweed in East Asia. According to the Food and Agricultural Organization, laver is a nutritious seaweed that contains more than 30% proteins, and about 75% of that is digestible. Moreover, laver is low in sugar and contains high amounts of vitamins A, B, and C (Fleurence and Levine, 2016). *Porphyra* spp. (*P. tenera* and *P. yezoensis*) are processed into many commercial food products, such as dried seasoned laver and roasted laver for sushi (Park et al., 2014), both of which are in considerable demand in Korean food markets as well as in the international market due to the high nutritional value, texture, compactness, and pleasant taste of processed *Porphyra* spp. (Park et al., 2014; Cho et al., 2015). Usually, gim is consumed in a dried form. Gimbugak (snack) and gim-bap are excellent examples of processed gim (Oh and Choi, 2015).

Gracilariopsis chorda is a red seaweed popular for its extensive medicinal benefits and its use as a food ingredient in Korea, Japan, and China (Mohibbullah et al., 2016). *G. chorda* is considered a valuable and important seaweed as it can be used as a raw material to extract agar.

Gelidium amansii is a popular edible red seaweed commonly used as a food ingredient in Asian countries such as Korea, China, and Japan (Kang et al., 2016b). This seaweed is a rich source of carbohydrates, especially galactose (23%) and glucose (20%) (Wi et al., 2009). *G. amansii* is considering a cheap source of agar. Thus, this red seaweed is commonly cultivated for agar production (Kang et al., 2013).

15.3.3 Edible Brown Seaweed

Hizikia fusiforme **(tot)** is a large, annual brown seaweed that naturally grows in Korea, China, and Japan; it has been used as an ingredient in traditional Chinese medicine for thousands of years (Chen et al., 2012). *H. fusiformis* is widely consumed by people who live near the coastal regions of Korea. In addition to Korea, tot is also a popular edible seaweed in Japan and China (Choi et al., 2009). It grows from the bottom of the eulittoral to the top of the sublittoral zone, around the Korean peninsula. *H. fusiformis* is consumed as a seaweed salad and often is used as an ingredient in covered rice and bi-bim-bap a mixture of rice with seasoned vegetables and chili pepper paste. During the last two decades, the market demand for hijiki has increased due to the proved nutritional and health effects of this seaweed (Hu et al., 2013). However, to avoid unsustainable harvesting, currently harvesting it from October to January along the Jeju coastal waters is prohibited by government laws (Ko et al., 2010).

Laminaria japonica **(da-si-ma)** has been commonly consumed as a sea vegetable in Pacific and Asian countries. Moreover, Korean people use this seaweed in traditional medicine to promote postnatal maternal health. Da-si-ma is commercially cultivated in the temperate seaside areas of the northwest Pacific region (Islam et al., 2013). Da-si-ma sliced into 5 ~ 6 cm long strips and boiled with hot water or dried da-si-ma can be eaten as cookies with green tea; sometimes, it is pickled in vinegar.

Undaria pinnatifida **(mi-yeok)** has a long history as a food resource and is popular as a food ingredient in Korea, which is one of its largest commercial cultivators (Choi et al., 2007b). The coastal area of the southern Korean peninsula is a popular area for growth and cultivation of this seaweed. *U. pinnatifida* is generally served with soup, salad, and side dishes (Kim, 2010). In addition, it is a popular food supplement among Korean mothers. Especially, a soup prepared from this seaweed is served to Korean mothers who given birth because Koreans traditionally believed that the soup prepared from *U. pinnatifida* has a potential to help postpartum convalescence and cleans the blood (Cho et al., 2007).

Sargassum fulvellum **(mo-ja-ban)** is a cheap and popular sea vegetable in Korean food markets. This seaweed is widely grown from the southern to the eastern coast of Korea. Especially, people on Jeju Island use this seaweed as a cooked vegetable, salad, and soup (mom-guk) or consume it as a side dish (Choi et al., 2007b; Hwang et al., 2007b). In addition to the food value, in traditional medicine *S. fulvellum* biomass can be used as an ingredient to treat inflammatory diseases such as a lump, dropsy, swollen and painful scrotum, and to treat urinary problems (Gwon et al., 2013).

Pelvetia siliquosa **(tum-bu-gi)** is a brown seaweed belonging to the family Fucaceae and endemic to the Korean peninsula, where it grows on the rocky surfaces of the southern seashores. *P. siliquosa* has been utilized as an important source of alginic acid. Traditionally, Korean people consume tum-bu-gi as a soup, salad, or seasoned vegetable (Lee et al., 2002; Yoon et al., 2003).

15.4 Bioactive Compounds

15.4.1 Polysaccharides

Sulfated polysaccharides are interesting macromolecules present in seaweed with a diverse range of bioactive properties to use in medical, pharmaceutical, functional food, and biotechnological applications including anticoagulant, anti-inflammatory, antioxidant, immunostimulatory, and antitumor agents (Groth et al., 2009). Studies have reported that polysaccharides present in seaweed are safer than the mammalian polysaccharides for drug discovery and applications in other potential industries. Other than the safety, the ability of mass production with low cost is another major advantage of seaweed polysaccharides (Blondin and de Agostiniz, 1995; Senni et al., 2011).

15.4.1.1 Fucoidans

Fucoidans (Figure 15.3) in brown seaweed represent a class of fucose-enriched sulfated polysaccharides found in brown seaweed cell walls with interesting bioactive properties such as antioxidant, anticancer, anticoagulant, and immunity modulation. Fucoidan is built up with a substantial amount of L-fucose, galactose, and sulfate with small amounts of guluronic acid, rhamnose, arabinose, and xylose (Synytsya et al., 2010). The main skeleton of fucoidans primarily consists of $(1 \rightarrow 3)$-linked α-L-fucose. However, this structure contains repeating sequences of alternating $\alpha(1 \rightarrow 3)$ and $\alpha(1 \rightarrow 4)$ glycosidic bonds. Due to the significant differences in fucoidan structure,

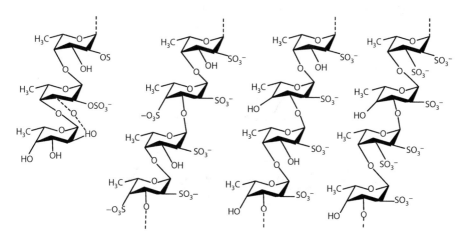

FIGURE 15.3
Chemical structures of fucoidans separated from brown seaweed.

fucoidans are very diverse in nature and structure heavily depends on the seaweed source. Moreover, bioactive properties of fucoidans depend on their structural properties (Berteau and Mulloy, 2003).

15.4.1.2 Laminarin

Laminarin is the most abundant storage polysaccharide present in brown seaweed (Figure 15.4), representing 35% of seaweed dry weight. However, the percentage of laminarin in seaweed depends on seaweed species, harvesting season, habitat, and extraction method (Kadam et al., 2015). Laminarin is a linear polysaccharide composed of (1,3)-β-D-glucan with β(1,6) branching. According to the reducing end, laminarins divided into two groups as M- and G-chains. M-chains end with a mannitol residue and G-chains end with a glucose residue (Rioux et al., 2007). Laminarin has many reported bioactivities such as anticancer, anti-inflammatory, anticoagulant, and antioxidant activities (Kadam et al., 2015).

15.4.1.3 Alginic Acid

Alginic acids are high molecular weight polysaccharides present in the brown seaweed cell wall and in the mucilage or intercellular matrix. Alginic acids are alkali-soluble polysaccharides, where the other cell wall constituents, such as fucoidan and laminarin, are water soluble. Moreover, seaweed contains 10% ~ 40% of alginic acid from their dry weight. The amount of alginic acid closely related to growing depth and season (Rioux et al., 2007). The structure of alginic acid is composed of linear polysaccharides containing 1,4-linked β-D-mannuronic and α-L-guluronic acid residues arranged

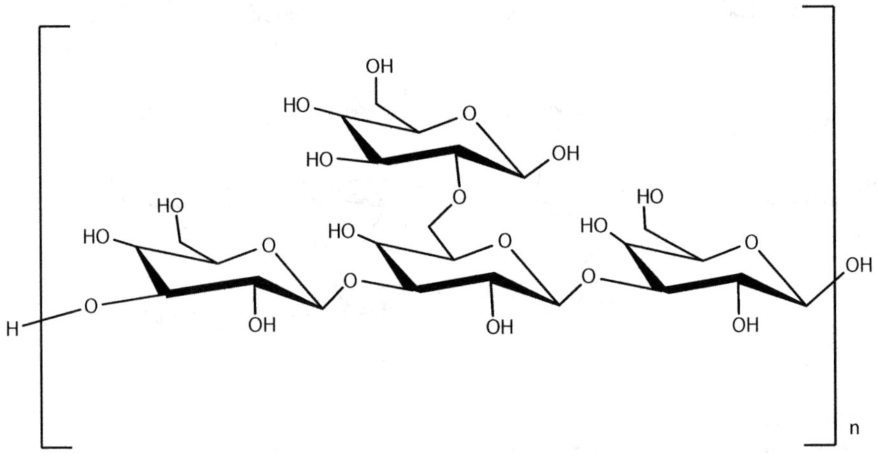

FIGURE 15.4
General structure of laminarin, a storage polysaccharide present in brown seaweed.

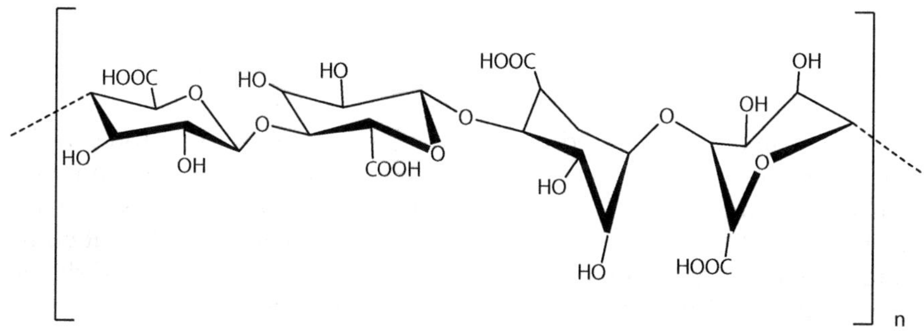

Edible Korean Seaweed 369

FIGURE 15.5
The chemical structure of the repeating unit's alginic acids.

simultaneously along the chain (Figure 15.5). Alginates are importantly used as an ingredient in food products as thickening agents or metal ion chelators (Gupta et al., 2011).

15.4.1.4 Carrageenans

Carrageenans are linear hydrophilic sulfated polysaccharides of D-galactose and 3,6-anhydro-D-galactose present in red seaweed (Figure 15.6). Most red seaweed produces carrageenans as the main cell-wall material. However, there is not considerable information about the biosynthesis of carrageenans and the genetics of the red seaweed cell wall (De Ruiter and Rudolph, 1997). In the food industry, carrageenans are used as an ingredient due to their important physical and functional properties. They are also commonly used as a thickening, stabilizing, or gelling agent (Campo et al., 2009). According to McHugh (2003), the total market for carrageenans was more than 300 million dollars in 2003.

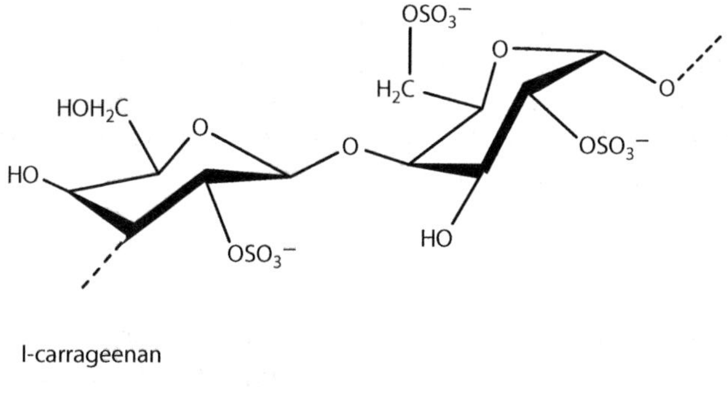

l-carrageenan

FIGURE 15.6
Repeating unit of the red seaweed polysaccharide, carrageenans.

15.4.1.5 Ulvan

Ulvan is a complex polysaccharide present in the green seaweed cell wall. Ulvans represent about 8%~29% of seaweed dry weight. The structure of ulvans is mainly composed of rhamnose, glucuronic and iduronic acids, and xylose. In addition, type A ulvanobiuronic acid 3-sulfate (A3s) and type B ulvanobiuronic acid 3-sulfate (B3s) are the major repeating units of ulvan (Robic et al., 2008). Partially sulfated xylose residues at the O-2 position in uronic acids and glucuronic acid can branch at the O-2 position of rhamnose 3-sulfate (Robic et al., 2009). Studies have reported that ulvans possess bioactive properties such as antioxidant, anticoagulant, immunomodulatory, antiviral, antihypercholesterolemic, antihyperlipidemic, and anticancer activities. Purified ulvans are used to form biomaterials such as microparticles, nanofibrous membrane, nanofibers, and molecular sponges for cell culture (Coste et al., 2015).

15.4.2 Polyphenols

Phenolic compounds are water-soluble plant substances naturally present in cell vacuoles that carry interesting bioactive activities such as anticancer, anti-inflammatory, and antioxidant properties (Harborne 1998; Manach et al., 2005). Chemical structures of phenols can be defined as an aromatic ring of carbon that bears one or more hydroxyl substituents. According to the Handique and Baruah (2002) model, polyphenol compounds are capable of pairing or reacting with one-electron oxidants formed during biological processes. As a result of this mode of action, polyphenol compounds are believed to be the major bioactive compounds found in biological systems (Handique and Baruah, 2002). Terrestrial polyphenols are polymers of flavonoids and gallic acid, and polyphenols in seaweed phlorotannins (reported only in brown seaweed) are chains of 1,3,5-trihydroxybenzene formed in the acetate–malonate pathway (Ragan 1973; Ragan et al., 1986; Sithranga and Kathiresen, 2010). Phlorotannins isolated from brown seaweed represent the most exclusively studied class of marine secondary metabolites (Fernando et al., 2016). Phlorotannins are considered as naturally occurring secondary metabolites with potential uses in economically important industries such as pharmacology and the functional food industry (Xiaojun et al., 1996; Mohamed et al., 2012). Figure 15.7 illustrates the chemical structures of some phlorotannins isolated from brown seaweed.

15.4.3 Carotenoids

Carotenoids are orange, purple, red, or yellow light-absorbing isoprenoid polyene pigments existing in chloroplast, reported from bacteria, fungi, seaweed, and higher plants. The main roles of carotenoids in photosynthetic organisms are light absorption functions, which help photosynthesis,

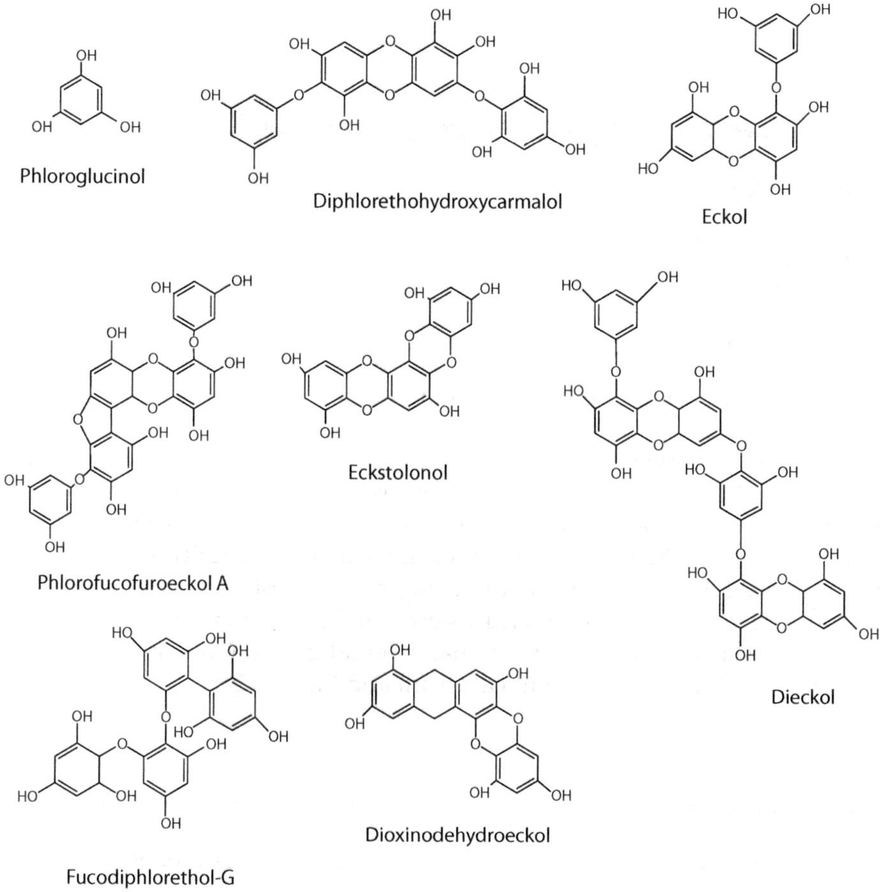

Edible Korean Seaweed 371

FIGURE 15.7
Bioactive phlorotannins from brown seaweed.

photoprotection, phototropism, and photoreception, or act as a repellent for their natural enemies (Matsuno, 2001; Dembitsky and Maoka, 2007). The bioactive properties of carotenoids depend on the polyene chains. A number of conjugated double bonds and the nature of cyclic end groups located in polyene chains determine the singlet oxygen-quenching properties and free radical scavenging activities of carotenoids (Britton, 1995).

Fucoxanthin is a major carotenoid present in brown seaweed. It is the most abundant of all carotenoids, accounting for more than 10% of the estimated total natural production of carotenoids (Matsuno, 2001). Due to the proved bioactive properties of fucoxanthin, it is currently used as a functional material in industries like functional foods, cosmeceuticals, and nutraceuticals (Peng et al., 2011). Figure 15.8 shows a general chemical structure of fucoxanthin isolated from seaweed.

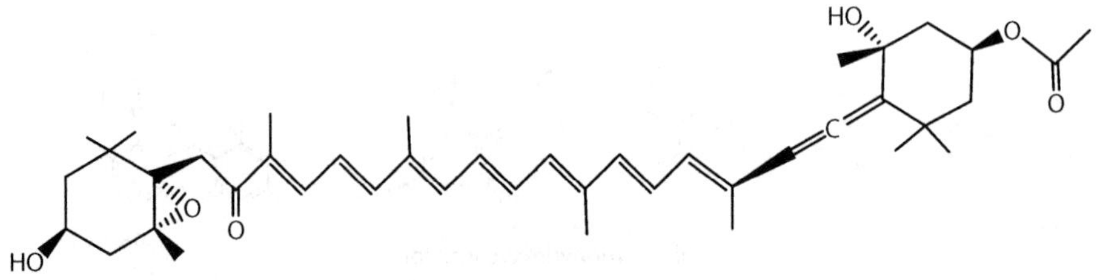

FIGURE 15.8
Chemical structure of fucoxanthin.

15.4.4 Sterols

Sterols are one of the important compounds in eukaryotic cell membranes. Moreover, cholesterols are major sterols of vertebrate organisms and a mixture of phytosterols is contained in photosynthetic organisms. Conversion of farnesyl diphosphate into squalene activates the isoprenoid pathway, which stimulates the sterol production in biological systems (Hartmann, 1998; Lopes et al., 2013). Seaweed is an important source of bioactive sterols. It has been reported that sterol biosynthesis in green (ergosterol), red (cholesterol and its derivatives), and brown (fucosterols and its derivatives) seaweed has the potential to develop as a functional material in different industries such as functional foods or nutraceuticals (Kim and Van Ta, 2011).

15.5 Potential Bioactive Properties as Functional Ingredients

Functional foods are one of the major food categories for the global health and wellness market. The term "functional" is used for food products that can possess tertiary functions other than "primary" and "secondary" functions that are related to nutritional value and preference. In general, functional food items are directly involved in the modulation of physiological systems including immune, endocrine, nerve, circulatory, and digestive systems (Arai, 1996). Thus, according to the aforementioned definition, secondary metabolites found in edible seaweed with bioactive properties such as antioxidant, anticancer, anti-inflammatory, antidiabetic, and antiobesity properties might potentially be developed as ingredients due to their therapeutic value. Here we discuss some interesting bioactive properties studied from edible Korean seaweed. Table 15.1 represents the seaweed with its bioactive properties.

15.5.1 Antioxidant

Being exposed to the environment of varying light and oxygen conditions induces the production of free radicals and oxidizing agents such as

TABLE 15.1

Reported Bioactive Compounds and Bioactivities of Edible Korean Seaweed

Name	Food Types	Bioactive Compound	Bioactivities	Ref.
Capsosiphon fulvescens	Soup	Polysaccharides	Anticancer and Anticoagulant	Kim et al., 2013; Synytsya et al., 2015
Caulerpa lentillifera	Salad	Polyphenols, omega-3-fatty acids	Anticancer, antioxidant, and antidiabetic	Nguyen et al., 2011; Sharma and Rhyu, 2014
Enteromorpha linza	Soup	Crude extracts	Antimicrobial and antifungal	Cho et al., 2011a
Enteromorpha prolifera	Soup, vegetable, snack, and flavoring agent	Pheophorbide	Anticancer, antioxidant, and anti-inflammation	Hiqashi-Okaj et al., 1999; Cho et al., 2011a
Gelidium amansii	Agar	–	–	Kang et al., 2016b
Gracilariopsis chorda	Agar	Arachidonic acid	Antioxidant	Mohibbullah et al., 2015
Porphyra tenera	Laver, gimbab, and kimbugak	Methanolic and water extracts	Anticancer	Kim et al., 2006
Porphyra yezoensis	Laver, gimbab, and kimbugak	–	Anticancer	Park et al., 2014; Cho et al., 2015
Hizikia fusiformis	Soup and salad	Organic solvent extracts	Antioxidant, anti-inflammation	Siriwardhana et al., 2003; Choi et al., 2009
Sargassum spp.	Cooked vegetable, salad, and soup	Fucoidan	Antioxidant, anticancer, and antiinflammation	Yang et al., 2013
Laminaria spp.	Salad, soup, and used as a condiment	Enzymatic extracts	Anti-inflammation and antioxidant	Cho et al., 2007; Kasimala et al., 2015
Pelvetia siliquosa	Alginic acid	Methanol extract	Hepatoprotective and antidiabetic	Lee et al., 2002
Undaria pinnatifida	Soup, salad, and side dishes	Fucoidan and phlorotaninns	Antioxidant and anticancer	Kim, 2010; Synytsya et al., 2010

hydrogen peroxide (H_2O_2), the hydroxyl radical (HO·), and the superoxide anion $\left(O_2^{\bullet-}\right)$. Seaweed produces antioxidant compounds to protect itself against oxidative damage as it is continuously exposed to hazardous environmental conditions.

Recently, a number of studies have reported that compounds and crude extracts collected from Korean edible seaweed have promising antioxidant properties in *in vitro* and *in vivo* conditions. Mohibbullah et al. (2015) reported that ethanol extract from *Gracilariopsis chorda* (GCE) had the highest neuroprotective effect against hypoxia/reoxygenation (H/R)-induced oxidative stress. Furthermore, the authors suggested that the active compound in the ethanol extract is arachidonic acid, which is responsible for neuroprotection against H/R-induced oxidative stress. Tong et al. (2014) reported antioxidant properties of the four extracts separated from *Hizikia fusiforme, Capsosiphon fulvescens, Undaria pinnatifida sporophyll*, and *Undaria pinnatifida* blades collected from Wando, Korea. According to the authors, among the tested seaweed extracts, *H. fusiforme* had best DPPH radical scavenging activity (90.12%, at a concentration of 0.32 mg/mL), followed by the *U. pinnatifida* blade. In addition, reducing power values are also high in *H. fusiforme* and *U. pinnatifida* extracts compared to the others. The promising antioxidant activity of a chlorophyll compound, pheophorbide, separated from *Enteromorpha prolifera* (green seaweed) was reported by Cho et al. (2011a). According to the results, the extracts had significantly high DDPH radical scavenging, hydroxyl radical scavenging, and reducing power compared to commercial antioxidants such as BHA and α-tocopherol.

Attempts made by Kim (2010) to evaluate antioxidant activities of two seaweed (*Undaria pinnatifida* and *Capsosiphon fulvescens*) yielded positive results. According to the author, DPPH radical scavenging activity and phlorotannins contents were higher in the extracts collected from the vacuum drying method compared to the hot air drying method (Kim, 2010). Cha et al. (2012) documented promising antioxidant effects of phlorotannins isolated from *Ecklonia cava* collected from the coast of Jeju Island, Korea. According to the results, phlorotannins isolated from *E. cava* demonstrated significant photoprotective effects following UV-B exposure in zebrafish embryo without showing any toxic effect. In addition, Siriwardhana et al. (2003) reported that water and organic extracts (diethyl ether, chloroform, ethyl acetate, acetone, ethanol, and methanol) collected from *Hizikia fusiformis* indicated antioxidant properties.

15.5.2 Anticancer

Cancer-associated diseases are considered a principal cause of death all around the world. Within the last few decades, the rate of new cancer incidence has dramatically increased with unusual eating habits and the changing lifestyles of humans. Some studies report that the phytochemicals isolated from marine organisms have a potential to develop as anticancer drugs with

Edible Korean Seaweed 375

lighter side effects compared to those of synthetic drugs (Sithranga and Kathiresen, 2010). Programmed cell death (apoptosis) is a natural process of cell death and is controlled by a group of intercellular proteases known as caspases. However, failures occurring in the normal apoptosis pathway are considered as the major cause for diagnosing cancer. Especially, deregulated levels of apoptosis in cancer cells are the principal barrier for eliminating them in an effective manner. Therefore, the compounds capable of restoring apoptosis are known to be a promising strategy for combating cancer cells (Fesik, 2005).

Kim et al. (2015b) reported that the ethanol extract prepared from laver, *Porphyra tenera* (PTE), has an anticancer effect on human oral squamous carcinoma YD-10B cells. According to the results, incubation of YD-10B cells with PTE (50–200 µg/mL) for 24 or 48 h had a potential to induce apoptotic cell death in those cells. According to Western blot protein expressions, down-regulation of procaspase3, procaspase9, BCL-2, and AIF and up-regulation of cleaved-PARP and cytochrome c might be responsible for inducing apoptosis in YD-10B cells (Kim et al., 2015b). Synytsya et al. (2010) attempted to evaluate the anticancer effect of fucoidan isolated from *Undaria pinnatifida* (mi-yeok) on four cancer cell lines. According to the results, commercial fucoidan and isolated fucoidan had similar anticancer properties (HeLa; cervical cancer cell, PC-3; prostate cancer cell, A549; carcinomic human alveolar basal epithelial cell and HepG2; hepatocellular carcinoma cell) under the tested concentrations (0.0~1.0 mg/mL).

However, Lee at al. (2012) reported that fucoidan purchased from Sigma-Aldrich has an anticancer effect on A549 cells with IC_{50} values with <200 µg/mL. Cho et al. (1997) reported the antimutagenic and anticancer properties of the methanol extracts collected from nine Korean seaweed (sea lettuce, chlorella, sea tangle, sea mustard, sporophyll of sea mustard, fusiforme, seaweed papulosa, purple laver, and Ceylon moss). According to the authors, almost all seaweed extracts showed promising antimutagenic activity against aflatoxin B1 (AFB1) and N-methyl-N'-nitro-N-nitrosoguanidine (MNNG) in the *Salmonella typhimurium* TA100. In addition, sea tangle, sea mustard, and sporophyll of sea mustard extracts possess promising anticancer activity on AGS human gastric adenocarcinoma cells and HT-29 human colon carcinoma cells at a 0.2 mg/mL concentration.

15.5.3 Anti-Inflammation

The word "inflammation" is commonly used to define the complex biological responses of infected or damaged cells to protect host cells from offending agents such as bacteria, viruses, and other pathogens. However, studies have been revealed that prolong and uncontrolled inflammatory responses have a potential to induce disease conditions such as Alzheimer's disease, rheumatoid arthritis, inflammatory bowel disease, and cancer. The term "anti-inflammation" refers to the property of a treatment or substance that has the ability to modulate inflammatory responses in a host (Thun et al., 2004). Interestingly, a large number of studies have reported that secondary metabolites present in seaweed have potential anti-inflammatory activities in *in vitro* and *in vivo* models (Kim et al., 2015c; Lee et al., 2016b).

Nuclear factor kappa B (NF-κB) and mitogen-activated protein kinases (MAPK) are the two known sell-signaling pathways associated with inflammatory responses. In general, first, macrophage cells are activated by offending agents such as bacterial lipopolysaccharides (LPS). Under normal conditions, NF-κB protein in the cytosol stays in an inactivated form; activation of this protein is controlled by another protein known as IκBα. However, when the macrophage cells exposed to the LPS IκBα quickly phosphorylates into pIκBα. Due to the sudden reduction of IκBα, the activation of the NF-κB protein and its translocation to the nucleus happens. The translocation induces the transcription of genes related to iNOS and COX-2 proteins. Finally, iNOS stimulates NO production and COX-2 induces PGE_2 production (Yamamoto and Gaynor, 2001; Wang et al., 2012). In addition, accumulating evidence suggests that the MAPK signaling cascade has an important role in activation of the NF-κB signaling cascade and meditates proinflammatory cytokine expression in macrophage cells such as interleukin 1β (IL-1β), IL-6, and tumor necrosis factor alpha (TNF-α) (Beyaert et al., 1996; Wu et al., 2015). Thus, regulation or inhibition of MAPK and NF-κB signaling cascades is found to be the key function of anti-inflammatory drugs.

Previously, *in vivo* (BALB/c mice) anti-inflammatory activity of *U. pinnatifida* and *L. japonica* was documented by Cho et al. (2007). Their results demonstrated that ethanol extract and the dichloromethane (0.4 mg/ear) extracts had strongly protective effects against mouse ear edema induced by phorbol 12-myristate 13-acetate (PMA) without showing any acute toxicity on the tested animals. Importantly, the authors proposed that the protective effect of their extracts was similar to those of the commonly used drugs indomethacin and acetyl salicylic acid (5 g/kg bw) (Cho et al., 2007). Khan et al. (2009) performed a similar study to Cho et al. using a methanol extract collected from *U. pinnatifida*. According to the results, this extract from the seaweed was active against mouse ear edema induced by PMA, with an IC_{50} of 10.3 mg/mL. However, according to the Cho et al. (2007) ethanol extracts are more effective than methanol as at a concentration 0.4 mg/ear, ethanol extract inhibited the ear edema by 95.3%. In addition, Kang et al. (2016a) attempted to isolate bioactive compound from *U. pinnatifida* through supercritical fluid extraction and evaluate the *in vivo* anti-inflammatory activity on a mouse model. The essential oil from *U. pinnatifida* was active against mouse ear inflammation induced by PBA, with IC_{50} values of 87, 134, and 158 µg per ear for edema and erythema.

Jung et al. (2013) reported *in vitro* anti-inflammatory activities of fucosterol and seven phlorotannins collected from edible brown seaweed *Eisenia bicyclis*. According to the results, all phlorotannins effectively inhibited LPS-induced NO production via down-regulating iNOS and COX-2 gene expression. In

Edible Korean Seaweed 377

addition, fucosterol also inhibited *tert*-butylhydroperoxide (*t*-BHP)-induced reactive oxygen species generation and suppressed the expression of iNOS and COX-2. In addition to this significant observation, Sevevirathne et al. (2012) reported that enzymatic hydrolysates collected from *Laminaria japonica* also possess antioxidant and anti-inflammatory activities under *in vitro* conditions.

15.5.4 Antidiabetic and Antiobese

Diabetes mellitus is a leading cause of mortality and increased disability-adjusted life years worldwide. This is a complex and chronic metabolic disease, which disturbs the glucose metabolism with abnormally high plasma glucose levels. In Korea, the prevalence of diabetes increased from 8.6% in 2001 to 11.0% in 2013. In addition, at the same period prevalence of adult obesity, considered the most important risk factor for diabetes mellitus, increased 2.5% (from 29.2% to 31.8%) (Ha and Kim, 2015). Obesity is a metabolic disorder that can be defined as increased body weight caused by excessive fat accumulation. Obesity presents a risk to health with an increase in health problems and reduced life expectancy by inducing other chronic disease conditions. Therefore, it is important to control obesity to reduce the risk of diabetic and other conditions such as cardiovascular and renal diseases associated with diabetes (Lee et al., 2016a). Recently, a number of studies have reported that compounds and extracts isolated from edible seaweed possess promising antidiabetic and antiobesity properties. In this section, recent findings of antidiabetic and antiobesity properties reported from Korean edible seaweed are briefly introduced.

Recently, Kang et al. (2016a) evaluated the *in vitro* and *in vivo* antidiabetic effects of 70% ethanol extract from *Gelidium amansii* (GAE). According to the authors, under *in vitro* conditions GAE suppressed differentiation of 3T3-L1 adipocyte through down-regulation of adipogenesis and lipogenesis. In addition to this significant finding, their *in vivo* experiment on obesity induced by a high-fat diet (HFD) mouse model also yielded promising results. GAE decreased the body weight gain and adipose cell size in HFD-induced obesity in mice. Oh et al. (2016) reported that extracts from *L. japonica* have the potential to induce insulin resistance in HFD-induced obesity in C57BL/6N mice. Thus, the group administered *L. japonica* extract showed resistance against HFD-induced obesity. Kim et al. (2014) reported that fucoidan obtained from a commercial dealer (Haewon Biotech, Seoul, Korea) had promising antiobesity activity on HFD-induced obesity in C57BL/6 mice. According to the results, HFD + 1% fucoidan and HFD + 2% fucoidan down-regulated mRANA expression of PPARγ, aP2, and ACC in epididymal fat tissues compared to the group administered HFD alone. Kim and Lee (2012) investigated the antiobesity effect of fucoidan extracted from *U. pinnatifida*. The authors assessed the obesity-specific therapeutic action of fucoidan in 3T3-L1 adipocytes. They demonstrated that fucoidan possesses antiobesity properties on 3T3-L1 cells via suppressing proliferator-activated receptor γ, CCAAR/enhancer-binding protein α, and adipocyte protein 2, which decreased the expression of inflammatory genes during adipogenesis in 3T3-L1 adipocytes.

15.6 Conclusion

As a food and medicine, seaweed has a long history in Asian countries such as Korea, China, and Japan. In contrast to Asians, most Europeans have neglected seaweed as a food source. Thus, seaweed is not a popular food in Western countries. Korea is one of the biggest consumers and producers of edible seaweed. Traditionally, Koreans have consumed seaweed as salads or boiled soup with water. In addition, dried seaweed has been used to prepare gim-bap, condiments or snacks to drink with tea. In addition to the nutritional value, with the advancement of science and technology, numerous studies have highlighted bioactive properties associated with secondary metabolites present in Korean edible seaweed. Thus, consumption of seaweed provides long-term health benefits in addition to its nutritional value. In this chapter, we discussed edible seaweed types in Korea and their bioactive effects, such as anticancer, anti-inflammatory, antioxidant, and antidiabetic properties. Therefore, the content in this chapter might be useful to increase consumption of seaweed as functional materials in the near future, not only in Asia but also in the rest of the world.

References

Aguilera-Morales, M., M. Casas-Valdez, S. Carrillo-Domínguez, B. González-Acosta, and F. Pérez-Gil. 2005. Chemical composition and microbiological assays of marine algae *Enteromorpha* spp. as a potential food source. *J Food Compos Anal* 18:79–88.

Arai, S. 1996. Studies on functional foods in Japan—State of the art. *Biosci Biotechnol Biochem* 60:9–15.

Berteau, O., and B. Mulloy. 2003. Sulfated fucans, fresh perspectives: Structures, functions, and biological properties of sulfated fucans and an overview of enzymes active toward this class of polysaccharide. *Glycobiology* 13:29–40.

Beyaert, R., A. Cuenda, W. Vanden Berghe et al. 1996. The p38/RK mitogen-activated protein kinase pathway regulates interleukin-6 synthesis response to tumor necrosis factor. *EMBO J* 15:1914–1923.

Blondin, C., and A. de Agostiniz. 1995. Biological activities of polysaccharides from marine algae. *Drugs Future* 20:1237–1249.

Britton, G. 1995. Structure and properties of carotenoids in relation to function. *FASEB J* 9:1551–1558.

Campo, V. L., D. F. Kawano, D. B. d. Silva, Jr., and I. Carvalho. 2009. Carrageenans: Biological properties, chemical modifications and structural analysis—A review. *Carbohydr Polym* 77:167–180.

Cha, S.-H., C.-I. Ko, D. Kim, and Y.-J. Jeon. 2012. Protective effects of phlorotannins against ultraviolet B radiation in zebrafish (*Danio rerio*). *Vet Dermatol* 23:51–56.

Chen, X., W. Nie, G. Yu et al. 2012. Antitumor and immunomodulatory activity of polysaccharides from *Sargassum fusiforme*. *Food Chem Toxicol* 50:695–700.

Cho, E.-J., S.-H. Rhee, and K.-Y. Park. 1997. Antimutagenic and cancer cell growth inhibitory effects of seaweeds. *Prev Nutr Food Sci* 2:348–353.

Cho, H.-B., H.-H. Lee, O.-H. Lee et al. 2011a. Clinical and microbial evaluation of the effects on gingivitis of a mouth rinse containing an *Enteromorpha linza* extract. *J Med Food* 14:1670–1676.

Cho, J.-Y., J.-Y. Kang, M. N. A. Khan et al. 2007. Anti-inflammatory activities of *Undaria pinnatifida* and *Laminaria japonica* (Phaeophyta). *Fish Aquat Sci* 10:127–132.

Cho, M., H.-S. Lee, I.-J. Kang, M.-H. Won, and S. You. 2011b. Antioxidant properties of extract and fractions from *Enteromorpha prolifera*, a type of green seaweed. *Food Chem* 127:999–1006.

Cho, S., J. Kim, M. Yoon et al. 2015. Monitoring and optimization of the effects of the blending ratio of corn, sesame, and perilla oils on the oxidation and sensory quality of seasoned laver pyropia spp. *Fish Aquat Sci* 18:27–33.

Choi, D.-S., Y. Athukorala, Y.-J. Jeon et al. 2007a. Antioxidant activity of sulfated polysaccharides isolated from *Sargassum fulvellum*. *Preventive Food Sci Nutr* 12: 65–73.

Choi, E.-Y., H.-J. Hwang, I.-H. Kim, and T.-J. Nam. 2009. Protective effects of a polysaccharide from *Hizikia fusiformis* against ethanol toxicity in rats. *Food Chem Toxicol* 47:134–139.

Choi, H. G., Y. S. Kim, J. H. Kim et al. 2007b. Effects of temperature and salinity on the growth of *Gracilaria verrucosa* and *G. chorda*, with the potential for mariculture in Korea. *Eighteenth International Seaweed Symposium: Proceedings of the Eighteenth International Seaweed Symposium*, held in Bergen, Norway, 20–25 June 2004. R. Anderson, J. Brodie, E. Onsøyen and A. T. Critchley. Dordrecht, Springer Netherlands: 43–51.

Coste, O., E.-j. Malta, J. C. López, and C. Fernández-Díaz. 2015. Production of sulfated oligosaccharides from the seaweed *Ulva* sp. using a new ulvan-degrading enzymatic bacterial crude extract. *Algal Res* 10:224–231.

Dembitsky, V. M., and T. Maoka. 2007. Allenic and cumulenic lipids. *Prog Lipid Res* 46:328–375.

De Ruiter, G. A., and B. Rudolph. 1997. Carrageenan biotechnology. *Trends Food Sci Technol* 8:389–395.

Dhargalkar, V., and N. Pereira. 2005. Seaweed: Promising plant of the millennium. *Science and Culture* 71:60–65.

FAO. 2014. Fishery and Aquaculture Statistics. Aquaculture production 1950–2012 (FishstatJ). In: FAO Fisheries and Aquaculture Department [online or CD-ROM]. Rome. Updated 2014. http://www.fao.org/fishery/statistics/software/fishstatj/en

Fernando, I. S., M. Kim, K.-T. Son, Y. Jeong, and Y.-J. Jeon. 2016. Antioxidant activity of marine algal polyphenolic compounds: A mechanistic approach. *J Med Food* 19:615–628.

Fesik, S. W. 2005. Promoting apoptosis as a strategy for cancer drug discovery. *Nat Rev Cancer* 5:876–885.

Fleurence, J., and I. Levine. 2016. *Seaweed in health and disease prevention.* San Diego: Academic Press.

Groth, I., N. Grünewald, and S. Alban. 2009. Pharmacological profiles of animal- and nonanimal-derived sulfated polysaccharides—Comparison of unfractionated heparin, the semisynthetic glucan sulfate PS3, and the sulfated polysaccharide fraction isolated from *Delesseria sanguinea. Glycobiology* 19:408–417.

Gupta, S., and N. Abu-Ghannam. 2011. Bioactive potential and possible health effects of edible brown seaweeds. *Trends Food Sci Technol* 22:315–326.

Gwon, W. G., M. S. Lee, J. S. Kim et al. 2013. Hexane fraction from *Sargassum fulvellum* inhibits lipopolysaccharide-induced inducible nitric oxide synthase expression in RAW 264.7 cells via NF-kappaB pathways. *Am J Chin Med* 41:565–584.

Ha, K. H., and D. J. Kim. 2015. Trends in the diabetes epidemic in Korea. *Endocrinol Metab* 30:142–146.

Handique, J. G., and J. B. Baruah. 2002. Polyphenolic compounds: An overview. *React Funct Polym* 52:163–188.

Harborne, J. B. 1998. *Phytochemical methods: A guide to modern techniques of plant analysis.* Springer Science & Business Media.

Hartmann, M. A. 1998. Plant sterols and the membrane environment. *Trends Plant Sci* 3:170–175.

Hiqashi-Okaj, K., S. Otani, and Y. Okai. 1999. Potent suppressive effect of a Japanese edible seaweed, *Enteromorpha prolifera* (sujiao-nori) on initiation and promotion phases of chemically induced mouse skin tumorigenesis. *Cancer Lett* 140:21–25.

Holdt, S. L., and S. Kraan. 2011. Bioactive compounds in seaweed: Functional food applications and legislation. *J Appl Phycol* 23:543–597.

Hu, Z.-M., J. Zhang, J. Lopez-Bautista, and D.-L. Duan. 2013. Asymmetric genetic exchange in the brown seaweed *Sargassum fusiforme* (Phaeophyceae) driven by oceanic currents. *Mar Biol* 160:1407–1414.

Huh, M. K., H. Y. Lee, B. K. Lee, and J. S. Choi. 2004. Genetic diversity and relationships between wild and cultivated populations of the sea lettuce, *Enteromorpha prolifera*, in Korea revialed by RAPD markers. *Protistology* 3.

Hwang, E. K., J. M. Baek, and C. S. Park. 2007a. Assessment of optimal depth and photon irradiance for cultivation of the brown alga, *Sargassum fulvellum* (Turner) C. Agardh. *J Appl Phyco* 19:787–793.

Hwang, E. K., C. S. Park, and J. M. Baek. 2007b. Artificial seed production and cultivation of the edible brown alga, *Sargassum fulvellum* (Turner) C. Agardh: Developing a new species for seaweed cultivation in Korea. *Eighteenth International Seaweed Symposium: Proceedings of the Eighteenth International Seaweed Symposium,* held in Bergen, Norway, 20–25 June 2004. R. Anderson, J. Brodie, E. Onsøyen and A. T. Critchley. Dordrecht, Springer Netherlands: 25–31.

Hwang, H.-J., M.-J. Kwon, I.-H. Kim, and T.-J. Nam. 2008. The effect of polysaccharide extracted from the marine alga *Capsosiphon fulvescens* on ethanol administration. *Food and Chemical Toxicology* 46:2653–2657.

Islam, M. N., I. J. Ishita, S. E. Jin et al. 2013. Anti-inflammatory activity of edible brown alga *Saccharina japonica* and its constituents pheophorbide a and pheophytin a in LPS-stimulated RAW 264.7 macrophage cells. *Food Chem Toxicol* 55:541–548.

Jibril, S. M., B. H. Jakada, H. Y. Umar, and T. A.-Q. Ahmad. 2016. Importance of some algal species as a source of food and supplement. *Int J Curr Microbiol App Sci* 5:186–193.

Jung, H. A., S. E. Jin, B. R. Ahn, C. M. Lee, and J. S. Choi. 2013. Anti-inflammatory activity of edible brown alga *Eisenia bicyclis* and its constituents fucosterol and phlorotannins in LPS-stimulated RAW264.7 macrophages. *Food Chem Toxicol* 59:199–206.

Kadam, S. U., B. K. Tiwari, and C. P. O'Donnell. 2015. Extraction, structure and biofunctional activities of laminarin from brown algae. *Int J Food Sci Tech* 50:24–31.

Kang, J.-Y., B.-S. Chun, M.-C. Lee et al. 2016a. Anti-inflammatory activity and chemical composition of essential oil extracted with supercritical CO2 from the brown seaweed *Undaria pinnatifida*. *J Essent Oil Bear Pl* 19:46–51.

Kang, M., S. W. Kim, J.-W. Kim, T. H. Kim, and J. S. Kim. 2013. Optimization of levulinic acid production from Gelidium amansii. *Renew Energ* 54:173–179.

Kang, M.-C., N. Kang, S.-Y. Kim et al. 2016b. Popular edible seaweed, *Gelidium amansii*, prevents against diet-induced obesity. *Food Chem Toxicol* 90:181–187.

Kasimala, M. B., L. Mebrahtu, P. P. Magoha, G. Asgedom, and M. B. Kasimala. 2015. A review on biochemical composition and nutritional aspects of seaweeds. *Cari J SciTech* 3:789–797.

Khan, M. N. A., S.-J. Yoon, J.-S. Choi et al. 2009. Anti-edema effects of brown seaweed (*Undaria pinnatifida*) extract on phorbol 12-myristate 13-acetate-induced mouse ear inflammation. *Am J Chin Med* 37:373–381.

Kılınç, B., E. Koru, G. Turan, H. Tekogul, and S. Cirik. 2013. Seaweeds for food and industrial applications, INTECH Open Access Publisher.

Kim, K.-J., and B.-Y. Lee. 2012. Fucoidan from the sporophyll of *Undaria pinnatifida* suppresses adipocyte differentiation by inhibition of inflammation-related cytokines in 3T3-L1 cells. *Nutr Res* 32:439–447.

Kim, K. N., K. W. Lee, C. B. Song, C. B. Ahn, and Y. J. Jeon. 2006. Cytotoxic activities of red algae collected from jeju island against four tumor cell lines. *Prev Nutr Food Sci* 11:177–183.

Kim, K. O. 2015. Re-orienting cuisine: East Asian foodways in the twenty-first century. Berghahn Books.

Kim, M., and J. Chun. 2005. Bacterial community structure in kimchi, a Korean fermented vegetable food, as revealed by 16S rRNA gene analysis. *Int J Food Microbiol* 103:91–96.

Kim, M.-J., J. Jeon, and J.-S. Lee. 2014. Fucoidan prevents high-fat diet-induced obesity in animals by suppression of fat accumulation. *Phytother Res* 28:137–143.

Kim, S. C., J. R. Lee, and S. J. Park. 2015b. *Porphyra tenera* induces apoptosis of oral cancer cells. *Korea J Herbol* 30:25–30.

Kim, S.-K., and Q. Van Ta. 2011. Potential beneficial effects of marine algal sterols on human health. *Adv Food Nutr Res* 64:191–198.

Kim, S. M. J. 1999. Iodine content of human milk and dietary iodine intake of Korean lactating mothers. *Int J Food Sci Nutr* 50:165–171.

Kim, Y. K. 2010. Total phenolic contents and antioxidant activities of *Undaria pinnatifida* and *Capsosiphon fulvescens*. *Korean J Food Cook Sci* 26:499–502.

Kim, Y. M., I. H. Kim, and T. J. Nam. 2013. *Capsosiphon fulvescens* glycoprotein reduces AGS gastric cancer cell migration by downregulating transforming growth factor-β1 and integrin expression. *Int J Oncol* 43:1059–1065.

Kim, Y. T., J.-H. Lee, J.-Y. Ko et al. 2015c. Isolation of eckol from *Ecklonia cava* via centrifugal partition chromatography (CPC) and characterization of Its anti-inflammatory activity. *Korean J Fish Aquat Sci* 48:301–307.

Ko, J.-Y., G. A. Jones, M.-S. Heo, Y.-S. Kang, and S.-H. Kang. 2010. A fifty-year production and economic assessment of common property-based management of marine living common resources: A case study for the women divers communities in Jeju, South Korea. *Mar Policy* 34:624–634.

Lee, Y.-S., S.-H. Jung, S.-H. Lee, Y.-J. Choi, and K.-H. Shin. 2002. Hepatoprotective and anti-diabetic effects of *Pelvetia siliquosa*, a marine algae, in rats. *Biomol Ther* 10:165–169.

Lee, H., J.-S. Kim, and E. Kim. 2012. Fucoidan from seaweed *Fucus vesiculosus* inhibits migration and invasion of human lung cancer cell via PI3K-Akt-mTOR pathways. *PLoS ONE* 7:e50624.

Lee, J.-C., M.-F. Hou, H.-W. Huang et al. 2013. Marine algal natural products with anti-oxidative, anti-inflammatory, and anti-cancer properties. *Cancer Cell Int* 13:1–7.

Lee, J. H., K. D. Han, H. M. Jung et al. 2016a. Association between obesity, abdominal obesity, and adiposity and the prevalence of atopic dermatitis in young Korean adults: The Korea National Health and Nutrition Examination Survey 2008–2010. *Allergy Asthma Immunol Res* 8:107–114.

Lee, J.-H., J.-Y. Ko, E.-A. Kim et al. 2016b. Identification and large isolation of an anti-inflammatory compound from an edible brown seaweed, *Undariopsis peterseniana*, and evaluation of its anti-inflammatory effect in *in vitro* and *in vivo* zebrafish. *Journal of Applied Phycology*: 1–10, DOI: 10.1007/s10811-016-1012-3.

Lobban, C. S., and P. J. Harrison. 1994. *Seaweed ecology and physiology*. Cambridge University Press.

Lopes, G., C. Sousa, P. Valentão, and P. B. Andrade. 2013. *Sterols in algae and health. Bioactive compounds from marine foods*, 173–191. New York: John Wiley & Sons Ltd.

Mabeau, S., and J. Fleurence. 1993. Seaweed in food products: Biochemical and nutritional aspects. *Trends Food Sci Technol* 4:103–107.

MacArtain, P., C. I. Gill, M. Brooks, R. Campbell, and I. R. Rowland. 2007. Value of edible seaweeds. *Nutr Rev* 65:535–543.

Manach, C., G. Williamson, C. Morand, A. Scalbert, and C. Rémésy. 2005. Bioavailability and bioefficacy of polyphenols in humans. I. Review of 97 bioavailability studies. *Am J Clin Nutr* 81:230–242.

Matanjun, P., S. Mohamed, N. M. Mustapha, and K. Muhammad. 2009. Nutrient content of tropical edible seaweeds, *Eucheuma cottonii, Caulerpa lentillifera* and *Sargassum polycystum. J Appl Phycol* 21:75–80.

Matsuno, T. 2001. Aquatic animal carotenoids. *Fish Sci* 67:771–783.

McHugh, D. 2003. A guide to the seaweed industry. FAO Fisheries Technical Paper 441. Food and Agriculture Organization of the United Nations, Rome.

Mohamed, S., S. N. Hashim, and H. A. Rahman. 2012. Seaweeds: A sustainable functional food for complementary and alternative therapy. *Trends Food Sci Technol* 23:83–96.

Mohibbullah, M., M. A. Hannan, J.-Y. Choi et al. 2015. The edible marine alga *Gracilariopsis chorda* alleviates hypoxia/reoxygenation-induced oxidative stress in cultured hippocampal neurons. *J Med Food* 18:960–971.

Mohibbullah, M., M. Abdul Hannan, I.-S. Park, I. S. Moon, and Y.-K. Hong. 2016. The edible red seaweed *Gracilariopsis chorda* promotes axodendritic architectural complexity in hippocampal neurons. *J Med Food* 19:638–644.

Mouritsen, O. G. 2009. Plants from the sea. In *SUSHI food for the eye, the body & the soul*, 86–91. Boston, MA: Springer US.

Nautiyal, O. H. 2013. Natural products from plant, microbial and marine species. *Int J Sci Technol* 10:611–646.

Nguyen, V. T., J.-P. Ueng, and G.-J. Tsai. 2011. Proximate composition, total phenolic content, and antioxidant activity of seagrape (*Caulerpa lentillifera*). *J Food Sci* 76:950–958.

Oh, J.-H., J. Kim, and Y. Lee. 2016. Anti-inflammatory and anti-diabetic effects of brown seaweeds in high-fat diet-induced obese mice. *Nutr Res Pract* 10:42–48.

Oh, K.-H., and Y.-S. Choi. 2015. Development of a pasting and garnishing machine for manufacturing kimbugak. *Jf Biosystems Eng* 40:320–326.

Oum, Y. R. 2005. Authenticity and representation: Cuisines and identities in Korean-American diaspora. *Postcolonial Studies* 8:109–125.

Park, M. H. 2005. The efect of *Capsosiphon fulvecense* extract on inhibition of platelet aggregation and serum lipid level in ovariertomized rats. *J Life Sci* 15:1028–1033.

Park, S. Y., H.-H. Song, and S.-D. Ha. 2014. Synergistic effects of NaOCl and ultrasound combination on the reduction of *Escherichia coli* and *Bacillus cereus* in raw laver. *Foodborne Pathog Dis* 11:373–378.

Peng, J., J.-P. Yuan, C.-F. Wu, and J.-H. Wang. 2011. Fucoxanthin, a marine carotenoid present in brown seaweeds and diatoms: Metabolism and bioactivities relevant to human health. *Mar Drugs* 9:1806.

Ragan, M. 1973. *Handbook of phycological methods—Physiological and biochemical methods*, Eds. J. A. Hellebust, J. S. Craigie. Cambridge University Press.

Ragan, M. A., and K.-W. Glombitza. 1986. Phlorotannins, brown algal polyphenols. *Progress in Phycological Res* 4:129–141.

Rioux, L. E., S. L. Turgeon, and M. Beaulieu. 2007. Characterization of polysaccharides extracted from brown seaweeds. *Carbohydr Polym* 69:530–7.

Robic, A., C. Rondeau-Mouro, J. F. Sassi, Y. Lerat, and M. Lahaye. 2009. Structure and interactions of ulvan in the cell wall of the marine green algae *Ulva rotundata* (Ulvales, Chlorophyceae). *Carbohydr Polym* 77:206–216.

Robic, A., J. F. Sassi, and M. Lahaye. 2008. Impact of stabilization treatments of the green seaweed *Ulva rotundata* (Chlorophyta) on the extraction yield, the physico-chemical and rheological properties of ulvan. *Carbohydr Polym* 74:344–352.

Sanjeewa, K. K. A., E.-A. Kim, K.-T. Son, and Y.-J. Jeon. 2016. Bioactive properties and potentials cosmeceutical applications of phlorotannins isolated from brown seaweeds: A review. *J Photochem Photobiol B* 162:100–105.

Senni, K., J. Pereira, F. Gueniche et al. 2011. Marine polysaccharides: A source of bioactive molecules for cell therapy and tissue engineering. *Mar Drugs* 9:1664–1681.

Sevevirathne, M., K.-H. Lee, C.-B. Ahn, P.-J. Park, and J.-Y. Jeon. 2012. Evaluation of antioxidant, anti-Alzheimer's and anti-inflammatory activities of enzymatic hydrolysates from edible brown seaweed (*Laminaria japonica*). *J Food Biochem* 36:207–216.

Sharma, B. R., and D. Y. Rhyu. 2014. Anti-diabetic effects of *Caulerpa lentillifera*: Stimulation of insulin secretion in pancreatic β-cells and enhancement of glucose uptake in adipocytes. *Asian Pac J Trop Biomed* 4:575–580.

Siriwardhana, N., K.-W. Lee, Y.-J. Jeon, S.-H. Kim, and J.-W. Haw. 2003. Antioxidant activity of *Hizikia fusiformis* on reactive oxygen species scavenging and lipid peroxidation inhibition. *Food Sci Technol Int* 9:339–346.

Sithranga, B. N., and K. Kathiresan. 2010. Anticancer drugs from marine flora: An overview. *J Oncology* 2010, Article ID 214186, 18 pp.

Synytsya, A., D. J. Choi, R. Pohl et al. 2015. Structural features and anti-coagulant activity of the sulphated polysaccharide SPS-CF from a green alga *Capsosiphon fulvescens*. *Mar Biotechnol* 17:718–735.

Synytsya, A., W.-J. Kim, S.-M. Kim et al. 2010. Structure and antitumour activity of fucoidan isolated from sporophyll of Korean brown seaweed *Undaria pinnatifida*. *Carbohydr Polym* 81:41–48.

Thun, M. J., S. J. Henley, and T. Gansler. 2004. Inflammation and cancer: An epidemiological perspective. Novartis Foundation Symposium, Chichester: John Wiley.

Tong, T., J. Li, D.-O. Ko et al. 2014. Effects of the addition of *Hizikia fusiforme, Capsosiphon fulvescens,* and *Undaria pinnatifida sporophyll* on antioxidant and inhibitory potential against enzymes related to type 2 diabetes of vegetable extract. *Korean J Food Preserv*, 21:460–467.

Wang, L., Y. Zhang, Z. Wang et al. 2012. Inhibitory effect of ginsenoside-Rd on carrageenan-induced inflammation in rats. *Can J Physiol Pharmacol* 90:229–236.

Wi, S. G., H. J. Kim, S. A. Mahadevan, D.-J. Yang, and H.-J. Bae. 2009. The potential value of the seaweed Ceylon moss (*Gelidium amansii*) as an alternative bioenergy resource. *BioresTechnol* 100:6658–6660.

Wu, Z., D. Pan, Y. Guo, and X. Zeng. 2015. N-acetylmuramic acid triggers anti-inflammatory capacity in LPS-induced RAW 264.7 cells and mice. *J Funct Foods* 13:108–116.

Xiaojun, Y., L. Xiancui, Z. Chengxu, and F. Xiao. 1996. Prevention of fish oil rancidity by phlorotannins from *Sargassum kjellmanianum*. *J Appl Phy* 8:201–203.

Yamamoto, Y. and R. B. Gaynor. 2001. Role of the NF-kB pathway in the pathogenesis of human disease states. *Current Molecular Medicine* 1:287–296.

Yang, E.-J., Y. M. Ham, W. J. Lee, N. H. Lee, and C.-G. Hyun. 2013. Anti-inflammatory effects of apo-9'-fucoxanthinone from the brown alga, *Sargassum muticum*. *DARU J Pharmaceutical Sci* 21:1–7.

Yang, H., K. Jung, K. Gang et al. 2005. Physicochemical composition of seaweed fulvescens (*Capsosiphon fulvescens*). *Korean J Food Sci Technol* 37:912–917.

Yoon, J. J., Y. J. Kim, S. H. Kim et al. 2010. Production of polysaccharides and corresponding sugars from red seaweed. *Adv Mater Res* 93/94:463–466.

Yoon, J. T., Y. G. Gong, and G.-H. Chung. 2003. Development and morphology of *Pelvetia siliquosa* Tseng et Chang (Phaeophyta) in culture. *J Aquaculture* 16:37–43.

Yuan, Y. V., and N. A. Walsh. 2006. Antioxidant and antiproliferative activities of extracts from a variety of edible seaweeds. *Food Chem Toxicol* 44:1144–1150.

16

Namul, the Korean Vegetable Dish

Young-Eun Lee

CONTENTS

16.1   Introduction 386
16.2   History 387
16.3   Meaning of Namul 389
16.4   Preparation 389
     16.4.1   Classification of Edible Vegetables 391
     16.4.2   Preparation of Namul Dishes 391
          16.4.2.1   Seasoned, Cooked-Vegetable Dish 393
          16.4.2.2   Seasoned, Fresh-Vegetable Dish 394
16.5   Food Composition 394
     16.5.1   Water-Soluble Vitamins 395
     16.5.2   Carotenoids 396
     16.5.3   Vitamin K 396
     16.5.4   Minerals 396
     16.5.5   Dietary Fiber 397
16.6   Health Benefits 397
     16.6.1   Antioxidative Effects 404
          16.6.1.1   Bioflavonoid (Quercetin) 404
          16.6.1.2   Lutein and Zeaxanthin 404
     16.6.2   Antidiabetic Effects 404
     16.6.3   Immunoenhancing Effects 405
     16.6.4   Anticancer Effects 406
          16.6.4.1   Carotenoids 407
          16.6.4.2   Chlorophyll 407
          16.6.4.3   Folic Acid 408
          16.6.4.4   Sulforaphane 408
          16.6.4.5   Dietary Fiber 408
     16.6.5   Cardiovascular Disease 409
     16.6.6   Blood Pressure 410
16.7   Conclusion 410
References 410

16.1 Introduction

Collectively, namul means all the kinds of edible vegetables from mountains and fields as well as the banchan (side dish) prepared with them. While wild greens are called pusae, the namul cultivated by man is differentiated by calling it namsae or chaema (National Institute of Korean Language, 2017). The Korean vegetable dish namul is prepared as fresh (saengchae), cooked by blanching, or stir-frying with small amount of oil (sukchae) with various seasonings. Dried vegetables cooked after rehydration are called jinchae.

Since diverse terms and cooking methods have been used for vegetables and the daily vegetable consumption of Koreans ranked first among 29 OECD countries according to the "OECD Health at a Glance 2015" (Figure 16.1), Koreans have developed a unique vegetable food culture—namul—with diverse vegetables.

For namul as a dish, virtually any types of vegetables can be used; the ingredients include leaves, stems, sprouts, roots, and fruits. Although in most cases the vegetables are blanched before being seasoned, the method of preparation can also vary; they may be served fresh (raw), boiled, stir-fried with a small amount of oil, or sautéed. Especially in Korea, most of san-namul (mountain herbs) are dried for preservation and rehydrated before being cooked and seasoned.

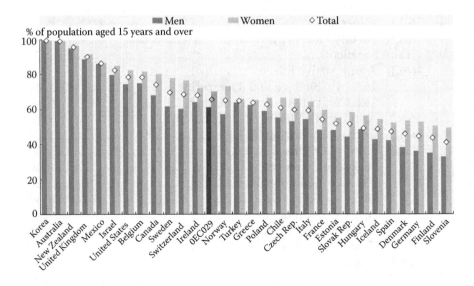

FIGURE 16.1
Daily vegetable eating among adults, 2013 (or nearest year). Nearly 100% of the population aged 15 years and over in Korea ate vegetables every day. (OECD. 2015. Health at a glance 2015: OECD indicators. Paris: OECD Publishing.)

Namul, the Korean Vegetable Dish

Traditional Korean meals are composed of cooked rice (bap), soup (guk) or pot stew (jjigae), kimchi, and several banchans. Everyday banchan is made up with vegetables and legumes, occasionally with fish, and rarely with meats. Namul is typically served accompanying the staples, usually bap. It is possible to have more than one type of namul dish made with seasonal vegetables served as banchan at a single meal. Many Koreans feel that, along with rice, kimchi, and guk or jjigae, no meal is complete without a namul dish.

16.2 History

Humans have used vegetables as food since time immemorial. Different type of vegetables, depending on the place and the season, have been part of the human diet since prehistoric times. Originally, vegetables were collected from the wild by hunter–gatherers and entered cultivation in several parts of the world, probably during the period from 10,000 to 7000 BC, when a new agricultural way of life developed. Nowadays, most vegetables are grown all over the world as climate permits (National Geographic, accessed on 2016). Mostly, the wild greens, which taste bitter and contain more nutrients and phytochemicals, are the native plants in Korean peninsula.

Traces of edible vegetables have been found in ancient Egyptian archaeological sites. Some edible vegetables were historically documented in ancient Greece (1,100~146 BC), in ancient Rome, in ancient Sri Lanka, and in the Middle Ages (Andah et al., 1994).

The first record in history of edible vegetables in Korea is from the foundation myths in *Samguk-yusa* (*The Story of Three Kingdoms*, Il-yeon, 1281). They are the Korean mugwort and garlic. It is as follows:

> Hwanung (son of God) gave the bear a bundle of Korean mugwort and twenty cloves of garlic and said, "You may become a human if you only eat them and survive for 100 days." The bear endured the pain and transformed into a woman. The bear woman married the son of God and gave birth to Dangun, who opened Korea's first nation, Gojoseon, in 2333 BC.

The etymology of the word namul goes back to the Silla dynasty. According to *Dongun-goryak* (Anonymous), namul comes from the object from the Silla. It may be inferred that the vegetable dish namul had begun to be served alongside the cooked rice bap from the time of the Three Kingdoms, when the basic structure of the Korean diet "bansang" (Korea's traditional meal setting) began to be established. In another document, *Myungmul-girak* (Hwang, 1870), which identified the name of various objects, namul means "silk-like food" because "na [pronounced as 'la' if it locates at the back]" means the silk in the kanji character, and a vegetable dish in the Korean diet is as important and precious as silk. The vegetarian diet of the Goryeo dynasty diversified and developed the namul dishes, influenced by Buddhism.

According to the poem of Gapoyukyoung of *Donggukyisanggukjip* (1241) written by Gyu-bo Lee, six vegetables—cucumber, eggplant, turnip, scallion, curled mallow, and calabash—were cultivated in the garden of the house in Goryeo dynasty.

Even though Koreans are an herbaceous people, there are not many vegetables originating from Korea. Koreans became the best known consumers of namul by cooking and eating many types of vegetables that were imported through exchanges. The ancient civilization of the Middle East is known to be the most communal area of vegetables, and many vegetables from this region were brought to East Asia and Europe (Figure 16.2). The propagation of vegetables to East Asia was carried out through the East–West trading routes like the Silk Road, the Siberian Route, the Tibet Route, and the Ocean Route (Chung, 2017). Korean angelica tree shoot, Java water dropwort, Korean wild chive, giant butterbur, and East Asian wild parsley originated in Korea, which can be regarded as an area mainly used for young shoots and young leaves.

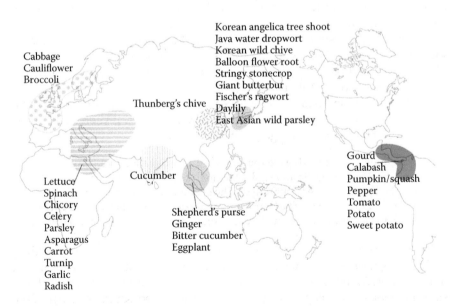

FIGURE 16.2
Origins of vegetables. Modified from Lee, S.W., Research on the Dietary Life Before Goryeo Dynasty. Seoul: Hyangmunsa, 1978.

16.3 Meaning of Namul

For Koreans, namul dishes have been a symbol of a life of peace and no greed, or a symbol of simple happiness with family. But namul has also been a symbol of hunger and poverty.

In Analects (~475–221 BC), a collection of sayings and ideas attributed to the Chinese philosopher Confucius, written by Confucius's followers, namul is a concept of confrontation with meat, and a symbol of a clear life without greed. In the Chosun dynasty, when Confucianism was followed, namul was a symbol of a satisfying life without greed to Koreans. A poem in Analects says,

> Eat namul dishes and drink water.
> Lay down on my arms.
> Pleasure is in it.
> The unfair advantage of wealth, it is like a frosty cloud to me.

Namul is also a pleasant food, which means simple happiness with family. In his poem, Dasan Jung Yak-Yong recalled the summer of 1797, when he spent a pleasant 3 days in Cheonjinam near his home with his brothers and family members, eating 56 fragrant wild vegetables such as Shepherd's purse, Korean angelica tree shoot, and eastern bracken fern, and creating and enjoying more than 20 poems with harmonious families together.

However, in the Chosun dynasty, picking the herbaceous plants also meant that people began to starve to death because of no more food to eat. Famine is called gi-geun as a kanji. The hunger for lack of grains is called gi and the hunger for lack of vegetables called geun. In thousands of years of Korean dietary history, vegetables are just as important as the staple food grains (Lee, 2005).

We do not know that namul picked by women in the fields or mountains in spring is a symbol of life of no greed, a symbol of poverty, or a simple food ingredient for a happy family dinner. But recently, namul has become neither a symbol of poverty nor of no greed. Some people argue that vegetarianism is the only way to save people and to save the planet. In any case, namul must be the healthiest food for Koreans because of its nutrients and phytochemicals.

16.4 Preparation

Culinary use of edible vegetables is very diverse in Korea. Mostly they are used to make various namul dishes (Figure 16.3a,b,c) and kimchi. They can be an ingredient for boiled guk (Figure 16.3d) and jjigae, stir-fried buchimgae (Korean pancake) and jeon (Figure 16.3e), deep-fat fried bugak, and jangajji

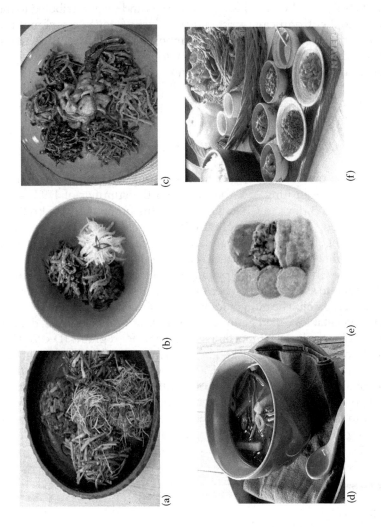

FIGURE 16.3
Representative Korean dishes prepared with vegetables. (a) Fresh namul, "saengchae"; (b) cooked namul, "sukchae"; (c) dried, rehydrated, and stir-fried namul, "jinchae"; (d) guk (soup); (e) pan-fried jeon; (f) ssam (vegetable wrap).

Namul, the Korean Vegetable Dish 391

(pickled vegetables in jang such as soy sauce, soybean paste, or chili paste). Leafy greens can be used to wrap other ingredients such as bap, fish, and meat with jang into an edible package called ssam (vegetable wrap) (Figure 16.3f), similar to how a tortilla is used (Cho, 1998; Korean Food Foundation, 2014).

16.4.1 Classification of Edible Vegetables

According to the WHO (2003), the classification of vegetables can vary from country to country. The reason for this differentiation is related to the inclusion or exclusion of starchy roots, tubers, and legumes within the vegetable groups. In addition to the related differences between vegetables and legumes, the USDA (2010) classifies all of them within one category—namely, "vegetable group." This category has been divided into five subgroups: (1) dark green vegetables; (2) red and orange vegetables; (3) starchy vegetables; (4) beans and peas (legumes); and (5) other vegetables (Fabbri and Crosby, 2016). Usually, dark green, red and orange, and other vegetables are used for namul dishes in Korea.

In Korea, edible vegetables are usually classified as leafy vegetables, bulb and stem vegetables, root and tuberous vegetables, or fruit vegetables according to the main parts for culinary use.

- Leafy vegetables are a green or dark green color. Green leafy vegetables that Koreans most often use are lettuce, perilla leaves, spinach, chard, curled mallow, daylily, stringy stonecrop, Fischer's ragwort, East Asian wild parsley, Korean mugwort, crown daisy, etc.
- Bulb and stem vegetables are Korean wild chive, Thunberg's chive, scallion, garlic, Java water dropwort, eastern bracken fern, giant butterbur, etc.
- Root and tuberous vegetables used most for namul dishes are balloon flower root, bamboo shoot, burdock, lotus root, carrot, radish, turnip, ginger, etc.
- Fruit vegetables used most are cucumber, calabash, Korean zucchini, eggplant and hot pepper, soybean, mung bean, etc. Soybean and mung bean are used as namul after sprouting throughout the year, regardless of the season.

In Korea, flower and flower buds like cauliflower and broccoli traditionally are not often used as namul. But they have been consumed a lot since their health benefits have become known to Koreans.

16.4.2 Preparation of Namul Dishes

Namul is a dish prepared by seasoning wild herbs, roots, sprouts, or vegetables (either fresh or cooked). There are two types of methods for preparing namul: One is to mix fresh or blanched and presqueezed vegetables with seasonings; the other is to stir-fry with a small amount of oil. Table 16.1 shows

TABLE 16.1

How to Prepare Representative Korean Namul Dishes

Classification	Namul Dishes	Method
Saengchae (seasoned fresh vegetable dish)		Balloon flower roots saengchae: 1. Peel the bellflower root and cut it into a size proper to eat. 2. Remove the bitter taste by steeping the cut bellflower root in salt water. 3. Make a sauce with kochujang, vinegar, sugar, salt, red pepper powder, sesame seed, minced garlic, and chopped scallion. 4. Drain the water from bellflower roots and mix with prepared kochujang and vinegar sauce.
	Muchim namul (mix with sauce and seasonings)	Soybean sprout namul: 1. Wash bean sprouts cleanly by removing dirt. 2. Put one cup water and one-half teaspoon salt in a pot and add bean sprouts. Cover the lid of the pot and boil it for 3–4 minutes. Drain the water and squeeze out the extra water lightly. (Adjust the boiling time according to the thickness of the bean sprouts.) 3. Mix salt, red pepper powder, minced garlic, chopped scallion, and sesame oil in the bowl. 4. Sprinkle sesame seeds evenly on it.
Sukchae (seasoned cooked vegetable dish)		Spinach namul: 1. Wash spinach cleanly by removing dirt. 2. Put one cup water and one-half teaspoon salt in a pot and add spinach without lid on for 30 seconds, then rinse in cold water. 3. Drain the water and squeeze out the extra water thoroughly. 4. Mix ganjang, minced garlic, chopped scallion, and sesame oil in the bowl. 5. Sprinkle sesame seeds evenly on it.
	Bokkeum namul (stirfry with sauce and seasonings)	Eastern bracken fern namul (jinchae): 1. Rehydrate dried eastern bracken fern overnight. 2. Boil well more than 30 minutes to soften. 3. Drain the water and squeeze out the extra water thoroughly. 4. Cut into bite size (about 4–5 cm). 5. Mix ganjang, minced garlic, chopped scallion, and sesame oil (or perilla oil) in the bowl. 6. Stir-fry with a small amount of oil and add a cup of water or stock, cover with lid, and boil with low fire until the water disappears. 7. Sprinkle sesame seeds evenly on it.

Namul, the Korean Vegetable Dish

how to prepare the representative namul dishes such as balloon flower root saengchae (doraji-saengchae), bean sprout namul (kong-namul), spinach namul (sigeumchi-namul), and eastern bracken fern namul (gosari-namul).

16.4.2.1 Seasoned, Cooked-Vegetable Dish

The seasoned cooked-vegetable dish (sukchae) is a representative cooking method of namul in Korea. Unlike Western countries, Koreans eat cooked-vegetable dishes rather than fresh-vegetable ones. To minimize destroying vitamins from cooking, vegetables are blanched in a short period of time.

Sukchae is prepared by blanching and presqueezing vegetables and then seasoning them with sauces and spices. The most commonly used sauce for namul is soy sauce (kanjang), sometimes salt, doenjang (soybean paste), or kochujang (red chili pepper paste), according to the color and flavor of the vegetables. Some wild vegetables, especially mountain herbs (san-namul) with a bitter taste, often are seasoned with doenjang or kochujang instead of soy sauce or salt. In addition to the basic saltiness, namul is seasoned with chopped scallion, minced garlic, and crushed sesame seed. A few drops of sesame oil or perilla oil are added as a finishing touch for a heavenly aroma that lingers on the palate. Squeezing is a very important step to making sukchae more delicious because this prevents the seasonings from being diluted by the extra water. Soybean and mung bean sprouts, spinach (refer to Table 16.1), crown daisy, and Java water dropwort are representative of the blanched and seasoned (Muchim) namul.

The other way of making sukchae is stir-frying vegetables with small amounts of cooking oil (Bokkeum), seasoned with soy sauce, scallion, garlic, sesame seed, and sesame oil. If meat is added, the taste becomes better. Eastern bracken fern (refer to Table 16.1), balloon flower root, mushroom, and dried vegetables such as radish green, Korean zucchini, and eggplant are representative of vegetables cooked in this way.

Especially during the winter, seasonal vegetables are dried for preservation. Dried vegetables are boiled well to soften them, and some of them are steeped to let the bitter taste out; the excess water is squeezed out and then the vegetables are stir-fried in a small amount of oil. Sometimes a little bit of water or stock is added and then the mixture is covered with a lid and boiled softly with low heat. Koreans enjoyed special delicacies with dried vegetables called jinchae. Some people prefer to use perilla oil instead of sesame oil to make jinchae with dried wild vegetables.

On the day of the first full moon of the year, nine boreum namul ("full-moon namul") dishes with five-grain rice are prepared. It is believed that boreum namuls help to get through the hot weather and stay healthy in the coming summer. These boreum namul dishes are called a jinchae meal.

The three namul dishes cooked with white balloon flower root, green spinach, and black eastern bracken fern must be prepared for New Year's Day, Thanksgiving Day, and the ancestral ritual ceremony. These are the most highly used vegetables for namul dishes in Korea and have a meaning in addition to the harmony of colors and taste. The white balloon flower root symbolizes the ancestor as the root of the family, the black bracken the parents as the stem, and the greens spinach the siblings as the leaf.

16.4.2.2 Seasoned, Fresh-Vegetable Dish

Saengchae (seasoned fresh vegetables) is seasoned usually with kochujang or mustard and vinegar. Radish, cucumber, and balloon flower roots (refer to Table 16.1) have been used as raw materials for the saengchae dish. Fresh, newly sprouted five spring herbs, such as mountain mustard greens, Korean angelica tree shoot, radish sprout, Java water dropwort, and scallion grown underneath the thin ice have been prepared as saengchae to supplement vitamins and minerals insufficiently taken in during the long winter and renew the strong vitality that endures over the cold winter to bring a new energy into the body. Moreover, the scent and taste of spring vegetables bring back lost appetite and recover energy for the spring.

16.5 Food Composition

Food ingredients of a Korean diet consist of vegetables and meat in an 8:2 "golden" ratio, which is considered healthy because it is low in fat and calories and balanced in nutrition compared to a Western diet (Oh et al., 2014a). Eating five variously colored vegetables helps to reduce the risk of lifestyle diseases by inducing a balanced intake of phytochemicals in addition to nutrients such as vitamins, minerals, and dietary fibers.

The philosophy of cosmic dualism (yin and yang) and the five elements principle can be understood as the basis of constructing the Korean meal. Among vegetables, the duality of yin and yang exists; for example, most summer vegetables with cooling sensations belong to yin and the hot-tasting, sulfur-containing *Allium* genus and Cruciferae family vegetables to yang.

According to the five elements theory, five different colors are considered to affect the five different organs in the body and possess different health benefits. The vegetables with five different colors (green, red, yellow, white, and black)—matching five different tastes (sour, bitter, sweet, hot, and salty, respectively)—make an extraordinary combination. These tastes are combined together in harmony (Cha et al., 2006):

- Sweet and hot tastes belong to the positive attribute (yang); sweetness helps the body to protect and harmonize, and the hot and spicy taste helps energy to move out and circulate the blood
- Salty, sour, and bitter tastes belong to the negative attribute (ying); the salty taste turns the hard textured ones to soft, the sour taste encourages energy to contact, and the bitter taste drops a fever and makes things harden (or stiffen)

The balanced combination of five elements ranks as outstanding because there is nothing that is left out in terms of health benefits. Various phytochemicals are all there: green with chlorophyll, red with lycopene and capsaicin, yellow with carotenoids, white with quercetin and sulforaphane, and black with anthocyanins. Additionally, the colors are pleasing to the eye.

Korean traditional vegetables are mainly green, white, and purple. There are very few red and yellow vegetables, which are filled with spices and seasonings (chili pepper for red and sesame seed for yellow) used to prepare namul dishes, and they make the namul dish balanced nutritionally and in terms of phytochemical aspects.

Similar to the five elements theory in Korea, healthy eating patterns recommended by the USDA include a variety of vegetables from all of the five vegetable subgroups—dark green, red and orange, beans and peas, starchy, and other. The recommended amount of vegetables in the Healthy U.S.-Style Eating Pattern at the 2,000-calorie level is 2.5 cup-equivalents of vegetables per day. In addition, weekly amounts from each vegetable subgroup are recommended to ensure variety and meet nutrient needs. Vegetables supply many nutrients, including dietary fiber, potassium, vitamin A, vitamin C, vitamin K, copper, magnesium, vitamin E, vitamin B6, folate, iron, manganese, thiamin, niacin, and choline. Each of the vegetable subgroups contributes different combinations of nutrients, making it important for individuals to consume vegetables from all the subgroups. For example, dark-green vegetables provide the most vitamin K, red and orange vegetables the most vitamin A, legumes the most dietary fiber, and starchy vegetables the most potassium. Vegetables in the "other" vegetable subgroup provide a wide range of nutrients in varying amounts (USDA, 2015).

16.5.1 Water-Soluble Vitamins

With the typical four seasons of a temperate zone, Korea produces a variety of seasonal vegetables. Spring is the season of new life, when nature generously provides fragrant vegetables and herbs such as mugwort, Shepard's purse, wild chive, and angelica tree shoots. Most spring vegetables are high in vitamin B complexes, especially thiamin and riboflavin, which are required by the body for energy metabolism. Dark green leafy vegetables are the rich source of folic acid which has an integral role in DNA methylation and DNA synthesis in conjunction with vitamin B6 and vitamin B12.

All the steps included before vegetable consumption can directly affect nutritional quality. The Korean meal, which is predominantly made up of seasonal vegetables and namul dishes, is filled with nutrients and phytochemicals. There are many benefits to eating vegetables in season. They are more likely to be fresher and taste better when consumed closer to harvesting and are higher in nutritional value then.

Some antioxidants, such as vitamin C, folate, and carotenes, will rapidly decline when stored for periods of time. In the process of cooking, water-soluble or susceptible nutrients such as vitamin B1, niacin, folic acid, vitamin C, and minerals may be lost, and the vitamin C content may vary depending on the cooking method. Vegetables are 80% to 90% water of their weight, so they can be cooked with their own water without the water addition. When cooked in a large amount of water, 75%~80% of vitamin B1 is lost, whereas when low moisture cooking is adapted, only 5%~20% of vitamin B1 is lost and 50% of vitamin C is lost. In order to reduce the cooking loss, it is necessary to select the proper cooking method according to the nature of the vegetable. Fabbri and Crosby (2016) reviewed on the relationship between the cooking methods and the nutritional quality of vegetables, steaming seems to be the best method to maintain the nutritional quality of total antioxidant capacity (TAC), carotenoids, glucosinolates, sulforaphane, folate, and phytochemicals.

16.5.2 Carotenoids

Dark green vegetables are high in beta-carotene, which improves immune function considerably once it is converted into vitamin A. Vitamin A keeps eyes and skin healthy and helps protect against infections.

16.5.3 Vitamin K

The vitamin K content of green leafy vegetables such as spinach, mustard green, perilla leaves, radish green, crown daisy, and Swiss chard is particularly high, since these are photosynthetic tissues and phylloquinone is involved in photosynthesis (Kessler and Glauser, 2014; Korean Nutrition Society, 2011).

High levels of vitamin K in green vegetables make it an ideal and natural way to prevent bone problems. Vitamin K mediates the γ-carboxylation of glutamyl residues on several bone proteins, notably osteocalcin. High serum concentrations of undercarboxylated osteocalcin and low serum concentrations of vitamin K are associated with lower bone mineral density and increased risk of hip fracture. The addition of green leafy vegetables to the diet considerably decreases the chances of hip fractures in middle-aged women (Feskanich et al., 1999).

16.5.4 Minerals

Green leafy vegetables are high in magnesium and have a low glycemic index, thus proving to be helpful for patients with type 2 diabetes (Barbagallo and Dominguez, 2015). Eating at least one serving of green leafy vegetables each day will considerably lower the risks of diabetes. Green vegetables are also rich in iron and calcium, except for Swiss chard and spinach, since they are high in oxalic acid and inhibit mineral absorption.

16.5.5 Dietary Fiber

According to the Institute of Medicine, Food and Nutrition Board (IOM, 2005), dietary fiber intake could lower the risk of coronary disease and cancer.

The World Health Organization (WHO/FAO, 2005) recommends a minimum of 400 g of fruit and vegetables per day (excluding potatoes and other starchy tubers) for the prevention of chronic diseases, as well as for the prevention and alleviation of several micronutrient deficiencies. Epidemiologic and intervention studies have suggested that an intake of 14 g of dietary fiber per 1000 kcal would promote heart health (Storey and Anderson, 2014).

The contents of total dietary fiber (TDF) in 15 Korean vegetables showed 1.20%~7.11% on a fresh weight basis and a great portion of TDF was from the insoluble dietary fiber. Garlic, burdock, and chili pepper leaves showed relatively higher contents of TDF than other vegetables (Kye, 2014).

Dietary fiber absorbs the extra water in the colon and thereby retains the moisture content in the fecal matter. This prevents chronic constipation, diarrhea, and colon cancer. Vegetables also tend to make a person feel full for longer and thus stop unnecessary snacking, which can help reduce weight.

16.6 Health Benefits

Vegetables are generally lower in fat and higher in dietary fiber than other foods and, in addition, contain numerous phytochemicals that protect against many diseases. The five subgroups of distinctive and brightly colored vegetables are rich sources loaded with various phytochemicals.

A diet rich in vegetables offers the benefit of abundant antioxidants that keep away diseases like diabetes, coronary heart disease, strokes, and cancer. Moreover, vegetables deliver ample amounts of vitamins, including folate, vitamins A, K, and B6, and carotenoids like beta-carotene, lutein, and zeaxanthin from dark green vegetables. Vegetables also help in keeping weight under control and promoting healthy skin and hair. Innumerable research has been conducted that strongly suggests that consuming fresh, green vegetables on a regular basis is far better than taking supplementary tablets to get the wholesome nutrition needed (Willet et al., 2013).

Among 150,000~200,000 bioactive compounds known in the plant kingdom (Vijayakumar et al., 2013), many Korean traditional vegetables and herbs used for namul possess numerous bioactive compounds, which have physiological functions, including antioxidant, antidiabetic, immune-enhancing, and anticancer activities. These are summarized in Table 16.2.

TABLE 16.2

Health Benefits of Color Vegetables Commonly Used for Namul Dishes in Korea

Color	Vegetables	Effectiveness	Ref.
Green	Shepherd's purse (*Capsella bursa-pastoris*)	Dried whole plants, including roots, used for Korean traditional medicine for treatment of detoxification and diabetes, dysentery, high blood pressure, and excessive bleeding after birth Enhance and improve eyesight and vision Anti-inflammatory activity, antibacterial and antisuperbacterial activity	Choi et al., 2014; Lim and Yun, 2009; Kim and Kim, 2002
	Korean wild chive (*Allium monanthum*)	Effective in stomachache, normalizing intestinal function, and tranquillization of nerves on Korean traditional medicine Hepatoprotective effects on ethanol-induced liver damage High antioxidant activity, cancer cell growth inhibition, and highest antiproliferation effect in hexane fraction Antibacterial effect (allicin, methyl alliin, scorodose) Reduces total blood cholesterol and blood glucose	Choi et al., 2004; Oh et al., 2014b
	Thunberg's chive (*Allium tuberosum*)	Representative spring vegetable to give stamina and to be good for liver according to *Donibogam* because slightly warm in character Shows antioxidant and antibacterial activity Thiosulfinates inhibit the cell proliferation in HepG2 via apoptosis	Park et al., 2009
	Shoot of Korean angelica tree (*Aralia elata*)	Triterpenoid saponin helps blood circulation, lowers blood sugar and blood lipids Water extract lowers the HbA1c in diabetic rats Cytotoxic effect on human breast cancer cells via apoptosis through caspase-dependent cascade pathway	Shin, 2006; Ryu and Chung, 2015
	Korean zucchini (*Cucurbita moschata*)	Pectin improves cardiovascular health, lower cholesterol, improve arterial health and reduce disease-causing inflammation, so it might also offer protection against diabetes and insulin resistance	Jang et al., 2002

(Continued)

TABLE 16.2 (CONTINUED)

Health Benefits of Color Vegetables Commonly Used for Namul Dishes in Korea

Color	Vegetables	Effectiveness	Ref.
Green	Swiss chard (*Beta vulgaris*)	2'Vitexin-2"O-rhamnoside strongly inhibits DNA synthesis in MCF-7 breast cancer cells, whereas 2"-xylosylvitexin and isorhamnetin 3-gentiobioside are activators; combinations of activators and inhibitors maintain the overall inhibitory effect	Pyo et al., 2004; Ninfali et al., 2007
	Korean mugwort (*Artemisia* spp.)	Effective in alleviating metabolic dislipidemia, insulin resistance, and adipokine dysregulation induced by a high-fat diet Antiamnesic and neuroprotective effects (phenolics [eupatilin, jaceosidin]) Antioxidant and anticancer activities in various *Artemisia* are very promising: *A. princeps* Pampanini and *A. Argyi* H. extracts inhibit growth of MCF cells greater than 80% Antimutagenic effect against aflatoxin B1 (myrcene, cineole, camphor, caryophyllene, coumarin, farnesol)	Kim et al., 2016b; Ha et al., 2015; Kim et al., 2012a; Kim and Lee, 1992
	Spinach (*Spinacia oleracea*)	Effective in accelerating the healing process of ulcers, especially diabetic ulcers because of antioxidative and anti-inflammatory activities Decreases blood glucose and increases insulin level Effective against reducing osteoclast differentiation through the NF-κB-mediated pathway	Rahati et al., 2016; Bonari, 2011; Kim et al., 2015
	Water dropwort (*Oenanthe javanica*)	Antioxidants; decreasing oxidative stresses in the liver (persicarin and isorhamnetin). Improved hepatic fat accumulation, hyperglycemia, and dyslipidemia induced by high-fat, high-cholesterol diet, suggesting their potential use for the prevention and treatment of NAFLD Anti-inflammatory effect; the ethyl acetate fraction effectively reduced protein expression of iNOS and COX-2, and production of proinflammatory cytokines	Jang et al., 2016; Sim et al., 2015; Lee et al., 2015; Ku et al., 2013; Jeong et al., 2009; Lee et al., 2005a,b; Han et al., 1993; Kim et al., 1993

(Continued)

400 — Korean Functional Foods

TABLE 16.2 (CONTINUED)

Health Benefits of Color Vegetables Commonly Used for Namul Dishes in Korea

Color	Vegetables	Effectiveness	Ref.
Green		Antimutagenic effect against aflatoxinB1and anticancer effect in HT-29 colon cancer cells Decrease blood pressure by inhibiting angiotensin I converting enzyme (adenosine)	
	Fischer's ragwort (*Ligularia fischeri*)	Prevent diabetic neurodegeneration: decrease intracellular ROS, whereas increasing neuronal cell viability against high glucose/H_2O_2-induced cytotoxicity Decrease atherogenic index: increase HDL cholesterol by total cholesterol ratio Alleviate hepatic damage: enhance superoxide dismutase activity of liver tissues	Park et al., 2016; Yu et al., 2015; Bae et al., 2009; Ham et al., 1998
	Crown daisy (*Glebionis coronaria*)	Potential antiangiogenic action of campesterol via an inhibition of endothelial cell proliferation and capillary differentiation Antibacterial effects against the Gram-positive bacteria Antiproliferative properties towards different human cancer cell lines, of which colon cancer was the most sensitive to the essential oil treatment	Bardaweel et al., 2015; Choi et al., 2007
	Godeulbaegi (*Ixeris sonchifolia, Youngia sonchifokia*)	Antimutagenic and preventing cancer via apoptosis Activate immune cells Decreasing hyperlipidemia Antioxidant Preventing hepatotoxicity	Shin et al., 2016; Chon and Kang, 2013; Rhu et al., 2008; Sohn et al., 2001; Bae et al., 1998, 1997; Lim et al., 1997
	Perilla leaves (*Perilla frutescens*)	Phytol and eicosatrienoic acid of perilla leaves play a role on the growth inhibition of human colon, osteosarcoma, and gastric cancer cells	Lee et al., 1999; Ham et al., 2003
	Mustard green (*Brassica juncea*)	Excellent source of phenolic antioxidants, especially caffeic acid and ferulic acid; contains flavonoids such as isorhamnetin, quercetin, and kaempferol	Walia et al., 2011; Cha and Jung, 1998; Lee et al., 1997

(Continued)

TABLE 16.2 (CONTINUED)

Health Benefits of Color Vegetables Commonly Used for Namul Dishes in Korea

Color	Vegetables	Effectiveness	Ref.
Green		Lowers the risk of atherosclerosis, and provides help in the regulation of blood lipid levels, including levels of total cholesterol, LDL cholesterol, and HDL cholesterol; cooked mustard greens may provide more bile-acid-binding ability than raw ones Increased long-term intake of sinigrin decreased formation of molecules in the body called AGEs (advanced glycation end-products) related to increased oxidative stress Pet ether and ethanolic leaf extract show hepatoprotective effect with reduction of ALT, AST ALP, and total bilirubin level	
	Dried radish green (*Raphanus sativus*)	Cooked siraegi with seasoning shows better antioxidant and antibacterial activities than raw material Inhibits cell proliferation via the ErbB-Akt pathway in MDA-MB-231 human breast cancer cell Shows strong antioxidant and anti-inflammatory potential and, in consequence, profound effects on ulcerative colitis	Park et al., 2014; Kim et al., 2011b; Ji, 2011
	Scallion (*Allium* spp.)	Used as a seasoning for namul Et-OH extract of *Allium wageki* has protective effect on the increase of TG, total cholesterol, insulin level, and blood pressure in fructose-induced hypertensive rats	Kang et al., 2002
Red	Red chili pepper (*Capsicum annuum*)	Used as a seasoning for namul Plays a beneficial effect on analgesia, cardiovascular system, diabetes, gastroprotection, urological disorders, and weight reduction	Fattori et al., 2016; Chang et al., 2003; Oh, 2004
Yellow	Soybean sprout (*Glycine max*)	Asparagine and isoflavone produced during cultivation of bean sprouts lower blood alcohol levels, inhibit absorption of alcohol, and speed up the recovery from hangover	Chon et al., 2013; Jeong et al., 2009; Kim et al., 2003, 2005

(*Continued*)

TABLE 16.2 (CONTINUED)

Health Benefits of Color Vegetables Commonly Used for Namul Dishes in Korea

Color	Vegetables	Effectiveness	Ref.
Yellow	Sesame seed or its oil (*Sesamum indicum*)	Used as a seasoning for namul The effect of sesame oil on serum triglyceride and LDL-cholesterol is greater than that of olive oil. Lignans have various physiological activities such as cholesterol-lowering action, inhibition of cancer cell proliferation, aging, and blood pressure increase	Namayandeh et al., 2013; Aldercreutz, 2007; Coulman et al., 2005
White	Radish (*Raphanus sativus*); turnip (*Brassica napa*)	Used for diuretic, digestive, and curative for jaundice in Korean traditional medicine Water extract improves bowel function and constipation Et-OH extract of turnip shows hepatoprotective effect on liver damage Et-OH extract of turnip decreases TC, PL and TG, β-sitosterol exert antihyperlipidemic activity	Baik et al., 2004; Choi et al., 2006; Rhee et al., 2005
	Balloon flower root (*Platycodon grandifloras*)	Platycodin, oleanane-type pentacyclic triterpenoid saponins alleviate phlegm and protect the bronchi, and have immunological, antiasthmatic, anti-inflammatory, antioxidant, antitumor, antiobesity and hepatoprotective effect Animal experiments show lower cholesterol and blood sugar	Kim and Kang, 2017; He et al., 2015; Choi et al., 2001a, 2001b
	Garlic (*Allium sativum*)	Used as a seasoning for namul Onions and leeks, sulfur compounds break down more slowly than allicin in garlic, and the amount of active sulfur is lower than that of garlic because amount of sulfamic acid is small The scorodin component warms the internal organs and smooths the blood circulation and metabolism, so the penis is filled with the corpus cavernosum, which is effective in strengthening the tongue	Lu et al., 2012; Hirasa and Takemasa, 1998; Fukushima et al., 1997
	Lotus root (*Nelumbo nucifera*)	Lotus diet prevents the development and progression of NAFLD in diabetic patients by suppressing the expression of lipogenic and inflammatory genes as a result of the higher serum adiponectin level Antidiabetic effect: decreased blood sugar level	Yang et al., 2016; Tsuruta et al., 2012; Huang et al., 2011; Mukherjee et al., 1997

(Continued)

Namul, the Korean Vegetable Dish

403

TABLE 16.2 (CONTINUED)
Health Benefits of Color Vegetables Commonly Used for Namul Dishes in Korea

Color	Vegetables	Effectiveness	Ref.
White	Bamboo shoot (*Bambusa vulgaris*, and *Phyllostachys edulis*)	Cholesterol lowering effect (phytosterol) Antidiabetic effect: inhibits obesity associated chronic systemic inflammation	Chongtham et al, 2011; Koidea et al., 2011; Park and Jhon, 2009, 2010; Han and Koo, 1993
	Burdock root (*Arctium lappa*)	Prevent cancer, cure diabetes, lower blood pressure and overcome hangovers Diuretic principles, which help expel toxic products from the blood through urine Cynarin-riched ethylacetate fraction shows antioxidative and tyrosinase inhibitory activity	Im and Lee, 2014; Kim et al., 2012b; Lee, 2011; Lin et al., 2002; Han and Koo, 1993; Park et al., 1992
Violet (black)	Eggplant (*Solanum melongena*)	Eggplant peel inhibits xanthine oxidase and ACE (phenolics and flavonoids compounds) Antioxidant: delphinidin (nasunin) against free-radical–induced oxidative stress and melanogenesis by UV-B Ameliorate ROS-induced oxidative stress via hepatic xanthine oxidase activity Anti-inflammatory effect (solanoflavone) Inhibit immunologic and nonimmunologic stimulator-mediated anaphylactic reactions Hypolipidemic effect Highest inhibitory effect against the mutagenicity of Trp-P-1, Trp-P-2, B[a] P, AB1, and MNNG among dialyzate vegetables	Lee et al., 2017a; Ko et al, 2016; Jo et al., 2012; Kim et al, 2011a; Beik et al., 2009; Shen et al., 2005; Lee et al., 2001; Sudheesh et al., 1997; Shinohara et al., 1988
	Eastern bracken fern (*Pteridium aquilinum*)	Exhibit anti-inflammatory and/or antioxidative properties (chlorogenic acid, caffeic acid, p-coumaric acid, ferulic acid, kaempferol and apigenin) Western people do not eat ferns because of ptaquiloside, which is known as a carcinogen and thiaminase, but fern namul is safe and has excellent physiological effects if it is eaten cooked as namul after eliminating more than 90% by boiling in baking soda to soften and eliminate astringent taste and then stir-fried	Dion et al., 2015
	Perilla seed or its oil (*Perilla frutescens*)	Blood pressure reduction, prevention of arteriosclerosis, inflammation and allergy (α-linolenic acid) suppression of colon tumorigenesis and hepatotoxicity	Lee et al., 2014; Philip, 2010; Takano et al., 2004

404 Korean Functional Foods

16.6.1 Antioxidative Effects

Free radicals, such as reactive oxygen and nitrogen species, are produced as by-products of aerobic metabolism and have been implicated in the pathogenesis of many diseases, including cancer, atherosclerosis, diabetes, hypertension, inflammation, and aging (Lobo et al., 2010; Park and Kim, 2014; Singh et al., 2015). Antioxidant phytochemicals neutralize free radicals (unstable molecules) that are associated with oxidative stress.

One of the most powerful wild greens, purslane (*Portulaca oleracea* L.), is high in omega-3 fatty acids, antioxidants, vitamins E, C, and K, beta-carotene, glutathione, and psoralens. Psoralens have powerful antioxidant properties that, besides fighting cancer, are particularly beneficial for normalizing skin pigmentation. Although purslane is considered a weed in the United States, it has been eaten as saengchae with kochujang and vinegar dressing in Korea.

16.6.1.1 Bioflavonoid (Quercetin)

Vegetables have abundant levels of antioxidants that prevent the growth of cancerous cells. Dark green vegetables have lots of phenolic flavonoid antioxidants and minerals. Moreover, antioxidants boost the body's immunity and keep it from developing infections and diseases.

Leafy green vegetables and wild greens have a bioflavonoid known as "quercetin" (Trichopoulou et al., 2000). Along with its unique anticancer properties, it is responsible for the antioxidant and anti-inflammatory activities of vegetables. Quercetin also effectively cuts down the flow of substances that lead to allergies. This compound plays the role of an inhibitor of mass cell secretion, thereby decreasing the release of interleukin-6.

16.6.1.2 Lutein and Zeaxanthin

The antioxidants lutein and zeaxanthin likely play a role in preventing cataracts. Eating dark green vegetables can also keep the eyes healthy and may help prevent two common aging-related eye diseases—cataracts and macular degeneration—that afflict millions of Americans over age 65 (Brown et al., 1999; Cho et al., 2004; Moeller et al., 2004; Christen et al., 2005). In fact, a study demonstrated that higher dietary intake of lutein, zeaxanthin and vitamin E was associated with a significantly decreased risk of cataract formation (Christen et al., 2008). Beyond reducing the risk of eye disease, separate studies have shown that lutein and zeaxanthin improve visual performance in age-related macular degeneration patients, cataract patients and people in good health (Stringham and Hammond, 2005).

16.6.2 Antidiabetic Effects

The global prevalence of diabetes among adults over 18 years of age has risen from 4.7% in 1980 to 8.5% in 2014 (WHO, 2017). Diabetes is generally not

Namul, the Korean Vegetable Dish

considered to be curable through medical treatment, including drugs and surgeries. Dietary factors are important and are potentially modifiable risk factors.

A recent meta-analysis concluded that greater intake of green leafy vegetables was associated with a 14% reduction (hazard ratio 0.86, 95% confidence interval 0.77 to 0.97) in risk of type 2 diabetes (p = 0.01). Estimates of this study showed no significant benefits of increasing the consumption of vegetables, fruit, or fruit and vegetables combined (Carter et al., 2010).

In a study of over 70,000 female nurses aged 38–63 years who were free of cardiovascular disease, cancer, and diabetes, research showed that consumption of green leafy vegetables and fruit was associated with a lower risk of diabetes. While not conclusive, research also indicated that consumption of fruit juices may be associated with an increased risk of diabetes among women (Bazzano et al., 2008). Rats fed a diet that contains water extracts of angelica tree shoot (*Aralia elata*) significantly decreased blood glucose level, restored insulin level that had decreased due to diabetes, and significantly lowered HbA1c (Shin, 2006).

16.6.3 Immunoenhancing Effects

During the past several decades, much attention has been devoted to various traditional Korean vegetables and herbs for their immunocompetent and therapeutic effects (Park and Kim, 2014). Many *in vivo* experiments have been performed in rodent models that were administered water extracts (Kim and Kim, 2002; Kim et al., 2009; Ryu et al., 2008).

Aster scaber water extract in lipopolysaccharide (LPS)-stimulated animals increased peritoneal macrophage tumor necrosis factor (TNF)-α production and splenocyte proliferation (Kim and Kim, 2002). Activated macrophages release various products (i.e., proteases, neutrophil, cytokines, and growth factors) that result in the destruction of tissue. Thus, increased cytokine production from the activated macrophages after administration of certain materials would indicate that the materials are effective immune enhancers in the early stage of inflammation response (Park and Kim, 2014). Studies with hesperidin (Lee et al., 2011) and quercetin (Jung et al., 2012) indicated that Korean traditional vegetables and herbs that contain these compounds might relieve inflammation triggered by radiation.

As seen in previous studies, naturally occurring components of individual namul plants might enhance immune function. However, there have not been enough studies in which components actually led to pharmacological activities. They could be plant alkaloids or terpenoids. Further studies are needed to identify the active compounds from Korean traditional vegetables and herbs (Park and Kim, 2014). Green vegetables have high levels of beta-carotene, which improves immune function considerably once it is converted into vitamin A.

Water-soluble vitamins B and C rich in Korean traditional vegetables are also known to have immune-enhancing effects. In an experiment using athymic nude mice, vitamin B supplementation caused increased response of B lymphocytes with lipopolysaccharide (LPS), but did not inhibit the development of human malignant melanoma (M21-HPB) xenografts. This evidence suggests that tumor inhibition by high dietary vitamin B may be mediated by T-lymphocyte-dependent mechanisms (Moriguchi et al., 2003). Vitamin C is also an essential nutrient playing a role in protecting against carcinogenesis. In one of its inhibitory actions against carcinogenesis, enhancement of cellular immunity is involved. However, when stable immunoenhancement is desired, a high-level intake of vitamin C more than 1000 mg per day is needed (Anderson et al., 1980).

16.6.4 Anticancer Effects

An European study tracked 142,605 men and 335,873 women for an average of nearly 9 years. Eating more vegetables was associated with a small but statistically significant reduction in cancer risk. The data translated into a 4% lower risk of cancer for every two extra servings of vegetables a day per person (Key, 2011).

A more likely possibility is that some types of vegetables may protect against certain cancers. A report by the World Cancer Research Fund and the American Institute for Cancer Research suggested that nonstarchy vegetables—such as lettuce and other leafy greens, bok choy, and cabbage, as well as garlic, onions, and the like "probably" protected against several types of cancers, including those of the mouth, throat, voice box, esophagus, and stomach (Wiseman, 2008).

Block et al. (1992) reviewed on the relationship between vegetable and fruit consumption and risk of cancer by examining 206 human epidemiologic studies and 22 animal studies. They verified that 128 of 156 dietary studies presented a statistically significant protective effect with vegetables and fruit intake. The evidence for a protective effect of greater vegetable and fruit consumption is consistent for cancers of the stomach, esophagus, lung, oral cavity and pharynx, endometrium, pancreas, and colon. The types of vegetables or fruit that most often appear to be protective against cancer are raw vegetables, followed by allium vegetables, carrots, green vegetables, cruciferous vegetables, and tomatoes. Substances present in vegetables and fruit that may help protect against cancer and their mechanisms were dithiolthiones, isothiocyanates, indole-3-carbinol, allium compounds, isoflavones, protease inhibitors, saponins, phytosterols, inositol hexaphosphate, vitamin C, D-limonene, lutein, folic acid, beta-carotene, lycopene, selenium, vitamin E, flavonoids, and dietary fiber.

16.6.4.1 Carotenoids

Dark green vegetables containing carotenoids may protect against lung, mouth, and throat cancer (Wiseman, 2008). But more research is needed to clarify the exact relationship among vegetables, carotenoids, and cancer. Foods high in beta-carotene include dark green vegetables. Other than beta-carotene, they also contain canthaxanthin phytoene, lutein, xanthophylls, and lycopene, many of which may offer greater anticarcinogenic effects than beta-carotene (Stahl and Sies, 2005).

Vitamin A is the nutrient with the most impact on both tumor incidence and growth and host immune system (Moriguchi et al., 2003). Epidemiological studies have demonstrated that a high intake of food rich in beta-carotene is associated with reduced risk of certain types of cancers, especially lung cancer (Le Marchand et al., 1989). Since other carotenoids lacking provitamin A activity had a similar anticancer effect as that of beta-carotene, it has been suggested that the anticancer and antibacterial effects of beta-carotene are not considered to be due to provitamin A functions but rather to antioxidant and immunomodulatory functions (Bendich and Shapiro, 1986). Proliferation of peripheral blood lymphocytes with PHA or ConA was 1.4- to 1.9-fold higher in the beta-carotene supplemented group compared to the control group, whereas there was no significant difference in NK cell activity between both groups (Moriguchi et al., 1996). In addition, the study on *in vitro* effects of beta-carotene could induce higher tumoricidal activity of human monocytes following short-term and lower concentration incubation compared to those of beta-carotene (Moriguchi and Kishino, 1990). Since many other reports support the action of beta-carotene against inhibition of tumorigenesis and tumor cell growth and the enhancement of immune responses, it is believed that beta-carotene is a nutrient for improving conditions in cancer patients and aged people showing decreased cellular immunity (Moriguchi et al., 2003).

16.6.4.2 Chlorophyll

Chlorophyll and its derivatives in all green vegetables are very effective at binding carcinogens like polycyclic aromatic hydrocarbons, heterocyclic amines, aflatoxin, and other hydrophobic molecules. The chlorophyll–carcinogen complex is much harder for the body to absorb, so most of it is swept out with the feces (Donaldson, 2004). A prospective randomized controlled trial conducted in Qidong, China, showed the anticarcinogenic effects of chlorophyll against liver cancer. A 55% reduction in aflatoxin–DNA adducts was found in the group that took 100 mg of chlorophyllin three times a day (Egner et al., 2001). Dark leafy green vegetables are high in chlorophyll and other anticarcinogenic compounds and should be eaten daily, both raw and cooked (Lee and Park, 1993).

16.6.4.3 Folic Acid

Many studies have found a significant reduction in colon, rectal, and breast cancer with folate consumption. Folic acid has an integral role in DNA methylation and synthesis. If sufficient folic acid is not available, uracil is substituted for thymidine in DNA, which leads to DNA strand breakage. Alcohol is an antagonist of folate, so, drinking alcoholic beverages greatly magnifies the cancer risk of a low-folate diet (Donalson, 2004). Genetic polymorphisms (common single DNA base mutations resulting in a different amino acid encoded into a protein) in the methylenetetrahydrofolate reductase and the methionine synthase genes, which increase the relative amount of folate available for DNA synthesis and repair, also reduce the risk of colon cancer (Giovannucci 2002; Hubner and Houlston, 2009). Cravo et al. (1998) used 5 mg of folic acid a day (a supraphysiological dose) in a prospective, controlled, crossover study of 20 patients with colonic adenoma polyps. They found that the folic acid could reverse DNA hypomethylation in 7 of 12 patients who had only one polyp.

Folate may be more important for rapidly dividing tissue, like the colonic mucosa. Therefore, the cancer risk associated with low folate intake is probably higher for colon cancer than for breast cancer. Most breast cancer studies only found a protective effect of folate among women who consumed alcohol. However, among women residents of Shanghai who consumed no alcohol or vitamin supplements and ate unprocessed, unfortified foods, there was a 29% decreased risk of breast cancer among those with the highest intake of folate (Shrubsole et al., 2001). Thus, there may be a true protective effect that is masked in Western populations by so many other risk factors. Two studies showed that the risk of cancer due to family history can be modified by high folate intake, so a prudent anticancer diet would be high in dark green, leafy vegetables (Donalson, 2004).

16.6.4.4 Sulforaphane

The cruciferous vegetables that Koreans consume much through kimchi and namul dishes contain a potent, cancer-fighting compound, sulforophane. The latest study has also suggested a potentially higher anticancer benefit of eating vegetables for people who regularly drink alcohol.

Cruciferous family vegetables were investigated by measuring the activity of natural killer (NK) cells, which play an important role in protecting the body from bacterial and viral infections, as well as in excluding transformed cells and suppressing carcinogenesis (Baraz et al., 1999; Cooley et al., 1999). Furthermore, since vegetables are great antioxidants, they also alleviate the chances of fatal diseases like cancer.

16.6.4.5 Dietary Fiber

The majority of investigative evidence supports the notion that a higher fiber diet reduces the risk of colon cancer. The first hypothesis is that fiber increases

Namul, the Korean Vegetable Dish 409

bulk and in turn dilutes fecal bile acids, which are thought to promote cancer of the colon. Second, dietary fiber may reduce the action of certain colonic bacteria, which are responsible for the transmission of primary bile acids into secondary bile acids. These secondary bile acids are thought to promote tumorigenesis in the colon. Third, increased dietary fiber is thought to dilute the contents in the lumen of the colon, which will decrease the exposure of mucosal tissue to potential carcinogens.

The mechanism by which fiber is thought to decrease the risk of breast cancer is less complex. When breast cancer cannot be attributed to genetic predisposition, an increased level of circulating estrogen is suspected. Dietary fiber is speculated to bind the estrogen excreted into the digestive tract and block its reabsorption. Also, compounds such as phytoestrogens found in fiber-containing food may compete with estradiol for estrogen receptors in breast tissue and in this manner beneficially affect breast cancer risk. Another proposed mechanism is that fiber may positively influence the formation of mammalian lignin, which protects against breast cancer.

16.6.5 Cardiovascular Disease

There is compelling evidence that a diet rich in vegetables can lower the risk of heart disease and stroke (Hung et al., 2004; Dauchet et al., 2006; He et al., 2006, 2007). Although the pathways involved remain uncertain, the results in a mouse model of atherosclerosis indicated that a diet rich in green and yellow vegetables inhibits the development of atherosclerosis and may therefore lead to a reduction in the risk of coronary heart disease (Adams et al., 2006).

According to the Harvard-based Nurses' Health Study and Health Professionals Follow-up Study, which included almost 110,000 men and women for 14 years, the higher the average daily intake of vegetables was, the lower were the chances of developing cardiovascular disease. Although all fruits and vegetables likely contribute to this benefit, green leafy vegetables such as lettuce, spinach, Swiss chard, and mustard greens and cruciferous vegetables such as cabbage and bok choy make important contributions (Hung et al., 2004).

When researchers combined findings from the Harvard studies with several other long-term studies in the United States and Europe, and looked at coronary heart disease and stroke separately, they found a similar protective effect: Individuals who ate more than five servings of fruits and vegetables per day had roughly a 20% lower risk of coronary heart disease (He et al., 2007) and stroke (He et al., 2006), compared with individuals who ate less than three servings per day.

Another meta-analysis of cohort studies indicated that fruit and vegetable consumption is inversely associated with the occurrence of coronary heart disease (CHD). The risk of CHD was decreased by 4% for each additional portion per day of fruit and vegetable intake, by 7% for fruit intake, and by 11% for vegetable intake (Dauchet et al., 2006).

16.6.6 Blood Pressure

The dietary approaches to stop hypertension (DASH) diet, rich in fruits, vegetables, and low-fat dairy products, restricted the amount of saturated and total fat, reduced the systolic blood pressure by about 11 mm Hg and the diastolic blood pressure by almost 6 mm Hg—as much as medications can achieve (Appel et al., 1997).

A randomized trial known as the Optimal Macronutrient Intake Trial for Heart Health (OmniHeart) showed that this fruit- and vegetable-rich diet lowered blood pressure even more when some of the carbohydrate was replaced with healthy unsaturated fat or protein (Appel et al., 2005). In 2014 a meta-analysis of clinical trials and observational studies found that consumption of a vegetarian diet was associated with lower blood pressure (Yokoyama et al., 2014).

16.7 Conclusion

Korean traditional food culture was close to nature, and the vitality of nature is permeated with the simple beauty of food. From a long time ago, Koreans have described the importance of food life with the expression "medicine and foods are from the same origin." This means the food we eat is closely related to keeping our health and curing diseases. Based on the humanitarian and welfare spirit during the Chosun dynasty, food was considered a medicine, and the practice to cure with food became conventional.

Namul is the iconic banchan made with cultivated or nondomesticated vegetables. The consumption of wild vegetables has often been perceived to have a medicinal character. Recently, a number of phytochemicals or bitter-tasting compounds have been compiled that possibly exert health benefits. Some people argue that vegetarianism is the only way to save people and to save the planet. According to nutrient contents and health benefits of Korean traditional vegetables and herbs, namul would be one of the healthiest food in the world.

References

Adams, M.R., D.L. Golden, H. Chen, T.C. Register, and E.T. Guggery. 2006. A diet rich in green and yellow vegetables inhibits atherosclerosis in mice. *Nutr Disease* 136:1886–1889.

Analects. Confucius' followers. 475~221 BC. Beijing: China.

Andah, B.W., T. Shaw, P. Sinclair, and A.I. Okpoko. 1994. *The Archaeology of Africa: Food, Metals and Towns.* London: Routlege.

Anderson, R., R. Oosthuizen, R. Maritz, A. Theron, and A.J. Van Rensburg. 1980. The effects of increasing weekly doses of ascorbate on certain cellular and humoral immune function in normal volunteers. *Am J Clin Nutr* 33:71–76.

Anonymous. Production time unknown. *Dongun-goryak*. Seoul: Korea.

Appel, L.J., T.J. Moore, E. Obarzanek et al. 1997. A clinical trial of the effects of dietary patterns on blood pressure. DASH collaborative research group. *New England J Med* 336:1117–1124.

Appel, L.J. et al. 2005. Effects of protein, monounsaturated fat, and carbohydrate intake on blood pressure and serum lipids: Results of the OmniHeart randomized trial. *JAMA* 294(19):2455–2464.

Bae, J.H., S.O. Yu, Y.M. Kim, S.U. Chon, B.W. Kim, and B.G. Heo. 2009. Physiological activity of methanol extracts from *Liguralia fischeri* and their hyperplasia inhibition activity of cancer cell. *J Bio-Environ Control* 18:67–73.

Bae, S-J., N-H. Kim, B-J. Ha, B-M. Jung, and S-B. Roh. 1997. Effects of godulbaegi leaf extracts on CCl_4-induced hepatotoxicity in rats. *J Kor Soc Food Sci Nut* 26:137–143.

Bae, S-J., S-B. Roh, and B-M. Jung. 1998. Effects of godulbaegi extracts on the stability and fluidity of phospholipid liposomal membranes. *J Kor Soc Food Sci Nut* 27:508–517.

Baik, S-O., H-Y. Kim, Y-H. Lee, and Y-S. Kim. 2004. Preparation of active fractions from radish water extracts for improving the intestinal functions and constipation activities. *J Korean Soc Appl Biol Chem* 47:315–320.

Bailey, C.J., and C. Day. 1989. Traditional plant medicines as treatments for diabetes. *Diabetes Care* 12:553–564.

Baraz, M., E. Khazanov, R. Condiotti, M. Kotler, and A. Nagler. 1999. Natural killer (NK) cells prevent virus production in cell culture. *Bone Marrow Transplan* 24:179–189.

Barbagallo, M., and L.J. Dominguez. 2015. Magnesium and type 2 diabetes. *World J Diabetes* 6:1152–1157.

Bardaweel, S.K., M.M. Hudaib, K.A. Tawaha, and R.M. Bashatwah. 2015. Studies on the *in vitro* antiproliferative, antimicrobial, antioxidant, and Acetylcholinesterase inhibition activities associated with *Chrysanthemum coronarium* essential oil. ECAM, Article ID 790838:1-6. http://dx.doi.org/10.1155/2015/790838

Bazzano, L.A., Y.L. Tricia, J.J. Kamudi, and B.H. Frank. 2008. Intake of fruit, vegetables, and fruit juices and risk of diabetes in women. *Diabetes Care* 31:1311–1317.

Beik, K-Y., S-I. Lee, J-S. Kim et al. 2009 Antioxidative effects of extracts of various cultivars and different plant parts of eggplant. *J East Asian Soc Dietary Life* 19:195–201.

Bendich, A., and S.S. Shapiro. 1986. Effect of beta-carotene and canthaxanthin on the immune responses of rat. *J Nutr* 116:2254–2262.

Block, G., B. Patterson, and A. Subar. 1992. Fruit, vegetables, and cancer prevention: a review of the epidemiological evidence. *Nutr Cancer* 18:1–29.

Boeing, H., A. Bechthold, A. Bub et al. 2012. Critical review: Vegetables and fruit in the prevention of chronic diseases. *Eur J Nutr* 51:637–663.

Bonari, R.A.K. 2011. Effect of the spinach (*Spinacia oleracea*) on blood glucose and insulin levels in diabetic rats. In: *12th Iranian Congress of Biochemistry and 4th International Congress of Biochemistry & Molecular Biology*. September 9, Mashhad University of Medical Sciences, Mashhad, Iran.

Brown, L., E.B. Rimm, J.M. Seddon et al. 1999. A prospective study of carotenoid intake and risk of cataract extraction in US men. *Am J Clin Nutr* 70:517–524.

Carter, P., L. Gray, J. Troughton, K. Khunti, and M.J. Davies. 2010. Fruit and vegetable intake and incidence of type 2 diabetes mellitus: Systematic review and meta-analysis. *BMJ* 341:c4229. doi:10.1136/bmj.c4229.

Chang, U.J., D.G. Kim, J.M. Kim, H.J. Suh, and S.H. Oh. 2003. Weight reduction effect of extract of fermented red pepper on female college students. *J Korean Soc Food Sci Nutr* 32:479–484.

Cha, G-H., Y-J. Song, and H-G. Lee. 2006. The Kimi theory on vegetables: Focused on *Sikgamchalyo* of *Jeongjoji* in *Limwonsibyukji* and *Tangaekpyeon* in *Donguibogam*. *Korean J Food Cookery Sci* 23:690–701.

Cha, Y-S., and B-M. Jung. 1998. Effect of leaf mustard (*Brassica juncea*) on lipid metabolism of rat chroethanol administration. *J Korean Soc Human Ecol*. 1:94–102.

Cho, E., J.M. Seddon, and B. Rosner. 2004. Prospective study of intake of fruits, vegetables, vitamins, and carotenoids and risk of age-related maculopathy. *Arch Ophthalmol* 122:883–892.

Cho, H-J. 1998. The traditional method for preparing Korean vegetable dishes—Especially about *na mul, seng chae, ssam*. *J Korean Soc Food Sci* 14:339–347.

Choi, C.Y., J.Y. Kim, Y.S. Kim et al. 2001a. Aqueous extract isolated from *Platycodon grandiflorum* elicits the release of nitric oxide and tumor necrosis factor-α from murine macrophages. *Intl Immunopharmacol* 1:1141–1151.

Choi, C.Y., J.Y. Kim, Y.S. Kim et al. 2001b. Augmentation of macrophage functions by an aqueous extract isolated from *Platycodon grandiflorum*. *Cancer Lett* 166:17–25.

Choi, H.J., M.J. Han, I.B. Nam, D.H. Kim, H.G. Jung, and N.J. Kim. 2006. Hepatoprotective effects of *Brassica rapa* (turnip) on D-galatosamine induced liver injured rats. *Kor J Pharmacogn* 37:258–265.

Choi, H-S., M-Y. Lee, Y. Jeong, and G-M. Shin. 2004. Hepatoprotective effects of *Allium monanthum* max. extract on ethanol-induced liver damage in rat. *J Food Sci Nutr* 9:245–252.

Choi, J-M., E-O. Lee, H-J. Lee et al. 2007. Identification of campesterol from *Chrysanthemum coronarium* L. and its antiangiogenic activities. *Phytother. Res* 21:954–959.

Choi, W.J., S.K. Kim, H.K. Park, U-D. Sohn, and W. Kim. 2014. Anti-inflammatory and anti-superbacterial properties of sulforaphane from Shepard's purse. *Korean J Physiol Pharmacol* 18:33–39. http//dx.doi.org/10.4196/kjpp.2014.8.1.33.

Chon, S-U., and J-G. Kang. 2013. Phenolics level and antioxidant activity of methanol extracts from different plant parts in *Youngia sonchifolia*. *Korean J Crop Sci* 58:20–27.

Chon, S-U., D-K. Kim, and Y-M. Kim. 2013. Phenolics content and antioxidant activity of sprouts in several legume crops. *Korean J Plant Res* 26:159–168.

Chongtham, N., M.S. Bisht, and S. Haorongbam. 2011. Nutritional properties of bamboo shoots: Potential and prospects for utilization as a health food. *Compreh Rev Food Sci Food Safety* 10:153–169.

Christen, W.G., S. Liu, D.A. Schaumberg, and J.E. Buring. 2005. Fruit and vegetable intake and the risk of cataract in women. *Am J Clin Nutr* 81:1417–1422.

Christen, W.G., S. Liu, R.J. Glynn, J.M. Gaziano, and J.E. Buring. 2008. Dietary carotenoids, vitamins C and E, and risk of cataract in women: A prospective study. *Arch Ophthalmol* 126:102–109.

Chung, H.K. 2017. *Humanities of vegetables*, Seoul: Ddabi.

Cooley S., L.J. Burns, T. Repka, and J.S. Miller. 1999. Natural killer cell cytotoxicity of breast cancer targets is enhanced by two distinct mechanisms of antibody-dependent cellular cytotoxicity against LFA-3 and HER2/neu. *Exp Hematol* 27:1533–1541.

Coulman, K.D., Z. Liu, W.Q. Hum, J. Michaelides, and L.U. Thompson. 2005. Whole sesame seed is as rich a source of mammalian lignan precursors as whole flaxseed. *Nutr Cancer* 52:156–165.

Cravo, M.L. et al. 1998. Effect of folate supplementation on DNA methylation of rectal mucosa in patients with colonic adenomas: correlation with nutrient intake. *Clin Nutr.* 17:45–49.

Dauchet, L., A. Philippe, S. Hercberg, and J. Dallongeville. 2006. Fruit and vegetable consumption and risk of coronary heart disease: A meta-analysis of cohort studies *J Nutr* 136: 2588–2593.

Dion, C., C. Haug, H. Guan et al. 2015. Evaluation of the anti-inflammatory and anti-oxidative potential of four fern species from China intended for use as food supplements. *Nat Prod Commun* 10:597–603.

Donaldson, M.S. 2004. Nutrition and cancer: A review of the evidence for an anti-cancer diet. *Nutrition J* 3(19):1–21, doi:10.1186/1475-2891-3-19.

Egner, P.A., J.B. Wang, Y.R. Zhu et al. 2001. Chlorophyllin intervention reduces aflatoxin-DNA adducts in individuals at high risk for liver cancer. *Proc Natl Acad Sci USA* 98:14601–14606.

Fabbri, A.D.T., and G.A. Crosby. 2016. A review of the impact of preparation and cooking on the nutritional quality of vegetables and legumes. *Intl J Gast Food Sci* April:2–11. https://doi.org/10.1016/j.ijgfs.2015.11.001.

Fattori, V., M.S. Hohmann, A.C. Rossaneis, F.A. Pinho-Ribeiro, and W.A. Verri. 2016. Capsaicin: Current understanding of its mechanisms and therapy of pain and other pre-clinical and clinical uses. *Molecules* 21:844, doi:10.3390/molecules21070844.

Feskanich, D., P. Weber, W.C. Willett et al. 1999. Vitamin K intake and hip fractures in women: A prospective study. *Am J Clin Nutr* 69:74–79.

Fukushima, S., N. Takada, T. Hori, and H. Wanibuchi. 1997. Cancer prevention by organosulfur compounds from garlic and onion. *J Cell Biochem Suppl* 27: 100–105.

Giovannucci, E. 2002. Epidemiologic studies of folate and colorectal neoplasia: a review. *J Nutr.* 132:2350S–2355S.

Ha, G-J., D.S. Lee, T.W. Seung et al. 2015. Anti-amnesic and neuroprotective effects of *Artemisia argyi* H. (*Seomae* mugwort) extracts. *Korean J Food Sci Technol* 47:380–387.

Ham, S-S., S-Y. Lee, D-H. Oh et al. 1998. Antimutagenic and antigenotoxic effects of *Ligularia fischeri* extracts. *J Korean Soc Food Sci Nutr* 27:745–750.

Han, K-S., E-H. Cheong, S-S. Ham et al. 1993. Antimutagenicity of small water drop-wort juice on the microbial mutagenicity induced by 2-aminofluorene. *Korean J Food Hyg* 8:225–230.

Han, S.H. Result announcement on Attitude Survey for the Healthy Eating Habits of Koreans http://sports.chosun.com/news/ntype.htm?id=201705160100125010000 8918&servicedate= 20170516 (accessed on May 20, 2017).

Han, S.J., and S.J. Koo. 1993 Study on the chemical composition in bamboo shoot, lotus root and burdock. *Korean J Soc Food Sci* 9:82–87.

He, F.J., C.A. Nowson, M. Lucas, and G.A. MacGregor. 2007. Increased consumption of fruit and vegetables is related to a reduced risk of coronary heart disease: Meta-analysis of cohort studies. *J Hum Hypertens* 21:717–728.

He, F.J., C.A. Nowson, and G.A. MacGregor. 2006. Fruit and vegetable consumption and stroke: Meta-analysis of cohort studies. *Lancet* 367(9507):320–326.

He, J-Y., N. Ma, S. Zhu, K. Komatsu, Z-Y. Li, and W-M. Fu. 2015. The genus *Codonopsis* (Campanulaceae): A review of phytochemistry, bioactivity and quality control. *J Nat Med* 69:1–21.

Hirasa, K. and M. Takemasa. 1998. *Spice science and technology*. New York: Marcel Dekker.

Hubner, R.A., and R.S. Houlston. 2009. Folate and colorectal cancer prevention. *Br J Cancer* 100:233–239. doi:10.1038/sj.bjc.6604823.

Hung, H.C., K.J. Joshipura, R. Jiang et al. 2004. Fruit and vegetable intake and risk of major chronic disease. *J Natl Cancer Inst* 96:1577–1584.

Hwang, P-S. 1870. *Myunmul-giryak*. Seoul: Korea.

Il-yeon. 1281. *Samguk-yusa*. Seoul: Korea.

Im, D.Y., and K.I. Lee. 2014. Antioxidative activity and tyrosinase inhibitory activity of the extract and fractions from *Arctium lappa* roots and analysis of phenolic compounds. *Kor J Pharmacogn* 45:141–146.

IOM (Institute of Medicine), Food and Nutrition Board. 2005.

Jang J-H., H-W. Cho, B-Y. Lee, K-Y. Yu, and J-Y. Yoon. 2016. Anti-inflammatory effects of *Oenanthe javanica* ethanol extract and its fraction on LPS-induced inflammation response. *J Korean Soc Food Sci Nutr* 45:1595–1603.

Jang, J-H., K.S. Lee, and J-S. Seo. 2011. Effect of dietary supplementation of β-carotene on hepatic antioxidant enzyme activities and glutathione concentration in diabetic rats. *J Korean Soc Food Sci Nutr* 40:1092–1098.

Jang, S-M., J-B. Lee, and H. Ahn. 2002. The effect of pumpkin and medical herb extract supplement on blood composition of women delivered of a child. *Food Ind. Nutr* 7:45–49.

Jeong, Y-S., K.H. Dhakal, and Y-H. Hwang. 2009. Effects of soy-sprout asparagine on hangover. Agric Rex Bull Kyungpook Natl Univ 27:53–58.

Ji, S.J. 2011. Antioxidant and anti-inflammatory activities of dried *Raphanus sativus* L. and *Angelica keiskei* L. Master's thesis. Seoul: Danguk University.

Jo, J-O., and I-C. Jung. 2000a. Analysis of flavonoids in raw and blanching of several green-yellow vegetables. *J East Asian Soc Dietary Life* 10:42–47.

Jo, J-O., and I-C. Jung. 2000b. Changes in carotenoid contents of several green-yellow vegetables by blanching. *Korean J Soc Food Sci* 16:17–21.

Jo, Y-N., H.R. Jeong, J-H. Jeong, and H.J. Heo. 2012. The skin protecting effects of ethanolic extracts of eggplant peels. *Korean J Food Sci Technol* 44:94–99.

Jung, J-H., J-I. Kang, and H-S. Kim. 2012. Effect of quercetin on impaired immune function in mice exposed to irradiation. *Nutr Res Pract* 6:301–307.

Kang, D.G., E.J. Sohn, A.S. Lee et al. 2002. Effects of the ethanol-extract of *Allium wageki* on the fructose-induced hypertensive rats. *Korean J Pharmacognosy* 33:384–388.

Kessler, F., and G. Glauser. 2014. Prenylquinone profiling in whole leaves and chloroplast subfractions. *Plant Isoprenoids* 1153:213–226. doi:10.1007/978-1-4939-0606-2_15.

Key, T.J. 2011. Fruit and vegetables and cancer risk. *British J Cancer* 104:6–11.

Kim, D-G., M-H. Kim, M.J. Kang, and J.H. Shin. 2015. Effect of spinach extract on RANKL-mediated osteoclast differentiation. *J Korean Soc Food Sci Nutr* 44:532–539.

Kim, E.M., K-J. Kim, J-H. Choi, and K.M. Chee. 2005. Bioavailability assessment of isoflavones between soybean and soybean sprout in rat. *J Korean Soc Nutr* 38:335–343.

Kim, H-J., and S-H. Kang. 2017. Ethnobotany, phytochemistry, pharmacology of the Korean Campanulaceae: A comprehensive review. *Korean J Plant Res* 30: 240–264.

Kim, H.Y., Y.J. Cho, N. Yamabe, and E.J. Cho. 2011a. Free radical scavenging activity and protective effect from cellular oxidative stress of active compound from eggplant (*Solanum melongena* L.). *CNU J Agric Sci* 38:625–629.

Kim, J., and H.S. Kim. 2002. The immunomodulating effects of *Aster scaber* Thunb extracts in mice. *Nutr Sci* 5:203–210.

Kim, J., C-S. Park, Y. Lim, and H-S. Kim. 2009. *Paeonia japonica, Houttuynia cordata,* and *Aster scaber* water extracts induce nitric oxide and cytokine production by lipopolysaccharide-activated macrophages. *J Med Food* 12:365–373. https://doi .org/10.1089/jmf.2008.1013.

Kim, J-O., Y-S. Kim, J-H. Lee et al. 1992. Antimutagenic effect of the major volatile compounds identified from mugwort (*Artemisia asitica* Nakai) leaves. *J Korean Soc Food Nutr* 21:308–313.

Kim, K-H, M-W. Chang, K-Y. Park et al. 1993. Effects of phytol and small water drop-wort extract on the T subset in the sarcoma 180-tranplanted mice. *J Korean Soc Food Nutr* 22:405–411.

Kim, R-J., M-J. Kang, C-R. Hwang, W-J. Jung, and J-H. Shin. 2012a. Antioxidant and cancer cell growth inhibition activity of five different varieties of *Artemisia* cul-tivars in Korea. *J Life Sci* 22:(6):844–851.

Kim, S.H., M.S. Kim, M.S. Lee et al. 2016a. Korean diet: Characteristics and historical background. *J Ethnic Foods*. 3:26–31.

Kim, S.M., and S.W. Lee. 1992. The bibliographical study on the famine relief food of Chosun dynasty. *J East Asian Dietary Life* 2:26–55.

Kim, W.K., J.H. Kim, D.H. Jeong et al. 2011b. Radish (*Raphanus sativus* L. leaf) eth-anol extract inhibits protein and mRNA expression of ErbB2 and ErbB3 in MDA-MB-231 human breast cancer cells. *Nutr Res Pract* 5:288–293.

Kim, Y-H., Y-H. Hwang, and H-S. Lee. 2003. Analysis of isoflavones for 66 varieties of sprouting beans and bean sprouts. *Korean J Food Sci Technol* 35:568–575.

Kim, Y-H., C-M. Park, and G-A. Yoon. 2016b. Amelioration of metabolic disturbances and adipokine dysregulation by mugwort (*Artemisia princeps* P.) extract in high-fat diet-induced obese rats. *J Nutr Health* 49:411–419.

Kim, Y.J., S.C. Kang, S. Namkoong, M.G. Choung, and E.H. Sohn. 2012b. Anti-inflammatory effects by *Arctium lappa* L. root extracts through the regulation of ICAM-1 and nitric oxide. *Korean J Plant Res* 25:1–6.

Ko, H-J., T.Y. Sun, and J-A. Han. 2016. Nutritive and antioxidative properties of egg-plant by cooking conditions. *J Korean Soc Food Sci* 45:1747–1754.

Ko, S-H., S-W. Choi, S-K. Ye et al. 2008. Comparison of anti-oxidant activities of sev-enty herbs that have been used in Korean traditional medicine. *Nutr Res Pract* 2:143–151.

Koidea, C.L.K., A.C. Collierb, M.J. Berrya, and J. Panee. 2011. The effect of bamboo extract on hepatic biotransforming enzymes—Findings from an obese–diabetic mouse model. *J Ethnopharmacol* 133:37–45.

Korean Food Foundation. 2014. *Bapsang of the people of Joseon.* Seoul: Hallym Publishing Co.

Korean Nutrition Society. 2011. CAN (Computer Aided Nutritional Analysis Program) PRO 4.0. 176E8F12.

Kye, S-K. 2014 Studies on composition of dietary fiber in vegetables. *J East Asian Soc Dietary Life* 24:28–41.

Le Marchand, L. Meat intake, metabolic genes and colorectal cancer. *IARC Sci Publ.* 2002;156:481–5.

Le Marchand, L., C.N. Yoshizawa, L.N. Kolonel, J.H. Hankin, and M.T. Goodman. 1989. Vegetable consumption and lung cancer risk: a population-based case-control study in Hawaii. *J Natl Cancer Inst* 81:1158–1164.

Lee, E., Y.H. Park, and S.C. Lim. 2005a. Effects of *Oenanthe javanica* sap on lipid composition, liver function and oxidative capacity in oxidized fat and ethanol fed rats. *Korean J Plant Resour* 18:343–350.

Lee, G-B. 1241. *Dongguk-yisangguk-jip*. Seoul: Korea.

Lee, H-K., H-S. Choi, K-A. Cho et al. 2017a. Effect of *Solanum melongena* extract on the xanthine oxidase inhibitory, nitrite scavenging, and angiotensin I-converting enzyme inhibitory activities. *J Adv Eng Technol* 10:23–27.

Lee, K-I., S-H. Rhee, and K-Y. Park. 1999. Anticancer activity of phytol and eicosatrienoic acid identified from perilla leaves. *J Korean Soc Food Sci Nutr* 28:1107–1112.

Lee, K-I., S-H. Rhee, and K-Y. Park. 2005b. The antimutagenic activity and the growth inhibition effect of cancer cells on methanol extracts from small water drop-wort. *Korean J Commun Living* 16:3–9.

Lee, M.S. 2011. Antioxidant and antimutagenic effects of *Arctinum lappa* ethanol extract. *Korean J Food Nutr* 24:713–719.

Lee, M.Y., J-H. Han, and M-H. Kang. 2016. Protective effect of Korean diet food groups on lymphocyte DNA damage and contribution of each food group to total dietary antioxidant capacity (TDAC). *J Nutr Health* 49:277–287.

Lee, M.Y., H.A. Kim, and M.H. Kang. 2017b. Comparison of lymphocyte DNA damage levels and total antioxidant capacity in Korean and American diet. *Nutr Res Pract* 11:33–42.

Lee, S-M., S-H. Rhee, and K-Y. Park. 1997. Antimutagenic effect of various cruciferous vegetables in *Salmonella* assaying system. *J Food Hygiene Safety* 12:321–327.

Lee, S.W. 1978. Research on the dietary life before Goryeo dynasty. Seoul: Hyangmunsa.

Lee, Y., B. Song, and J. Ju. 2014. Anti-inflammatory activity of *Perilla frutescens* Britton seed in RAW 264.7 macrophages and an ulcerative colitis mouse model. *Korean J Food Sci Technol* 46:61–67.

Lee, Y-E. 2005. Bioactive compounds in vegetables: Their role in the prevention of disease. *Korean J Food Cookery Sci* 21:380–398.

Lee, Y.R., J.H. Jung, and H.S. Kim. 2011. Hesperidin partially restores impaired immune and nutritional function in irradiated mice. *J Med Food* 14:475–482.

Lim, H-A., and S-I. Yun. 2009. Antimicrobacterial activities of *Capsella bursa-pastoris* extracts. *Korean J Food Preserv* 16:562–566.

Lim, S.S., H.O. Jung, and B. M. Jung 1997. Effect of *Ixeris Sonchifolia* H. on serum lipid metabolism in hyperlipidemic rats. *Korean J Nutr* 30:889–894.

Lin, S.C., C.H. Lin, Y.H. Lin et al. 2002. Hepatoprotective effects of *Arctium lappa* Linne on liver injuries induced chronic ethanol consumption and potentiated by carbon tetrachloride. *J Biomed Sci* 9:401–409.

Lobo, V., A. Patil, A. Phatak, and N. Chandra. 2010. Free radicals, antioxidants and functional foods: Impact on human health. *Pharmacogn Rev* 4(8):118–126.

Lu, Y., Z. He, X. Shen, J. Fan, S. Wu, and D. Zhang. 2012. Cholesterol-lowering effect of allicin on hypercholesterolemic ICR mice. *Oxid Med Cell Longev*. Article ID 489690, 6 pages. http://dx.doi.org/10.1155/2012/489690.

Moeller, S.M., A. Taylor, K.L. Tucker et al., 2004. Overall adherence to the dietary guidelines for Americans is associated with reduced prevalence of early age-related nuclear lens opacities in women. *J Nutr* 134:1812–1819.

Moriguchi S., and Y. Kishino. 1990. In vitro activation of tumoricidal properties of human monocytes by beta-carotene encapsulated in liposomes. *Nutr Res* 10:837–846.

Moriguchi S. et al.1996. Beta-carotene supplementation enhances lymphocyte proliferation with mitogens in human peripheral blood lymphocytes. *Nutr Res* 16:211–218.

Moriguchi, S., S. Yamashita, and E. Shimizu. 2003. Nutrient to stimulate cellular immunity: Role in cancer prevention and therapy. In *Functional Foods & Nutraceuticals in Cancer Prevention*, ed. R.R. Watson. Iowa State Press. Blackwell Publishing Co., Iowa.

Mukherjee, P.K., K. Saha, M. Pal, and B.P. Saha. 1997. Effect of *Nelumbo nucifera* rhizome extract on blood sugar level in rats. *J Ethnopharmacol* 58:207–213.

Namayandeh, S.M., F. Kaseb, and S. Lesan. 2013. Olive and sesame oil effect on lipid profile in hypercholesterolemic patients, which better? *Int J Prev Med* 4:1059–1062.

National Geographic. The development of agriculture. https://genographic.national geographic.com/development-of-agriculture (accessed on May 14, 2017).

National Institute of Korean Language. Standard Korean dictionary. http://stdweb2 .korean.go.kr/search/List_dic.jsp (accessed on May 14, 2017).

Ninfali, P., M. Bacchiocca, A. Antonelli et al. 2007. Characterization and biological activity of the main flavonoids from Swiss chard (*Beta vulgaris* subspecies *cycla*). *Phytomedicine: Intern J Phytother Phytopharm* 14:216–221.

OECD. 2015. Health at a glance 2015: ECD indicators. Paris: OECD Publishing.

Oh, S-H., K.W. Park, J.W. Daily III, and Y-E. Lee. 2014a. Preserving the legacy of healthy Korean food. *J Med Food* 17:1–5.

Oh, T-S., C-H. Kim, Y-K. Cho, S-M. Kim, P-H. Kim, and D-I. Shin. 2014b. *Allium monanthum* flavors biological activity and characteristics according to collecting in different region. *J Korea Acad-Indus Coop Soc* 15:51776–51785.

Oh, T-W. 2004. Effect of ingested capsaicin on serum and leptin mRNA in genetically obese and lean Zucker rats. *Korea Sport Res* 15:1233–1240.

Omara-Alwala, T.R., T. Mebrahtu, D.E. Prior, and M. O. Ezekwe. 1991. Omega-three fatty acids in purslane (*Portulaca oleracea*) tissues. *J Am Oil Chem Soc* 68:198–199.

Osakabe, N., A. Yasuda, M. Natsume et al. 2002. Rosmarinic acid, a major polyphenolic component of *Perilla frutescens* reduces lipopolysaccharide (LPS)-induced liver injury in D-galactosamine (D-GalN)-sensitized mice. *Free Radical Bio Med* 33:798–806.

Park, C-H., K-H. Kim, and H-S. Yook. 2014. Comparison of antioxidant and antimicrobial activities in *Siraegi* (dried radish greens) according to cooking process. *Korean J Food Nutr* 27:609–618.

Park, E.J., and D.Y. Jhon. 2009. Effects of bamboo shoot consumption on lipid profiles and bowel function in healthy young women. *Nutrition* 25:723–728.

Park, E.J., and D.Y. Jhon . 2010. The antioxidant, angiotensin converting enzyme inhibition activity, and phenolic compounds of bamboo shoot extracts. *Food Sci Techn* 43:655–659.

Park, H., and H-S. Kim. 2014. Korean traditional natural herbs and plants as immune enhancing, antidiabetic, chemopreventive, and antioxidative agents: A narrative review and perspective. *J Med Food* 17:21–27.

Park, K-Y., K-I. Lee, and S-H. Rhee. 1992. Inhibitory effect of green–yellow vegetables on the mutagenicity in *Salmonella* assay system and on the growth of AZ-521 human gastric cancer cells. *J Korean Soc Food Nutr* 21:149–153.

Park, S.H., S.K. Park, J.S. Ha et al. 2016. Effect of gomchwi (*Ligularia fischeri*) extract against high glucose- and H2O2-induced oxidative stress in PC12 cells. *Korean J Food Sci Technol* 48:508–514.

Park, S-Y., J-Y. Kim, K-W. Park, K-S. Kang, K-H. Park, and K-I. Seo. 2009. Effects of thiosulfinates isolated from *Allium thuberosum* L. on the growth of human cancer cells. *J Kor Soc Food Sci Nutr* 38:1003–1007.

Philip, C.C. 2010. Omega-3 fatty acids and inflammatory processes. *Nutrients* 2:355–374.

Pyo, Y-H., T-C. Lee, L. Logendra, and R.T. Rosen. 2004. Antioxidant activity and phenolic compounds of Swiss chard (*Beta vulgaris* subspecies *cycla*) extracts. *Food Chem* 85:19–26.

Rahati, S., A. Ebrahimi, M. Eshraghian, and H. Pishva. 2016. Effect of spinach aqueous extract on wound healing in experimental model diabetic rats with streptozotocin. *J Sci Food Agric* 96:2337–2343.

Rhee, Y.H., E.O. Lee, S.Y. Park et al. 2005. Effect of *Brassica rapa* L. extracts and β-sitosterol on hyperlpidemic rats. *Korean J Oriental Phrm Pathol* 19:1528–1533.

Ryu, H.S., J.H. Kim, and H.S. Kim. 2008. Effects of plant water extract mixture *Ixeris sonchifolia* Hance, *Oenanthe javanica*, *Fagopyrum esculentum* Moench, *Hisikia fusiforme*, *Zingiber officinele* Roscoe on mouse immune cell activation *ex vivo*. *Kor J Nutr* 41:141–146.

Ryu, M.J., and H.S. Chung. 2015. Effect of *Aralia elata* on apoptosis in MDA-MB-231 human breast cancer cells. *Food Eng Prog* 19:235–242.

Shen, G., P.V. Kien, X-F Cai et al. 2005. Solanoflavone, a new bioflavonol glycoside from *Solanum Melongena*: Seeking for anti-inflammatory components. *Arch Pharm Res* 28:657–659.

Shin, K-H. 2006. Effect of Araliaceae water extracts on blood glucose level and biochemical parameters in diabetic rats. *Korean J Nutr* 39:721–727.

Shin, S-A., H-N. Lee, G-S. Choo et al. 2016. Induction of apoptosis in human cancer cells with extracts of *Taraxacum coreanum*, *Youngia sonchifolia* and *Ixeris dentate*. *J Food Hyg Saf* 31:51–58.

Shinohara, K., S. Kuroki, M. Miwa, Z-L. Kong, and H. Hosoda. 1988. Antimutagenicity of dialyzates of vegetables and fruits. *Agric Biol Chem* 52:1369–1375.

Sim, H-J., S-M. Kim, Y-J. Jeon, and Y-E. Lee. 2015. Antioxidant activity of dropwort (*Oenanthe javanica* DC) fermented extract and its hepatoprotective effect against alcohol in rats. *J Korean Soc Food Cult* 30:97–104.

Singh, R., S. Devi, and R. Gollen. 2015. Role of free radical in atherosclerosis, diabetes and dyslipidaemia: larger-than-life. *Diabetes Metab Res Rev* 31:113–126.

Sohn, H.S., B.M. Jung, and Y.S. Cha. 2001. Effect of *Ixeris Sonchifolia* H. Fiet on lipid metabolism and liver function of rats administered ethanol. *Korean J Nutr* 34:493–498.

Stahl, W., and H. Sies. 2005. Bioactivity and protective effects of natural carotenoids. *Biochimica et Biophysica Acta* 1740:101–107.

Stringham, J.M., and B.R. Hammond. 2005. Dietary lutein and zeaxanthin: Possible effects on visual function. *Nutr Rev* 63:59–64.

Storey, M., and P. Anderson. 2014. Income and race/ethnicity influence dietary fiber intake and vegetable consumption. *Nutr Res* 34:844–850.

Takano, H., N. Osakabe, C. Sanbongi et al. 2004. Extract of *Perilla frutescens* enriched for rosmarinic acid, a polyphenolic phytochemical, inhibits seasonal allergic rhinoconjunctivitis in humans. *Exp Biol Med* 229:247–254.

Trichopoulou, A., E. Vasilopoulou, P. Hollman et al. 2000. Nutritional composition and flavonoid content of edible wild greens and green pies: A potential rich source of antioxidant nutrients in the Mediterranean diet. *Food Chemistry* 70:319–323.

Tsuruta, Y., K. Nagao, B. Shirouchi et al. 2012. Effects of lotus root (the edible rhizome of *Nelumbo nucifera*) on the deveolopment of non-alcoholic fatty liver disease in obese diabetic *db/db* mice. *Biosci Biotechnol Biochem* 76:462–466.

United States Department of Agriculture—USDA. 2010. Item clusters, percent of consumption, and representative foods for typical choices food patterns. http://www.cnpp.usda.gov/sites/default/files/usda_food_patterns/TableA 1ListOfTypicalRepFoodsWithPercentages.pdf (accessed on Jan. 17, 2015).

United States Department of Agriculture—USDA. 2015. Dietary guidelines for Americans 2015–2020. 8th ed. https://health.gov/dietaryguidelines/2015 /guidelines/ (accessed on May 17, 2017).

Vijayakumar, R., A. Pameerselvam, and N. Thajuddin. 2013. Marine actinobacteria: A potential source of antifungal compounds. In *Marine parmacognosy: Trends and applications*, ed. S-K. Kim, 233. Boca Raton, FL: CRC Press.

Walia, A., R. Malan, S. Saini, V. Saini, and S. Gupta. 2011. Hepatoprotective effects from the leaf extracts of *Brassica juncea* in CCl4 induced rat model. *Der Pharmacia Sinica* 2:274–285.

Willett, W., H. Sesso, and E. Rimm. 2013. Demystifying nutrition: The value of food, vitamins and supplements Longwood Seminars. Boston: Harvard Health Publications

Wiseman, M. 2008. The second World Cancer Research Fund/American Institute for Cancer Research expert report. Food, nutrition, physical activity, and the prevention of cancer: A global perspective. *Proc Nutr Soc* 67:253–256.

World Health Organization—WHO. 2003. Fruit and vegetable promotion initiative— A meeting report, Geneva, Switzerland, August 25–27. http://www.who .int/dietphysicalactivity/publications/fandv_promotion_initiative_report .pdf?ua¼1 (accessed on Nov. 15, 2016).

World Health Organization. 2017. WHO fact sheet. Diabetes. http://www.who.int /mediacentre/factsheets/fs312/en/ (accessed on August 1, 2018).

World Health Organization and Food and Agriculture Organization of the United Nations. 2005. Fruit and vegetables for health: Report of a joint FAO/WHO workshop, Kobe, Japan, September 1–3, 2004. http://www.who.int/dietphysicalactivity /publications/fruit_vegetables_report.pdf (accessed·on May 17, 2017).

Yang, Y., J. Sun, J. Xie, T. Min, L-M. Wang, and H-X. Wang. 2016. Phenolic profiles and antioxidant activity of lotus root varieties. *Molecules* 21:863, doi:10.3390 /molecules21070863.

Yokoyama, Y., K. Nishimura, N.D. Barnard, D. Neal et al. 2014. Vegetarian diets and blood pressure: A meta-analysis. *JAMA Intern Med* 174:577–587.

Yu, K-H., S-Y. Lee, H-M. Yang et al. 2015. Effect of fermented water extracts from *Ligularia fischeri* on hepatotoxicity induced by D-galactosamine in rats. *J Korean Soc Food Sci Nutr* 44:1422–1430.

17

Bibimbap as a Balanced One-Dish Meal

Youn-Soo Cha

CONTENTS

17.1 Introduction 421
17.2 Background 423
    17.2.1 Origin 424
        17.2.1.1 Royal Court Food 425
        17.2.1.2 Community Cuisine 425
        17.2.1.3 Convenience 425
    17.2.2 Philosophical Background 426
    17.2.3 Provincial Background 428
    17.2.4 Transitions in Bibimbap's Name 428
17.3 Varieties and Characteristics 429
    17.3.1 Based on Toppings 429
    17.3.2 Based on Geographical Locations 430
    17.3.3 Based on Sauces or Condiments (Jang) 430
17.4 Health Benefits 430
    17.4.1 Science of Yin–Yang and Five Elements Theory 430
    17.4.2 Health Benefits 431
17.5 Strategy for Modernization and Globalization 433
    17.5.1 Industrialization 435
17.6 Conclusion 436
References 436

17.1 Introduction

Bibimbap is rice mixed with meat and assorted vegetables (Figure 17.1). It is served as a bowl of warm white rice topped with namul (sautéed and seasoned vegetables) and kochujang (chili pepper paste), soy sauce, or doenjang (a fermented soybean paste) (Wikipedia). Bibimbap is one of the definitive Korean dishes in the eyes of both Koreans and international enthusiasts (Korean Food Foundation, 2013).

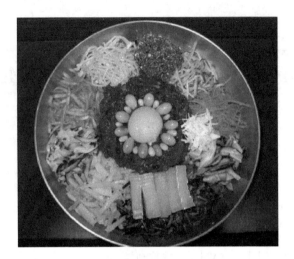

FIGURE 17.1
Bibimbap.

Korean gastronomy has evolved through centuries of social and cultural changes on the Korean peninsula. Originating from ancient times by interaction with surrounding countries, Korean cuisine has evolved through a complex interaction of the natural environment and various cultural drifts (Figure 17.2). Among Korean delicacies, bibimbap is a healthy, well-balanced, native cuisine that is considered an iconic Korean dish. It originated and evolved for more than a thousand years; a well-known ethnic food of Korea, it is also popular among people from all over the world (Chung et al., 2015). The Korean word "bibimbap" means mixed rice; it is

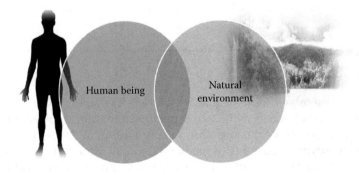

FIGURE 17.2
Harmony between human being and natural environment.

mixed with fresh bean sprouts and then topped with more than 30 different vegetables along with gingko seeds, fried egg, pine nuts, chestnuts, walnuts, and other similar ingredients (Wikipedia). Bibimbap contains many ingredients that offer a balance of proteins, vitamins, minerals, carbohydrates, and fat.

"Hansik," the traditional Korean meal, not only refers to the food but also to the etiquette, manners, and procedures in serving the food charmingly and exquisitely. Hansik is generally made of four constituents: the cooked rice (bap), then the kuk (soup), followed by side dishes (banchan), and finally sauce (jang, yangnyum). The rice provides calories whereas the soup helps in chewing and swallowing the rice, in turn supporting the digestive system. The palatable side dishes make the taste of the food better and also replenish the body with nutrients. And sauce stimulates appetite (Hwang et al., 2005; Kwon et al., 2015).

The normal Korean meal consists of various outside dishes that make it a bountiful feast. The composition of rice and various ingredients makes an appropriately balanced meal, providing many nutrients that are required for an average healthy person; this adds one more reason to include hansik in a healthy daily diet. The harmony between the people and the food is richly supported by the beautiful land of Korea, which is bordered on three sides by water, and therefore has plentiful marine products as well as rich resources of herbs and wild vegetables, which are appropriately used in Korean cuisine.

Bibimbap as a meal has characteristics differing from the usual Korean traditional meal. Westerners often serve a single dish during a meal and bibimbap resembles that, which has made it very favored and loved. Jeonju bibimbap is the most popular bibimbap in Korea as well as in the world. Bibimbap reflects the philosophy and foresight of ancient Korea and now is approved and much appreciated by the world.

Bibimbap has been a favorite dish since ancient times and has improved time over time, making it a favorite dish in modern times also. It is indicated as one of three popular dishes of the Chosun era and is a famous dish among foreigners (Bang, 1921). Depending on personal preferences, dietary needs, and creativity one can substitute several ingredients when preparing the dish and make it a more colorful, beautiful, edible, and distinctive meal.

17.2 Background

Korea has several similarities with Japan and China as it shares many historical and cultural backgrounds with these nations. But, over the ages

Korea has developed its own unique cuisine. The Korean peninsula, with its abundance of marine resources and mountainous regions, maintains the harmony between humans and nature. A traditional Korean meal consists of rice and various side dishes that provide adequate amounts of all nutrients required for a healthy individual. Korean side dishes not only consist of vegetables but also meat, fish, and other seafood that maintain a perfect harmony with nature and also contain balanced nutrients essential for a healthy human body.

Bibimbap is a typical example of hansik. Korea not only sustains the harmony with nature geographically but also in its food habits. The Korean climate and geographical features are favorable for the growth of large varieties of vegetables and herbs. Once primarily an agricultural nation, rice became the staple food of Korea.

17.2.1 Origin

With an abundance of health benefits, bibimbap has soul of ancient Korea. As mentioned earlier, it originated from the Korean traditional meal setting (Figure 17.3). Korean's common meal structure—bap, guk, and banchan—generates the bibimbap consisting of bap and banchan. Bibimbap has been chosen by the people because it is good to eat (Joo, 2010). It is claimed that bibimbap was developed in the sixteenth century because there are records in Chinese literature of that time regarding bibimbap. However, considering that the traditional Korean meal setting is the origin of bibimbap (Chung et al., 2015; Kwon et al., 2015), it could be stated that bibimbap has been made since the tenth century (Hwang et al., 2005), when there was no Korean language. There are many tales regarding the origin of bibimbap and some are mentioned next.

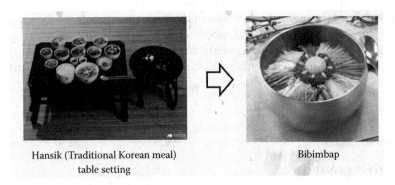

Hansik (Traditional Korean meal) table setting   Bibimbap

FIGURE 17.3
Bibimbap originated from Korean traditional meal settings.

17.2.1.1 Royal Court Food

The royal meal consisted of various dishes that were rich in nutrients and beneficial for health because it was served to rulers of the country in various periods. Special women cooks were appointed to conserve and take great care in the preparation and serving of food. A well-known tale behind the origin of bibimbap is that it is originated from the royal court. People may have tried to find a way to make delicious food to serve for important guests and dignitaries. They created a dish that had vegetables, rice, and meat and mixed it with kochujang (red chili paste) in a bowl. Ancient literature shows that bibimbap was a famous dish among the rich and high-ranking officials and dignified guests (Lee, 1967; Chung et al., 2015).

17.2.1.2 Community Cuisine

Korea has a tradition of commemorating family ancestors and lineages on important or special occasions. In the ancestral ceremonies that took place in traditional society, meals and vegetables were kept as an offering for the spirits of departed souls. All the family members would gather together to show their veneration of and respect for their ancestors. After the ceremony the whole family shared the same food by mixing it all together and then shared the fellowship that physically expressed the closeness of the clan.

Another interesting story behind the origin of bibimbap is that it may have been created by the wives of farmers during busy harvest seasons when they had no time or convenience to serve the meal properly. The farmers' wives would bring abundant available ingredients in their provisions and mix the ingredients together with what others had brought. Then they would serve it along with the rice as a community, sharing the food. The variety of food sources ensured that diversity in tastes and nutrients was maintained and balanced well.

17.2.1.3 Convenience

In ancient times, when the people did not have enough time or space to have a traditional meal, they may have looked for a method for preparing a food that could provide them with all nutrients without consuming much of their time. Thus, bibimbap might have originated as a way of consuming healthy food in comparatively easier ways (Choi, 1977; Chung et al., 2015). Someone could easily prepare bibimbap and serve it as a healthy, convenient food (Joo, 2010).

Although there are many theories about the origin of bibimbap, no substantial evidence confirms one particular theory. Based on the previously mentioned explanations, it can be assumed that bibimbap naturally originated through the Korean bapsang culture, which consisted of rice and various side dishes.

17.2.2 Philosophical Background

Korean food culture is based on a system of philosophy: the yin–yang and five elements principles; also, Koreans have given colors symbolic meanings according the yin–yang and five elements principles (Lee and Yun, 2011). In Chinese philosophy the yin and yang, which means two halves that together complete wholeness, portray how two seemingly opposite yet complementary energies balance and rebalance to form a state of perfect harmony. In the principle of this philosophy of yin–yang, yang means coming to the outside, such as sky above, sun, male, as well as strong and conative; yin means "behind things," such as ground, bottom, moon, female, as well as weak and passive (Lee and Yun, 2011). Neither yin nor yang can survive alone and they cannot exist in an unbalanced state. They complement and balance each other.

In traditional Chinese medicine, a person's health is maintained by the balance of these vitalities, yin and yang. When there is balance and equilibrium, there is good health and when there is imbalance between the energies it causes illness. Similarly, the foods we eat also have either a yin or yang nature within them (Kim, 2012). The five elements theory is an implementation of the yin–yang philosophy. This theory has been used to explain interactions and relationships in various domains.

All the ingredients used in bibimbap form a harmony of taste and colors based on the yin–yang concept and five elements theory. All the ingredients for bibimbap are carefully chosen based on the yin–yang and five elements principle and they are in great harmony not only in appearance but also in taste and feel.

There is an order of presentation in the five elements theory known as the "mutual generation" sequence, which is the order of "mutually overcoming" each other. The five elements theory is the implementation of yin–yang philosophy in the Korean table setting, and they consist of fire (red), wood (green or blue), water (black), earth (yellow), and metal (white) (Figure 17.4a). According to this theory, each food color is associated with the function of specific organs in the body (Figure 17.4b). For example, the function of liver is associated with wood (green foods). Similarly, the function of lungs is associated with metal (white), heart to fire (red), kidneys to water (black), and stomach to earth (yellow). The consumption of various colors of foods is greatly encouraged based on this idea (Chung et al., 2015).

Modern nutritional research also supports eating a "rainbow" of foods, which provides a balanced range of nutrients. Consuming different colored foods plays a role in ensuring consumption of all—essential nutrients, vitamins, minerals, antioxidants, fiber, and more. Eating this way can help to overcome illnesses like flu, cancers, digestive issues, declining vision, loss of bone density, and even help with weight and fat management. Also,

Bibimbap as a Balanced One-Dish Meal 427

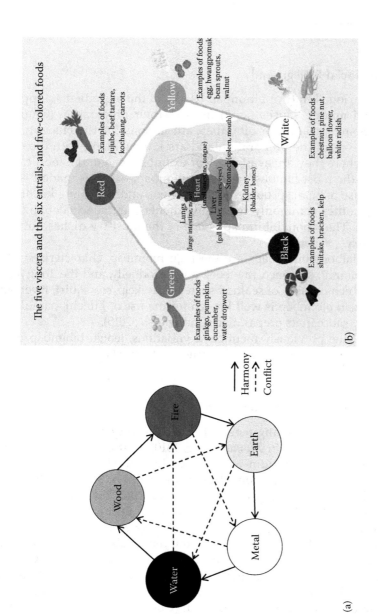

FIGURE 17.4
(a) Mutual relationships among the five elements; (b) the inter-relationships among the five colored-foods in the human body.

the mood will most likely be lifted when one is served a variety of visually alluring bright colored foods versus foods that are dull, white, and plain and suggest weakness. Brightening up the plate with colorful bibimbap can brighten up one's health.

17.2.3 Provincial Background

There are various kinds of bibimpap based on the ingredients, toppings, regions, and mixing sauces (jang) used in their preparation (Chung et al., 2015). Some varieties of bibimpap are famous for the characteristic ingredient used in the preparation and are known along with the name of the city where they are available. For example, Jeonju, the food capital of Korea, is the most famous place for bibimbap, which is made distinctive by the use of bean sprouts, sliced raw beef, and Sunchang kochujang along, with other commonly used ingredients (Bibimpap Globalization Foundation). The Jeonju bibimpap is one of the must-try dishes during a visit to Korea.

Yet other famous bibimbaps are the Jinju bibimbap, characterized with green bean namul, seasoned raw beef, and blood jelly, and the Tongyeong bibimbap, which consists of seafood such as raw kelp, sea squirt, laver, and seaweed. Haeju bibimbap is well known for the use of kimchi, namul, and seasoned soy sauce in its preparation (Chung et al., 2015).

Among all the previously mentioned variations, Jeonju bibimbap is the most famous and unique among the varieties of bibimbap.

17.2.4 Transitions in Bibimbap's Name

In Hangul (the written language of Korea), the very first mention about bibimbap is found in *Mongyupyun* (Jang, 1810). In this book, the old form of bibim, known as bubuium was written in both Hangul and Chinese characters. However, while considering the origin of bibimbap to be the traditional Korean meal setting (Chung et al., 2015; Kwon et al., 2015), it could be stated that bibimbap had been made since the tenth century, when there were no Hangul characters (Hwang et al., 2005). In Chinese literature of the 16th century, there are references about bibimbap, which is mentioned as bubuiumbap. Three ways were used to write it in Chinese characters: hondonban, referring to the meaning (Park, 1590); bubiban, referring to the sound (Hwang, nineteenth century); and koldongban, borrowing its name from a Chinese dish (Dong, 1590). Considering these references in Chinese literature, it could be suggested that bibimbap derived its name in Hangul, known as bubium, from one of the Chinese ways, bubiban, which was used to mention bibimbap when Hangul did not exist (Figure 17.5).

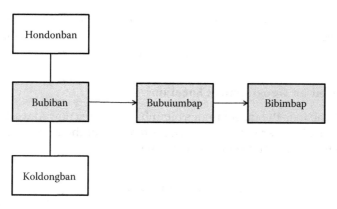

FIGURE 17.5
Transitions in the name of bibimbap.

17.3 Varieties and Characteristics

Bibimbap's ingredients can be divided into three major parts, (1) Base where cooked rice function as base parts. (2) Topping included namul, nuts, vegetables, meat, etc. (3) Condiments, sauce oil, Jang belongs to third part. Customers can select their own favorite ingredients according to their health status and taste preference.

There are many varieties of Bibimbap based on the toppings used in the preparation, province of origin, and "jang," or the sauce used in the process of making that particular bibimpap. A few classifications of bibimpap are mentioned next (Chung et al., 2015).

17.3.1 Based on Toppings

Many types of bibimbap can be made during mealtime in the home: dolsotbibimbap (stone pot bibimbap), sanchaebibimbap (vegetarian bibimbap), yeolmubibimbap (young summer radish kimchi bibimbap), nakjibokkeumbibimbap (stir-fried octopus bibimbap), meonggebibimbap (sea squirt bibimbap), etc. Bibimbap's structure of <bap + banchan + yangnyeom> easily makes a simple but complete Korean meal (Joo, 2010).

Several bibimbaps are named based on the vegetables and toppings used in making the dish. Some examples include bean sprout, green pumpkin, eggplant, wild vegetable, thistle, raw beef, sliced raw fish, sea squirt, and laver bibimbaps. Ancient literature shows that these varieties were named long ago (Chung et al., 2015).

The more than 30 vegetables that can be added as namul include soybean sprouts, bracken, spinach, white radish, balloon flower, carrot, pumpkin, shiitake, water dropwort, and cucumber. Pine nuts, chestnuts, and ginkgo nuts are some of the nuts used while making bibimbap. Raw beef, egg yolk, hwangpomuk, and jujube comprise a few of the other ingredients used to decorate the bibimbap at the end of its preparation. These ingredients are full of nutrition and look colorful on top of the bibimbap.

17.3.2 Based on Geographical Locations

Jeonju bibimbap is the most famous bibimbap in Korea nowadays. In spite of its popularity, there are some other places famous for their unique bibimbap. Pyeongyang, Haeju, and Jinju are a few of them.

17.3.3 Based on Sauces or Condiments (Jang)

The sauces used in every kind of bibimbap are entirely different from each other. In Jeonju bibimbap, kochujang is the main sauce. Haeju bibimbap is seasoned with soy sauce and raw fish bibimbap uses vinegar (kochujang) (Chung et al., 2015). Each bibimbap has different and unique sauces and ingredients, which produce different tastes. Sauces used in bibimbap show the historical, geographical, and cultural characteristics of Korea.

Jang, or condiments, is the third part in the preparation of bibimpap. Kochujang, doenjang, and cheonggukjang are the three most used condiments in bibimbap. Sesame oil and perilla oil can also be used and soybean sprout soup is usually served with bibimbap.

17.4 Health Benefits

Bibimbap has unlimited possibilities for variation depending on the types of rice and toppings used in a personalized diet to protect against some metabolic diseases (Oh et al., 2013). Bibimbap is part of a healthy diet for people who need a balanced meal. People who suffer from weak health can adapt the recipe to their dietary requirements by selecting different vegetables and rice.

17.4.1 Science of Yin–Yang and Five Elements Theory

All ingredients that are used in bibimbap form a harmony of the taste and style of five colors and five tastes based on yin–yang and the five elements theory. Green, red, yellow, white, and black are the five colors associated with the health of different parts of the body, such as liver, heart, stomach, lungs, and kidneys, respectively (Figure 17.4b) (Chung et al., 2015). All these colors not only are a pleasure to the eye but also have deep philosophical meaning. The ingredients in bibimbap can be divided by these colors, for example:

- Cucumber, ginkgo nut, squash, and water parsley (green)
- Korean style raw beef, carrots, red pepper paste, and jujube (red)
- Bean sprouts, egg, yellow mung bean jelly, and walnuts (yellow)
- Pine nuts, white radish, balloon flower root, and chestnuts (white)
- Shiitake, bracken, and kelp (black)

The five colors in bibimbap represent not only the importance of harmony between the body and soul, but also the harmony of nature and humankind. The five elements theory is also applicable to the taste of food. The five tastes—sweet, salty, sour, bitter, and spicy—are well balanced in bibimpap. The blending of colors and tastes in this Korean dish is an ideal practice in meal preparation.

17.4.2 Health Benefits

One can select one's own favorite ingredients according to health status and preference for making a unique version of bibimpap. Various types of rice and vegetables can be substituted according to the taste and preference of the consumer. Using different vegetables may help people to manage their health and body weight and maintain the nutritional status of the body. At present, a nutritionist or a registered dietitian can help to choose the ingredients to make bibimbap. The ingredients of bibimbap and their health benefits are listed in Tables 17.1 and 17.2.

Vegetables in bibimbap are rich in vitamin C, carotenoids, minerals, dietary fibers, and other nutraceuticals that have hypoglycemic, anti-inflammatory, antioxidant, neuroprotective, and hepatoprotective effects (Table 17.1). The condiments for bibimbap have protective effects against obesity-related metabolic disorders by reducing fat accumulation and by improving systemic inflammation, glucose homeostasis, and blood cholesterol levels (Table 17.2). In animal study, oral administration of freeze-dried bibimbap (500 mg/kg body weight) for 4 weeks to BALB/c mice significantly increased splenic B- and T-cells, and thymic (Th)-lymphocyte subpopulations compared to hamburger-treated group. Furthermore, the bibimbap group increased serum IFNγ and enhanced hemaggluthination tiers that affect immune activities (Kim et al., 2013). A recent clinical study reported that bibimbap, a rice-based Korean meal, significantly lowered glycemic responses and postprandial-triglyceride concentrations than energy-matched a Western meal, pork cutlet, in participants with and without metabolic syndrome (Figure 17.6) (Jung et al., 2015). High content of carbohydrate meals has been reported to increase the risk of metabolic syndrome. However, bibimbap, high in carbohydrate, showed beneficial effects in lowering the risk of metabolic response. These results indicate that bibimbap is a well-balanced diet with many health benefits and offer a chance to modernize and globalize bibimbap according to the flavors and tastes of people from other national, cultural, and nutritional affiliations.

432 *Korean Functional Foods*

TABLE 17.1

Health Benefits of Toppings

Toppings	Effectiveness	Ref.
Soybean sprouts	Hypoglycemic effect by inhibiting alpha glucosidase activity	Kim et al., 2003
Spinach	Diabetic mellitus–induced ulcer regenerating effect and decreased blood glucose and increased insulin concentrations Protection against chemical-induced neuronal cell death, and may be useful in treatment of neurodegenerative diseases	Rahati et al., 2016; Park et al., 2007; Bonari, 2011
Balloon flower roots	Inhibited the development of atopic dermatitis-like skin symptoms by regulating cytokine mediators Reduced vascular cell injury and prevented high-fat diet-induced dyslipidemia and oxidative stress Inhibited the tumor necrosis factor-induced expression of adhesion molecules in human endothelial cells	Choi et al., 2014; Chung et al., 2012; Kim et al., 2010
Shiitake	Anti-inflammatory effect and improved antioxidant enzyme activities Decreased concentrations of LDL cholesterol and reduced risk factors for cardiovascular disease in patients with type 2 diabetes	Zembron-Lacny et al., 2013; Drori et al., 2016; Chang et al., 2007
Water dropwort (Oenanthe javanica)	Antioxidants; decreasing oxidative stresses in the liver Improved hepatic fat accumulation, hyperglycemia, and dyslipidemia induced by high-fat, high-cholesterol diet, suggesting potential use for prevention and treatment of NAFLD	Lee et al., 2015; Jeong et al., 2009
Pumpkin (zucchini)	Includes pectin, which improved cardiovascular health, the ability to lower cholesterol naturally, improve arterial health, and reduce disease-causing inflammation, so it might also offer protection against diabetes and insulin resistance	Brouns et al., 2012
White radish	Diminished hepatic damage by toxic agents such as CCl4 and protective effects on galactosamine (GalN)-mediated nephrotoxicity; this may be related to action of the antioxidant content of the extract	Lee et al., 2012b; Bojan et al., 2016
Carrot	Beta-carotene; great antioxidative potential for preventing damage to lymphocyte DNA in smokers and decreased risk of cardiovascular disease and some cancers, and some, notably ß-carotene, act as precursors to vitamin A	Lee et al., 2011a

(Continued)

Bibimbap as a Balanced One-Dish Meal

TABLE 17.1 (CONTINUED)

Health Benefits of Toppings

Toppings	Effectiveness	Ref.
Bracken	Contains a thiaminase that converts thiamine into products that cannot replace the intact vitamin in mammalian nutrition	Williams and Evans, 1959
Cucumber	Used for skin treatment and natural beautification and to bring relief to the eyes in summer Cucumber extract can be incorporated into first aid treatment of corneal acid burn Presence of flavonoids and tannins in the extract might be responsible for free radical scavenging and analgesic effects	Uzodike and Onuoha, 2009; Kumar et al., 2010
Pine nut	Ameliorates status of HDL and LDL cholesterol in high-cholesterol diet-fed rats Korean pine nut polyunsaturated fatty acid suppresses appetite and consequently may affect food intake	Baek et al., 2011; Pasman et al., 2006
Chestnuts	Anti-inflammatory effect induced by polyphenols; COX inhibition in chestnuts	Sato et al., 2006
Ginkgo nuts	Heat-stable antioxidant components present in the nuts accounted for 60% of their antioxidant capacity Lipid-soluble fraction was responsible for decreased hepatic cholesterol and prevention of cardiovascular diseases, while water-soluble fraction may contribute to increased serum cholesterol	Goh and Barlow, 2002; Mahadevan et al., 2008
Hwangpomuk	Contains Mung bean; protective effect against alcohol-induced liver injury A potential insulin-sensitizing agent in type 2 diabetes mellitus with insulin resistance	Liu et al., 2014; Chen et al., 2014
Jujube	Includes vitamins, flavonoids, amino acids, organic acids, microelements, and polysaccharides Hepatic protective effects and cytotoxic activity on different tumor cell lines Reduced intestine MDA level and increased antioxidant enzyme activities	Pareek, 2013; Shen et al., 2009; Vahedi et al., 2008; Wang, 2011

17.5 Strategy for Modernization and Globalization

Bibimpap can be made more popular and consumer friendly by modifying the shape and size of the food. Usually, bibimpap is served as a full meal, so the size of food portions makes it inconvenient to be used as a snack and inappropriate as a takeout item. Therefore, in order to make bibimpap more well known among foreigners and travelers, the shape,

TABLE 17.2

Health Benefits of Condiments

Condiment	Effectiveness	Ref.
Kochujang	Improved glucose homeostasis by reducing insulin resistance Improvement associated with decreased hepatic fat storage Hypocholesterolemic effect and improved blood cholesterol levels in subjects at high risk for cardiovascular disease	Kwon et al., 2009; Lim et al., 2015
Doenjang	Reduced body weight and visceral fat in overweight adults and ameliorated systemic inflammation and oxidative stress in obesity via inhibition of inflammatory signals of adipose tissue Promoted gut health by regulating gut microbiota and its LPS concentrations and suppressing harmful enzyme production	Cha et al., 2012; Lee et al., 2012a; Nam et al., 2015; Jang et al., 2014b
Chenggukjang	Reduced accumulation of body fat and improved serum lipids in high-fat diet fed mice Antiasthmatic dietary supplement candidate for histamine-mediated asthma	Soh et al., 2008; Bae et al., 2014
Sesame oil	Inhibited activation of NADPH oxidase-dependent inflammatory mechanism due to 6-hydroxydopamine (6-OHDA)-induced neurotoxicity in mice; 6-OHDA-induced Parkinson's disease model in mice Improved hyperglycemia; synergistic effect with glibenclamide (antidiabetic medication) Mitigated deoxycorticosterone acetate and 1% NaCl induced chronic kidney disease and inhibited renal fibrosis in rats	Ahmad et al., 2012; Sankar et al., 2011; Liu et al., 2015
Perilla oil	Affected hepatic lipid accumulation, inhibited platelet aggregation, and delayed thrombosis following oxidative arterial wall injury Protected airways, lungs, and spleen from allergic inflammation	Lee et al., 2011b; Chang et al., 2012; Jang et al., 2014a

size, and plating of the food should be modified so that it can look more attractive and appetizing as well as handy and convenient during travel and busy times.

The plating of the meal is also an important factor to make the food unique and noticeable to people. A characteristic feature of bibimpap is that the toppings and vegetables used in the dish can be varied according to the choices of the one making or purchasing it. Therefore, if restaurants and food courts can prepare bibimbap with a varied selection of colorful and flavorful ingredients that can appeal to a wide range at food requirements and preferences, it should appeal to many people.

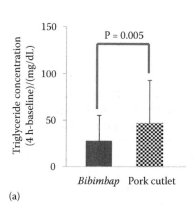 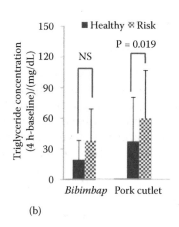

FIGURE 17.6
Change of postprandial plasma triglyceride concentrations 4 hours after test meals. (a) Postprandial plasma triglyceride concentrations of all participants. (b) Postprandial plasma triglyceride concentrations of participants with and without metabolic syndrome.

With this innovative idea, customers will find bibimbap more attractive and impressive because of its nutritional values and recognize it as a healthy yet highly palatable food. Replacing the ingredients according to the region, climate, availability of toppings, and culture may also help in globalizing bibimbap. For example, substituting noodles or bread for rice may help people to try it as a variety dish. For those who do not prefer a particular sauce, it can be replaced with the sauce of their choice. To attract connoisseurs with other tastes, making rolls of bibimbap in naan, roti, dosa, etc. also can be tried.

17.5.1 Industrialization

In this fast-paced world, people rarely get time to cook and prepare healthy food at home. Convenience foods have become very popular these days because of the short time for meal preparation. Bibimpap can possibly be one of the best options for a healthy and balanced convenience food. Providing bibimpap as an easily prepared or ready-to-eat food will help more to industrialize its production. Bibimbap can be customized according to health requirements, food intolerances, religious constraints, and personal preferences. For example, rather than using big plates and bowls, using a small cup or roll-type packing would be more convenient for travelers. Even carrying it in baggage would be possible with this type of plating conversion. Therefore, changing the plating style and size would make bibimpap more consumer friendly. Also, replacing the ingredients according to differences in tastes and health situations (e.g., rice to noodle, bread, variety of sauces and toppings, etc.) would make it more popular. Industrial adaptations such as ready to eat, packet, and takeout packages also would be helpful for promoting the usage of bibimbap.

17.6 Conclusion

Bibimbap is rice mixed with meat and assorted vegetables and is considered the iconic Korean dish. Bibimbap has the soul of ancient Korea, originating from the Korean traditional meal setting. There are various kinds of bibimpap, based on the ingredients, toppings, regions in which it is made, and the mixing sauces (Jang) used in preparation of the dish. Bibimbap's ingredients can be divided into four major parts: base (cooked rice), namul, nuts, and condiments. All the ingredients used in bibimbap form a harmony of the taste and style of five colors and five tastes based on yin–yang and the five elements theory. Because of its health benefits, it would be of great interest to modernize and globalize bibimbap according to the flavors and tastes of people from other national, cultural, and nutritional affiliations.

References

Ahmad, S., M. B. Khan., M. N. Hoda et al. 2012. Neuroprotective effect of sesame seed oil in 6-hydroxydopamine induced neurotoxicity in mice model: Cellular, biochemical and neurochemical evidence. *Neurochem Res* 37(3), 516–526.

Bae, M. J., H. S. Shin, H. J. See, O. H. Chai, and D. H. Shon. 2014. Cheonggukjang ethanol extracts inhibit a murine allergic asthma via suppression of mast cell-dependent anaphylactic reactions. *J Med Food* 17(1), 142–149.

Baek, J., T. W. Kim, J. Kim, T. H. Kim, and M. Choe. 2011. Effects of pine nuts oil supplementation on serum cholesterol concentration. *FASEB J* 25(1 supplement 582.10).

Bang, S. Y. 1921. *Chosun-yorijebup* (recipe book for Chosun dynasty). Seoul, Korea.

Bibimbap Globalization Foundation. http://www.koreancuisine.kr/en (jeon ju bibimbap—features (Accessed August 30, 2016).

Bojan, M. S., R. Rajappa, D. R. K. Vijayakumar, and J. Gopalan. 2016. Protective effect of Raphanussativus on D-galactosamine induced nephrotoxicity in rats. *Nutr Clin Metab* 30(1), 22–28.

Bonari, A. R. K. 2011. Effect of the spinach (Spinaciaoleracea) on blood glucose and insulin levels in diabetic rats. *Clin Bio chem* 44(13), S331–S331.

Brouns, F., E. Theuwissen, A. Adam, M. Bell, A. Berger, and R. P. Mensink. 2012. Cholesterol-lowering properties of different pectin types in mildly hypercholesterolemic men and women. *Eur J Clin Nutr* 66(5), 591–599.

Cha, Y. S., J. A. Yang, H. I. Back et al. 2012. Visceral fat and body weight are reduced in overweight adults by the supplementation of doenjang, a fermented soybean paste. *Nutr Res Prac* 6(6), 520–526.

Chang, H. H., C. S. Chen, and J. Y. Lin. 2012. Protective effect of dietary perilla oil on allergic inflammation in asthmatic mice. *Eur J Lipid Sci Tech* 114(9), 1007–1015.

Chang, J. H., M. S. Kim, J. Y. Kim, W. H. Choi, and S. S. Lee. 2007. Effects of mushroom supplementation on blood glucose concentration, lipid profile, and antioxidant enzyme activities in patients with type 2 diabetes mellitus. *J Nutr Health* 40(4), 327–333.

Chen, Y. I., Y. W. Cheng, C. Y. Tzeng et al. 2014. Peroxisome proliferator-activated receptor activating hypoglycemic effect of Gardenia jasminoides Ellis aqueous extract and improvement of insulin sensitivity in steroid induced insulin resistant rats. *BMC Complem Altern Med* 14, 1472–6882.

Choi, J. H., S. W. Jin, E. H. Han et al. 2014. Platycodon grandiflorum root-derived saponins attenuate atopic dermatitis-like skin lesions via suppression of NF-kappaB and STAT1 and activation of Nrf2/ARE-mediated heme oxygenase-1. *Phytomedicine* 21(8–9), 1053–1061.

Choi, S. B. 1977. Lannokgi, Seoul, Korea. Sewoonmunhwasa. 104–105.

Chung, K. R., H. J. Yang, D. J. Jang, and D. Y. Kwon. 2015. Historical and biological aspects of bibimbap, a Korean ethnic food. *J Ethnic Foods* 3(2), 163–164, 2352–6181.

Chung, M. J., S. H. Kim, J. W. Park, Y. J. Lee, and S. S. Ham. 2012. Platycodon grandiflorum root attenuates vascular endothelial cell injury by oxidized low-density lipoprotein and prevents high-fat diet-induced dyslipidemia in mice by upregulating antioxidant proteins. *Nutr Res* 32(5), 365–373.

Dong, K. C. 1590. Koldong-sipsangsol. China, sixteenth century.

Drori, A., Y. Shabat, A. Ben-Ya'acov et al. 2016. Extracts from Lentinula edodes (Shiitake) edible mushrooms enriched with vitamin D exert an anti-inflammatory hepatoprotective effect. *J Med Food* 19(4), 383–389.

Goh, L. M., and P. J. Barlow. 2002. Antioxidant capacity in ginkgo biloba. *Food Res Int* 35(9), 815–820.

Hwang, H. S., B. R. Han, and B. J. Han. 2005. *Korean Traditional Foods*. Kyomunsa, 16–29.

Hwang, J. S. Late nineteenth century. Myungmul-kiryak, Korea.

Jang, H. 1810. *Mongyupyun*. Korea.

Jang, J. Y., T. S. Kim, J. Cai et al. 2014a. Perilla oil improves blood flow through inhibition of platelet aggregation and thrombus formation. *Lab Anim Res* 30(1), 21–27.

Jang, S. E., K. A. Kim, M. J. Han, and D. H. Kim. 2014b. Doenjang, a fermented Korean soybean paste, inhibits lipopolysaccharide production of gut microbiota in mice. *J Med Food* 17(1), 67–75.

Jeong, Y. Y., Y. J. Lee, K. M. Lee, and J. Y. Kim. 2009. The effects of oenanthejavanica extracts on hepatic fat accumulation and plasma biochemical profiles in a non-alcoholic fatty liver disease model. *J Korean Soc Appl Bi* 52(6), 632–637.

Joo, Y. H. 2010. A study on evolution and discourse of bibimbap. *Society and History* 87, 5–38.

Jung, S. J., M. G. Kim, T. S. Park, Y. G. Kim, W. O. Song, and S. W. Chae. 2015. Rice-based Korean meals (bibimbap and kimbap) have lower glycemic responses and postprandial-triglyceride effects than energy-matched Western meals. *J Ethnic Foods* 2(4), 154–161.

Kim, H. G., T. T. Hien, E. H. Han, Y. C. Chung, and H. G. Jeong. 2010. Molecular mechanism of endothelial nitric-oxide synthase activation by *Platycodon grandiflorum* root-derived saponins. *Toxicol Lett* 195(2–3), 106–113.

Kim, J. I., M. J. Kang, and S. Y. Bae. 2003. Hypoglycemic effect of the methanol extract of soybean sprout in streptozotocin-induced diabetic rats. *J Korean Soc Food Sci Nutr* 32(6), 921–925.

Kim, N. S., M. K. Cho, S. H. Oh et al. 2013. The effects of several types of bibimbaps on immune activities in mice. *J East Asian Soc Dietary Life* 23(1), 023–030.

Kim, Y. G. 2012. Yin-yang of foods. *Hwalcheon* 698(1), 70–71.

Korean Food Foundation. 2013. Great food, great stories from Korea. http://terms .naver.com/entry.nhn?docId=3384587&cid=42701&categoryId=58382 (accessed August 2, 2017).

Kumar, D., S. Kumar, J. Singh et al. 2010. Free radical scavenging and analgesic activities of *Cucumissativus* L. fruit extract. *J Young Pharm* 2(4), 365–368.

Kwon, D. Y., K. R. Chung, H. J. Yang, and D. J. Jang. 2015. Gochujang (Korean red pepper paste): Korean ethnic sauce, its role and history, *J Ethnic Foods* 2, 29–35.

Kwon, D. Y., S. M. Hong, I. S. Ahn, Y. S. Kim, D. W. Shin, and S. Park. 2009. Kochujang, a Korean fermented red pepper plus soybean paste, improves glucose homeostasis in 90% pancreatectomized diabetic rats. *Nutrition* 25(7–8), 790–799.

Lee, C. H., J. H. Park, J. H. Cho et al. 2015. Effect of *Oenanthe javanica* extract on antioxidant enzyme in the rat liver. *Chinese Med J-Peking* 128(12), 1649–1654.

Lee, C. S. 1967. *Peoples' unofficial story of Jeonju*. Jeonju Press.

Lee, H. J., Y. K. Park, and M. H. Kang. 2011a. The effect of carrot juice, beta-carotene supplementation on lymphocyte DNA damage, erythrocyte antioxidant enzymes and plasma lipid profiles in Korean smoker. *Nutr Res Pract* 5(6), 540–547.

Lee, J. E., J. E. Seong, S. H. Hong, and Y. O. Song. 2011b. Inhibitory effect of perilla oil on hepatic lipid accumulation in the apoE knock-out mice fed high cholesterol diet. *P Nutr Soc* 70(Oce4), E142–E142.

Lee, M. S., S. W. Chae, Y. S. Cha, and Y. S. Park. 2012a. Supplementation of Korean fermented soy paste doenjang reduces visceral fat in overweight subjects with mutant uncoupling protein-1 allele. *Nutr Res Pract* 32(1), 8–14.

Lee, S. E., and M. H. Yun. 2011. A study on color appeared on modern Korean table arrangement. *J Korean Soc Design Culture* 17(3), 627–640.

Lee, S. W., K. M. Yang, J. K. Kim et al. 2012b. Effects of white radish (Raphanus sativus) enzyme extract on hepatotoxicity. *Toxicol Res* 28(3), 165–172.

Lim, J. H., E. S. Jung, E. K. Choi et al. 2015. Supplementation with *Aspergillus oryzae*-fermented kochujang lowers serum cholesterol in subjects with hyperlipidemia. *Clin Nutr* 34(3), 383–387.

Liu, C. T., S. P. Chien, D. Z. Hsu, S. Periasamy, and M. Y. Liu. 2015. Curative effect of sesame oil in a rat model of chronic kidney disease. *Nephrology (Carlton)* 20(12), 922–930.

Liu, T., X. H. Yu, E. Z. Gao et al. 2014. Hepatoprotective effect of active constituents isolated from mung beans (*Phaseolus radiatus* L.) in an alcohol-induced liver injury mouse model. *J Food Biochem* 38(5), 453–459.

Nam, Y. R., S. B. Won, Y. S. Chung, C. S. Kwak, and Y. H. Kwon. 2015. Inhibitory effects of doenjang, Korean traditional fermented soybean paste, on oxidative stress and inflammation in adipose tissue of mice fed a high-fat diet. *Nutr Res Practice* 9(3), 235–241.

Oh, S. H., J. J. Yul, S. G. Kim et al. 2013. Excellence and functionality of bibimbap. *Food Ind Nutr* 18(1), 16–36.

Pareek, S. 2013. Nutritional composition of jujube fruit. *Emir J Food Agr* 25(6), 463–470.

Park, D. R. 1590. *Kijae-jabki*. Vol. 1. *Yokjokumun*. Korea.

Park, J. Y., J. C. Heo, S. U. Woo et al. 2007. *Spinacia oleracea* extract protects against chemical-induced neuronal cell death. *Korean J Food Preserv* 14(4), 425–430.

Pasman, W. J., J. Heimerikx, C. M. Rubingh et al. 2006. Polyunsaturated fatty acids derived from Korean pine nuts affect appetite suppressing hormones and appetite sensations in overweight women. *Gastroenterology* 130(4), A451–A451.

Rahati, S., M. Eshraghian, A. Ebrahimi, and H. Pishva. 2016. Effect of spinach aqueous extract on wound healing in experimental model diabetic rats with streptozotocin. *J Sci Food Agric* 96(7), 2337–2343.

Sankar, D., A. Ali, G. Sambandam, and R. Rao. 2011. Sesame oil exhibits synergistic effect with anti-diabetic medication in patients with type 2 diabetes mellitus. *Clin Nutr* 30(3), 351–358.

Sato, I., H. Kofujita, T. Suzuki, H. Kobayashi, and S. Tsuda. 2006. Anti-inflammatory effect of Japanese horse chestnut (*Aesculus turbinata*) seeds. *J Vet Med Sci* 68(5), 487–489.

Shen, X. C., Y. P. Tang, R. H. Yang, L. Yu, T. H. Fang, and J. A. Duan. 2009. The protective effect of *Zizyphus jujuba* fruit on carbon tetrachloride-induced hepatic injury in mice by anti-oxidative activities. *J Ethnopharmacol* 122(3), 555–560.

Soh, J. R., D. H. Shin, D. Y. Kwon, and Y. S. Cha. 2008. Effect of cheonggukjang supplementation upon hepatic acyl-CoA synthase, carnitine palmitoyltransferase I, acyl-CoA oxidase and uncoupling protein 2 mRNA levels in C57BL/6J mice fed with high fat diet. *Genes Nutr* 2(4), 365–369.

Uzodike, E., and I. Onuoha. 2009. The effect of cucumber (*Cucumbis savitus*) extract on acid induced corneal burn in guinea pigs. *J Nigerian Optomet Assoc* 15(1), 3–7.

Vahedi, F., M. F. Najafi, and K. Bozari. 2008. Evaluation of inhibitory effect and apoptosis induction of *Zyzyphus jujuba* on tumor cell lines, an in vitro preliminary study. *Cytotechnology* 56(2), 105–111.

Wang, B. 2011. Chemical characterization and ameliorating effect of polysaccharide from Chinese jujube on intestine oxidative injury by ischemia and reperfusion. *Int J Bio l Macromol* 48(3), 386–391.

Wikipedia. https://en.wikipedia.org/wiki/Bibimbap (accessed August 30, 2016).

Williams, D. R., and R. A. Evans. 1959. Bracken (*Pteridium aquilinum*)—The effect of steaming on the nutritive value of bracken hay. *Brit J Nutr* 13(2), 129–136.

Zembron-Lacny, A., M. Gajewski, M. Naczk, and I. Siatkowski. 2013. Effect of shiitake (*Lentinus edodes*) extract on antioxidant and inflammatory response to prolonged eccentric exercise. *J Physiol Pharmacol* 64(2), 249–254.

18

Korean Alcoholic Beverages: Makgeolli/Yakju

Seok-Tae Jeong, Han-Seok Choi, and Ji-Eun Kang

CONTENTS

18.1 History of Korean Alcoholic Beverages 442
18.2 Characteristics and Categories...443
18.3 Manufacturing Method..443
18.4 Fermentation Agent, Nuruk 444
18.5 Composition of Nuruk 445
18.6 Functionality of Nuruk 446
    18.6.1 Cytotoxic and Anti-Inflammatory Activity..........................446
    18.6.2 Cholesterol and Activities of Hepatic Oxygen Free
            Radical Metabolizing Enzymes 446
    18.6.3 Bioactive Compounds 2,6-Dimethoxy-1,4-Benzoquinone
            (2,6-DMBQ)...449
18.7 Composition of Makgeolli 449
18.8 Functionality of Makgeolli 450
    18.8.1 Lactic Acid Bacteria..450
    18.8.2 Anticancer 450
    18.8.3 Improvement of Liver Function...452
    18.8.4 Cholesterol-Lowering Effect...452
    18.8.5 Improved Blood Flow Effect..452
    18.8.6 Removing Reactive Oxygen Species (Antioxidant Effect) ...453
    18.8.7 Inhibiting Hypertension (ACE-Inhibiting Effect).................453
18.9 Composition of Yakju 454
18.10 Functionality of Yakju 454
    18.10.1 Antioxidant Effect 454
    18.10.2 Anticarcinogenic Effects..455
    18.10.3 Anticancer Effects..455
    18.10.4 Fibrinolytic Activity 455
    18.10.5 Protecting the Liver 457
18.11 Conclusion...457
References...458

442   *Korean Functional Foods*

18.1 History of Korean Alcoholic Beverages

The origins of Korean alcoholic beverages are not known exactly. However, the opinion that they started naturally in agriculture is dominant. "Samgukji Wiji Dongijeon" recorded that people drank and danced in the ceremony of Buyeo (second century BC–AD 494) and Goguryeo (first century BC–AD 668).[*] In the Three Kingdoms period (fourth to seventh centuries), the method of making liquor using grains in earnest was complete and had spread to neighboring countries (S. H. Lee, 2009).

The Goryeo dynasty (918–1392) was a revolutionary era in the history of Korean alcoholic beverages, in which the basic recipes of the three representative liquor types—makgeolli, yakju, and soju—were completed and more various types of liquor were developed (Kim 2011). Among the records on makgeolli, "Goryeo dogyeong"[†] described it as a murky liquor, and "Dongguk Isangguk Jib"[‡] as a white liquor. In this period, too, it was largely favored by the commoners. Upon further advancement of liquor production technology, various drinks of fame including nokpaju and hwanggeumju came into being. Korea's own high-quality makgeolli, ihwaju, was also born during this period. As international trade largely increased, distilled soju from the Yuan dynasty was introduced (Kang 2014).

The Joseon dynasty (1392–1910) was the golden age of Korean alcoholic beverages. The main ingredient for liquor production shifted from nonglutinous rice to glutinous rice, which elevated the quality of ingredients. With the influence of Confucianism, every household applied varied ingredients and developed home-brewed liquor. Representative liquors that shaped the regional identity emerged as a result of the application of diverse ingredients and brewing techniques suitable for each region. In addition, honyangju, which is a mix of fermented liquor and distilled liquor, appeared around this time in addition to makgeolli, yakju, and soju, and a total of 340 types of recorded liquors were found in the literature (Kim et al., 2011).

The golden age of Korean alcoholic beverages enjoyed its blooming era in the Joseon dynasty, but started to decline when Japanese colonization (1910–1945) took effect. In 1916, a liquor tax law was enforced that considered home-brewed liquors illegal, and they became the target of crackdowns. Korean alcoholic beverages were put under the simpler categories of makgeolli, yakju, soju, and Japanese sake for taxation. The unique Korean liquor culture, jumak (Korean tavern), was abolished. Breweries were merged for

---

[*] A book (280–289) written by Jinsu of China, this records on the Goryeo and Buyeo included in the throne of the Three Kingdoms.

[†] A book written by Seo Geung, who came to Goryeo as an envoy from the Song dynasty in the first year of King Injong of Goryeo (1123) during the mid-Goryeo period.

[‡] A collection of poems written by Gyubo Lee (1168–241), a Goryeo official.

Korean Alcoholic Beverages 443

the sake of a stable taxation system for liquor consumption, and personal liquor production was banned. Licensed independent brewers numbered 370,000 in 1916; however, this number gradually declined along the course of coming years from 130,000 in 1926 to 265 in 1929. Independent brewers were completely gone by 1934 (S. H. Lee, 2009).

After the Korean War (1950–1953), liquor production was constrained due to food shortages, and the Korean liquor culture faced more hardships as the liquor taxation followed in the footsteps of the Japanese liquor administration for the advantages in budget collection (H. J. Lee, 2009). In 1965, the cereals regulation act banned the use of rice in liquor production, and imported ingredients including wheat flour were used for producing makgeolli. However, the craze for traditional liquor arose following the rise of Korean culture and the well-being trend after the mid-2000s, and it was reborn as people's liquor. Specialized shops for traditional liquors are recently on the rise, and a new culture has been shaped along with the releases of traditional liquor-based cocktails and premium makgeolli. Globalization of Korean cuisine is further fueling efforts to invent and promote high-quality liquors that can represent Korea worldwide (Jeong et al., 2012b).

18.2 Characteristics and Categories

The majority of Korean alcoholic beverages use rice as their ingredient, and they are categorized into makgeolli, yakju, and soju depending on the fermentation methods with steamed rice and nuruk. Makgeolli is made by pouring the liquor, which is completely fermented, into a sieve and roughly filtering the liquid with palms (Kang et al., 2014). Yakju is a clear liquor made by filtering completely fermented liquor with a bamboo yongsu (a sieve used for filtering soy sauce or liquor), whose other name is cheongju (Kang et al., 2015). Soju is a liquor made by distilling the completely fermented liquor through a sojutgori; it is also called hwaju. It is thought to have come from the Yuan dynasty at the end of Goryeo (fourteenth century) (Choi, 2016).

18.3 Manufacturing Method

The traditional manufacturing method of making makgeolli and yakju is as follows. Rice is prepared by cleaning, soaking it in water, drying at room temperature, and then steaming. Subsequently, water and steamed rice are added to nuruk. Fermentation is carried out at 20°C–30°C for 14 days, until the makgeolli

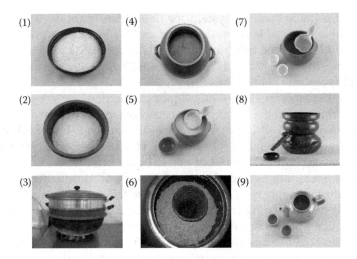

FIGURE 18.1
Manufacturing method of makgeolli, yakju, and soju; (1) cleaning rice, (2) soaking rice in water, (3) steaming rice, (4) water, steamed rice, nuruk put in the jar, and fermentation at 20–30°C, (5) mageolli, (6) filtering the makgeolli, (7) yakju, (8) distilled makgeolli or yakju, (9) soju.

is completed. Makgeolli is filtered to prepare yakju. Then, when the makgeolli or yakju is distilled, the soju is completed (Figure 18.1) (Kang et al., 2016).

18.4 Fermentation Agent, Nuruk

The most distinctive characteristic distinguishing Korean alcoholic beverages from Western liquors represented by wine, beer, and whiskey is the fermentation agent nuruk. Among Western liquors, beer is made through saccharification and fermentation of hops. Wine is a liquor made through saccharification straight from fruit. Korean alcoholic beverages utilize nuruk fungi to ferment cereals and produce liquor; therefore, the taste is more diversified depending on the environment of each nuruk production. Nuruk is defined as "fermentation agent used for brewing liquor" (Jeong, 2012a). In 1971, the National Tax Service in Korea said, "Nuruk is a fermentation agent in which natural enzymes included in raw cereals, mold fungi, yeast, and other fungi including *Rhizopus*, *Aspergillus*, *Lichtheimia*, and *Mucor* breed, produc[ing] a variety of enzymes" (Yu and Yu, 2011).

Nuruk is categorized into different uses for yakju, makgeolli, and soju depending on liquor type. In general, it is categorized into two different types according to the production method: traditional nuruk, which is made with wheat and wheat bran crushed and fermented in a mass like meju (blocks of fermented soybeans), and rice nuruk (Japanese koji), in which fungi grow on the grains (Jeong, 2012a).

18.5 Composition of Nuruk

Nuruk contributes to the unique characteristics of Korean alcoholic beverages. Most nuruks are composed of raw wheat grains (Shon et al., 1990; Yu et al., 2004). Other grains, such as rice, barley, sorghum, corn, soybeans, and rye are also used elsewhere (Yang et al., 2011). Naturally inoculated by airborne microorganisms, nuruk consists of useful fungi such as Aspergillus sp., Absidia sp., Rhizopus sp., Mucor sp., yeast, and lactic acid bacteria (Lee et al., 2012). Nuruk provides protease and proteolytic enzymes that play an important role in starch saccharification, dextrin production activity, and protein digestion. Through the process of alcohol fermentation, it produces a wide variety of organic acids and flavor compounds. Thus, it is responsible for the deep and complex taste of Korean alcoholic beverages (Yang et al., 2011).

Wheat, which is mainly used in Korean traditional nuruk, is an annual plant of terminal leaves distributed throughout temperate climates all over the world; it is cultivated as the most important food crop in the world. In oriental medicine, it is known that it replenishes insufficient energy, assists the activity of the internal organs, relieves fatigue, and improves blood circulation (Vaaler et al., 1986). The compounds isolated from wheat include alkaloids (allantoin, biotin, gramine, vitamin B1, etc.), flavonoids (apigenin, quercetin, tricin, etc.), flavonoid glycosides (orientin, schaftoside, isoschaftoside, etc.), phenylpropanoids (caffeic acid, ferulic acid, vanillic acid, cinnamic acid, etc.), terpenoids (citrinin, tocopherol, etc.), steroids (ergosterol, cholesterol, β-sitosterol, etc.), and the like (Wu et al., 1999; Raoul et al., 2003). Their functional properties include antioxidant activity and antimicrobial activity (Lankisch et al., 1998). *Rhizopus oryzae* is isolated mainly in the traditional nuruk made by wheat, which is a strain mainly used in the fermentation process when making traditional alcohol beverages in Korea, Japan, China, and Indonesia. Many studies have been reported on the production of lactic acid (Spiricheva et al., 2007). In Korea, it is a common fungus in meju and it regulates this strain to make deonjang (Korean traditional soybean paste) and soy sauce (Kwak et al., 2008).

Rice nuruk made from rice is mainly used to make fermented foods such as sake, shochu, and miso. Generally, fungi isolated from rice nuruk are mainly *Aspergillus kawachii* and *Aspergillus oryzae* (Bentley, 2006; Miyake et al., 2007; Suganuma et al., 2007; Machida et al., 2008), which are mainly used for antioxidant, tyrosinase inhibition, and glycolysis activities. In particular, *A. oryzae* has been reported to be an ideal microorganism for nuruk fermentation because it is responsible for the synthesis of amino acid metabolism and acts as a sugar uptake transporter (Bentley, 2006; Machida et al., 2007). In addition, representative secondary metabolites have been used as cosmetic and food additives to prevent skin lightening and enzyme browning with kojic acid (Burdock et al., 2001; Bentley, 2006). *A. oryzae* contains several enzymes, such as α-amylase, aminopeptidase, amyloglucosidase, lactase,

446   *Korean Functional Foods*

and lipase (Bentley, 2006; Suganuma et al., 2007). These enzyme activities can be changed based on the rice composition (Kim et al., 2012).

18.6 Functionality of Nuruk

18.6.1 Cytotoxic and Anti-Inflammatory Activity

To evaluate the cytotoxicity of the fatty acid compounds derived from nuruk (made with *Rhizopus oryzae* KSD-815 in wheat) to cancer cells, the cell survival rate of human breast cancer (MDA-MB-231) and liver cancer (SK-HEP-1) was evaluated by the MTT (3-[4,5-dimethylthiazol-2-yl]-2,5-diphenyl tetrazolium bromide) method (Mosmann, 1983). Compounds 1 (linolenic acid methyl ester) and 3 (linoleic acid) for breast cancer cells showed 49% and 43% cytotoxicity at a concentration of 50 µM, respectively. Compounds 1 and 3 for liver cancer cell lines induced 47% and 38% cytotoxicity at 50 µM, respectively (Figure 18.2). It has been reported that the intake of unsaturated fatty acids inhibits lipogenic enzymes such as fatty acid synthase (FAS) and induces the death of cancer cells (Clark et al., 1990; Menendez et al., 2004). Compounds 1 and 3, which are unsaturated fatty acids, are thought to regulate the growth of cancer cells through signal transduction and regulation of lipogenic enzymes (Kwak et al., 2008).

Nitrogen oxide (NO) is produced from L-arginine by nitric oxide synthase (NOS) and is known to be involved in various physiological processes (Moncada et al., 1991; Miyasaka and Hirata, 1997). The inclusive NOS (iNOS) detected by LPS (lipopolysaccharide) or cytokine has been reported to produce a large amount of NO in the calcium-dependent manner and to participate in inflammation reaction and tumor development (Nathan and Wie, 1994). The effect of nuruk-derived fatty acid compounds on NO production, which plays an important role in inflammation induction, was evaluated. The NO produced was determined using the Griess reagent to determine the form of NO_2^- present in the cell culture medium. As a result, concentration-dependent inflammation inhibitory activity was confirmed in compound 3 (Figure 18.3)—especially at the concentration of 5 µg/mL (Kwak et al., 2008).

18.6.2 Cholesterol and Activities of Hepatic Oxygen Free Radical Metabolizing Enzymes

Free radical metabolism enzyme activity and serum cholesterol levels in liver tissues of rats fed with nuruk containing *Aspergillus terreus* or wheat bran were observed. Nuruk or wheat bran intake groups showed higher feed efficiency than the control group during the growth period (Yoon et al., 1999).

Korean Alcoholic Beverages

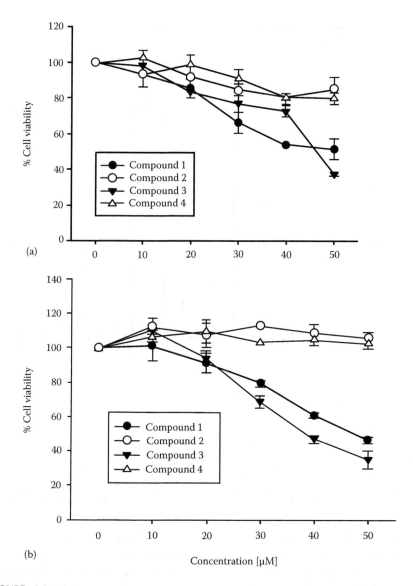

FIGURE 18.2
Inhibitory effects of compounds from nuruk on cancer cell cytotoxicity. MDA-MB-231 and SK-HEP-1 cells (2 × 10^4 cells/well) were incubated and doses of compounds purified from nuruk for 24 h and treated with MTT solution for 4 h. The extent of the reduction of MTT to formazan within cells was quantitated by the measurement of absorbance at 540 nm. (a) Human breast cancer cells, MDA-MB-231; (b) human hepatocarcinoma, SK-HEP-1.

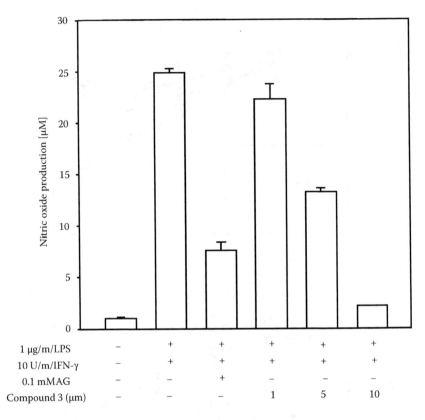

FIGURE 18.3
Inhibitory effects of compound 3 on the production of nitric oxide in RAW264.7 cells. The production of nitric oxide was assayed from culture medium of RAW264.7 cells stimulated with LPS (1 µg/mL) and IFN-γ (10 U/mL) in the presence of compound 3. RAW264.7 cells were plated at a density of 2×10^5 cells/mL. Nitrite accumulation was measured by Griess reaction in culture medium. The values are the means ± standard deviation of three independent experiments.

The liver tissue glutathione (GSH) content, which is a physiologically active substance acting as an antioxidant (Boyland and Chasseud, 1969) in the nuruk-containing group was lower than that in the control group, but the glutathione S-transferase (GST) activity was higher in all experimental groups grown in the nuruk-containing diet than in the control group. In addition, the activity of aniline hydroxylase activity by cytochrome P-450, which is involved in the toxic substance and drug detoxification in liver (Haugen and Coon, 1976), was also increased in all nuruk-containing diet groups. Superoxide dismutase activity in liver tissues involved in oxygen free radical detoxification (Halliwell, 1978) was not different in all experimental groups and the control group, but xanthine oxidase activity involved in the defense of biological cells (Yoon, 1980) was decreased in the nuruk-containing group without *Asp. terreus*.

Serum LDL-cholesterol activity, which is involved in arteriosclerosis induction, was significantly lower in the other groups than in the control group, except for the *Asp.* sp. (3-6, 12-1), *Pen.* sp. HDL-cholesterol, which is a lipoprotein involved in the transport of cholesterol, was significantly higher in the diets containing the nuruk and wheat bran than in the control group.

In the case of rats, the ingestion of nuruk containing *Asp. terreus* and wheat bran would improve toxicity and detoxification of harmful oxygen. In addition, the effect of lowering serum cholesterol content can be observed when nuruk is consumed.

18.6.3 Bioactive Compounds 2,6-Dimethoxy-1,4-Benzoquinone (2,6-DMBQ)

Quinone is a class of bioactive compound that may be components of anticancer chemotherapy drugs (Dandawate et al., 2010). 2,6-DMBQ exerts significant in vitro cytotoxicity against human tumor cell lines and also exhibits antibacterial activities (Tomoskozi-Farkas and Daood, 2004; Lana et al., 2006; Kim et al., 2010). Nuruk contains 2,6-DMBQ, also found in fermented wheat germ extract, and has anticancer and immunity-supporting effects. The presence of 2,6-DMBQ was confirmed by high-performance liquid chromatography and mass spectrometry. Among the five traditional nuruks tested, 2,6-DMBQ content of 0.38 ± 0.01–1.16 ± 0.07 mg/50 g was obtained from nuruk. 2,6-DMBQ was hypothesized to be produced by the actions of microbial β-glucosidases in nuruk. The specific microorganisms present in different nuruks and their enzymes may play important roles in converting the glycone form of 2,6-DMBQ to its aglycone form (Yoo et al., 2011).

18.7 Composition of Makgeolli

The alcohol content of makgeolli is lower than that of beer at 6%–8% (Kim et al., 2012). The protein content of makgeolli is about 1.7%–1.9% and includes amino acids that are produced by protein breakdown during the fermentation process. Valine, leucine, isoleucine, methionine, threonine, lysine, and phenylalanine are especially important amino acids since they are necessary components of the cell (Park, 2016).

The organic acids in makgeolli are either secreted from nuruk or synthesized during the fermentation process by microorganisms. A low organic acid content causes the lack of sour flavor, while a high organic acid content produces strong sourness and rancidity (Kim et al., 2012). The organic acid content of makgeolli is 0.15%–0.3%; however, an organic acid content higher than 0.5% turns the liquor rancid and therefore undrinkable.

The main organic acids in makgeolli are succinic acid, citric acid, and malic acid (Lee et al., 2011).

It is known that 75%–80% of rice is composed of starch, which is degraded into polysaccharides and oligosaccharides by the α-amylases contained in nuruk. These products are further metabolized by glucoamylases to produce glucose. Amylases hydrolyze most complex sugars into glucose. The transglucosidases present in nuruk produce oligosaccharides with altered structures. These sugars are not easily degraded by glucoamylases and remain in makgeolli, causing a sweet flavor (Bae, 2008).

Alcohols are common aroma compounds in liquors that are responsible for producing their basic fragrance. Many of the fragrances in makgeolli are produced by yeast. Higher alcohols and esters from intermediate fatty acids produce a peculiar fragrance in makgeolli. Since the compounds mentioned before are stable, their activity is high during the initial fermentation process, while it decreases afterwards. Phenyl alcohol is an important aroma compound in liquors, exhibiting a rose-like fragrance that smoothes the liquor flavor (Kim, 2016b).

Nitrogen compounds are metabolized by yeast during the fermentation process to produce higher alcohols, which give the fragrance to the liquor and affect its flavor. Amino acids are usually involved in liquor's umami flavor. A high concentration of amino acids causes a greasy flavor, while a low concentration produces a bland flavor. However, the appropriate levels of amino acids in liquors have not yet been defined (Kang et al., 2015).

18.8 Functionality of Makgeolli

18.8.1 Lactic Acid Bacteria

Lactic acid bacteria in makgeolli and other fermented food promote the peristalsis of the intestines, preventing constipation and carcinogenesis. Furthermore, they contribute to the hematopoiesis and the formation of vitamin B. During the manufacturing process of makgeolli, lactic acid bacteria are produced in the fermentation step by acidification of lactic acid. Such bacteria can prevent the growth of harmful pathogens and bacteria (Kim et al., 2012).

18.8.2 Anticancer

Recently, it was found that makgeolli contains about 150–500 ppb of the anticancer agent farnesol (Ha et al., 2013). The maximum content was 25 times more compared to 15–20 ppb in wine or beer. Farnesol is the substance that gives the flavor to fruit wines. It is a substance exhibiting anticancer and

Korean Alcoholic Beverages

antiulcer effects even with a very little amount of about 5–7mg/L. The solid content of makgeolli, particularly, holds more farnesol, and it can be more effectively ingested if makgeolli is consumed after a proper shake. It was also found that makgeolli contains squalene (Ha et al., 2014). Wine contains 10–20 µg/kg of it, and makgeolli 1260–4560 µg/kg (Table 18.1). It is thought that squalene is produced by the yeast used in the makgeolli production process. Squalene is a substance mainly extracted from the livers of sharks living in deep sea. It is a functional substance with antioxidant and anticancer effects, and its benefits are globally recognized (Ha et al., 2014).

Recent findings confirmed that makgeolli has the effect of containing the growth of cancer cells in the stomach (Shin et al., 2016). When stomach cancer cells originating in the human body were treated with makgeolli with its water and alcohol contents removed, the growth of cancer cells was limited, and the expression of the tumor suppressor gene phosphatase and tensin homolog (PTEN) increased. In animal testing, makgeolli was orally administered to mice to which stomach cancer cells originating from the human body had been transplanted, and the growth of ulcers was constrained. It was found that the major substance with an anticancer effect was beta

TABLE 18.1

Concentration[a] of E,E-Farnesol and Squalene in Several Makgeollis

Sample	E,E-farnesol (ng/mL)	Squalene (ng/mL)
1	92.3 ± 0.3	583.2 ± 0.7
2	73.6 ± 0.2	1205.5 ± 0.6
3	62.7 ± 0.6	1068.2 ± 0.3
4	41.4 ± 0.5	514.3 ± 0.6
5	44.9 ± 0.3	616.9 ± 0.5
6	103.2 ± 0.5	1919.7 ± 0.2
7	78.3 ± 0.8	572.4 ± 0.6
8	46.2 ± 0.6	794.3 ± 0.6
9	78.9 ± 0.4	1423.2 ± 0.8
10	73.2 ± 0.2	7431.1 ± 0.7
11	142.4 ± 0.4	1704.0 ± 0.2
12	33.6 ± 0.5	615.5 ± 0.3
13	68.2 ± 0.6	513.2 ± 0.3
14	71.7 ± 0.2	2756.7 ± 0.4
15	60.5 ± 0.2	562.7 ± 0.4
16	94.8 ± 0.6	3568.3 ± 0.3
Min[b]	33.6 ± 0.5	513.2 ± 0.3
Max[c]	142.4 ± 0.4	7431.1 ± 0.7
Average	72.6	1610.7

[a] Value represents the mean of the triplicate analyses ± the standard deviation.
[b] Maximum value.
[c] Minimum value.

452 *Korean Functional Foods*

sitosterol, which is mainly found in rice. This had been previously known for its health benefits for prostate and cholesterol control.

In addition, the evidence of cancer cell growth control by makgeolli fractions and the increased activation of quinone reductase confirmed its anticancer effects (Shin et al., 2008).

18.8.3 Improvement of Liver Function

The amino acids present in makgeolli are necessary nutrients for improving liver function by protecting it and promoting its regeneration (Kim et al., 2001). Toxic liver markers include alkaline phosphatase (ALP), alanine aminotransferase (ALT), and aspartate aminotransferase (AST). These enzymes exist in both liver and heart at high concentrations and react very sensitively to organ damage. Therefore, they are widely used as markers for hepatitis and cirrhosis. Hepatitis, cirrhosis, jaundice, and liver cancer lead to an increase in the level of these enzymes. It was found that when a specific amount of makgeolli was administered to a male white mouse over a 6-week period, the corresponding ALP, ALT, and AST levels in its blood significantly decreased and were further reduced with increasing densities of makgeolli.

18.8.4 Cholesterol-Lowering Effect

LDL (low-density lipoprotein) and HDL (high-density lipoprotein) cholesterol are two forms of cholesterol that exist in the blood. The LDL level increases with the consumption of animal-derived products with a high content of saturated fats and can cause atherosclerosis by depositing in the walls of blood vessels. HDL transfers the cholesterol deposits from the blood vessels to the liver, decreasing the risk of atherosclerosis (Bae, 2010). In a recent study, the ovaries of a female mouse were removed to artificially induce menopause, and then fractions of makgeolli were administered at different concentrations. The results indicated that the blood triglyceride and total cholesterol levels decreased by 5%–10%, while the HDL-cholesterol blood level significantly increased (37%) (Kim et al., 2001).

18.8.5 Improved Blood Flow Effect

A concentrate of makgeolli was administered to a group of female white mice that had undergone ovary removal, and it was observed that their blood flow was faster than that of the control group. Fat deposits in the blood vessels slow down the blood flow and can even cause coronary artery disease in extreme cases. The consumption of appropriate amounts of makgeolli can increase the speed of the blood flow and therefore improve it (Shin et al., 2010). Furthermore, platelet aggregation examinations revealed that the group treated with makgeolli exhibited a decreased platelet aggregation of about 11% compared to the control group. Thus, the consumption of appropriate amounts of makgeolli can decrease platelet aggregation, which is responsible for coronary artery disease, and improve blood flow. Therefore, makgeolli produces positive effects in the prevention of cardiovascular diseases (Shin et al., 2010).

18.8.6 Removing Reactive Oxygen Species (Antioxidant Effect)

As a result of comparison with the control group, the active oxygen removal efficiency was increased according to the increase of concentration in the makgeolli methanol fraction layer, and the concentration of active oxygen was increased by SIN-1 (3-morpholinosyndnonimine). The removal of active oxygen from the makgeolli concentrate and hexane layer was followed by the similar trends (Bae, 2010).

18.8.7 Inhibiting Hypertension (ACE-Inhibiting Effect)

The precursor compound angiotensinogen present in the blood is hydrolyzed by renin, which is formed in the kidneys, to produce angiotensin I. Angiotensin I is cleaved by ACE (angiotensin converting enzyme) to produce angiotensin II, which causes constriction of the blood vessels and consequentially increases blood pressure. The addition of makgeolli to a hydrolysate interferes with the mechanism of ACE and inhibits the increase of blood pressure. Compared to the control group, 82.6%, 68.9% of the group treated with makgeolli showed inhibition of ACE and the antihypertensive properties were confirmed (Figure 18.4) (Shin et al., 2010).

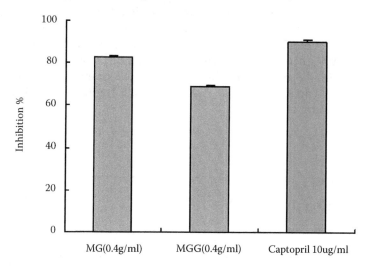

FIGURE 18.4
In vitro inhibitory effects of the MG and MGG on ACE (angiotensin-converting enzyme) activities. The assay procedure was described in experimental methods. Values are mean ± standard deviation of triplicated experiments. MG: makgeolli; MGG: makgeolli gigemi (by product of makgeolli).

18.9 Composition of Yakju

The alcohol content of yakju is higher than that of makgeolli at 13%–15% (Shin et al., 1999). The organic acid contents of succinic acid, malic acid, and citric acid are contained in yakju in equal concentrations and they make up 80% of the total organic acid content. As yakju rots, both the lactic acid and acetic acid levels increase, while the malic acid level decreases. Succinic acid possesses a savory sour taste and is one of the main components of yakju. The organic acids are produced by yeast during the metabolism of the raw materials (Huh et al., 2013).

The sweet taste of yakju is determined by its glucose content. Besides free sugars, amino acids such as D-tryptophan (35 times sweeter than sucrose), phenylalanine (7 times sweeter than sucrose), and tyrosine (5.5 times sweeter than sucrose) produce a strong sweetness in liquors (Lee, 2015).

Higher alcohols such as isoamyl alcohol or isobutanol are produced by the metabolism of amino acids promoted by yeast (Selli et al., 2006). These higher alcohols are the main aroma compounds of yakju and makgeolli. Although they contribute to the fragrance of these liquors, they are 15–30 times more toxic than alcohol and are known to cause hangovers (Kwon et al., 2010). An increase in the rice milling ratio during yakju manufacturing produces liquors with good isoamyl acetate and ethyl caproate balance (Bae, 2008).

Concerning the nitrogen compound content of yakju, its sweetness mostly originates from glucose, which is produced by the degradation of starch. Glucose is converted into alcohols during fermentation and the remaining sugars and sweet flavor producing amino acids (alanine, arginine, glycine, and proline) are responsible for the sweetness of the liquor (Choi et al., 2015). Tyrosine and tryptophan in yakju produce brown-colored compounds when exposed to sunlight, causing browning of the liquor. Sugars and amino acids undergo the Maillard reaction when the liquor is fermented for a long time. The Maillard reaction produces diverse flavors, fragrances, and coloring compounds (Kang et al., 2016).

18.10 Functionality of Yakju

18.10.1 Antioxidant Effect

It was found that makgeolli and yakju contained a higher volume of antioxidants than other types of liquor (Lee et al., 2013). In Korean traditional alcoholic beverages, the average content of antioxidant polyphenol was 21.7 mg/L TAE (tannic acid equivalent, conversion unit for antioxidants) in yakju, 18.7 mg/L TAE in makgeolli, 17.9 mg/L TAE in fruit wine, and 5.8 mg/L TAE in distilled liquor.

Korean Alcoholic Beverages

The average content of flavonoid was 6.27 mg/L QDE (conversion unit for antioxidants) in yakju, the highest of all. Then, followed fruit wine with 3.58 mg/L QDE, makgeolli with 3 mg/L QDE, and distilled liquor with 2.7 mg/L QDE. Polyphenol is effective for cancer, dementia, cardiovascular diseases, and prevention of skin aging. Flavonoid is known for its antivirus, anticancer, antiallergic, and antibacterial effects. These two substances are found in rice, vegetables, and flower, fruit, trunk, and root of plants. Minerals and substances for physiological functions, such as calcium, magnesium, and copper, were found most in volume in yakju and makgeolli. The average content of calcium was 4.8 mg per 100 g of both makgeolli and yakju, and that of magnesium was 4.67 mg and 3.11 mg in yakju and makgeolli, respectively. Copper content was 0.004 mg in makgeolli and 0.003 mg in yakju.

18.10.2 Anticarcinogenic Effects

The cytotoxicities of yakju containing 10 different medicinal herbs (ginseng, schisandra, goji berries, ball leaves, cinnamon, dried ginger, Cynanchum wilfordii, tuckahoe, liquorice, and *Astragalus*), yakju containing buckwheat and Morus alba L., red wine, white wine, beer, and sake were investigated (Chung et al., 1998). Cytotoxicity causes direct damage on the cancer cells with increased toxicity by stimulating cytotoxic cells. The medicinal herb containing yakju exhibited a cytotoxicity on cancerous colon cells that was three times lower than that of red wine, while other liquors had negligible cytotoxic effects. Red wine, medicinal herb yakju, and buckwheat yakju showed similar cytotoxicity on cancerous liver cells. Cytotoxicities on cancerous lymphocytes were similar for medicinal herb yakju (91.26%), buckwheat yakju (88.61%), and red wine (90.48%). Cytotoxicities on cancerous breast cells were also similar for medicinal herb yakju (90.54%), buckwheat yakju (88.61%), and red wine (90.19%) (Kim et al., 2004).

18.10.3 Anticancer Effects

Some mice were injected with cancer cells in order to test the effect on the growth and metastasis of cancer cells of the solid content in yakju brewed by the raw rice brewing technique (Chung et al., 1998). The mouse group fed with the traditional yakju showed a relatively slower growth of cancer cells compared to the control group 19 days after the injection. It is thought that the solid deposit of the yakju stimulated nearby immunocytes and other diverse cells and vitalized anticancer activity in the surrounding environment of cancer cells (Figure 18.5).

18.10.4 Fibrinolytic Activity

The fibrinolytic activities of self-prepared samheju (made from rice and nuruk, with a fermentation period of 30–100 days) and five different types of

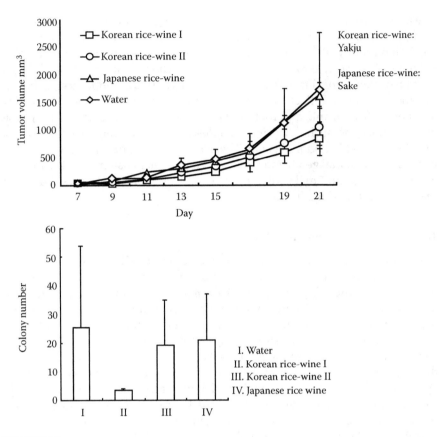

FIGURE 18.5
Inhibitory effects of rice wine on *in vivo* growth of B16BL6 mouse melanoma cells. Tumor cells were inoculated into foot pads of the mice, were daily fed with a solution of rice wine solids. Tumor growth was monitored to day 21 after tumor inoculation, and lung colonization was measured on day 35.

yakju sold in the Korean market were compared (Lim et al., 2009). Fibrinolysis is the breakdown of fibrin clots in the blood and, therefore, compounds with fibrinolytic activity can prevent vascular diseases in the brain and blood flow blockages. The fibrinolytic activity of samheju is high at 13.8–17.6 units/Ml, while the yakju sold in the market showed an activity of 7.3–10.4 units/Ml. The ABTS (2,2′-azino-bis(3-ethylbenzothiazoline-6-sulphonic acid) radical removing effects and cytotoxicity on cancerous cervical cells (HeLa: human cervix adenocarcinoma; A549: human lung carcinoma; L-132: human fetal lung cell) of samheju were significantly higher than those of commercial yakju. It is inferred that the pharmacological ingredients, which affect cancerous cells and physiological functions, were formed in samheju by nuruk during the long fermentation process (100 days).

Korean Alcoholic Beverages

TABLE 18.2

Effects of Korean Rice Wine (Yakju) on Absolute Ethanol-Induced Gastric Lesions in Rats

Treatment	Dose (mg/kg, p.o.)	No. of Animals	Gastric Lesion (mean ± SEM, mm²)	Inhibition Ratio (%)
Control	–	10	131.50 ± 64.18	–
Korean rice Wine	250	10	89.60 ± 57.94	31.9
	500	10	75.50 ± 49.82[a]	42.6
	1000	10	46.10 ± 26.23[b]	64.9
Cimetidine	150	10	22.40 ± 22.61[b]	83.0

[a] Significantly different from each control ($p < 0.05$).
[b] Significantly different from each control ($p < 0.01$).

18.10.5 Protecting the Liver

Yakju containing 10 different medicinal herbs (ginseng, schisandra, goji berries, ball leaves, cinnamon, dried ginger, Cynanchum wilfordii, tuckahoe, licorice, and *Astragalus*) was concentrated under high pressure and the residue was administered to mice to confirm the liver-protecting effects and ulcer/gastritis-inhibiting effects of yakju (Kim et al, 2004). Low-density yakju at 250 mg/kg inhibited the damage on the gastric mucosa, while high-density yakju at 1000 mg/kg showed an inhibition rate of 80.51%. The observed inhibition was 1.4 times more effective than that of 150 mg/kg of cimetidine, which was used as reference compound. Furthermore, 250–1000 mg/kg of yakju was orally administered in mice that were fasted for 24 h, followed by administration of ethanol after 30 min. The group treated with yakju showed significantly lower rates of gastric diseases compared to the control group. When 30% of alcohol was administered every 12 h for 7 days, the effects of yakju on gastric disease inhibition were confirmed (Table 18.2).

18.11 Conclusion

Recently, a new era has begun with the interest in and consumption of Korean traditional alcohol beverages. Nuruk is a traditional fermented agent made of naturally occurring microorganisms, or is artificially microbially inoculated, and has various functions. Typically, it contains cytotoxic and anti-inflammatory activity, lowers cholesterol, inhibits free radical activity, anticancer substances, etc. Utilization methods such as functional food or drug development are being explored.

Korea's representative traditional alcoholic beverages, makgeolli and yakju, are made of rice and recognized as health foods because they have lower calories than wine, soju, and whiskey. Especially, the discovery of farnesol, an anticancer substance, has greatly increased the consumption of makgeolli. And yakju contains various kinds of herbal ingredients and acts to protect the liver while alcohol beverages are drunk. Based on the results of the studies discussed, it can be developed as a global fermented food if Korean traditional alcohol beverages are recognized as health foods, not merely alcohol.

References

Bae, S.J. 2010. *Traditional well-being liquor makgeolli*. Hanam Publishing.

Bae, S.M. 2008. *Sake manufacturing technology*. Design Plus Co.

Bentley, R. 2006. From miso, sake and shoyu to cosmetics: A century of science for kojic acid. *Nat Prod Rep* 23: 1046–1062.

Boyland, E., and L.F. Chasseud. 1969. The role of glutathione and glutathione S-transferase in mercapturic acid bio-synthesis. *Adv Enzymol* 32: 173.

Burdock, G.A., M.G. Sony, and I.G. Carabin. 2001. Evaluation of health aspects of kojic acid in food. *Regul Toxicol Pharmacol* 33: 80–101.

Choi, H.S. 2016. The water of life, spirit (Interrobang No.168), ed. S.T. Jeong, and J.E. Kang, 1–2. Rural Development Administration.

Choi, H.S., J.E. Kang, S.T. Jeong, C.W. Kim, and M.K. Kim. 2015. Changes observed in doenjang (soybean paste) with added fermented Rhus verniciflua extract during aging. *Korean J Food Sci Technol* 47: 599–607.

Chung, K.S., W.T. Oh, S.M. Nam, B.S. Son, and Y.S. Park. 1998. Effect of Korean rice-wine (yakju) on in vitro and in vivo progression of B16BL6 mouse melanoma and HRT18 human colon adenocarcinoma cells. *Korean J Food Sci Technol* 30: 1470–1475.

Clark, B.A., M.K. Armstrong, and D.B. Jump. 1990. Nutritional control of rat liver fatty acid synthase and S14 MNA abundance. *J Nutr* 120: 218-224.

Dandawate, P.R., A.C. Vyas, S.B. Padhye, M.W. Singh, and J.B. Baruah. 2010. Perspectives on medicinal properties of benzoquinone compounds. *Mini Rev Med Chem* 10: 436–454.

Ha, J.H., Y.S. Shim, D.W. Seo, and H.J. Jang. 2014. Analysis of e,e-farnesol and squalene in makgeolli using stir bar sorptive extraction coupled with gas chromatography-mass spectrometry. *Analytical Sci Technol* 27: 60–65.

Ha, J.H., Y. Wang, H.J. Jang, H.M. Seong, and X. Chen. 2013. Detection of E, E-farnesol in makgeolli (rice wine) using dynamic headspace sampling and stir bar sorptive extraction coupled with gas chromatography-mass spectrometry. *Food Chem* 142: 79–86.

Halliwell, B. 1978. Biochemical mechanism accounting for the toxic action of oxygen on living organism: The key role of superoxide dismutase. *Cell Biol Int Rep* 2: 113.

Haugen, D.A., and M.J. Coon. 1976. Properties of electrophoretically homogenous phenobarbital-inducible and A-naphthoflavone-inducible form of liver microxomal cytochrome P-450. *J Biol Chem* 251: 7929.

Huh, C.K., J.W. Lee, and Y.D. Kim. 2013. Comparison of the organic acids, fusel oil contents and antioxidant activities of yakju with the additions of various rice cultivars. *Korean J Food Preserv* 20: 365–371.

Jeong, D.H. 2012a. *Science of nuruk*. Yuhansa Publishing.

Jeong, S.T. 2012b. Traditional liquor story (interrobang no. 50), ed. J.E. Kang, and H.S. Choi, 17–18. Rural Development Administration.

Kang, J.E. 2014. Makgeolli story (Interrobang No.124), ed. H.S. Choi, and J.H. Choi, 1-2, 6-9. Rural Development Administration.

Kang, J.E., H.S. Choi, J.H. Choi, S.H. Yeo, and S.T. Jeong. 2014. Physicochemical properties of Korean non-sterilized commercial makgeolli. *Korean J Community Living Sci* 25: 636–372.

Kang, J.E., H.S. Choi, J.W. Kim, C.W. Kim, S.H. Yeo, and S.T. Jeong, 2016. Quality characteristics of yakju with nuruk extracts. *Korean J Food Sci Technol* 48: 1–8.

Kang, J.E., J.W. Kim, H.S. Choi, C.W. Kim, S.H. Yeo, and S.T. Jeong. 2015. Effect of the addition of protein and lipid on the quality characteristics of yakju. *Korean J Food Preserv* 22: 361–368.

Kim, A.J., J.N. Choi, J.Y. Kim, H.Y. Kim, S.B. Park, S.H. Yeo, J.H. Choi, K.H. Liu, and C.H. Lee. 2012. Metabolite profiling and bioactivity of rice *koji* fermented by *Aspergillus* strains. *J Microbiol Biotechnol* 22: 100–106.

Kim, H.R. 2016a. The composition of Korean liquor, ed. G.C. Song, and S.T. Jeong, 19, 24. National Institute of Agricultural Science.

Kim, J.W. 2016b. Correlation of physicochemical characteristics and sensory properties commercial makgeoll. Master's thesis, Chonbuk Univ.

Kim, K.W. 2012. Makgeolli and yakju; science and application, ed. J.H. Kim, and B.S. Noh, 16–26, 226–232. Ministry for Food, Agriculture, Forestry and Fisheries.

Kim, M.H., S.H. Jo, K.S. Ha, J.H. Song, H.D. Jang, and Y.I. Kwon. 2010. Antimicrobial activities of 1,4-benzoquinones and wheat germ extract. *J Microbiol Biotechnol* 20: 1204–1209.

Kim, M.H., W.H. Kim, and S.J. Bae. 2001. The effects of makkoil on serum lipid concentration in male rate. *Journal of Nat Sci of Silla Univ* 9: 73–84.

Kim, S.J., J.Y. Baek, C.K. Park, and G.W. Kim. 2004. Gastroprotective effect of Korean rice-wine (yakju). *Korean J Food Sci Technol* 36: 818–822.

Kim, T.Y. 2011. Korean liquor story (interrobang no.3), ed. S.T. Jung, and H.S. Choi, 4–7. Rural Development Administration.

Kwak, H.Y., S.J. Lee, D.Y. Lee, L.K. Jung, N.H. Bae, S.Y. Hong, G.W. Kim, and N.I. Baek. 2008. Cytotoxic and anti-inflammatory activities of lipids from the nuruk (*Rhizopus oryzae* KSD-815). *J Korean Soc Appl Biol Chem* 51: 142–147.

Kwon, Y.H., S.J. Jo, J.H. Kim, and B.H. Ahn. 2010. Fermentation characteristics and volatile compounds in yakju made with various brewing conditions; glutinous rice and pre-treatment. *Korean J Microbiol Biotechnol* 38: 46–52.

Lana, E.J., F. Carazza, and J.A. Takahashi. 2006. Antibacterial evaluation of 1,4-benzoquione derivatives. *J Agric Food Chem* 54: 2053–2056.

Lankisch, M., P. Layer, R.A. Rizza, and E.P. DiMagno. 1998. Acute postprandial gastrointestinal and metabolic effects of wheat amylase inhibitor (WAI) in normal, obese, and diabetic humans. *Pancreas* 17: 176–181.

Lee, H.J. 2009. *Korean traditional liquor*. Press Hanyang.

Lee, J.G. 2015. Distilled spirits, ed. S.H. Moon, and G.H. Bae, 422-425. Ministry for Food, Agriculture, Forestry and Fisheries.

Lee, M.K., J.T. Kim, B.H. Lee, G.M. Yum, B.Y. Lee, B.H. Yun, Y.J. Yu, and P.G. Min. 2013. Study on excellence of traditional liquors. *Chungbuk Provincial Institute of Health Environment* 22: 33–55.

Lee, S.H. 2009. *Liquor culture of Korea.* Sun Press.

Lee, S.J., S.W. Cho, Y.Y. Kwon, H.S. Kwon, and W.C. Shin. 2012. Inhibitory effects of ethanol extracts from *nuruk* on oxidative stress, melanogenesis, and photo-aging. *Mycrobiology* 40: 117–123.

Lee, S.J., J.H. Kim, Y.W. Jung, S.Y. Park, W.C. Shin, C.S. Park, S.Y. Hong, and G.W. Kim. 2011. Composition of organic acids and physiological functionality of commercial makgeolli. *Korean J Food Sci Technol* 43: 206–212.

Lim, C.L., H.J. Son, I.Y. Jo, G.W. Kim, S.J. Choi, I.S. Kim, K.Y. Han, J.Y. Choi, and B.S. Noh. 2009. Physiological functionality and cytotoxic effect of Korean traditional noble wine, samhaeju, and commercial rice wine on various tumor cell lines. *Korean J Food Sci Technol* 41: 687–693.

Machida, M., O. Yamada, and K. Gomi. 2008. Genomics of *Aspergillus oryzae*: Learning from the history of koji mold and exploration of its future. *DNA Res* 15: 173–183.

Menendez, J.A., S. Ropero, I. Mehmi, E. Atlas, R. Colomer, and R. Lupu. 2004. Overexpression and hyperactivity of breast cancer-associated fatty acid synthase (oncogenic antige-519) is insensitive to normal arachidonic fatty acid-induced suppression in lipogenic tissue but it is selectively inhibited by tumoricidal α-linolenic acid and γ-linolenic acid fatty acid: A novel mechanism by which dietary fat can alter mammary tumorigenesis. *Inter J Onchol* 24: 1369–1383.

Miyake, Y., C. Ito, M. Itoigawa, and T. Osawa. 2007. Isolation of the antioxidant pyranonigrin-A from rice mold starters used in the manufacturing process of fermented foods. *Biosci Biotechnol Biochem* 71: 2515–2521.

Miyasaka, N., and Y. Hirata. 1997. Nitric oxide and inflammatory arthritides. *Life Sci* 61: 2073–2081.

Moncada. S., R.M. Palmer, and E.A. Higgs. 1991. Nitric oxide: Physiology, pathophysiology, and pharmacology. *Pharmacol Rev* 43: 109–142.

Mosmann, T. 1983. Rapid colorimetric assay for cellular growth and survival: Application to proliferation and cytotoxicity assays. *J Immunol Methods* 65: 55–63.

Nathan, C., and Q.W. Xie. 1994. Nitric oxide synthases: Roles, tolls and controls. *Cell* 78: 915–918.

Park, Y.D. 2016. Comparative study on the physicochemical and sensory properties of heat treated and draft makgeolli. Master's thesis. Chonbuk Univ.

Raoul, R., L.R.M. Nike, P. Geraldine, C. Patrice, L.D. Dominique, M.D. Nathalie, M. Marc, and Q.L. Joelle. 2003. Phytosterol analysis and characterization in spelt (Triticum aestivum spelta L.) and wheat (T. aestivum L.) lipids by LC/APCI-MS. *J Cereal Sci* 38: 189–197.

Selli, S., A. Canbas, T. Cabaroglu, H. Erten, and Z. Günata. 2006. Aroma components of cv Muscat of Bornova wines and influence of skin contact treatment. *Food Chem* 94: 319–326.

Shin, E.J., J.H. Kim, K.S. Seong, S.K. Yum, and J.T. Hwang. 2016. Effect of commercial makgeolli on tumor growth in tumor xenograft mice. *Korean J Food Presrv* 23: 104–109.

Shin, K.R., B.C. Kim, J.Y. Yang, and Y.D. Kim. 1999. Characteristics of yakju prepared with yeast from fruits: 1. Volatile compounds in yakju during fermentation. *J Korean Soc Food Sci Nutr* 28: 794–800.

Shin, M.O., D.Y. Kang, M.H. Kim, and S.J. Bae. 2008. Effect of growth inhibition and quinone reductase activity stimulation of makgeoly fractions in various cancer cells. *J Korean Soc Food Sci Nutr* 37: 288–293.

Shin, M.O., M.H. Kim, and S.J. Bae. 2010. The effect of makgeolli on blood flow, serum lipid improvement and inhibition of ACE in vitro. *Journal of Life Science* 20: 710–716.

Shon, S.K., Y.H. Rho, H.J. Kim, and S.M. Bae. 1990. Takju brewing of uncooked rice starch using *Rhizopus koji. Korean J Appl Microbiol Bioeng* 18: 506–510.

Spiricheva, O.V., O.V. Senko, D.V. Veremeenko, and E.N. Efremenko. 2007. Lactic acid production by immobilized cells of the fungus *Rhizopus oryzae* with simultaneous product extraction. *Theor Found Chem Eng* 41: 150–153.

Suganuma, D., K. Fujita, and K. Kitahara. 2007. Some distinguishable properties between acid-stable and neutral types of α-amylases from acid-producing *Koji. J Agric Food Chem* 56: 11612–11620.

Tomoskozi-Farkas, R., and H.G. Daood. 2004. Modification of chromatographic method for the determination of benzoquinones in cereal products. *Chromatographia* 60: S227–230.

Vaaler, S., K.F. Hansen, K. Dahl-Jorgensen, W. Frolich, J. Aaseth, B. Odegaard, and O. Aagenaes. 1986. Diabetic control is improved by guar gum and wheat bran supplementation. *Diabet Med* 3: 230–223.

Wu, H., T. Haig, J. Pratley, D. Lemerle, and M. An. 1999. Simultaneous determination of phenolic acids and 2,4-dihydroxy-7-methoxy-1,4-benzoxazin-3-one in wheat (*Triticum aestivum* L.) by gas chromatography–tandem mass spectrometry. *J Chromatogr A* 864: 315–321.

Yang, S.Y., J.K. Lee, J.K. Kwak, K.H. Kim, M.J. Seo, and Y.W. Lee. 2011. Fungi associated with the traditional starter cultures used for rice wine in Korea. *J Korean Soc Appl Biol Chem* 54: 933–943.

Yoo, J.G., D.H. Kim, E.H. Park, J.S. Lee, S.Y. Kim, and M.D. Kim. 2011. Nuruk, a traditional Korean fermentation starter, contains the bioactive compound 2,6-dimethoxy-1,4-benzoquinone (2,6-DMBQ). *J Korean Soc Appl Biol Chem* 54: 795–798.

Yoon, C.G., S.N. Chae, N.E. Huh, H.S. Kim, and T.S. Yu. 1999. Effects of nuruk or wheat bran supplemented diet on the serum levels of cholesterol and activities of hepatic oxygen free radical metabolizing enzymes in rats. *J Korean Soc Food Sci Nutr* 28: 212–217.

Yoon, J.G. 1980. Changes in liver and serum xanthine oxidase activity following administration of carbon tetrachloride in rats. *J Inst Life Sci* 6: 75.

Yu, T.S., S.H. Yeo, and H.S. Kim. 2004. A new species of hyphomycetes, *Aspergillus coreanus* sp. nov., isolated from traditional Korean nuruk. *Korean J Microbiol Biotechnol* 14:182–187.

Yu, T.S., and H.Y. Yu. 2011. *Traditional Korean fermenter, nuruk, of origin form and excellency.* Korean Society for Biotechnology and Bioengineering.

19

Clinical Trials of Some Korean Functional Foods

Soo-Wan Chae and Su-Jin Jung

CONTENTS

19.1 Introduction 464
19.2 Basics in Functional Foods 465
19.3 Types of Studies...466
    19.3.1 Preclinical and Clinical Study..466
        19.3.1.1 Preclinical Study 466
        19.3.1.2 Clinical Study 467
    19.3.2 Challenge of Customized Nutrition in Clinical Study 470
19.4 Understanding Clinical Study of Foods and Procedures 470
19.5 Strategy for Developing Healthy Functional Foods 474
19.6 Successful Development Strategy for Healthy Functional Foods
    and Clinical Practices 476
    19.6.1 Application of Successful Strategy for Clinical Studies of Foods...476
        19.6.1.1 Stress Loading Methods 476
        19.6.1.2 Pilot Clinical Study for Increasing Success Rate
            of a Preclinical Study......................................478
19.7 Clinical Trial Center for Functional Foods (CTCF2) for Chonbuk
    National University Hospital 479
    19.7.1 Overview 479
19.8 Clinical Cases in Some Korean Healthy Functional Foods 480
    19.8.1 Development of Healthy Functional Foods............................480
        19.8.1.1 Pomegranate 480
        19.8.1.2 Fermented Curcuma Longa.......................483
        19.8.1.3 Persimmon Leaves and Yuja.....................485
        19.8.1.4 Muju Gastrodiae Rhizome.........................487
        19.8.1.5 *Cordyceps sinensis* 490
    19.8.2 Verification of Clinical Excellence in Korean Foods 492
        19.8.2.1 Intake of Korean Foods and Generative Function ...492
        19.8.2.2 Korean Foods and NCD Dietetic Treatments 492
        19.8.2.3 Bibimbap and Kimbap and Metabolic Diseases.....494
        19.8.2.4 Rice-Oriented Meals: Mixed Grains (Improving
            Memory) 494

463

| 19.8.3 | Traditional Soy Bean Fermented Products | 495 |

19.8.3 Traditional Soy Bean Fermented Products 495
      19.8.3.1 Cheonggukjang 495
      19.8.3.2 Doenjang 496
      19.8.3.3 Gochujang 497
19.9 Conclusion 498
References 498

19.1 Introduction

Noncommunicable diseases (NCD) caused by changes in modern lifestyles, cancer, cardiovascular disease, diabetes, dementia, respiratory disease, etc., are responsible for 60% of deaths throughout the world. Also, it is estimated that NCDs are constantly increasing. National medical expenses in the United States increased from 5% of the GDP in the 1960s to 17% in 2010, and the nation's obesity rate rose by more than 30%. Also, there were no significant achievements in the war against cancer. In the 2000s—the age of the new millennium—the United States faced many difficulties due to increases in diseases and medical expenses, even though R&D expenses and investments have been continuously increased.

Although an NCDs reaches a limit as they are treated by conventional methods, it has been shown that 80% of NCDs can be prevented through improving dietary life. In the United States, NCCIH (the National Center for Complementary and Integrative Health), which is an affiliate of the National Institutes of Health (NIH) will increase investments for the field of nutraceuticals as an alternative plan for preventing and managing diseases. In general, pharmaceutical and nutraceutical markets increase by about 5% and 15% every year, respectively. It is expected that the scale of nutraceutical markets will exceed the that of pharmaceutical markets in 2025. Also, it has been shown that our living environments, including dietary life, play a more important role than inherited genes in NCDs.

In addition, the effects of dietary life on preventing and managing diseases have been attracted to the point of view of epigenetics that various gene expressions occur according to the food we eat. Different animal tests and clinical research show the reasons for this (Kontou et al., 2011; Gardener et al., 2012). For instance, Waterland, and Jirtle (2003) reported that a brown colored slender rat was born because of the change in gene phenotypes as folic acid, vitamin B_6, betain, and choline that supply a methyl group to cells were applied to a yellow colored fat rat, which has a fat genotype of agouti, during pregnancy. In addition, Ornish et al. (2003) showed that the expression of genes related to cancer was inhibited as dietetic treatments were applied to prostate cancer patients denied chemical, radiation, and surgical treatments in which the size of the prostate cancer was decreased.

As mentioned before, the theory of epigenetics that our fate is determined by our dietary life is more convincing than what is in the order of genes.

Therefore, it represents that the food we are eating includes substances of changing gene phenotypes, and the good food should include not only vitamins and minerals, but also bioactives (phytochemicals) abundantly. Genetic nutritioneering is presented as a study of investigating the relationship between phytochemicals and genes. The phytochemicals familiar to people are catechins in green teas, genistein in beans, resveratrol in grapes, curcumin in turmeric, and so on. In actuality, these substances are included in different plants with more than 10,000 species. It has been known that foods supply basic calories and nutrients as a primary function and satisfy tastes and flavors as a secondary function. Health functional foods are determined by the fact that bioactives included in foods contribute to health beyond the values of the basic nutrients as a tertiary function and the effects are scientifically proven. For the conditions of satisfying such health functional foods, the effects of foods on health are objectively evaluated and the safety and functionality of the bioactive substances are to be proven scientifically.

19.2 Basics in Functional Foods

For presenting functionalities in functional foods, it is necessary to preferentially acquire the evaluation of the functionalities in raw materials from the Ministry of Food and Drug Safety (MFDS) in Korea. The functionalities represent useful effects in the human body through taking substances and compositions of the raw materials in foods and are to be proven scientifically. A study on the evaluation process of the functionalities can be classified according to the type and quality of the study and the classification is based on the scale, consistency, and applicability of the study.

The fundamental principles for evaluating the presentation of functionalities in MFDS are determined as follows:

1. Verifying the characteristics of the applied functional raw materials and the correlation between the characteristics and the study
2. Verifying the functionalities based on the functional raw materials (or compositions)
3. Classifying individual materials according to study types and evaluating the type and quality of individual studies
4. Examining the scale, consistency, and applicability of the applied materials and evaluating the degree of scientific facts for presenting the functionalities

Thus, a systematic consideration based on research results allows presenting the relationship between food compositions and functionalities through an evidence-based evaluation process. This process evaluates individual research materials after obtaining proper materials based on examining related scientific data. Then, the consistency of data is to be verified based on examining the amount of data, the results of individual studies, the relations to subject groups, and the relationship between food compositions and functionalities. The evaluated consistency is reflected in the presentation of functionalities.

19.3 Types of Studies

The data for proving functionalities in foods include the results of clinical trials, animal studies, *in vitro* studies, epidemiological investigations, and related references. The functionalities in the raw materials of foods are to be verified in the human body scientifically and are determined by aggregating different study results. A clinical trial in the stage of evaluating functionalities is divided into intervention and observed studies. The tests performed by the randomized controlled double-blind trial and methods in the intervention study are recognized as the most excellent data in functionalities. Although the data obtained from animal studies, *in vitro* studies, reviews, meta-analyses, and traditional application materials may represent difficulties in determining functionalities in the human body, they become desirable data not only to describe raw materials to be verified, mechanisms in compositions, and dose responses, but also to verify the results of clinical study scientifically (Figure 19.1).

19.3.1 Preclinical and Clinical Study

An animal study is the easiest way to determine the causal relationship in treating and preventing diseases through foods, due to the usefulness of samples and the autonomy of controls. The ultimate goal in the study is to investigate a scientific basis in preventing diseases based on nutrients and functionalities in foods. Thus, it is essential to apply clinical trials for achieving this goal.

19.3.1.1 Preclinical Study

A researcher in an experimental study is able to directly design and control experimental conditions. *In vitro* studies have the advantages of searching the effects of different samples in a short time and of determining operational mechanisms in samples even though there is a limit in evaluating *in vivo* responses. An animal study is able to evaluate the effects of samples using an appropriate disease model and can easily obtain test animals.

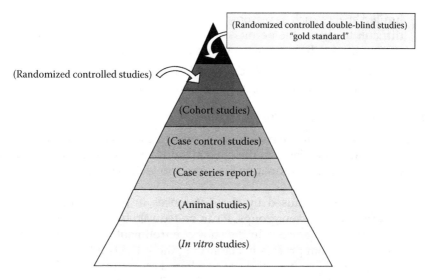

FIGURE 19.1
Assessment level of functional foods. Studies follow a hierarchy in terms of the quality of evidence that they can provide. Randomized double-blind placebo control (RDBPC) studies are considered the gold standard of epidemiologic studies. "Gold standard" can refer to the criteria by which scientific evidence is evaluated. Randomization is considered the most powerful experimental design in clinical trials.

Also, it is possible to implement consistent observations in a limited space. Although the animal study has a disadvantage in that the metabolic system of the animal is not the same as that found in the human body, it allows more exact evaluations than *in vitro* studies in determining functionalities in organisms.

19.3.1.2 Clinical Study

There are several difficulties in applying evaluation of the functionalities in foods in clinical trials as a clinical method. The characteristics of the clinical study are summarized next.

19.3.1.2.1 Characteristics of Clinical Study of Humans

1. It is necessary to preferentially consider ethical issues.
2. As it is not possible in a specific disease model in clinical studies, the mechanism of diseases in the human body is difficult. Also, it is difficult and important to determine conditions of clinical studies and to select proper subjects.
3. It is difficult to consistently determine the evaluation of effects in a space that limits eating and sleeping. For example, although it is possible to control eating, sleeping, and environmental conditions in

limited spaces such as prisons, training camps, dormitories, etc., it is difficult to obtain the permission of the Institutional Review Board (IRB) if it contributes to improving their quality of life.

4. It may cause wrong results due to different biases.
5. It is difficult to apply some limited results to all subjects.

19.3.1.2.2 Biases in Clinical Study of Humans

The accuracy of the clinical trial depends on how the risk in biases is reduced and minimized. The biases in the clinical study of humans are determined as a selection bias, an information bias, and a detection bias.

- *Selection bias* is caused by the differences in basic characteristics between comparison groups. It can be reduced by a well performed randomization process. In the subject enrollment, it is necessary to follow a random process in classifying the subjects into control and experimental groups. Clinical trials based on foods are significantly affected by the dietary life of subjects. For instance, subjects may consume lots of food and drink on some holidays, such as New Year's Day or the Chuseok holiday, during the clinical study period compared to other regular days. In particular, as one of these two groups takes more food in the test period than on other regular days, it may cause selection bias. In addition, the selection bias largely affects the study on the functionality of improving triglycerides as an important external factor.

- *Information bias* is caused by the test products provided from the clinical trial based on foods. In applying a double-blind method to a study design process properly, the information of the subjects employed in the study is not to be released. Thus, it is important to develop placebo products in order not to recognize the shape, size, weight, color, taste, and flavor for the subjects in the control and experimental groups. If there are differences in the appearance between the placebo and test products or subjects are close to other subjects in these two groups, it may affect the results of the study that compares the placebo and test products according to control and experimental groups because the information of the products may be released by these familiar subjects.

- *Detection bias* is caused by the systematic difference between groups in measuring the outcome of evaluation variables. If the observer does not recognize the arrangement of control and experimental groups, this will reduce the detection bias, which is a subjective issue, as the observer measures the state of evaluation variables. If an observer is changed during the clinical study, this will cause detection bias.

Clinical Trials of Some Korean Functional Foods

19.3.1.2.3 Randomization or Random Allocation

Although a randomized control group configuration test is not an absolute way to prove functionalities, it has been largely used because it can be used as the most persuasive way and the important basis in the test. The randomization is a way of allocating subjects without any intentions in the configuration of control and experimental groups. That is, it randomly allocates subjects to these two groups in order to reduce biases in clinical trial. The details are as follows:

1. Simple randomization allocates subjects using the numbers produced by a dice or a table of random numbers.
2. Block randomization corrects imbalances in subjects between test groups by determining a table of random allocations in each block in which the blocks are predetermined by specific numbers.
3. Stratified randomization allocates subjects according to hierarchies in which the hierarchies are determined according to the prognosis that represents a high level of significances.

19.3.1.2.4 Method of the Randomization

A computer programming process is used to generate random numbers. The site of generating random numbers (http://www.randomization.com) can also be used.

19.3.1.2.5 Types of Clinical Studies

Clinical trials can be classified into intervention and observed studies. In the intervention study, a researcher is able to engage the expression of taking test materials of subjects. However, this is not allowed in the observed study.

- Intervention study. In the stage of evaluating functional health foods, the gold standard study shows a randomized controlled double-blind study. This study allocates subjects randomly based on the predetermined probability distribution and is considered the most excellent method of investigating the correlation between food compositions and functionalities because the predetermined mixing factors can be artificially controlled. For certifying functional health foods in Korea, it is necessary to perform clinical trials according to the Enforcement Rule of the Raw Materials of Health Functional Foods (Kim et al., 2010). Thus, the randomization comparative intervention study in the clinical trial is performed by a parallel or cross-over design.
- Parallel design. This design allocates the selected subjects to the control or experimental group randomly and is allocated to a single test group during the entire period of the clinical trial. It is the simplest

way of applying test products to the subjects and of applying placebo products to the comparative control group.

- Crossover design. In this design each researcher plays a role in his or her own control group. This is a method in which the subjects are divided into two different groups. The method is performed by parallel design in the initial stage, and a washout period is given to remove the effect of the preintake at a specific point. Then, the study is implemented as a parallel design in which treatments for all groups are changed. Therefore, this method allows taking all products and test and control (placebo) products for all subjects. Although this study design is the most reliable method to prove the cause and result of the study, it is now allowed to generalize the study results to the total population.

19.3.2 Challenge of Customized Nutrition in Clinical Study

In the clinical evaluation of foods, it is necessary to establish a study design of applying nutrigenomics and a strategy of differentiation according to implements of personal customized treatments and preventions. In practical clinical sites, there are many cases that represent no differences in validity between test and placebo products. In the case of the clinical evaluation performed by genetic variation types based on personal genetic polymorphisms, however, there exist significant differences in effects according to groups. Thus, it is necessary to conduct studies of tracing the degree of manifestation according to personal genetic polymorphism and of approaching this as a manner of specialization.

To achieve this, different methods and technologies, such as molecular biologic tools and technologies of metabolomics, nutrigenetics, nutrigenomics, and proteomics, are needed. Therefore, it is necessary to establish a customized nutrition information system connected to related diseases instead of recommending some foods or tracing metabolisms for nutrients in order to treat and prevent diseases. For implementing basic studies on different fields related to diseases, a convergence study of medical science, molecular biology, food and nutrition, exercise, chemistry, pharmacology, statistics, etc. is required.

19.4 Understanding Clinical Study of Foods and Procedures

Clinical trial implementation tests based on the human body require a very careful plan and examination because of the many costs, including human dignity. The experiment's plan designed before implementing the clinical trial is the most important step in the entire process. For deducing valuable results, the plan includes selection of a specialized clinical experiment group and of subjects, study design, determination of parameters to be observed, method of collecting and analyzing data, and so on.

- The clinical trials of health functional foods should be designed based on the principle of good clinical practice (GCP). GCP is an international standard for performing the design, implementation, recording, and reporting of clinical trials based on ethical and scientific fundamentals (Figure 19.2) (Kamarei and Trygstad, 2004). It protects the rights and safety of life of the subjects who participate and is required to ensure the reliability of experiment results. The procedure and method of clinical trials are presented in Figure 19.3. A specific study plan of clinical trial is to be submitted to IRB that includes informed consents of subjects in order to get the prequalification and agreement of the study from IRB. Then, the clinical trials are implemented based on the study plan after obtaining the informed consents of subjects. The entire process of the clinical trial is to be

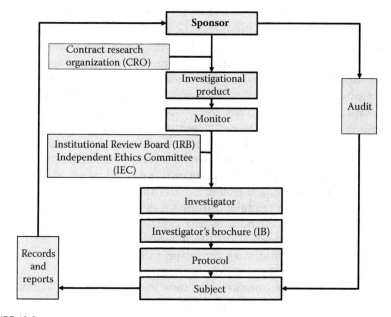

FIGURE 19.2
Designing clinical trials to substantiate claims upon good clinical practice (GCP). GCP is an international ethical and scientific quality standard for designing, conducting, recording, and reporting trials that involve the participation of human subjects. Compliance with this standard provides public assurance that the rights, safety and well-being of trial subjects are protected, consistent with the principles that have their origin in the Declaration of Helsinki, and that the clinical trial data are credible. Contract research organization (CRO) is a person or an organization (commercial, academic, or other) contracted by the sponsor to perform one or more of a sponsor's trial-related duties and functions. (See Reza and Carl, 2014 *Food Technology* 58(10):28–35, 2004.)

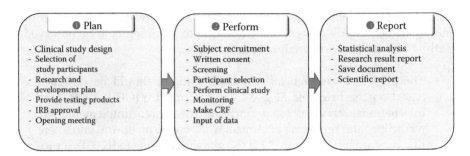

FIGURE 19.3
Method and procedure for clinical study.

monitored by a client or a contract research organization (CRO) in order to guarantee reliability of the process. A final report is prepared based on the results of the clinical trial, and the report is approved by IRB. In addition, a report on the collected data is prepared through a statistical analysis and is submitted to MFDA including the statement of examining the results that is reported to IRB.

- There are significant differences in clinical experiments between health functional foods and medical supplies. Clinical intervention studies based on foods are different from those of developing medical supplies. These may present some additional confusing factors in using foods compared to the clinical trial of medical supplies. For instance, some cases do not use control groups and may fail blind tests. Also, a study may present obscure results compared to the intervention study of medical supplies. In the case of medical treatments, evaluation may concern how swiftly subjects experiencing a syndrome recover from the onset point of a disease. However, the efficacy evaluation of the clinical trial of health functional foods verifies how the consistency is maintained from a state of managing the homeostasis or a bit out of the homeostasis, unlike drugs efficacy evaluation. Thus, these two processes are different (van der Greef et al., 2004) and it is important to minimize confusing factors that affect the results through a method that controls experimental environments in foods such as composition, quantity, and taste including dietary factors.
- The study of health functional foods includes healthy and semihealthy subjects. Toxicity studies in a clinical trial of health functional foods can be excused according to supplied foods compared to that of medical supplies. Although there are no differences in general clinical trials between foods and medical supplies, the clinical studies over phase 2 are applied to patients for evaluating the efficacy of medical supplies because the purpose of these studies is to treat diseases. However, the clinical trials of health functional foods

are applied to healthy or semihealthy subjects because it is aimed to help prevent diseases instead of treating diseases even though health functional foods affect treating specific diseases. For instance, in the case of health functional foods supplied to present health claims that help in maintaining blood pressure, the clinical trials are applied to semihealthy subjects who do not take any medicines and present borderline blood pressure (120–140 mg systolic blood pressure). Clinical trials of health functional foods applied to patients may cause serious medical and ethical problems as taking test food products is recommended only in order to verify the efficacy of these products without dosing the medical supplies for the patients. That is, if these food products are supplied to normal healthy subjects, this may help in maintaining blood pressure. However, in the case of patients who take medical supplies for treating their diseases, it should not to be recommended to the patients because it may cause serious medical and ethical problems.

- Estimation of the subjects in a clinical study of health functional foods. As medical supplies are developed based on specific mechanisms, there are clear boundaries in efficacies. There is a well-organized reference in doses based on much research and this allows an easy estimation of subjects who participate in clinical studies. In the case of clinical trials of health functional foods, however, this presents concerns in estimating the subjects for planning a protocol. In addition, it is not easy to select the patients, who represent specific signs in a disease, in the study. Also, it is difficult to expect presenting clinical effects similar to those of medical supplies. For verifying the significance of the results, the number of subjects in the study is estimated using a statistical method. Although there are differences in the functionalities to be evaluated, the subjects can be increased by more than an expected level for determining the significance of the results.

- It is necessary to investigate the dietary intake and diet in the clinical trials of health functional foods (KFDA, 2012). In the clinical trials of health functional foods, the importance of investigating the dietary intake and diet in subjects is stressed. Because these experiments are applied to subjects who are difficult to manage according to the study plan, there are difficulties in obtaining significant results. Thus, the investigation of the dietary intake and diet is required to design a serious study plan. That is, the detailed food intake is presented during the period of the experiments through the investigation of dietary intake and diet in subjects. In addition, it is necessary to control taking other food products similar to the functional health foods applied to the study in order to obtain accurate study results.

19.5 Strategy for Developing Healthy Functional Foods

As functional health raw materials obtain an individual certification from MFDS in efficacy and safety based on scientific data, it is expected that these materials present significant economic effects due to their reliability. The procedure of obtaining the individual certification of the functional health raw materials in health functional foods is as follows: (1) selecting individual elements, (2) standardization of manufacturing processes, (3) evaluating functionality/safety, (4) documentation of materials and data, and (5) certification of the products from MFDS. The certification requires the time and the money needed to perform the procedure. For developing such individually certified functional health raw materials, a proper strategy is required according to purposes and directions of the products. The strategy is summarized as follows (Figure 19.4):

1. Understanding market situations and consumer needs. For the successful development of health functional foods, it is necessary to preferentially establish a strategy that reflects market situations and consumer needs.
2. Strategy of the standardization of manufacturing processes. Manufacturing processes are important for presenting differentiations in products and for improving functionalities in addition to performing

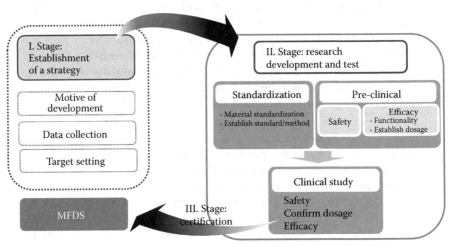

FIGURE 19.4
Procedure for individual certification for developing health functional foods. The procedure of obtaining the individual certification of functional health raw materials in health functional foods is as follows: Preferably, it must consider understanding market situations and consumer needs for the successful development of functional foods. (1) Market demand analysis, (2) standardization of manufacturing processes, (3) evaluating effectivity and safety, (4) documentation of the materials and data, and (5) certification of the products from MFDS.

standardization. Thus, it is possible to apply a solvent or a fermentation process in order to improve functionalities and safety. In addition, a special manufacturing process is used to reduce losses of materials and to improve yield rates of effective compositions in spite of increasing production costs.

3. Strategy of ensuring safety and functionality data. The evaluation of the functionality and safety of health functional foods is a process that needs the most money and time in developing such health functional foods. The safety data determined by MFDS requires the evaluations of all data submitted from manufacturers, including the origin, development processes, domestic and foreign certifications, manufacturing process, characteristics of raw materials, traditional usages, results of the numbers of intakes, results of the evaluation of nutrition, biological usefulness, results of clinical trials, and results of toxicity tests for the applied products. In addition, the data for the functionality of raw materials require not only the basis of traditional usage, meta-analyses, and reviews, but also *in vitro* animal study (preclinical) data and clinical study data. In the case of the process of mixing more than two raw materials, the functionalities of the mixed raw materials are to be verified and reasonable reasons and scientific bases are to be submitted. The submitted data will be evaluated as either individual items that include the quantity, quality, applicability, and consistency of the study or as a manner of overall evaluation. Then, the functionality is determined by the results of the evaluation. Thus, it is necessary to establish a strategy of considering the reference of the evaluation at the initial stage of planning the strategy.

   A. Ensuring data corresponding to the guidelines of MFDS. The preclinical data that can be accepted as the functionality data include domestic and foreign journals referenced in the Science Citation Index (SCI, SCIE) or Korea Citation Index (KCI). In the case of the clinical study, although the data referenced in domestic and foreign journals (SCI levels) or unpublished final reports on the clinical trial can be applied, the unpublished final reports are limited to the cases that are performed with the approval of the Institutional Review Board (IRB) according to the Guideline for Food Clinical Practice by International Conference on Harmonization (ICH GCP) in order to protect the rights of subjects and to guarantee the reliability of the study results.

   B. Using conventional data. In selecting candidate elements to be developed, it is necessary to establish a development strategy for targeting easily obtaining data of the manufacturing process and functionality through searching previously performed references. For instance, in developing a functionality element from pomegranates, if the largest amount of data related to alcoholic extracts is searched, and many data sets related to antioxidants and reducing body fat are also searched, the strategy will be effective for the development of antioxidants using a manufacturing process of alcoholic extracts. However, it should be noted that a strategy of considering market conditions and economic effects is also required.

19.6 Successful Development Strategy for Healthy Functional Foods and Clinical Practices

In general, in the case of the pharmaceutical clinical study, the mutual interaction is simplified by one compound and a single application point in order to evaluate biomarkers. Then, it carries out an investigational new drug (IND) application for patients. In the case of the clinical study, however, it is necessary to implement a proper evaluation not only for the single effect, but also for the complex effect of effective compositions in complex compounds based on different application points and interactions in organisms. In addition, it is very difficult to obtain significant results because the clinical studies of foods are applied to semihealthy subjects instead of patients. That is, it may be possible to properly evaluate the effectiveness of foods even though the clinical trial of health functional foods represents disadvantages in selecting subjects and in evaluating proper biomarkers compared to that of the pharmaceutical clinical study. For complementing these disadvantages, different evaluation methods are to be investigated by developing new biomarkers and clinical trial technologies in order to evaluate clinical efficacies in foods.

19.6.1 Application of Successful Strategy for Clinical Studies of Foods

19.6.1.1 Stress Loading Methods

The efficacy evaluation of health functional foods verifies how the consistency is effectively maintained based on a state of managing the consistency or a bit out of the consistency. However, the efficacy evaluation of the clinical trial based on natural foods shows difficulties in the evaluation because dozens and hundreds of bioactive substances are connected through a complex network (Jan et al., 2004). For instance, in the case of blood pressure or blood glucose level in average healthy subjects, it is difficult to deduce significant results in the evaluation of functionalities because it is operated as a way of maintaining the consistency of organisms. If it is possible, it will be presented by a very low level of less than 10%~20%. In particular, there are several difficulties in a proper evaluation because the samples obtained from the human body are very limited, such as blood or excretions.

In this study, an effective and useful method for solving such difficulties in the clinical evaluation of the human body is proposed. In general, chronic diseases, such as obesity, diabetes, hypertension, cardiovascular diseases, cancers, etc., are closely related to chronic inflammations caused by continuous oxidative stresses. As the antioxidant system in the human body is degraded, or the antioxidant defense system is not properly operated, unbalances in the human body occur and that increases the oxidative stresses and inflammations. Based on these responses in the human body, it is possible to find the factors or biomarkers related to recovering the antioxidant function and consistency through applying an artificially induced low-level stress to the human body. Then, it may allow the increase in the success rate of the evaluation. For instance, in a study, some methods of evaluating the functionalities based on a stress load method are introduced. The study includes evaluations of the efficacy of natural materials in recovering antioxidant functions after applying stresses through high-fat diet and of the adaptability of heart rate variability and relaxing capability through a blood vessel occlusion test.

- High-fat diet. Excessive oxidative stresses in the human body cause lipid oxidation in biological membranes, metamorphosis of proteins, and damage in DNA, which inhibits normal functions of cells and tissues. Then, it brings chronic diseases related to chronic inflammations. In clinical evaluations, there is a method that verifies changes in both oxidative stress–related chronic diseases and factors related to inflammation by applying functional materials (blueberry products) after generating oxidative stress through the high-fat diet (Ono-Moore et al., 2016). For instance, the effects of blueberry supplementation on high-fat-diet–induced postprandial inflammation and endothelial vasodilator function in humans have been observed. That is, it causes oxidative stresses after applying the high-fat diet (breakfast) to subjects. Then, it verifies the efficacy of the test product (blueberry products or others) by measuring biomarkers, which represent the capabilities of maintaining and recovering consistency in the human body.

- Heart rate variability (HRV). A decrease in heart rate variability has emerged as the single most common risk factor for many chronic diseases, such as diabetes, chronic fatigue, chronic heart failure, neurological disorders, and many other conditions. As humans are continuously stressed, it decreases the stress control ability in the human body decreases, which causes a degradation of the autonomous nervous system. As the autonomous nervous system is degraded, the reactivity and adaptability of the human body from external stimulations are decreased and that shows a decrease in the HRV (Maria et al., 2003). By applying the change in HRV to clinical study, it is possible to measure the biomarkers in HRV in order to determine how fast the response against an external stimulation needs to be as subjects take functional substances.

- Blood vessel occlusion test. Vascular occlusion is the blockage of a blood vessel, usually with a clot. It differs from thrombosis in that it can be used to describe any form of blockage, not just one formed by a clot. When it occurs in a major vein, it can, in some cases, cause deep vein thrombosis. The condition is also relatively common in the retina and can cause partial or total loss of vision. An occlusion can often be diagnosed using Doppler sonography (a form of ultrasound).

19.6.1.2 Pilot Clinical Study for Increasing Success Rate of a Preclinical Study

In developing medical supplies, clinical studies should be performed after implementing preclinical studies (i.e., animal tests for ensuring its functionality and safety to be performed as phase 1, phase 2, and phase 3 clinical studies according to cases). However, in the case of clinical studies of functional health foods, the animal test is not an essential process or a prerequisite condition for clinical trials. In general, the development process of health functional foods is determined as a standardization → a preclinical study (*in vitro*/animal tests) → a clinical study. In the case of the clinical trial of health functional foods, it represents a very low success rate because of inappropriate selections of biomarkers and subjects, wrong doses, and improper intake period. In practice, clinical trials are allowed to use nontoxic materials, which have the basis of traditional usage. Thus, a pilot study can be used to verify the functionality of test products before implementing animal tests. That is, the pilot clinical study is a human experiment for verifying the efficacy, duration, and effective dose of supplies. It is a method of screening the proper biomarkers to be measured in preclinical or clinical studies through configuring the dosage based on two or three different supplies. In particular, this method is useful in a case where there are difficulties in selecting biomarkers related to evaluating the functionalities in elements or targets that show lacks of references on effective doses and low efficacies in supplies. This makes it possible to determine an exact direction in studies and to establish a proper strategy for increasing the success rate of studies (Figure 19.5).

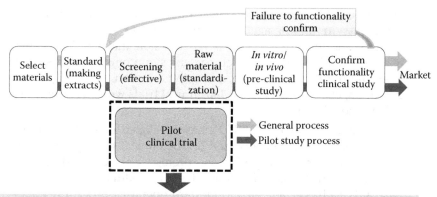

FIGURE 19.5
The concept of the pilot clinical study. Clinical trials are allowed to use nontoxic materials, which have the basis of traditional usage. Development processing (subject of exemption on good laboratory practice toxicity evaluation) for functional foods. A pilot clinical study can be used to verify the functionality of test products before implementing animal study. That is, the pilot clinical study is a human experiment for verifying the efficacy, duration, and effective dose of supplies. It is a method of screening the proper biomarkers to be measured in preclinical or clinical studies through configuring the number of doses based on two or three different supplies.

19.7 Clinical Trial Center for Functional Foods (CTCF2) for Chonbuk National University Hospital

19.7.1 Overview

A one-stop solution for functional health foods, CTCF2 is the "Organization of Industry Infrastructure Projects in Korea" sponsored by the Ministry of Trade, Industry, and Energy in December 2004 at Chonbuk National University Hospital in order to systematically and scientifically evaluate the products of functional health foods and their efficacy. This supported total services for functional health foods. Few organizations verify and manage effectiveness and clinical efficacy of the functional health foods developed in manufacturers before publishing the rule on the functional health foods in Korea (2003). It is a hurdle to develop functional health foods. For satisfying the social requirements, CTCF2 provides benefits to both consumers and producers based on reliable study results. In addition, CTCF2 supports a one-stop service to the manufacturers of functional health foods from developing products to the registration of the products to MFDS (http://www.ctcf2.com/).

- Effective system. For establishing a standard method in clinical trials for each functionality type, CTCF2 operates working groups based on expert pools in many fields, such as antiobesity, liver protection, antifatigue, immune system and allergy, improving climacteric symptoms in middle-aged women, bone and joint health care, stomach and intestinal function, hypertension, diabetes, improving blood circulation, improving climacteric symptoms in middle aged men, improving constipation, cognition function, retarding retrogradation, etc. A total of about 180 clinical trials were performed (as of December 2016).

- Project and service areas. CTCF2 has developed more than 30 different functional protocols based on the clinical trial system's corresponding various experiences, professional knowledge, and ICH-GCP in the fields of the clinical trials of health functional foods. Also, CTCF2 has established a standard operating procedure (SOP) in the field and provided one-stop services for the registration of products to MFDS.

A full array of services in all phases of studies on functional foods is offered. With these services, every step along a study's path can be supported to help in making critical decisions quickly.

CTCF2 provides specific services, including consultation of standardization and technology development, selection of health claim, methods of preclinical and nonclinical studies, data collection and analysis and documentation for the registration of individual certifications to MFDS. In addition, CTCF2 systematically performs clinical trials—the final stage of the certification of health functional foods—and makes efforts to support the clinical trials implemented in different ways.

19.8 Clinical Cases in Some Korean Healthy Functional Foods

19.8.1 Development of Healthy Functional Foods

CTCF2 certified 20 cases of health functional foods from MFDS, Korea. In these certified cases, eight that used Korean domestic materials for developing healthy functional food and its dietary types and diet interventions based on clinical trials are introduced as follows.

19.8.1.1 Pomegranate

19.8.1.1.1 Improving Climacteric Symptoms

Women reach the turning point of menopause when they are middle-aged. Sudden decreases in estrogen caused by menopause accelerate the human aging process and middle-aged women experience different physical and mental changes called climacteric symptoms (Schindler, 2006). The initial stage in climacteric symptoms causes light symptoms, such as hot flushes and night sweats, but the symptoms are developed as physical aging, bone density deterioration, cognitive decline, and cardiovascular diseases according to the passage of time (Collins et al., 2007). Although estrogen replacement therapy in women after menopause decreases these physical changes, the use of estrogen in a short period of time causes vaginal bleeding. Also, it increases risks of breast cancer, apoplexy, and cardiovascular diseases (Beral, 2003). Therefore, the phytoestrogen included in natural foods has largely been of interest as a botanical estrogen. The botanical estrogen, phytoestrogen, usually includes isoflavones and lignans and is similar to the compound of naturally generated estrogen from beans, fruits, vegetables, peanuts, grains, and so on (Boker et al., 2002). It was verified that taking isoflavones (Cheng et al., 2007) and γ-linolenic acid (Abraham et al., 1990) related to women's health represented some effects of improving menopausal symptoms and bone density and of decreasing serum lipid density compared to conventional estrogen treatments.

Recently, pomegranate has emerged as a type of phytoestrogen that helps women's health. The pomegranate includes not only estrogen, but also some different hormones, such as testosterone, β-sitosterol, and coumesterol; these have been used as folk remedies for curing menopausal symptoms (Jurenka, 2008; Ahn et al., 2010a). Research showed that dosing pomegranate extracts to climacteric symptom-induced animal models improved such climacteric symptoms. Also, it was reported that dosing pomegranate extracts, 40 mL/day, for 12 weeks to women who have climacteric symptoms improves the symptoms significantly (Ahn et al., 2010b). In a recent study, estrogen-like activities were verified in clinical study (CTCF2, clinical result report, January 6, 2014) in which dosing the functional pomegranate extract (P-estroHL) developed by a specially designed process, 10 mL/day, for 8 weeks to women aged 40–60 ($N = 60$) who have climacteric symptoms shows significant improvements in the symptoms (the scale of women's climacteric symptoms, KI) and MRS (menopause rating scale) compared to that of the placebo groups.

In particular, 11 items in KI, such as hot flush, night sweats, insomnia, nervous temperament, depression, vertigo, fatigue, arthralgia/myalgia, headache, palpitation, and vaginal dryness, were improved after 4 weeks of taking the P-estroHL and the MRS was also improved significantly (Figure 19.6). In the experiments of climacteric symptom-induced animal models, the representative climacteric fat index (49% weight loss, 57% belly fat loss) was improved after 12 weeks of taking P-estroHL as an oral administration; it also showed improvements in blood lipid (decreasing total cholesterol [TC] and low-density lipoprotein cholesterol [LDL-C] and increasing high-density lipoprotein cholesterol [HDL-C]) and bone density (increased by 7%). Also, the estrogen-like activity was verified (Kang et al., 2017). In the case of the human experiments in taking P-estroHL, it showed no significant changes in estrogen levels (E2; estradiol) before and after 8 weeks of taking it, representing the fact that side effects from its

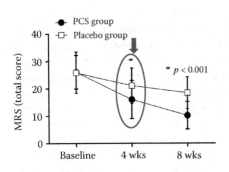 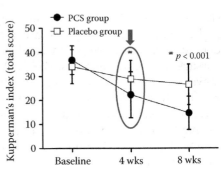

FIGURE 19.6
Change in menopause rating scale (MRS) and Kupperman's index of PCS. Changes of MRS and Kupperman's index during 8 weeks" administration of pomegranate (10 ml./day), and placebo in postmenopausal women. Data are shown as mean ± SD. **$p < 0.001$ versus placebo, $n = 60$.

excessive intake will be minimized. The functional pomegranate extract product (P-estroHL; 10 mL/day) was registered as a commercial product in MFDS because "it helps the health of climacteric women" (Certification, 2014-22, May 22, 2014 MFDS; HL SCIENCE Co. Ltd., Korea).

19.8.1.1.2 Skin Moisturizing Effect of Pomegranate Extracts (P-estroHL)

It was verified that the pomegranate extract (P-estroHL) shows significant increases in moisture density dependently and the ICR mouse model represents increases in moisture in animal tissues by increasing hyaluronic acids and collagens (Kang et al., 2015a). In addition, it was shown that dosing of the pomegranate extract (P-estroHL) shows improvements in skin moisturizing through composed increases in hyaluronic acids based on increases in the expression of the mRNA protein of hyaluronan synthase 1, 2, and 3. In the dosing of the pomegranate extract (P-estroHL), it was verified that the composed increases in collagen by increasing the mRNA expression of COL_1A_1 and COL_1A_2 contributed to producing alpha-1 and -2 chains in the collagen (Kang et al., 2016). In the case of the clinical trial, it showed different effects—not only increasing skin moisture, resilience, and tone, but also decreasing transepidermal water loss (TEWL) and skin keratin according to dosing the pomegranate extract (P-estroHL) to 60 women aged 25–60 for 8 weeks (Kyung Hee University Skin Biotechnology Center, clinical result report, June 20, 2014).

The improvement effects of the pomegranate extract increase the composition of hyaluronic acids, which are a natural moisturizing factor in the skin, the skin moisture by the composed increase in type I collagen, and the TGF-β1 that induces the composition of hyaluronic acids and the composition enzyme of HAS 1, 2, and 3 and COL_1A_1 and COL_1A_2, respectively. Thus, it is considered that increases in the composition of the hyaluronic acid, which is

Clinical Trials of Some Korean Functional Foods

a skin moisturizing element, and the composition of type I collagen contribute to decreasing TEWL and to increasing skin moisture and moisturizing effects. The functional pomegranate extract product (P-estroHL) was registered as a commercial product in MFDS because "it is a functional material for helping skin moisturizing" (Certification, August 2016 MFDS; HL SCIENCE Co. Ltd. Korea).

19.8.1.2 Fermented Curcuma Longa

Studies of developing functional materials for warm-temperature crops according to changes in climate environments in Korea have been continuously conducted. *Curcuma longa*, a warm-temperature crop, is classified as a genus of *Curcuma* in a family of Zingiberaceae. The curcumin largely included in the *Curcuma longa* is a representative bioactive composition and a functional food raw material that has been studied throughout the world. It is known that the *Curcuma longa* shows effects of improving cognitive ability, antimutagenicity, antivirus, anti-inflammatory, liver protection, antibiotics and antioxidant properties, immunomodulation, and so on (Mazumder et al., 1995; Gupta and Ghash, 1999; Ha et al., 2015). Although various manufacturing processes of *Curcuma longa* have been developed to increase its functionalities and its bioactivity has been verified in different studies, there still exist difficulties in using it in organisms because of its bitter taste and nasty smell (Kang and Hyun, 2007).

In Jindo-Gun, South Jeolla Province, a fermentation technology was applied to the *Curcuma longa* using *Aspergillus oryzae*. The fermented *Curcuma longa* improved in its taste and smell and the rate of using organisms increased. In addition, it has effects of controlling liver functions and blood neutral fats. Dosing the fermented *Curcuma longa* represents effects of protecting liver cell damages from the oxidative stress caused by alcohol. In comparing the fermented *Curcuma longa* dosing group and the positive control group (dosing silymarin), the AST/ALT activity, which is an index of the liver, was decreased (Sung et al., 2016). Using the fermented *Curcuma longa* showed the same results as in the clinical trial. The fermented *Curcuma longa* powder was given to subjects with liver damage in an amount of 3 g/day for 12 weeks. Serum ALT and AST values decreased significantly compared to those of the placebo group, as well as the blood TC, LDL-C, and triglyceride (TG) levels (Table 19.1). It is considered that the continuous intake of the fermented *Curcuma longa* powder improves liver function, which leads to improving blood neutral fats (CTCF2, clinical result report, 2012a). The fermented *Curcuma longa* (dosing 3 g/day) was registered as a commercial product in KFDA because "it may help liver health but is not enough to use it as a functional material (bioactivity material, class 3) due to lacks of human experiments" (Certification, 2013, MFDS; Inspharm Co. Ltd. Korea).

TABLE 19.1

Changes in Effective Evaluation Items before and after Taking Products for Human Experiments

	Active Group ($n = 26$)			Placebo Group ($n = 22$)			
	Baseline	12 Weeks	p-Value[a]	Baseline	12 Weeks	p-Value[a]	p-Value[b]
ALT (IU/L)	61.08 ± 25.1	44.92 ± 15.5	0.0006*	55.68 ± 15.1	53.82 ± 26.3	0.661	0.019**
AST (IU/L)	36.27 ± 13.8	27.96 ± 8.0	0.002***	35.59 ± 8.8	34.77 ± 10.9	0.662	0.020**
ALP (IU/L)	85.04 ± 19.3	80.04 ± 22.0	0.048**	71.73 ± 13.5	68.95 ± 13.2	0.125	0.471
γ-GT (IU/L)	86.31 ± 71.5	66.96 ± 45.6	0.068	104.2 ± 69.0	100.77 ± 68.4	0.696	0.254
Total bilirubin (mg/dL)	0.98 ± 0.5	0.88 ± 0.4	0.192	0.89 ± 0.3	0.84 ± 0.3	0.461	0.664
Triglyceride (~200 mg/dL)	215.7 ± 111.9	216.76 ± 126.1	0.674	180.9 ± 87.4	203.73 ± 152.2	0.026*	0.043*
LDL-cholesterol (0 ~ 140 mg/dL)	123.0 ± 29.1	119.31 ± 27.7	0.553	133.00 ± 38.8	118.90 ± 31.2	0.002***	0.055

Notes: Values are presented as mean ± SD. ALT: alanine aminotransferase; AST: aspartate aminotransferase; ALP: alkaline phosphatase; γ-GT: gamma-glutamyl transferase.

[a] Paired t-test.

[b] Linear mixed model for repeated measures of data.

*p < 0.001; ** p < 0.05; ***

Clinical Trials of Some Korean Functional Foods

19.8.1.3 Persimmon Leaves and Yuja

Although modern science has made significant progress, it still cannot cure diabetes. Treatments of diabetes usually depend on medicines, exercise, and dietetic treatments. In the case of medicines, it focuses on the prevention and treatment in minimizing the side effects of medicines. Thus, materials that represent inhibiting increases in blood glucose levels, including antioxidant effects, and the effects and mechanisms of these materials based on some natural materials such as fruits, vegetables, and herbs that represent excellent improvements in diabetes have been investigated.

19.8.1.3.1 Persimmon Leaf Extracts

Persimmon leaf teas are usually considered as functional health teas in Korea and Japan; interest in and need for the teas have increased. The main components of persimmon leaves are glycosides such as astragalin and myricitrin; tannin; polyphenol; organic acid; chlorophylls; vitamins A, C, and B_1; pantothenic acid; and folic acid (Moon and Park, 1995). The bioactivities known at the present time are antioxidant effects (Jeong et al., 2001; Hong et al., 2008), antimutagenicity and anticancer effects (Park et al., 1995), immunomodulatory effects (Jiang et al., 2010), blood pressure improvement (Kawakami et al., 2011), and body fat decrease (Jung et al., 2011). Based on the recent report on a mouse with streptozotocin-induced diabetes (C57BLS/J-m), Bae et al. (2015), dosing with aqueous extracts of persimmon leaves (PLE; 250 mg/kg and 1,000 mg/kg), showed significant decreases in the impaired fasting glucose and glucose tolerance test (GTT) compared to those of the treatment and control groups. In the case of a db/db mouse (C57BLKS/db/db mice, type II diabetes model), it represented significant improvements in blood glucose, insulin concentration, and insulin resistivity in the oral glucose tolerance test (OGTT) as the persimmon extracts of 250 mg/kg were given for 8 weeks. It is considered that dosing with PLE maintains both the function of the pancreas β-cells normally and the blood level through inhibiting α-glucosidase and that leads to antidiabetic effects. It showed the same effects as dosing in a clinical study (CTCF2, clinical result report, February 1, 2015).

In the clinical trial applied to the subjects of impaired fasting glucose (IFG) and postprandial plasma glucose (PPG) by dosing with persimmon leaf extracts (Wanju, Chonbuk Province, Korea,) for 8 weeks, the groups taking the extracts showed decreases in the measurement of PPG 120 min from 171.4 to 160.9 mg/dL compared to the placebo groups. Therefore, it was verified that continuously taking the persimmon extracts showed effects of improving blood glucose levels (Table 19.2). Although the relationship between these cases may be estimated, its mechanism is to be investigated by additional studies. Thus, it is considered that the clinical study based on dosing with persimmon extracts contributed to determining the improvement of PPG.

TABLE 19.2

Changes in Blood Glucose Levels before and after 8 Weeks of Taking Test Products

		PLE Group (*n* = 34)			Placebo Group (*n* = 34)			
		0 Weeks	8 Weeks	p-Value[a]	0 Weeks	8 Weeks	p-Value[a]	p-Value[b]
FPG[c] (mg/dL)		100.52 ± 9.24	99.06 ± 10.59	0.432	101.70 ± 8.50	99.19 ± 9.35	0.030*	0.584
PPG[d] (mg/dL)	30 min	180.15 ± 28.19	177.72 ± 28.84	0.666	177.91 ± 36.10	178.38 ± 29.90	0.986	0.783
	60 min	199.45 ± 40.44	190.66 ± 44.62	0.261	193.79 ± 41.95	190.34 ± 38.66	0.538	0.621
	90 min	187.24 ± 46.94	182.28 ± 46.25	0.540	184.09 ± 38.83	185.47 ± 38.86	0.912	0.608
	120 min	$171.36 \pm 3\,8.38$	160.91 ± 35.62	0.133	164.73 ± 32.95	172.03 ± 33.61	0.126	0.029*

Note: Values are presented as mean ± SD.

[a] Paired t-test.

[b] Linear mixed model.

[c] FPG: fasting plasma glucose.

[d] PPG: postprandial plasma glucose.

*$p < 0.05$.

19.8.1.3.2 Yuja (Citrus junos)

Natural antioxidants have been highlighted in recent years for preventing oxidative damage in diabetes. Various vegetables, fruits, and herbs contain lots of polyphenol and flavonoid. The effects of these compositions have already been proven partially in the chronic complications in diabetes caused by oxidative stresses (Kwon et al., 2007; Morand et al., 2011; Rizza et al., 2011). In particular, yuja (*Citrus junos*), which is a kind of citrus, includes phenolic compounds such as rutin and quercetin and flavanones such as hesperidin and tangeretin, including vitamins (Chanet et al., 2012). Yuja includes three times more vitamin C than lemon and is considered an effective bioactive element because its flesh and peels can be used. In addition, use of yuja in beverages, sauces, cosmetic products, etc. has recently been increased because has been reevaluated as a raw material in foods and processing materials because it contains plenty of organic acids and antioxidants (James et al., 2007) for helping blood circulation and improving blood glucose levels and lipid metabolism.

Recently, it was verified that Goheung yuja (Jeollado Province, Korea) represents an effect of glucose control through different cell tests, animal tests, and clinical trials in preventing diabetes. A preclinical study examined the antidiabetic properties of tangeretin in mice on HFD (high-fat diet). The administration of HFD plus 200 mg/kg of tangeretin significantly altered weight gain, glucose tolerance, TC levels, and secretion of adipocytokines, such as adiponectin, leptin, resistin, IL-6, and MCP-1. Moreover, AMPK was activated by 200 mg/kg of tangeretin in mouse muscle tissue, as expected from the cell system (Kim et al., 2012).

These results suggest that *Citrus junos* Tanaka peel extract exerts antidiabetic effects in both cell culture and mouse models; these effects are necessary for activating AMPK (Kim et al., 2013a). Giving yuja peel extracts in human experiments showed the same effects as other tests (Hwang et al., 2015). As the clinical study applied to adult subjects with a diagnosis of increased glucose, using yuja peel extracts (4250 mg/day) for 8 weeks showed significant decreases in impaired glucose levels, impaired insulin levels, insulin resistance index (HOMA-IR), and waist measurements compared to the placebo group. This shows that yuja peel extracts represent effects not only of improving blood glucose, but also of proving its safety in the human body (Table 19.3).

19.8.1.4 Muju Gastrodiae Rhizome

Senile dementia is a high risk in about 10% of patients aged over 65, causing social and economic issues; however, treatments have still not been developed. The most effective way is to delay the outbreak of dementia through early diagnoses and preemptive therapies (Francis et al., 1999). Dementia brings serious decreases in cognitive functions because of significant damage to neuronal cells and makes daily life difficult. Alzheimer's disease (AD)

TABLE 19.3

Changes in FPI, Insulin, HOMA-IR, C-Peptide, and iAUC before and after 8 Weeks of Taking Yuja Peel Extracts

	Group Taking Yuja Peel Extracts (n = 35)			Placebo Group (n = 35)			
	Baseline	8 Weeks	p-Value[a]	Baseline	8 Weeks	p-Value[a]	p-Value[b]
FPI[c] (μU/mL)	8.02 ± 5.29	6.98 ± 3.59	0.062	6.99 ± 4.15	7.84 ± 5.20	0.195	0.038[e]
HOMA-IR[d]	2.11 ± 1.52	1.84 ± 1.07	0.098	1.79 ± 1.12	2.15 ± 1.65	0.076	0.019[e]
C-peptide (ng/mL)	2.05 ± 0.78	1.88 ± 0.62	0.015*	1.93 ± 0.73	1.98 ± 0.91	0.538	0.057
iAUC$_{0-2h}$ (h*mg/dL)	139.12 ± 44.95	131.09 ± 45.84	0.156	137.30 ± 43.82	119.89 ± 58.49	0.041*	0.321

Note: Values are presented as mean ± SD.

a Analyzed by paired t-test.

b Analyzed by linear effect model for repeated measure data.

c FPG: fasting plasma glucose.

d Homeostatic model assessment for insulin resistance.

*p < 0.05.

is a gradual degeneration and damage of neurons in the brain. Dementia is a nervous degradation associated with aging and is caused by a lack of acetylcholine because of degradation of cholinergic neurons. The dementia gets worse due to increases in the activity of acetylcholinesterase (AChE), which is an acetylcholine decomposition enzyme (Howes and Houghton, 2003). Treatments for dementia developed up to the present are an acetylcholine precursor, acetylcholine esterase inhibitor, etc.; however, applying this to practical treatments is controversial because there is little effect and some serious side effects and toxicities. Thus, interest in health functional foods related to such cognitive functions has increased.

The Gastrodiae rhizome, which is a mountain medicine from old times, is a perennial herb of the Orchidaceae family and its main composition is vanillyl alcohol, vanillin, glycoside, β-sitosterol, and mucin (Heo et al., 2006). The Gastrodiae rhizome in traditional Korean medicine has been used in treating hypertension, invigorant, dizziness, headache, nervous prostration, etc. (Kim et al., 1999). The functionalities of the Gastrodiae rhizome decrease triglyceride and cholesterol levels and improve hypertension, brain nervous cells, and memory and cognitive functions (Scholey et al., 2008; Huang et al., 2013; Kim et al., 2013b). In recent different studies, the Muju Gastrodiae rhizome (Muju Province, Jeonbuk, Korea) showed various positive effects, not only protecting nervous cell death caused by amyloid-beta, but also expressing activation of the generation and decomposition enzymes of acetylcholine in Alzheimer's model mice, including the recovery of space memory (Lee et al., 2012; Huang et al., 2013).

For determining these effects in the human body, the same Gastrodiae rhizome materials were applied to subjects ages 50–64. The results of a clinical trial based on dosing with Gastrodiae rhizome powder (12 g/day) for 12 weeks showed no significant improvements of cognitive functions such as subjective cognitive scale and biological marker (BDNF and C-reactive protein; CRP). In a BDNF genetic polymorphism analysis according to different types of genetic polymorphism (BDNF Val66Met polymorphism), however, the group with Val/Met heterozygotes by taking the Gastrodiae rhizome showed some significant improvements in linguistic short-term and visual long-term memory (CTCF2, clinical result report, April 4, 2012b). Kennedy et al. (2015) showed that the secretion of BDNF is varied according to types of genetic polymorphism. Although the effects were not presented in the subjects with the BDNF marker in the placebo group, this represented improvements in advanced word short-term memory (VLT B) and visual recognition long-term memory (NORT, numbers of correct answers) tests.

Therefore, in the analysis of the clinical trials based on the facts, the cognitive functions were improved in middle-aged and older subjects who have Val/Met heterozygotes (Egan et al., 2003) according to dosing the Gastrodiae rhizome, even though the effects were not presented in the analyses for all subjects regardless of BDNF genetic types. Thus, it is necessary to apply a nutrigenomics design and to make a plan of differentiation based on

490   *Korean Functional Foods*

customized treatments and preventions according to expressions of genetic polymorphism.

19.8.1.5 Cordyceps sinensis

Cordyceps sinensis has long been used as an important medicinal mushroom in China. The composition of natural *Cordyceps sinensis* is complex and includes cordycepin, cordycepin derivatives, cordycepic acid, ergosterol, polysaccharides, and nucleosides. The well-known compositions are cordycepin and cordycepic acid (Ng and Wang, 2005). In recent years, the artificial cultivation and mass production of *Cordyceps sinensis* have solved decreases in the supply of natural *Cordyceps sinensis* and its unevenness of compositions (Song et al., 1998). It has largely been used in various fields including medical supplies and functional health foods. It has been known that the medicinal action and functionality of *Cordyceps sinensis* cause immunomodulatory, antitumor, antimetastatic, antioxidant, anti-inflammatory, insecticidal, antimicrobial, hypolipidemic, hypoglycemic, antiageing, and neuroprotective or renoprotective effects (Shin et al., 2010; Chae et al., 2014; Jang et al., 2015, 2016).

In the oral medication of the extracts of *Cordyceps militaris* produced by the artificial cultivation technology of *Cordyceps militaris* in Korea to immune inhibited mice for 14 days, it was verified that the activation of immune cells (spleen and natural killer cells) and the increase in immune substance (cytokines) helped it to recover to a normal state (Kang et al., 2014). It can be estimated that the medication of the extracts of *Cordyceps militaris* increases the proliferation of spleen cells and causes increases in IL-2, which are the major cytokines in a T-cell reaction, tumor necrosis factor-alpha (TNF-α), and IFN-γ generation and contribute to increasing immune activations by enhancing the activity of natural killer cells. In addition, in dosing the extracts of *Cordyceps militaris* (1.5 g/day, two tablets, twice a day) to 78 healthy Korean males for 4 weeks, the dosed group showed significant increases in NK-cell activities, increasing immune activations compared to the placebo group (Kang et al., 2015a).

In addition, the *Cordyceps sinensis* mycelium powder (*Paecilomyces hepiali*, CBG-CS-2) developed by the artificial cultivation and mass production of the *Cordyceps sinensis* that originated from Tibet increases the NK-cell activity in cells (Jang et al., 2016) and immune-inhibited animal models (Chae et al., 2014; Jang et al., 2015), and that improves immune activation effects. Using the same *Cordyceps sinensis* mycelium powder (*Paecilomyces hepiali*, CBG-CS-2), the immune activation effects in the human body were evaluated. In dosing the extracts of *Cordyceps sinensis* mycelium (1.43 g/day) to 80 Korean males and females for 8 weeks, the group taking the extracts showed significant increases in NK-cell activity. Thus, it showed that the extracts represent excellent immune activation in clinical cases (Table 19.4) (CTCF2, Clinical Result Report, January 31, 2016b).

TABLE 19.4

Changes in NK-Cell Activity before and after Taking the Product for Human Experiments

	Cordyceps sinensis Group (*n* = 39)			Placebo Group (*n* = 40)			
	0 Weeks	8 Weeks	p-Value[a]	0 Weeks	8 Weeks	p-Value[a]	p-Value[b]
NK cell activity	33.7 ± 17.1	39.2 ± 17.5	0.016	37.9 ± 18.2	35.5 ± 19.9	0.282	0.013*

Note: Values are presented as mean ± SD.

[a] Paired t-test.

[b] Analyzed by linear mixed effect model for repeated measure data.

*p < 0.05.

19.8.2 Verification of Clinical Excellence in Korean Foods

In recent years, there have been increases in eating animal foods and fats, and decreases in eating rice due to the Westernization of dietary life in Korea; that has caused well-known common diseases such cancer, obesity, hypertension, and diabetes. Cardiovascular diseases and cancers accounted for about 50% of the major cause of mortality in Korea starting from the mid-1970s. It showed significant increases in NCD (Jang and Kim, 2010). Studies on the relationship between dietary types and diseases have been attracting attention throughout the world. Also, the correlation between the dietary life and chronic diseases such as obesity, hypertension, and diabetes has been largely investigated.

In addition, clinical studies on the relationship between the dietary life and health conditions including the generative condition have also been largely conducted. Korean foods are known as a healthy diet in which the composition between vegetable and animal foods is a ratio of 8:2, but its scientific basis is still not clear. In recent trends of studying Korean foods and health conditions, there is still a lack of long-term studies on tracing the correlation between the dietary life and disease, even though there is a lot of information on Korean food dietary patterns. In Korea, although there are many study results on the effects of single nutrients or single foods (kimchi, soy-fermented products) compared to foreign studies, there are few medical studies focusing on Korean foods related to the human body.

19.8.2.1 Intake of Korean Foods and Generative Function

The decreasing birth rate in Korea is becoming a major social issue. The infertility rate increase up to the present is largely due to the male (about 50%) and is based on decreasing sperm counts and sperm motilities, increasing deformed sperms, and malfunctions in the genital system including spermary and prostate diseases. The reason for the sudden increases in the infertility rate is due to changes in dietary patterns according to the Westernization of lifestyles, which causes nutrient imbalances. There are some reports that dietary life is closely related to the health condition of males, including the generative function. In the investigation of changes in the sperm motility for Koreans aged 19–30 based on eating Korean and Western foods regularly for 8 weeks, sperm motility was significantly increased in the group eating a Korean style diet (Figure 19.7) (CTCF2, Clinical Result Report, May 22, 2009).

19.8.2.2 Korean Foods and NCD Dietetic Treatments

Patients diagnosed with diabetes and hypertension at the same time changed their main diet of rice to grains, and other various foods such as soups, kimchi, cooked pot herbs, fermented foods, etc. that were supplied to the them for 12 weeks. The patients showed significant improvements in diseases caused

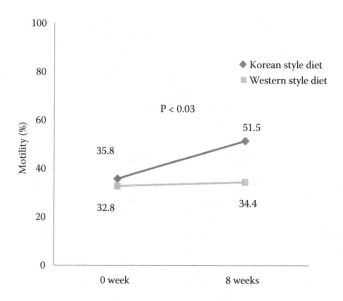

FIGURE 19.7
Sperm motility of subjects. Changes of the sperm motility for subjects of abnormal sperm motility based on following Korean and Western diets regularly for 8 weeks. Sperm motility was significantly increased in the group following the Korean diet style ($p < 0.03$).

by their lifestyles even though they took in lots of calories and sodium. In addition, the group eating Korean foods represented decreases not only in obesity and glycosylated hemoglobin, which is a glucose control index (Korean foods group: 0.72%, control group: 0.25%), but also significantly in heart rates (Korean foods group: −7.1 vs. control group: +1.6) (Jung et al., 2014) (Figure 19.8). It is considered that taking enough grains and vegetables, the

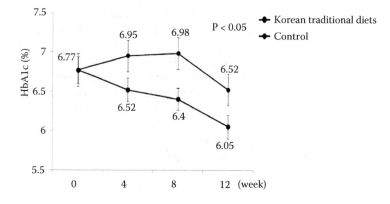

FIGURE 19.8
Change of HbA1c (%) of subject for 12 weeks. Changes of glycated hemoglobin during 12 weeks' administration of Korean traditional diets and control group on the patients with both type 2 diabetes and hypertension. Data are shown as mean ±SD, $p < 0.05$ versus control group, $n = 41$.

hyperglycemia generation is delayed due to slow digestion and absorption and this contributes to minimizing hunger and to reducing food intake. Also, the micronutrients included in foods, such as unsaturated fats, dietary fiber, magnesium, and calcium, represent well-known beneficial effects, and the bioactive substances in diet fiber, vitamins, inorganic matter, lignans, and other vegetable-induced compositions included in grains affected medical improvements significantly.

19.8.2.3 Bibimbap and Kimbap and Metabolic Diseases

In general, Koreans who live on rice take 65% of the total energy from carbohydrates. Although intensive carbohydrate meals represent high risks in metabolic diseases such as diabetes, obesity, and cardiovascular diseases, recent studies have shown that the qualitative aspects of carbohydrates is important as much as their quantitative aspects (Gaesser, 2007; McKeown et al., 2009). Although bibimbab and kimbap are recognized as one of representative complex diets in Korea, there is almost no solid information about metabolic reactions in the human body. In recent years, however, several reports have indicated that taking Korean foods such as bibimbap and kimbap results in improvements in some factors related to metabolic diseases more than taking Western style meals (in which Korean foods such as bibimbap and kimbap represent smaller levels of insulin indexes and postprandial triglyceride values than those of Western style meals such as pork cutlets and hamburgers) (Jung et al., 2015).

19.8.2.4 Rice-Oriented Meals: Mixed Grains (Improving Memory)

A clinical study based on mixed grains showed improvements in concentration by using such grains as a functional food instead of applying them as pills or refined substances. Recently, it was verified that the functional mixed grain (boiled brown rice cereal) developed by improving tastes and by considering that functionality and nutrition improve cognitive functions (improving concentration) (Chung et. al., 2012). In a study of applying mixed and general meals to the diets of Korean high school students for 8 weeks in order to investigate cognitive functions, students who took general meals showed decreases in correct responses and increases in incorrect responses in mental fatigue levels. However, students who also mixed grain meals represented no significant changes in the fatigue levels before and after taking the meals. In particular, the study showed that taking mixed grain meals decreases mental fatigue levels and increases task performance and linguistic capabilities significantly, including BDNF concentrations. Based on the results of these studies, it is expected that Korean rice-oriented dietary life using brown rice and mixed grains will be acknowledged as contributing to increasing concentration.

19.8.3 Traditional Soy Bean Fermented Products

19.8.3.1 Cheonggukjang

Cheonggukjang includes representative bioactive substances such as dietary fiber, phosphorlipids, isoflavones, phenolic acids, polyglutamic acids (gamma-PGA), saponins, trypsin inhibitors, and phytic acids including the nutrients in soy beans. The protein hydrolysate, dietary fiber, and indigestible glucose produced during the fermentation process of cheonggukjang prevent arteriosclerosis by increasing lipid excretion through inhibiting the absorption of intestinal postprandial triglyceride and cholesterol (Lae, 2005). A study of applying cheonggukjang powder to mature mice with hyperlipidemia through a high-fat diet for 5 weeks showed an effect of antiarteriosclerosis by decreasing serum TG, TC, LDL-C, and VLDL-C concentrations, arteriosclerosis indexes, and weight and body fat levels (Lee et al., 2001; Koh 2006). It showed that the dietary fiber and indigestible glucose in cheonggukjang represent an effect of controlling obesity by inhibiting the absorption of lipid in the intestine and by increasing excretions.

In a recent study, as uncooked cheonggukjang (dried weight of 26 g) was applied to overweight adults, who were overweight and had a BMI more than 23 kg/m^2, for 12 weeks, apolipoprotein B, which is an index of arteriosclerosis, was significantly decreased compared to the control group (Back et al. 2011). In the same application to the adults who had a symptom of impaired fasting glucose for 8 weeks, the concentration ratio of apolipoprotein B and apolipoprotein A1 was decreased significantly (Shin et al. 2011).

Recently, the apolipoproteins have been used as an important estimation factor in clinically diagnosing risk factors in arteriosclerosis and cardiovascular diseases. Apolipoprotein B is related to all types of arteriosclerosis and potentially occurring cardiovascular diseases. Also, it shows more excellent diagnosis capabilities in these diseases than LDL-C; the lower value of apolipoprotein B represents the lower occurring level of arteriosclerosis. As weight and BMI were decreased by applying cheonggukjang to mice with hyperlipidemia for 4 weeks, the dietary fiber and indigestible glucose of cheonggukjang showed an effect of controlling obesity by inhibiting the absorption of lipid in the intestine and by increasing excretions. As uncooked cheonggukjang—about 70 g (dried weight of 26 g)—was applied to overweight adults who showed overweight and BMI of more than 23 kg/m^2, for 12 weeks, significant decreases in intestinal fat areas occurred (Back et al., 2011).

Cheonggukjang includes a polynucleic acid produced by the ferment bacilli. This increases immunity by secreting in the Th1 lymphocyte in order to activate immune cells. Also, giving cheonggukjang pills of 35 g/d ($n = 30$, 27 g/d of uncooked cheonggukjang) to patients who had allergic skin troubles showed positive effects in immune control and in improving hypersensitive skin reactions. In particular, the size of wheal reactions caused by its antigens was decreased and the long-term intake of cheonggukjang increased immunity based on increasing some immune indexes (Baek et al., 2015).

19.8.3.2 Doenjang

It has been known that the genistein included in soy beans and soy bean fermented foods facilitates the fatty acid β-oxidation process and is beneficial to decreasing weight and body fat. The fact that the fermented soy bean paste, doenjang, is more effective to combat antiobesity than unfermented raw soy bean products has been proved by different animal tests and human clinical experiments. Also, doenjang shows that it decreases risks of cardiovascular diseases, which are caused by arteriosclerosis, by decreasing blood TC cholesterol and by inhibiting LDL-C oxidation as the isoflavone, glucosides, is changed to aglycone during the fermentation process of doenjang. In a recent clinical study, applying doenjang to overweight adults for 12 weeks showed no significant changes in lipid metabolism even though it showed a tendency of improving it. It is considered that taking doenjang affects the lipid metabolism positively by decreasing the composition of VLDL-C and LDL-C instead of composing HDL-C.

In addition, a study including doenjang in several animal tests showed improvements in hyperlipidemia based on decreasing blood TC and TG (Lee and Kim, 2002). In the case of clinical study, however, there were no specific improvements in lipid compared to the animal tests. This is due to the fact that the diet was not controlled and the subjects participating in the experiments showed no improvements in blood lipid levels because they represented normal levels of blood lipid and lipoprotein concentration. In particular, the isoflavone increases the receptor activity of LDL-C and decreases the LDL-C level. Also, it plays a positive role in preventing cardiovascular diseases by increasing HDL-C, which is effective in preventing vascular diseases. In applying a high-fat diet to animal models, applying doenjang showed more decreases in the sizes of intestinal fat accumulation and fatty cells than the group taking unfermented soy bean products (Kwak et al., 2012).

The case of the clinical study (Cha et al., 2012) showed the same results. Cheonggukjang pills of 9.9 g (about 40 g of uncooked doenjang) were given for 12 weeks to overweight adults who showed overweight and BMI of more than 23 kg/m^2, while their dietary life and activities were maintained. Significant decreases in weights and body fat rates occurred. In particular, the areas of intestinal belly fat were significantly decreased compared to the control group. In this case, the amount of doenjang was the same as three bowls of doenjang soup (similar to Japanese miso soup) every day. That is, a bowl of doenjang soup (about 13.3 g of uncooked doenjang) includes isoflavones—as much as about 20–30 mg/day (containing 8.57 mg aglycones) (Cha et al., 2012). This showed that a decrease in the intestinal fat (particularly in the belly fat) by taking doenjang for a long period of time suggested a high possibility of preventing arteriosclerosis.

19.8.3.3 Gochujang

There are different studies on the effects of gochujang on antiobesity, hyperlipidemia, and antistress. The capsaicinoid and isoflavones included in gochujang affect antiobesity effects by facilitating lipid metabolism in the human body. The effects are influenced by specific elements in gochujang, such as bioactive compositions, isoflavones, and capsaicin and capsioid compositions. Also, it was verified that the products generated in its fermentation process—red pepper powder and other ingredients—control energy and dextrose metabolism and decrease both the size of fatty cells and the fat accumulation. In addition, although the red pepper powder represents a decrease in body fats and a decomposition of fat, gochujang has larger bioactivities than the red pepper powder.

In particular, the capsaicin included in the red pepper powder activates metabolism by accelerating the secretion of the adrenalin in adrenal glands and uses both fatty cells and the glycogen accumulated in the liver by decomposing them as energy, including the decomposition and use of body fats (Koo et al. 2008; Soh et al. 2008). In animal tests, although applying fermented traditional gochujang showed decreases in weight and improved lipid metabolism, the groups taking unfermented gochujang and red pepper powder represented small decreases in the symptoms.

The fermentation of gochujang plays an important role in decreasing weight and fatty tissues (Choo and Shin, 1999). Also, it has been known that the nonglycoside isoflavone of meju included in gochujang and the capsaicin included in red pepper act as a synergy factor in presenting effects of gochujang. A study applying gochujang pills to adults who showed hyperlipidemia for 12 weeks showed significant decreases in serum TC and LDL-C and agrees with that of other animal tests (Lim et al., 2014). Gochujang pills of 32 g were given to overweight adults, who had BMIs of more than 23 kg/m^2, for 12 weeks. Results showed significant improvements in the intestinal area in the belly and the rate of intestinal fat/subcutaneous fat compared to the placebo group, which agrees with the animal tests (Cha et al., 2013). The major factor of the capsaicin activity increased the secretion of catecholamine in the adrenal medulla through activating the sympathetic nervous system, which contributed to improving energy and lipid metabolism (Diepvens et al., 2007).

Also, the study suggested that taking gochujang for a long period of time helped to prevent and improve coronary artery disease by preventing obesity and by controlling glucose. Obesity-induced mice with a high-fat diet that took gochujang showed improvements in lipid by decreasing blood TG and TC significantly. In particular, the results showed that the traditionally fermented gochujang represented dramatic decreases in blood TG compared to factory-made gochujang, in which the ingredients produced in its fermentation process were important Also, the fermented gochujang diet affected lipid metabolism based on decreasing TG and TC and removing lipid compositions through excrement. In addition, applying gochujang pills for 12 weeks to adults who showed hyperlipidemia showed significant decreases in blood TC and LDL-C compared to the placebo group, which agreed with animal tests Moreover, in applying gochujang pills (32.0 g/day) to overweight women with a BMI more than 23 kg/m^2, the serum TC and LDL-C were decreased; the isoflavone of meju included in gochujang contributes to improving lipids.

19.9 Conclusion

Lifestyle-caused diseases have increased dramatically in modern times. Thus, personal lifestyles are becoming the most important factor for a healthy life. In recent years, it has become apparent that our fate is not changed by the order of genes, but rather by our dietary life as an epigenetic organism in which the bioactive substances that change the phenotype of genes are included in our foods. The desirable foods for humans should include not only vitamins and minerals, but also enough bioactive substances (phytochemicals). It is necessary to prove the bioactive functions in foods based on clinical studies and to provide correct information on foods in order to prevent and manage diseases. The developing fields of functional health foods contribute to ensuring safety and functionality for humans by investigating the effects on the human body of bioactive substances and nutrients in foods and helping to produce new high-value-added benefits in industries including the farming and fishing industries. In addition, managing functional raw materials and ensuring them at a national level is desperately needed in order to produce high value-added benefits, including preparation of scientific competitiveness for both the public trust and the efficacy of functional health foods.

References

Abraham, R.D, R.A. Riemersma, R.A. Elton, C. Macintyre, and M.F. Oliver. 1990. Effects of safflower oil and evening primrose oil in men with a low dihomo-gamma-linolenic level. *Atherosclerosis* 81:199–208.

Ahn, K.H., K.W. Yi, H.T. Park et al. 2010a. The effect of pomegranate on postmenopausal syndrome: A randomized, double-blind, placebo-controlled trial. *Journal of Korean Society of Menopause* 16:99–106.

Ahn, K.H., K.W. Yi, H.T. Park et al. 2010b. The effect of pomegranate on postmenopausal syndrome in ovariectomized rats. *Korean Journal of Obstetrics and Gynecology* 53:354–359.

Back, H.I., S.R. Kim, J.A. Yang, M.G. Kim, S.W. Chae, and Y.S. Cha. 2011. Effects of chungkookjang supplementation on obesity and atherosclerotic indices in overweight/obese subjects: A 12-week, randomized, double-blind, placebo-controlled clinical trial. *Journal of Medicinal Food* 14:532–537.

Bae, U.J., S.H. Park, S.Y. Jung, B.H. Park, and S.W. Chae. 2015. Hypoglycemic effects of aqueous persimmon leaf extract in a murine model of diabetes. *Molecular Medicine Reports* 12:2547–554.

Baek, H.I., S.Y. Jung, K.C. Ha et al. 2015. Effect of chongkukjang on histamine-induced skin wheal response: A randomized, double-blind, placebo-controlled trial. *Journal of Ethnic Foods* 2:52–57.

Beral, V. 2003. Breast cancer and hormone-replacement therapy in the Million Women Study. *Lancet* 362: 419–427.

Boker, L.K., Y.T. van der Schouw, M.J. de Kleijn, P.F. Jasques, D.E. Grobbee, P.H. Peters. 2002. Intake of dietary phytoestrogens by Dutch women. *Journal of Nutrition* 132: 1319–28.

Cha, Y.S., S.R. Kim, J.A. Yang et al. 2013. Kochujang, fermented soybean-based red pepper paste, decreases visceral fat and improves blood lipid profiles in overweight adults. *Nutrition Metabplism* 10:1–5.

Cha, Y.S., J.S. Yang, H.I. Back et al. 2012. Visceral fat and body weight are reduced in overweight adults by the supplementation of doenjang, a fermented soybean paste. *Nutrition Research Practice* 6:520–526.

Chae, S.W., F. Mitsunaga, S.J. Jung et al. 2014. Nutrigenomic study on immunomodulatory function of cordyceps mycelium extract (*Paecilomyces hepiali*) in mitomycin C–treated mice. *Food and Nutrition Sciences* 5:2217–2224.

Chanet, A., D. Milenkovic, and C. Manach. 2012. Citrus flavanones: What is their role in cardiovascular protection? *Journal of Agriculture and food Chemistry* 60:8809–8822.

Cheng, G., B. Wilczek, M. Warner, J.A. Gustafsson, and B.M. Landgren. 2007. Isoflavone treatment for acute menopausal symptoms. *Menopause* 14:468–473.

Choo, J.J. and H.J. Shin. 1999. Body-fat suppressive effects of capsaicin through ß-adrenergic stimulation in rats fed a high-fat diet. *Korean Journal of Nutrition* 32:533–539.

Chung, Y.C., C.H. Park, H.Y. Kwon et al. 2012. Improved cognitive performance following supplementation with a mixed-grain diet in high school students: A randomized controlled trial. *Nutrition* 28:165–172.

Clinical Trial Center for Functional Foods (CTCF2) for Chonbuk National University Hospital. 2009. A randomized controlled trial of a Korean dietary intervention for male adult: Sexual and reproductive function for 8 weeks. Clinical result report May 22, 2009. Korea.

Clinical Trial Center for Functional Foods (CTCF2) for Chonbuk National University Hospital. 2012a. A randomized, double-blind, placebo-controlled trial to the efficacy and safety of fermented *Curcuma longa* L. powder on non-alcoholic fatty liver subjects for 12 weeks. Clinical result report March 20, 2012. Korea.

Clinical Trial Center for Functional Foods (CTCF2) for Chonbuk National University Hospital. 2012b. A randomized, double-blind, placebo-controlled trial to the efficacy and safety of cognitive function of *Gastrodia elata* Blume powder on elderly subjects for 12 weeks. Clinical result report April 30, 2012. Korea.

Clinical Trial Center for Functional Foods (CTCF2) for Chonbuk National University Hospital. 2014. A randomized, double-blind, placebo-controlled trial of safety and efficacy of pomegranate on postmenopausal syndrome for 8 weeks. Clinical result report, January 6, 2014. Korea.

Clinical Trial Center for Functional Foods (CTCF2) for Chonbuk National University Hospital. 2015. Efficacy and safety of glucose control of persimmon leaf extracts in pre- type 2 diabetes: A randomized, double-blind, placebo-controlled, cross-over trial 8 weeks. Clinical result report, February 1, 2015. Korea.

Clinical Trial Center for Functional Foods (CTCF2) for Chonbuk National University Hospital. 2016. Efficacy and safety of mycelium extract of cordyceps (*Paecilomyces hepiali*; CBG-CS-2) consumption improves immune function: A randomized, double-blind clinical trial 8 weeks. Clinical result report, January 31, 2016. Korea.

Collins, P., G. Rosano, and C. Casey. 2007. Management of cardiovascular risk in the perimenopausal women: A consensus statement of European cardiologists and gynecologists. *Climacteric* 10:508–526.

Diepvens, K., R. Westerterp, and M.S. Plantenga. 2007. Obesity and thermogenesis related to the consumption of caffeine, ephedrine, capsaicin, and green tea. *American Journal of Physiology—Regulatory Integrative and Comparative Physiology* 292:77–85.

Egan, M.F., M. Kojima, J.H. Callicott et al. 2003. The BDNF val66met polymorphism affects activity dependent secretion of BDNF and human memory and hippocampal function. *Cell* 112:257–269.

Francis, P.T., A.M. Palmer, M. Snape, and G.K. Wilcock. 1999. The cholinergic hypothesis of Alzheimer's disease: A review of progress. *Journal of Neurology and Neurosurgical Psychiatry* 66:137–147.

Gaesser, G.A. 2007. Carbohydrate quantity and quality in relation to body mass index. *Journal of the American Dietetic Association* 107:1768–1780.

Gupta, B. and B. Ghash. 1999. *Curcuma longa* inhibits TNF-α induced expression of adhesion molecules human umbilical vein endothelial cells. *International Journal of Immunopharmacology* 21:745–757.

Ha, Y., O.K. Kim, D.E. Nam et al. 2015. Effects of *Curcuma longa* L. extracts on natural killer cells and T cells. *Journal Korean Society Food Science Nutrition* 44:307–313.

Hwang, J.T., H.J. Yang, K.C. Ha, B.O. So, E.K. Choi, and S.W. Chae. 2015. A randomized, double-blind, placebo-controlled clinical trial to investigate the anti-diabetic effect of *Citrus junos* Tanaka peel. Journal of *Functional Foods* 18:532–537.

Heo, J.C., J. Park, S.M. An et al. 2006. Anti-oxidant and anti-tumor activities of crude extracts by *Gastrodia elata* Baume. *Korean Journal Food Preservation* 13:83–87.

Hong, J.H., H.J. Kim, Y.H. Choi, and I.S. Lee. 2008. Physiological activities of dried persimmon, fresh persimmon and persimmon leaves. *Journal of the Korean Society Food Science and Nutrition* 37:957–64.

Howes M.J. and P. Houghton. 2003. Plants used in Chinese and Indian traditional medicine for improvement of memory and cognitive function. *Pharmacologic and Biochemical Behavior* 75:513–527.

Huang, G.B., T. Zhao, M.S. Shrestha et al. 2013. Therapeutic potential of *Gastrodia elata* Blume for the treatment of Alzheimer's disease. *Neural Regeneration Research* 8:1061–1070.

James, M., C.N. Roza, and Xian-Liu. Zheng. 2007. Effect of citrus flavonoids and tocotrienols on serum cholesterol levels in hypercholesterolemic subjects. *Alternative Therapy* 13:44–48.

Jang, S.H., S.H. Kim, H.Y. Lee et al. 2015. Immune-modulating activity of extract prepared from mycelial culture of Chinese caterpillar mushroom, *Ophiocordyceps sinensis* (Ascomycetes). *International Journal of Medicinal Mushrooms* 17:1189–1199.

Jang, S.H., J.S. Park, S.H. Jang et al. 2016. In vitro stimulation of NK cells and lymphocytes using an extract prepared from mycelial culture of *Ophiocordyceps sinensis*. *Immune Network* 16:140–145.

Jang, S.N. and D.H. Kim. 2010. Trends in the health status of older Koreans. *Journal of American Geriatrics Society* 58:592–598.

Jeong, H.S., H.S. Chung, H.D. Lee, J.H. Seong, and J.U. Choi. 2001. Controlled atmosphere storage and modified atmosphere packaging of astringency-removed persimmons. *Food Science Biotechnol* 10:380–386.

Jiang, M.H., L. Zhu, and J.G. Jiang. 2010. Immunoregulatory actions of polysaccharides from Chinese herbal medicine. *Expert Opinion. Therapeutic. Targets* 14:1367–1402.

Jung, S.J., M.G. Kim, T.S. Park, Y.G. Kim, W.O. Song, and S.W. Chae. 2015. Rice-based Korean meals (bibimbap and kimbap) have lower glycemic responses and postprandial-triglyceride effects than energy-matched Western meals. *Journal of Ethnic Foods* 2:154–161.

Jung, S.J., S.H. Park, E.K. Choi et al. 2014. Beneficial effects of Korean traditional diets in hypertensive and type 2 diabetic patients. *Journal of Medicinal Food* 17:161–171.

Jung, U.J., J.S. Lee, S.H. Bok, and M.S. Choi. 2011. Effects of extracts of persimmon leaf, buckwheat leaf, and Chinese matrimony vine leaf on body fat and metabolism in rats. *Journal of the Korean Society Food Science and Nutrition* 40:1215–1226.

Jurenka, J.S. 2008. Therapeutic applications of pomegranate (*Punica granatum* L.): A review. *Alternative Medicine Review* 13:128–144.

Kamarei, R. and C. Trygstad. 2004. Designing clinical trials to substantiate claims. *Food Technology* 58:28–35.

Kang, H.J., H.W. Baik, S.J. Kim et al. 2015a. *Cordyceps militaris* enhances cell-mediated immunity in healthy Korean men. *Journal of Medicine Food* 18:1164–1172.

Kang, I.S., H.J. Kim, T.H. Lee et al. 2014. Effect of *Cordyceps militaris* on immune activity. *Yakhak Hoeji* 58:81–90.

Kang, S.J., B.R. Choi, S.H. Kim et al. 2015b. Inhibitory effects of pomegranate concentrated solution on the activities of hyalrunidase, tyrosinase, and metalloproteinase. *Journal of Cosmetic Science* 66:145–159.

Kang, S.J., B.R. Choi, S.H. Kim et al. 2016. Evaluation of the *in vivo* skin moisturizing effects and underlying mechanisms of pomegranate concentrate solution and dried pomegranate concentrate powder. *Journal of Korean Medicine* 37:12–22.

Kang, S.J., B.R. Choi, S.H. Kim et al. 2017. Anti-climacterium effects of pomegranate concentrated solution in ovariectomized ddY mice. *Experimental and Therapeutic Medicine* 13:1249–1266.

Kang, S.K. and K.H. Hyun. 2007. Optimization of curcumin extraction and removal of bitter substance from *Curcuma longa* L. *Korean Journal of Food Preservation* 14:722–726.

Kawakami, K., S. Aketa, H. Sakai, and Y. Watanabe. 2011. Antihypertensive and vasorelaxant effects of water-soluble proanthocyanidins from persimmon leaf tea in spontaneously hypertensive rats. *Bioscience Biotechnology Biochemistry* 75:1435–1439.

Kennedy, K.M., E.D. Reese, M.M. Horn et al. 2015. BDNF val66met polymorphism affects aging of multiple types of memory. *Brain Research* 1612:104–1617.

KFDA. 2012. Guide of the clinical trial of health functional foods.

Kim, C.M., M.G. Shin, and D.G. Ahn. 1999. *A complete translation encyclopedia of Chinese herbal medicine*. Seoul: Jungdam, 4105–4107.

Kim, J.H., J.Y. Kim, H.S. Won et al. 2010. Human studies on functional foods: How they are regulated. *Korean Journal of Nutrition* 43: 653–660.

Kim, M.S., H.J. Hur, D.Y. Kwon, and J.T. 2012. Tangeretin stimulates glucose uptake via regulation of AMPK signaling pathways in C2C12 myotubes and improves glucose tolerance in high-fat diet-induced obese mice. *Molecular Cellular Endocrinology* 358:127–134.

Kim, S.H., H.J. Hur, H.J. Yang et al. 2013a. *Citrus junos* Tanaka peel extract exerts antidiabetic effects via AMPK and PPAR-γ both *in vitro* and *in vivo* in mice fed a high-fat diet. *Evidence-Based Complementary and Alternative Medicine* 8 pp.

Kim, W.C., J.H. Jeong, J.S. Kim, and K.O. Kim. 2013b. The verify of memory improvement by *Gastrodia elata* Blume. *Journal of Oriental Neuropsychiatry* 24:27–44.

Koh, J. 2006. Effects cheonggukjang added to *Phellinus linteus* on lipid metabolism in hyperlipidemic rats. *Journal Korean Society Food Science Nutrition* 35:301–308.

Koo, B., S.H. Seong, D.Y. Kown, and Y.S. Cha. 2008. Fermented kochujang supplement shows anti-obesity effects by controlling lipid metabolism in C57BL/6J mice fed high fat diet. *Food Science and Biotechnology* 17:336–342.

Kontou, N., T. Psaltopoulou, D. Panggiotakos, M.A. Dimopoulos, and A. Linos. 2011. The mediterian diet in cancer prevention: A review. *Journal of Medicinal Food* 14:1065–1078.

Korean Ministry of Health & Welfare. Health Functional Foods Acts; 2010; https://ko.wikipedia.org/

Kwak, C.S., P. Park, and K.Y. Song. 2012. Doenjang, a fermented soybean paste, decreased visceral fat accumulation and adipocyte size in rats fed with high fat diet more effectively than nonfermented soybeans. *Journal of Medicinal Food* 15:1–9.

Kwon, Y.I., E. Apostolidis, Y.C. Kim, and K. Shetty. 2007. Health benefits of traditional corn, beans and pumpkin. In vitro studies for hyperglycemia and hypertension management. *Journal of Medicinal Food* 10:266–275.

Kyung Hee University Skin Biotechnology Center. 2014. Effects of oral administration of Pomegranate concentrated solution in the human skin: 8 week, randomized, double-blinded, placebo controlled trial (skin moisture, elasticity, color, and wrinkle. Clinical trial report, June 20, 2014.

Lae, P. 2005. The effect of fermented soybean powder on improvement of constipated patients receiving maintenance hemodialysis. M.S. thesis, KyungBuk National University Daegu (Korea).

Lee, G.H., H.R. Kim, S.Y. Han et al. 2012. *Gastrodia elata* Blume and its pure compounds protect BV-2 microglial-derived cell lines against β-amyloid: The involvement of GRP78 and CHOP. *Biological Research* 45:403–410.

Lee, I.K. and J.K. Kim. 2002. Effects of dietary supplementation of Korean soybean paste (deonjang) on the lipid metabolism in rats fed a high fat and/or a high cholesterol diet. *Journal Korean Public Health Association* 28:282–305.

Lee, J.C., H. Cho, J. Kim, J.Y. Kim, D.S. Kim, and H.B. Kim. 2001. Antioxidant activity of substances extracted by alcohol from chungkookjang powder. *Korean Journal Microbiology* 37:177–181.

Lim, J.H., E.S. Jung, E.K. Choi et al. 2014. Supplementation with *Aspergillus oryzae*-fermented kochujang lowers serum cholesterol in subjects with hyperlipidemia. *Clinical Nutrition* 34:383–387.

Mazumder, A., K. Raghavan, J. Weinstein, K. Kohn, and Y. Pommier. 1995. Inhibition of human immunodefiency virus type-1 integrase by curcumin. *Biochemical Pharmacology* 49:1165–1170.

McKeown, N.M., E. Liu, J.B. Meigs, G. Rogers, R. D'Agostino, and P. Jacques. 2009. Carbohydrate-related dietary factors and plasma adiponectin levels in healthy adults in the Framingham Offspring Cohort. *FASEB Journal* 23:229–235.

Moon, S.H. and K.Y. Park. 1995. Antimutagenic effects of boiled water extract and tannin from persimmon leaves. *Journal of the Korean Society Food Science and Nutrition* 24:880–888.

Morand, C., C. Dubary, D. Milenkovic, D. Lioger, J. Martin, A. Scalbert, and A. Mazur. 2011. Hesperidin contributes to the vascular protective effects of orange juice: A randomized crossover study in healthy volunteers. *American Journal Clinical Nutrition* 93:73–80.

Ng, T.B. and H.X. Wang. 2005. Pharmacological actions of Cordyceps, a prized folk medicine. *Jouranl of Pharmacy Pharmacology* 57:1509–1519.

Ono-Moore, K.D., R.G. Snodgrass, S. Huang et al. 2016. Postprandial inflammatory responses and free fatty acids in plasma of adults who consumed a moderately high-fat breakfast with and without blueberry powder in a randomized placebo-controlled trial. *Journal of Nutrition* 146:1411–1419.

Ornish, D., G. Weidner, W.R. Fair et al. 2003. Intensive lifestyle changes may affect the progression of prostate cancer. *Journal of Urology* 174:1065–1070.

Park, Y.J., M.H. Kang, J.I. Kim, O.J. Park, M.S. Lee, and H.D. Jang. 1995. Changes of vitamin C and superoxide dismutase (SOD)-like activity of persimmon leaf tea by processing method and extraction condition. *Korean Journal Food Science Technology* 27:281–285.

Reza, K. and T. Carl. 2004. Designing clinical trials to substantiate claims. *Food Technology* 58:28–35

Schindler, A.E. 2006. Climacteric symptoms and hormones. *Gynecological Endocrinol*ogy 22:151–154.

Scholey, A.B., N.T.J. Tildesley, C.G. Ballard et al. 2008. An extract of Saliva (sage) with anticholinesterase properties improves memory and attention in healthy older volunteers. *Psychopharmacology* 198:127–139.

Shin, S.K., J.H. Kwon, M. Jeon, J. Choi, and M.S. Choi. 2011. Supplementation of cheonggukjang and red ginseng cheonggukjang can improve plasma lipid profile and fasting blood glucose concentration in subjects with impaired fasting glucose. *Journal of Medicinal Food* 14:108–113.

Shin, S.M., J.H. Kwon, S.W. Lee et al. 2010. Immunostimulatory effects of *Cordyceps militaris* on macrophages through the enhanced production of cytokines via the activation of NF-κB. *Immune Network* 10:55–63.

Soh, J.R., D.H. Shin, D.Y. Kwon, and Y.S. Cha. 2008. Effect of cheonggukjang supplementation upon hepatic acyl-CoA synthase, carnitine palmitoyltransferase I, acyl-CoA oxidase and uncoupling protein 2 mRNA levels in C57BL/6J mice fed with high fat diet. *Genes and Nutrition* 2:365–269.

Song, C.H., Y.J. Jeon, B.K. Yang, K.S. Ra, and J.M. Sung. 1998. Anti-complementary activity of exo-polymers produced from submerged mycelial cultures of higher fungi with particular reference to *Cordyceps militaris*. *Journal of Microbiology and Biotechnology* 8:536–539.

Sung, H.M., Y.H. Lee, and W.J. Jun. 2016. *In vitro* hepatoprotective effects of fermented *Curcuma longa* L. by *Aspergillus oryzae* against alcohol-induced oxidative stress. *Journal Korean Society Food Science Nutrition* 45:812–818.

van der Greef, J., P. Stroobant, and R, van der Heijden. 2004. The role of analytical sciences in medical systems biology. *Current Opinion in Chemical Biology* 8:559–565.

Waterland, R.A. and R.L. Jirtle. 2003. Transposable elements: Targets for early nutritional effects on epigenetic regulation. *Molecular Cellular Biology* 23:5239–5300.

20

Functional Food Industry: Processing and Sanitation

Jin-Hee Lee

CONTENTS

20.1 Introduction: Background and History 505
20.2 Raw Materials 506
20.3 Standardization of Ingredients 508
20.4 Safety Assessment 508
20.5 Function Assessment 509
20.6 Functional Food Processing 511
20.7 Sanitation 518
20.8 Conclusion 519
References 521

20.1 Introduction: Background and History

Korean functional food has been established based on the regulation that designates the definition, raw ingredients available, processing conditions, and claims legally permitted. Food hygiene law and health functional food law comprise the detailed regulatory systems operating in Korea.

Industrial food research, development, processing, and communication are closely related to the regulatory system, which influences the overall production as well as designing the food. The reason why Korean food, especially functional food, has been tightly associated with regulatory affairs is that food and pharmaceuticals are legally incompatible with each other, where the definition of food in Korea is expressed as "food and drink edible except for those for pharmaceutical uses," and the definition of drugs in Korea are defined as "those used for diagnosis, treatment, alleviation, disposal and prevention purposes which influence the pharmacological structure and function in human and animals."

A new category of health functional food in Korea has been developed since 2004, when the regulation called the Health Functional Food Law came into effect, approved by the Korean government (Gwak et al., 2007).

The definition of Korean health functional food is designated as "food processed and made of ingredients or compounds which have functions beneficially available in humans," where the function in food is defined as that which can give beneficial health efficacy by means of regulating the nutrients against human structure and function, or physiological work.

Foods are composed of many compounds or ingredients. In Korea the components of raw food materials are classified into three major groups: food ingredients, food additives, and functional ingredients.

Food ingredients are edible raw materials and those processed from them, food additives are specific materials for food processing and preservation uses, and functional ingredients are ingredients claimed to have beneficial health uses. The criteria of judging food ingredients and food additives are based on safety, that of functional ingredients, on safety and efficacy scientifically proved and permitted as claimable and approved by the Korean government, especially the Korean Ministry of Food and Drug Safety.

The ingredients that can be used in Korean health functional foods are those described before, such as food ingredients, food additives, and functional ingredients, where functional ingredients are a must and where all of these are based on Korean health functional food law.

Together with the health functional foods, the other available functional foods in Korea are, even though restricted, those that comprise certain beneficial ingredients where the product of which the ingredient is composed should be proved as physiologically beneficial by scientific evidence officially published, based on Korean food hygiene law.

Strictly speaking, currently Korean regulation has two tracks that permit the function of food availably communicated. One is health functional food government approved, and the other is a little bit more restricted food whose beneficial effect is proved scientifically and its benefits can be communicated without government permission.

20.2 Raw Materials

Raw materials available in Korean functional food are mainly positively designated even though a few exceptions are present. There are positive lists, which are absolutely not permitted as food ingredients, and there are also positively listed ones which are absolutely not permitted as functional ingredients. These are the so-called negative lists not available in Korean food and functional food and they are totally different from those of other countries.

Ingredients incorporated into finished functional food products should be classified as one of the legal materials, food ingredients, food additives, and functional food ingredients, where those materials have been approved as available by the Korean Ministry of Food and Drug Safety. If not, the

Functional Food Industry

materials that have never been approved as available in food and functional food can be approved in advance as available ones by the Korean Ministry of Food and Drug Safety before usage.

The criteria of judging food materials as industrially available are summarized as safety first of all. If this is completed, the functionality should be proved scientifically by means of well-organized regulatory systems (Gwak et al., 2007). Food ingredients and food additives are allowed by means of only safety criteria, whereas functional food ingredients are concerned with functionality as well as safety.

The already allowed food ingredients are listed in a notification about food by the Korean Ministry of Food and Drug Safety. Food additives are addressed in another notification about food additives by the ministry, and functional food ingredients are covered in health and functional food notifications also by the ministry. Otherwise, for example, the food ingredients and additives that are not found in such government-published notification lists can be allowed to be available by the ministry by means of regulatory procedures by accepting the so-called temporary standards by which those materials are not to be utilized for commercial and industrial use until they have been approved.

Similarly, the functional food ingredients that are not found in legally published notifications about health and functional food lists can be allowed in advance as commercially and industrially available by the same government ministry by accepting the so-called individual authorization, which permits the function claim never been allowed before.

Table 20.1 shows the significant criteria for distinguishing raw materials incorporated in functional food. These strict limitations are present in

TABLE 20.1

Significant Criteria for Distinguishing Raw Materials Incorporated in Functional Food in Korea

	Food Ingredient	Food Additive	Functional Ingredient
Legal basis	Food hygiene law	Food hygiene law	Health functional food law
Criteria	Safety	Safety	Safety, function
Source	Food ingredient database approved by Ministry of Food and Drug Safety	Food additive database approved by Ministry of Food and Drug Safety	Functional food ingredient database approved by Ministry of Food and Drug Safety
Newly developed	Preapproval is required prior to industrial uses	Preapproval is required prior to industrial uses	Preapproval is required prior to industrial uses
Claim for health benefit	Not permitted	Not permitted	Permitted if approved
Application	Food, health functional food	Food, health functional food	Health functional food

Korean functional food because of the emphasis on food safety priority and the government's need to regulate the abuse of food materials as having medicinal effects.

20.3 Standardization of Ingredients

Standardization of functional ingredients is prerequisite prior to the evaluation of the ingredients' safety and function. The purpose of standardization is to ensure the quality constant and repeatability of the production of functional ingredients regardless of batches, ultimately guaranteeing the safety and function of the ingredients developed. The major considerations in the standardization of an ingredient are the accurate scientific name, accurately processed part, the origin, harvest times, processing conditions, and so forth.

Standardization includes the identification of function or marker compounds designating the characteristics of the functional ingredient candidates, the analytical method to detect them readily, harmful materials' specifications, and the establishment of standardized specifications of the ingredients. The marker compounds can be readily analyzed by common methods as much as possible. Economic analysis methods are to be adopted, and the marker compounds are to be as ingredient specific as possible, with representative compounds explaining the characteristics of the ingredients evaluated.

If the analytical methods adopted are more advanced than any others known before, they must be validated via appropriate methods described in Korean regulatory manuals. The definition of validation is the process of demonstrating or confirming the performance characteristics of a method of analysis, which involves the specificity; accuracy; precision, including repeatability and intermediate precision; limit of quantification; linearity; and range (Yang et al., 2008).

20.4 Safety Assessment

The assessment of safety of ingredients cannot be done until the standardization of ingredients evaluated has been established. We have to bear in mind that being of natural origin does not always mean safety in dealing with functional ingredients. The Korean Ministry of Food and Drug Safety adopts ingredients list that cannot be used in Korean functional food from the beginning. Those ingredients are prohibited as functional ingredients

Functional Food Industry

due to toxicity that may be harmful to humans or extreme medicinal action that is not accepted as food or functional food grade.

Ingredients permitted for medicinal purposes alone no doubt have rights to be used as functional ingredients as well. To prove the safety of a functional ingredient candidate before industrial use takes place, various kinds of evaluation data are needed for the candidate to be judged as safe. Prerequisite to the safety evidence is the experience of human intake of the ingredient, including historical records and scientific documents relating to the manufacturing procedure, application, and dose of daily intake.

Government-approved documents about safety and monographs, such as commission E, WHO, the natural medicine comprehensive database, and the natural standard database, meet the demand. Information about the safety of the active compounds or related components is also useful for proof of safety. This includes the database, documents and papers referring to toxicity, and monographs relating to the interactions between the multiple components.

Exposure assessments sometimes are needed to prove the safety of a certain ingredient due to the possibility for the same ingredient to be incorporated in various kinds of food matrices that may be taken simultaneously or within a given period. This is commonly analyzed by national nutrition survey results, research about the actual condition of daily intake of a certain ingredient, and so forth.

Additional requirements for proving safety include overall nutrition evaluation documents such as analyzed data for the effect of a certain ingredient on absorption, distribution, metabolism, excretion, and bioavailability and human clinical trials supporting the safety. Ultimately, the toxicity data elucidated by GLP (good laboratory practice)-based experiments, including single-dose toxicity, 3-month repeated oral toxicity studies, and genotoxicological safety estimates, are primary requirements. Otherwise, if not successfully proven yet, additional studies on reproductive toxicity, antigenicity, immunotoxicology, and carcinogenicity may be required (Park, 2010).

20.5 Function Assessment

The function of an ingredient in which active compounds or bioactivity may exist has to be elucidated scientifically and logically for a claim to be accepted. The claims are classified as concerning nutrition, function, or health.

- Nutrition claims deal with the potential benefits from action of nutrients such as vitamins, minerals, dietary fibers, amino acids, fatty acids, and so on, which are primarily nutrients in food before considering function.

- Function claims concern the potential benefits of reaction of a certain ingredient or compound (rather than nutritional ones) in affecting physiological conditions in the human body; they must be demonstrated scientifically.
- Health claims address the relationship between ingredients and diseases, supported by strong scientific evidence socially and scientifically agreed upon.

Prevention and cure of diseases are distinguished from the health benefits of functional food; if prevention and/or cure of diseases are claimed in functional food, punishment is based on violation of law, health functional food law, food hygiene law, and pharmaceutical law. The principle of evaluating the function of an ingredient is that it must be target population-based, showing relevance of a claimed function to human health. There must be scientific substantiation of the claimed effect.

For the development of industrial uses, investigations beforehand examine ease of use, economic efficiency, scale-up and mass production, patent restrictions, standardization, and imitation possibilities of the ingredient. Biomarkers representing the function evaluated must be established beforehand to show that the functions of ingredients are scientifically consistent enough to explain the *in vitro*, *in vivo*, and human clinical trials.

As shown in Table 20.2, the purpose of *in vitro* studies is to screen the materials with targeted function and to elucidate the action mechanism of those materials. *In vivo* animal studies identify the possible action mechanism and dose of intake of ingredients as well as *in vivo* screening of efficacy. The purpose of human clinical trials is to confirm the *in vivo* function evaluated in the human body; the human clinical experimental design should meet the ICH GCP (good clinical practice) guideline, followed by randomized, double-blinded and placebo-controlled studies.

Human clinical study alone without the support of *in vitro* and *in vivo* relevant evidence is not sufficient to prove the function of an ingredient. Instead, human clinical trial data together with other evidence must be considered in any evaluation. Intervention and observation studies can be used in

TABLE 20.2

Types of Studies for the Function Assessment

	In Vitro Study	*In Vivo* Animal Study	Human Clinical Study
Screening	O[a]	O	X[b]
Identification of action mechanism	O	O	X
Determination of dose of intake	X	O	X
Confirmation of *in vivo* function	X	X	O

[a] Appropriate for the purpose.
[b] Inappropriate for the purpose.

Functional Food Industry 511

evaluating those functions, and the resulting data should be suitable enough for analysis of statistical significance.

Major considerations for evaluation of functions of ingredients by means of human clinical trials include (Park, 2010):

- Characterization of the foodstuff
- All ingredients designated as being relevant are to be taken into account
- Effects have to be relevant to human health
- Practicable quantity to be consumed
- Studies with planned products should explain the matrix effect
- Subject population must match target group of the foodstuff
- Target group must be clearly defined
- Biomarkers must be based on the mechanism derived from *in vitro* and *in vivo* animal studies
- Significant results alone are not sufficient; placebo results are often significant as well
- Study design and statistical dimensions are required
- Backgrounds such as dietary habits, lifestyles, and physical activity are to be examined
- Long-term examination is sometimes required

20.6 Functional Food Processing

Korean functional food is based on ingredients originating from plants, animals, or microorganisms, and other processed materials that contain functional or marker compounds that are biologically active in human body. The characteristic of Korean functional food ingredients is that one or more compounds incorporated in them should be characterized and chemically identified as functional, or a marker compound rather than a functional one. If the specific functional compound in ingredients cannot be clearly identified, it can, instead, function as a marker compound, which plays a role as an index representing and guaranteeing the quality of the ingredients. Other than chemically identified compounds as markers, biological methods such as enzymatic activity and so on that can represent the characteristic of a certain ingredient as a functional one can also be designated as markers.

The common processing procedure for the development of functional food ingredients can be described as follows: extraction of plant-origin raw materials, followed by partial purification of the extracts, concentration of the extracts if diluted, and then further processing for the formation of standardized liquid or powder as a finished ingredient product. The solvent available for the extraction of raw materials is restricted to guarantee the safety of the ingredients produced. Although water, edible ethyl alcohol, and supercritical extraction methods are allowed to be used at any time, further chemical solvents such as ethyl acetate, hexane, and so on are selectively used according to Korean regulations for the available extraction solvents allowed for the treatment of functional ingredients.

If the usage of solvents for the extraction procedure is against its legal requirements, any further process for the industrial development and production of functional ingredients will be meaningless due to the illegality. The critical criteria for the decision depends on the safety secured.

Ingredients absolutely not permitted as functional ingredients in Korea are also the pre-checkpoints for the development and production of functional ingredients. Ephedra is a representative example of a prohibited ingredient as a functional ingredient in Korea. However, it is available in American nutraceuticals, indicating that the Korean functional food regulatory system is totally different from those of other countries in the world.

Not all plants can be candidates as functional ingredients if developed, because controversy may exist about the evidence of food experience of the plant from the past. Thus, a medicinal plant is to be examined thoroughly and may be excluded from the candidate for safety reasons. Biotechnology can also be utilized for development and production of functional ingredients; bioconversion, a process in which microorganisms convert a compound to a structurally related product, can be performed to produce specific functional ingredients (Wang et al., 1979).

Microorganisms utilized in the bioconversion process should be secured as safe for the production of food-grade ingredients. Genetically modified organisms and the enzymes originating from them should be deliberated by the committees necessary for approval of their safety before usage if this is the first time under consideration. Despite severe restrictions of microbial transformation, it is commonly used as a functional-ingredient–producing process for advantageous aspects of the technology: specificity of reaction, low-energy consumption, mild reaction condition, high yield, and eco-friendly condition.

One of the representative functional ingredient examples produced industrially by means of bioconversion technology is fructo-oligosaccharide. This has a health benefit as a prebiotic, produced by the process of converting the substrate, sucrose, into the bioconversion product, fructo-oligosaccharide, by enzymatic conversion using fructosyltransferase originated from *Aerobasidium pullulans*, with immobilized enzyme technology (Koh et al., 2011).

Aspergillus niger has been known to be able to function as a bioconversion catalyst to produce the same product. It has not been commercialized yet due to the difficulties in performing immobilized technology. The reaction

Functional Food Industry

model of fructosyltransferase to convert the substrate into the product is shown as follows, where G is the abbreviation of glucose and F of fructose:

$$GF + GF \rightarrow GF_2 + G \tag{20.1}$$

$$GF_2 + GF_2 \rightarrow GF_3 + GF \tag{20.2}$$

$$GF_3 + GF_3 \rightarrow GF_4 + GF_2 \tag{20.3}$$

The overall reaction model of the reaction of fructosyltransferase is expressed here, where n would be from 1 to 7 as a positive integer:

$$GF_n + GF_n \rightarrow GF_{n+1} + GF_{n-1} \tag{20.4}$$

Another example of biocatalytic conversion of a substrate into a bioavailable product is D-tagatose, a kind of sweetener, whose health benefit has been approved to be helpful for blood glucose level control. D-tagatose in the small intestine could inhibit the activity of sucrase and maltase, decreasing the absorption of the substrates. One of the overall procedures developed for its production is lactose; as a substrate, it is hydrolyzed and separated followed by its enzymatic conversion into the product, purified and crystallized in the long run (Figure 20.1).

The health benefit of D-tagatose has been established by the approval of the Korean Ministry of Food and Drug Safety through evaluation of standardization, safety, and function of the ingredient (Kwak et al., 2013). The safety assessment includes security for the safety of a living modified organism against human oral intake. The function assessment ultimately includes the human clinical trials performed based on randomized, double-blinded, placebo-controlled, and IRB (Institutional Review Board)-approved experimental design.

D-allulose, one of the substitutes for sweeteners, has been available for human diets in which the metabolic process is different from those of

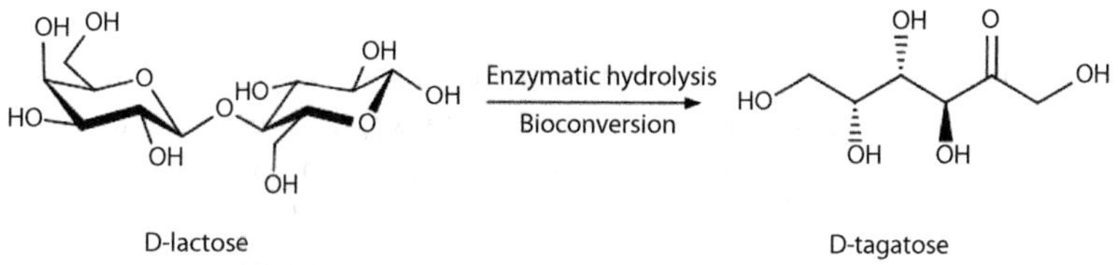

D-lactose

Enzymatic hydrolysis
Bioconversion

D-tagatose

FIGURE 20.1
Bioconversion of D-lactose to D-tagatose.

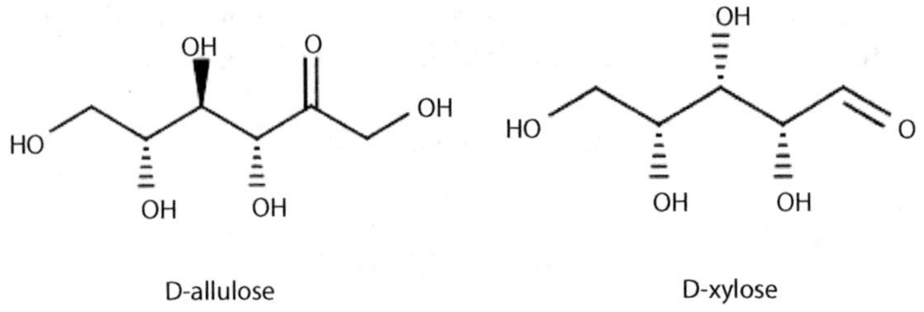

D-allulose   D-xylose

FIGURE 20.2
Molecular structure of D-allulose and D-xylose.

other traditional sweeteners such as glucose, fructose, and sucrose; this has resulted in less calorie intake after consumption, suggesting it may helpful for the prevention of obesity and diabetes (Figure 20.2). These health benefits are to be further proved scientifically and approved as the legal functional ingredient based on the safety for human oral intake.

D-xylose has proved to be an inhibitor of sucrase, and it has been found to be effective in the human body for the suppression of sucrose uptake by randomized, double-blinded, placebo-controlled, and IRB-approved human clinical trials (Figure 20.2). Currently it is commercially available in Korea as a sucrose uptake suppressor, based on the regulatory track, which permits the function of food communicated when its benefit can be communicated without government permission.

Another representative biomaterial approved as a functional ingredient whose health benefit is able to be claimed legally is probiotic; a specific example of a probiotic is the lactic acid bacteria, *Lactobacillus plantarum*, isolated from kimchi, the Korean traditional food. The legally permitted health benefit is, "It may be helpful for the prevention of hypersensitive immune response in the human body"—as well as the already approved traditional health benefit for the prevention of intestinal disorders.

One of the well-known animal-origin functional ingredients is the extract of hen comb, which contains hyaluronic acid as a marker compound whose health benefit has been approved to help in the moisturizing effect of human skin after oral intake based on the material's water-holding capacity being scientifically proved in physiological conditions. This material is currently utilized for cosmetic uses and as an eyewash as well as functional food ingredient.

Plant-origin materials come from various kinds of edible natural substances. They are be commonly extracted via legally appropriate methods such as usage of solvents, food additives, and so on, standardized by the characterization of marker compounds incorporated in them and established via specifications. The standardized ingredients are ready to be scientifically evaluated to prove the physiological function by means of *in vitro, in vivo*, and human clinical trials, along with the estimation of safety according

Functional Food Industry

to the GLP-based toxicity test as well as surveying additional scientific evidence supporting their safety.

Standardization, safety, and function evaluation are three major requirements for the acquiring approval of the ingredients' health benefits so that they are legally, industrially, and commercially available. The functional ingredients whose health benefits have already been approved are ready to be used in the processing of finished products. These are the so-called health functional foods, which are differentiated from food (the so-called conventional food to distinguish it from health functional food), where there are two methods used for the functional ingredients to be incorporated and processed into the finished product, health functional food.

The finished health functional food products, such as tablets, capsules, powders, granules, liquids, bead-like shapes, and so on whose legal meaning is based on daily intake dose have no further obligations to prove the finished products' safety and function. However, conventional foods have further obligations to prove that the safety and function have not been changed compared to those approved originally on the basis of the ingredients. The legal meaning implies that no further changes have occurred in the finished product during the processing conditions of food. It is an indisputable fact that the marker compounds should be stable enough to ensure the shelf life of health functional food during storage and supply chain structure.

An example of a health functional food developed in Korea is health functional cooked rice whose health benefit is to help to control blood glucose level after intake because it contains resistant starch that improves markers of endothelial function with reduction of postprandial blood glucose and oxidative stress in patients with prediabetes or newly diagnosed type 2 diabetes (Kwak et al., 2012). It is the first example to permit the health benefit of conventional food that adopted the regulatory basis to prove the safety and function had not been changed compared to those approved originally on the basis of ingredients.

Functional ingredients that are allowed are not always restricted to a single ingredient extract; mixed ingredients put together one by one also can be a functional mixed ingredient. The function of the total should be elucidated scientifically according to the same procedures and the bioactive markers of the mixed ingredients should be identified and characterized separately from one ingredient to another. One of the examples of the mixed functional ingredients is the mixed extracts of *Hibiscus*, which, specifically, consist of *Hibiscus* extract, modified chito-oligosaccharide, and L-carnitine and claim the health benefit of antiobesity.

One of the stereospecific isomers of HCA (hydroxy citric acid), (+)-allo-HCA lactone, has been identified as the marker compound of *Hibiscus* extract. HCA is commonly known as the citrate lyase inhibitor that can prohibit lipid biosynthesis from excess amounts of glucose absorbed in human blood (Figure 20.3).

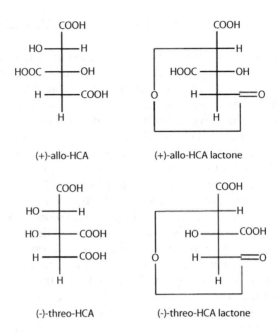

FIGURE 20.3
Comparison of the molecular structure of (+)-allo-HCA (hydroxy citric acid), its lactone form, and (−)-threo-HCA, its lactone form.

Chito-oligosaccharide is well known to form a complex with bile acid synthesized from blood cholesterol, resulting in the excretion of the complex rather than absorption of it in the intestinal environment. This implies the possibility of the complex molecule acting as a biomolecule to suppress the *in vivo* blood glucose level. However, this is not supported by many scientists by evidence of *in vivo* studies, suggesting that the intestinal environment is not appropriate to form a chito-oligosaccharide and bile acid complex mainly due to the neutral pH condition.

Prior to getting the modified chito-oligosaccharide molecule screened and pooled based on specific molecular weight range, treatment of the molecule with the enzymatic hydrolysis was performed, allowing the complex molecule to be bioactive in a human intestinal condition. The marker compound of chito-oligosaccharides has been characterized as the total glucosamine hydrolyzed. L-carnitine is the well-known biomarker compound that reacts with acyl-CoA in the cytosol to be transported through the mitochondrial membrane, which is destined to be oxidized to produce bioenergy. These ingredients together have been proved to have an antiobesity function, scientifically supported by the evidences of *in vivo* animal study and human clinical trials.

The biomarker compound identified as an index of a certain ingredient, if set up, should be stable enough to endure during the processing and storage

Functional Food Industry

to guarantee the quantitative amount of it per daily intake. If those compounds are chemically unstable during processing and storage, they cannot function as markers to control the quality of the products anymore, indicating that the stabilization of marker compounds in functional ingredients is the crucial point to be industrialized.

In the case of *Garcinia cambogia*, in which the active marker compound is known to be (–)-threo-HCA, an organic acid similar to citric acid found in citrus fruits such as oranges and lemons, the instability of the marker compound, (–)-threo-HCA, especially in acidic conditions, has been a critical problem limiting its application to various kinds of food. Commercial beverages are classified with two common groups according to their pH: the acidic beverage and the neutral beverage, where the pH of the finished product positions at acidic pH range and neutral pH range, respectively.

The Korean legal standard for the amount of the marker compound detected by an appropriate analysis method should range from 80% to 120% compared to the amount written on the package. The amount of (–)-threo-HCA analyzed during storage had been dramatically decreased. Specifically, the detected (–)-threo-HCA was free form rather than lactone form, which it can readily transform to during purification, processing, and storage at extremely acidic pH conditions (Figure 20.3). This compound is not appropriate for the role of a marker compound due to its variation and instability, resulting in illegal violation of the functional ingredient to the allowed specification.

Careful observation of the changes of the chemical profile of (–)-threo-HCA during storage of the beverage shows that the decrease of the amount of (–)-threo-HCA free form was roughly proportional to the increase of the amount of the (–)-threo-HCA lactone form generated from the original free form, indicating that chemical changes had happened in those beverage conditions. Considering these phenomena, the marker compounds indicating the quality of this functional ingredients would be better designated as the total amount of (–)-threo-HCA, containing the (–)-threo-HCA free form plus (–)-threo-HCA lactone form, the sum of which meets the specification level of the specific compounds during storage.

The whose health benefits of health functional food in Korea cannot be claimed until the functional ingredients incorporated in it are approved and permission given to communicate the health benefit based on the scientific proofs examined during the process of approval by the Ministry of Food and Drug Safety. One more channel to be able to communicate the functional benefit of an ingredient or the finished food product containing it is also available, in part based on the scientific proofs published or believed to be true by substantial social agreement in the field of food science regulated by food hygiene law.

One of the representative examples is the nutrient health benefit claims commonly recognized as natural to do, which include nutrients such as vitamins, minerals, dietary fibers, amino acids, fatty acids, and so forth.

The characteristic of the nutrient health benefit claim is that it is available regardless of the dose per day permitted to meet the legal claims defined by health functional food law, it is based on notification by self-determination rather than preapproval by government, and it is applicable to all kinds of conventional food.

Another aspect of such function claims corresponds to peculiar-use foodstuffs, one of the legal classification categories in conventional food other than health functional food. One of the subclassifications of the peculiar-use foodstuffs is the medical use of food whose application is confined to specific medical uses by which their definite uses are written as food for diabetes, food for specific diseases, etc.

One more available function expression notified by self-determination in conventional food is the food nutritional fact that is supported by objectively agreed upon means of scientific proof published in SCI (science citation index)-level papers, where the commercially available expressions are very restricted. An example of is the expression of sucrose uptake suppression via D-xylose, in which beneficial effects of xylose consumption on postprandial hyperglycemia in Koreans has been studied via randomized, double-blinded, crossover-designed human clinical trials (Jun et al., 2016).

20.7 Sanitation

Food and foodstuffs manufactured, preserved, and distributed should abide by the sanitation standards designated by the food hygiene law and related regulations; this regulation also applies to functional food. One of the major critical factors in the sanitation of functional food is the microbial parameters. *Coliform* bacteria, a marker of the sanitation index, and foodborne pathogens, such as *Bacillus* and *Clostridium* species, should be negative in the finished product. Except for RTC (ready to cook) food, RTE (ready to eat) functional food should be legally managed in order to ensure that sanitation factors are present. Microbial and chemical poisonous hazards should be carefully controlled according to regulations, assuring safe consumption for consumers.

Functional food mostly consists of functional ingredients; other ingredients may be needed to complete the food product and food additives are indispensable for the maintenance of quality. Hazardous chemicals not allowed to be used in functional food should be eliminated. Pathogen microbial strains also should be treated to be sterilized thoroughly enough to ensure security for consumers not to be contaminated by or exposed to them.

Raw materials that are to be combined and processed together should be managed according to the specifications that represent and ensure their quality. As for the microbial pathogens, they might be allowed to be present

Functional Food Industry

within a limit in a certain ingredient as long as such pathogens are to be sterilized during the processing operations or they do not proliferate during storage, thus inducing food poisoning. In cases of ingredients and foodstuffs containing them, the critical pathogenic microorganisms are different in origin; for example, for ingredients taken from the ground, *Bacillus subtilis* and *Clostridium perfringens* are major concerns and are difficult to sterilize by commercial methods. As for marine-origin fish, *Salmonella* may be the critical species causing foodborne pathogens.

To eliminate pathogens originating from various kinds of pathways, prolonged heat treatment can commonly be used as a sterilization method. The condition of heat treatment for sterilization depends on the environment of the foodstuffs processed, such as pH, temperature, and interaction between the ingredients incorporated in them causing the chemical reaction to produce some new compounds that may influence the quality of the food, etc.

Other than heat treatment, nonthermal methods such as high pressure, electric heat generation for a short time period; food grade cleansing agents; and radiation within limited conditions are representative of methods used. New, novel methods for the treatment of foodstuffs for sterilization by nonthermal means are currently being researched.

The first contamination originating from raw materials can be effectively eliminated from the foodstuffs treated. Another critical point to deal with pathogenic microorganisms is to protect the sterilized foodstuffs from secondary contamination that might result from the processing environment. Chemical poisoning, including agricultural chemicals, heavy metals, antibiotics, and new chemicals generated from the reaction during processing, should be regulated by appropriate methods do as not to be transferred to the finished foodstuffs. If it is impossible to perfectly eliminate those chemicals in foodstuffs, the residual permission limit is designated from case to case on the basis of elaborate safety assessment by the Ministry of Food and Drug Safety.

As for the overall process to produce functional food, GMP (good manufacturing practice) facilities, modified to apply to functional food rather than medicinal drugs, are (Moon et al., 2008). HACCP (hazard analysis and critical control points) management and operation also are available to regulate and guarantee the sanitation of the food, which is item based.

20.8 Conclusion

Korean industrial food research, development, processing, and communication are closely related to the regulatory system, which influences overall production as well as designing the food. The terminology "functional food" in Korea is not legal, but rather, conceptual. Functional food in Korea can be defined as a food category whose health benefit can be legally claimed by seeking appropriate permission procedures by the Korean government.

Korean functional food that claims health benefits is classified along two tracks. One is the conventional food with partial claims about its function; it is supported by scientific proof without preapproval by government. The other is health functional food totally preapproved by the government before its commercial usage.

Apart from conventional food, a new category of health functional food in Korea has been developed since 2004, when the regulatory basis called health functional food law came into effect, approved by the Korean government. Korean health functional food is approved on an ingredient basis, in which standardization of functional ingredients is a prerequisite prior to the evaluation of the ingredients' safety and function.

The purpose of standardization is to ensure the quality constant and repeatability of the production of functional ingredients regardless of batches, ultimately guaranteeing safety and function of the ingredients developed. To prove the safety of a functional ingredient candidate before industrial use, various kinds of evaluation data are needed for the food to be judged as safe.

Experience of human intake of the ingredient, including historical records and scientific documents relating to the manufacturing procedure, application, and dose of daily intake, is the prerequisite for the safety evidence. Exposure assessments sometimes are needed to prove the safety of a certain ingredient due to the possibility for the same ingredient to be incorporated in various kinds of food. Ultimately, the toxicity data elucidated by GLP-based experiments are required if needed.

To support the function of the food, biomarkers representing the function evaluated must be established prior to revealing the function of ingredients, where they must be scientifically consistent enough to explain the *in vitro*, *in vivo*, and human clinical trials, where the human clinical experimental design should meet the ICH GCP guideline.

The completed functional ingredients proved to be safe are ready to be used in the finished product of health and functional foods with various kinds of shapes and formulae. The maintenance of the standardized markers incorporated in the foodstuff is technically most crucial as well as meeting the sanitary requirements imposed on the food.

Manufactured, preserved, and distributed food and foodstuffs should abide by the sanitation standards designated by the food hygiene law and related regulations, where this regulation also applies to functional food in Korea. One of the major factors critical in the sanitation of functional food is the microbial parameters, where *Coliform* bacteria, a marker of the sanitation index, and foodborne pathogens such as *Bacillus* and *Clostridium* species should be negative in the finished product.

To eliminate the pathogens originating from various pathways, prolonged heat treatment can be used as a sterilization method. The condition of heat treatment for sterilization depends on the environment of the foodstuffs

Functional Food Industry

processed, such as pH, temperature, and interaction between the ingredients incorporated in them that is causing the chemical reaction to produce some new compounds that may influence the quality of the food, and so forth.

Other than heat treatment, nonthermal methods such as high pressure, electric heat generation over a short time period, food grade cleansing agents, and radiation within the limited conditions are representative methods developed. New, novel methods for the treatment of foodstuffs for sterilization by nonthermal means are currently being applied too.

Chemical poisoning, including agricultural chemicals, heavy metals, antibiotics, and new chemicals generated from the reaction during processing, should be regulated by appropriate methods.

References

Gwak, N.S., E.J. Kim, and Y.R. Kim. 2007. *A study on the definition of health functional food, scope of functionality, labeling and advertisement.* Administration of Food and Drug Safety.

Jun, Y.J., J.H. Lee, S.H. Hwang et al. 2016. Beneficial effect of xylose consumption on postprandial hyperglycemia in Korean: A randomized double-blind, crossover design. *Trials* 17:139–146.

Koh, J.H., K.M. Kim, S.M. Kim et al. 2011. Fermentation. Bomungak.

Kwak, J.H., J.K. Baek, H.I. Kim et al. 2012. Dietary treatment with rice containing resistant starch improves markers of endothelial function with reduction of postprandial blood glucose and oxidative stress in patients with prediabetes or newly diagnosed type 2 diabetes. *Atherosclerosis* 224:457–464.

Kwak, J.H., M.S. Kim, J.H. Lee et al. 2013. Beneficial effect of tagatose consumption on postprandial hyperglycemia in Koreans: A double-blind crossover designed study. *Food & Function* 4:1223–1228.

Moon, J.S. and C.S. Lee, 2008. Development on the general standard book and training program for the extension and globalization of good manufacturing practice (GMP). Korea Health Industry Development Institute.

Park, S.H. 2010. Metabolomics in disease diagnosis and drug toxicity assessment examples in hepatobiliary cancer and cisplatin toxicity. Korean Society of Applied Pharmacology.

Wang, D.I.C., C.L. Cooney, A.L. Demain et al. 1979. *Fermentation & Enzyme Technology,* New York: John Wiley & Sons, Inc.

Yang, J.H. and U.S. Kim. 2008. *Study on the model establishment of shelf-life for health functional food.* Administration of Food and Drug Safety.

21

Regulations of Korean Functional Foods

Ji Yeon Kim and Yeonkyung Lee

CONTENTS

21.1 Introduction 523
21.2 HFF Act and Its Subordinate Regulation—Legislation
  and Amendments 524
21.3 Ingredients for HFFs 526
  21.3.1 Nutrients 527
  21.3.2 Generic Functional Ingredients 529
  21.3.3 Product-Specific Functional Ingredients 531
21.4 Functional Ingredient/Product Approval 531
  21.4.1 Evaluation Process 531
  21.4.2 Standardization 531
  21.4.3 Safety Evaluation 533
  21.4.4 Efficacy Evaluation 534
  21.4.5 Specification Evaluation 535
21.5 Health Claims 535
21.6 Advertisement for HFFs 537
21.7 Management for Manufacturer 537
21.8 Postmarket Surveillance 537
References 537

21.1 Introduction

Since the late 1990s, the average life expectancy has been increasing and the prevalence of chronic diseases, including diabetes, cardiovascular disease, and cancer, will continue to rise. These worrying trends have compelled researchers to focus efforts on the identification of potentially useful bioactive components in food, and the relationship between diet and health has been receiving greater media attention. As a result, there have been rapid advances in scientific knowledge supporting the physiological role of food in health and disease. The increasing amount of public information available regarding the health benefits of foods has resulted in consumer interest in health issues becoming a major factor in purchasing decisions. Therefore, the labeling and advertising of products claiming health benefits have become the subject of regulations in order to avoid misunderstanding and exaggeration.

The need to protect consumers and ensure their right to accurate information on food functionality has led to strict labeling requirements for functional foods and dietary supplements in many nations since the 1990s, including the United States, Japan, and the European Union. The Health/Functional Food Act (HFFA) introduced in Korea in 2002 initially regulated only the supplement forms of health/functional foods (HFFs). The definition of HFF was then further expanded into various kinds of processed foods in a subsequent revision. Before the HFFAs, there were no ways to develop efficient brand product lines and marketing strategies regarding health issues and food ingredients in the perspective of industry. As for consumers, they were unable to assess the functionality of food products and easily misled by marketing and advertising.

This chapter deals with the scope of functional food regulations, the strength of evidence required for their efficacy, safety considerations, and future perspectives in Korea.

21.2 HFF Act and Its Subordinate Regulation—Legislation and Amendments

The Korean Health and Welfare Committee of the National Assembly proposed the HFFA in November 2000. In August 2002, the HFFA was enacted as a new regulatory framework for the safety, efficacy, and labeling of HFFs, and it went into effect starting January 2004. The ultimate goal of the act was to enhance public health by ensuring the safety of new bioactive ingredients. In 2004, the law defined HFFs as "food supplements such as pills, tablets, capsules and liquids"; in other words, conventional foods were not permitted to make any such claims. However, with increasing pressure from the food industry, after 2008 the definition of HFF was broadly expanded to encompass all types of processed foods. Now, HFFs are defined as "food manufactured or processed with ingredients or components that possess functionality useful for the human body." However, foods for special dietary usage remain under different regulations according to food hygiene laws (Figure 21.1) (MFDS, 2016a).

HFFs are divided into generic and product-specific HFFs according to the classification of functional ingredients. Generic HFFs are defined as products with generic ingredients that are functional ingredients as listed by the Ministry of Food and Drug Safety (MFDS). These products include vitamins, minerals, and various other functional compounds. All new ingredients that are not generic ingredients are subjected to efficacy evaluation before launch, on the basis of their ingredients or physiologically active components, to ensure accuracy

	Food	Health functional food
Act	Food sanitation act	Health functional food act
License		
- Manufacturer	O	O
- Importer	O	O
- Seller	X	O
Administrative disposition (punishment)	Weak	Strong (deceptive advertising)
Type	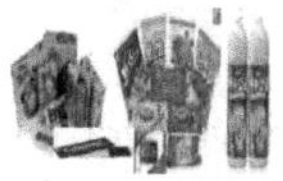	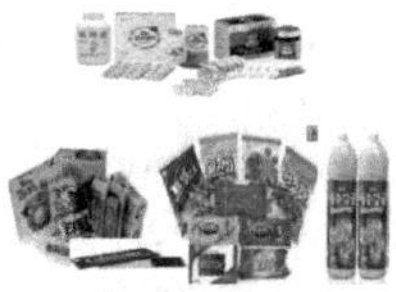
Others		Adverse event reporting mark (logo) for HFFs

FIGURE 21.1
Regulatory status of health functional foods compared to conventional foods.

of the health claims. Authorization is granted on a product-by-product basis by issuing a certificate without regulatory amendments. The HFFA does not define what constitutes "substantiation" for a claim made for an HFF. Instead, it gives the MFDS the exclusive authority to evaluate the safety and efficacy of HFFs prior to their introduction to the market, and it also keeps manufacturers and distributors responsible for providing all evidence regarding the advertised claims of their products, by developing a system for substantiation of claims or relying on existing information.

In 2004, when HFFA came into effect, there were 37 generic functional ingredients available, including 13 vitamins, 11 minerals, essential amino acids, proteins, dietary fiber, and essential fatty acids (MFDS, 2008a). The MFDS listed these generic HFFs in an HFF code. The categories were nutritional supplements, health supplements, and ginseng products; however, the HFFA at that time did not require scientific evaluation for functional claims. In other words, the list of HFF code in 2004 includes ingredients that have enough scientific evidence and ingredients that do not have enough evidence. Therefore, in order to balance with product-specific HFFs and meet the basic outline of the HFFA, a reevaluation of generic HFFs was needed. Based on these needs, from 2003 to 2007, the MFDS reevaluated the 37 generic HFFs for scientific substantiation of their claims. As a result, several generic HFFs, including royal jelly, yeast, bee pollen, digestive enzymes, turtles, and eels, were eliminated from the HFF category. These products were recategorized as conventional foods, which are not able to bear health claims (MFDS, 2010).

In 2015, MFDS created a plan to reevaluate functional ingredients because scientific evidence for efficacy and safety was gathered continuously.

According to the plan, they consider the various information, including adverse event analysis results, and select subjects for reevaluation.

21.3 Ingredients for HFFs

Ingredients used for HFFs comprise three kinds: nutrients, functional ingredients, and other ingredients (Figure 21.2). Nutrients mean ingredients to replenish deficiency, which can have occurred in diet, and include vitamins, minerals, dietary fiber, protein, and essential fatty acids. Functional ingredients mean substances to provide health benefits in products and are divided into generic functional ingredients and product-specific functional ingredients. Functional ingredients should be a substance providing health benefits and fall under any of the following: (a) processed raw material originating from animal, plant, or microorganism as it is; (b) extract or purified substance of any ingredient described in (a); (c) synthetic substance of purified substance of any ingredient described in (b); or (d) combinational substance of any ingredient described in (a), (b), or (c). The functional ingredients should also be specified by the standards and specifications of each functional ingredient of the code; or recognized under Article 15 of the Health

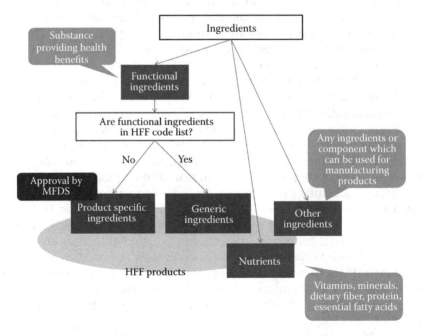

FIGURE 21.2
Ingredients for HFFs.

Regulations of Korean Functional Foods   527

Functional Food Act and Regulation on Approval of Functional Ingredient for Health Functional Food. In this case, only the business person who obtains the certificate can use it. Other ingredients are any ingredients that can be used for the manufacturing process such as excipients and flavors. They should be listed in the food additive code or be approved as food ingredients. HFF products can have nutrients or functional ingredients or both.

All ingredients can be used alone or together: nutrients and nutrients or nutrients and functional ingredients can be mixed for finished products, and their claims can be used together for finished products, too.

21.3.1 Nutrients

Nutrients in the HFF code include 14 vitamins, 11 minerals, dietary fiber, protein, and essential fatty acids (Table 21.1). All nutrients' ingredients should be listed in food additive code or be approved as food ingredients. The health functional foods with vitamins and/or minerals as functional ingredients are intended for use in supplementing the daily diet with vitamins and/or minerals. Therefore, these products neither substitute for a meal nor supplement other ingredients. The health functional foods with vitamins and/or minerals as functional ingredients should be manufactured in forms such as capsules, tablets, powders, granules, liquids or pills, etc. that are designed to be taken in measured, small-unit quantities but not in a conventional food form.

The health functional foods with vitamins and/or minerals as functional ingredients may contain all vitamins and minerals that comply with the code, a single vitamin and/or mineral, or an appropriate combination of vitamins and/or minerals. For vitamins and minerals, nutrient function claims and daily intake levels for individual nutrients are managed by MFDS and listed in the HFF code. Claims should be based on current, university-level nutritional texts as a source of evidence, and the review for nutrient function claims is led by the government. In terms of daily intake levels, minimum values of nutrients are 30% of nutrient reference value (NRV) and maximum values are given considering the safety of individual nutrients. Minimum values are compulsory, but maximum values are recommended (Table 21.1).

When a certain health functional product specifies the intended age group for consumption, the minimum level of each vitamin and/or mineral should be 30% of the intake levels recommended by the Korean dietary reference intakes for that particular age group. When there are more than two recommended intake levels for an age group, the higher level should be used. In the case when a certain health functional food contains vitamins and/or minerals at 30% or more of nutrient reference value, those vitamins and/or minerals should be presented in nutrition facts. However, it is not compulsory to describe all health claims of each nutrient (nutrient function claim) on the label. The sources or chemical forms of vitamins and minerals that are allowed in the manufacture or processing of health functional foods is listed

TABLE 21.1

Minimum and Maximum Daily Dose Levels of Nutrients

Nutrients		Daily Dose
Vitamins	Vitamin A	210~1,000 mcgRE
	Beta-carotene	–0.42~7 mg (processed oil that contains beta-carotene, which is extracted from algae, green plants, or carrot or syn.)
		–1.26 mg–no max (food ingredients that contain beta-carotene through grinding or water/fermented ethanol extraction)
	Vitamin D	1.5~10 mcg
	Vitamin E	3.3~400 mg alpha TE
	Vitamin K	21~1000 mcg
	Vitamin B1	0.36~100 mg
	Vitamin B2	0.42~40 mg
	Niacin	4.5~23 mg (nicotinic acid); 4.5~670 mg (nicotinamide)
	Pantothenic acid	1.5~200 mg
	Vitamin B6	0.45~67 mg
	Folic acid	120~400 mcg
	Vitamin B12	0.72~2000 mcg
	Biotin	9~900 mcg
	Vitamin C	30~1000 mg
Minerals	Calcium	210~800 mg
	Magnesium	94.5~250 mg
	Iron	3.6~15 mg
	Zinc	2.55~12 mg
	Copper	0.24~7.0 mg
	Selenium	16.5~135 mcg
	Iodine	45~150 mcg
	Manganese	0.9~3.5 mg
	Molybdenum	7.5~230 mcg
	Potassium	1.05~3.7g
	Chromium	0.015~9 mg
Dietary fiber		5 g or more as dietary fiber
Protein		12 g or more as protein
Fatty acid		4.0 g or more as linoleic acid or 0.6 g or more as linolenic acid

in the code. The purity criteria or specifications for each source of vitamins and/or minerals should conform with the food code or the food additive code.

Dietary fiber and essential fatty acids in nutrient categories are ingredients for the supplementation. With this point, they can be distinguished from functional dietary fiber and functional fatty acid ingredients in the functional ingredients category.

21.3.2 Generic Functional Ingredients

Functional ingredients are divided into generic functional ingredients and product-specific functional ingredients. Generic functional ingredients are listed in the HFF code by MFDS and can be used by anyone who has HFF business licenses, if their products are acceptable to standards and specifications in the HFF code. However, the number of generic functional ingredients in the HFF code is limited, so a new channel for ingredients that are not listed is required. When the new developed ingredient is needed to use for HFFs, the new ingredient can be registered from MFDS as a product-specific ingredient. When 6 years have passed after the correct registration and 50 products or more have been launched in the market, product-specific ingredients can be converted to generic ingredients by MFDS, because they can now be considered a general ingredient in the market.

The HFF code lists 67 generic functional ingredients including 14 functional dietary fibers. For example, functional dietary fibers such as Arabic gum and oat fiber have specific functions with dietary fiber besides dietary fiber supplements (Table 21.2).

In the HFF code, the standards and specifications for each generic functional ingredient are presented by MFDS. All information of ingredients such as the raw material, manufacturing process, information of marker compounds, specifications of contaminants, claims, and daily values are included.

TABLE 21.2

Functional Ingredients and Functional Dietary Fibers Listed in HFF Code

Function	Ingredients
Functional Ingredients	
Improvement of immunity	Ginseng, red ginseng, chlorella, aloe gel, alkoxyglycerol, *Phellinus linteus* extract
Recovery from fatigue	Ginseng, red ginseng, Japanese apricot extract
Blood circulation	Red ginseng, GLA, EPA/DHA, reishi fruit body extract, ginkgo leaf extract
Blood cholesterol	*Chlorella*, *Spirulina*, green tea extract, GLA, lecithin, phytosterol/phytosterol ester, chitosan/chito-oligosaccharide, red rice yeast, soy protein, garlic powder
Blood pressure	Coenzyme Q10
Blood triglyceride	EPA/DHA
Blood glucose	Guava leaf extract, banana leaf extract, evening primrose seed extract
Improvement of memory	Red ginseng, ginkgo leaf extract, EPA/DHA
Antioxidant	Red ginseng, plants containing chlorophyll, *Chlorella*, *Spirulina*, green tea extracts, propolis, coenzyme Q10, squalene, tomato extract

(Continued)

TABLE 21.2 (CONTINUED)

Functional Ingredients and Functional Dietary Fibers Listed in HFF Code

Function	Ingredients
Skin health (including skin moisture, hypersensitive skin)	Plants containing chlorophyll, *Chlorella*, *Spirulina*, phosphatidylserine, *N*-acetyl glucosamine, aloe gel, hyaluronic acid, konjac potato extract, GLA
Body fat reduction	Green tea extract, CLA, *Garcinia cambogia* extract, chitosan/chito-oligosaccharide
Intestine health (including bowel function, improvement of beneficial flora/ suppression of harmful flora)	Aloe gel, aloe leaf, probiotics, fructo-oligosaccharide, raffinose, agar
Joint/cartilage	Glucosamine, *N*-acetyl glucosamine, mucopolysscharide/protein, MSM
Bone health	Soy isoflavone
Stress relaxation	Milk protein hydrolysates, *Rhodiola* extract, theanine
Eye health (including fatigue, yellow pigment density, etc.)	Lutein, *Haematococcus* extract, bilberry extract
Liver health	Milk thistle
Prostate health	Saw palmetto fruit extract
Calcium absorption	Fructo-oligosaccharide, poly-gamma-glutamic acid
Cognitive function	Phosphatidylserine
Menopause	Red ginseng
Antibiotic activity of oral cavity	Propolis
PMS	GLA
Enhancement of endurance during exercise	Octacosanol
Exercise performance improvement during muscle training	Creatine
Functional Dietary Fibers	
Blood cholesterol	Guar gum/guar gum hydrolyte, glucomannan, oat, soy fiber, corn bran, inulin/chicory extract, psyllium husk
Blood glucose	Guar gum/guar gum hydrolyte, oat, digestion-resistant maltodextrin, soy fiber, wheat fiber, corn bran, inulin/chicory extract, seed of *Trigonella foenum-graecum*
Bowel movement	Guar gum/guar gum hydrolyte, glucomannan, digestion-resistant maltodextrin, soy fiber, *Auricularia auricula-judae*, wheat fiber, barley fiber, Arabic gum, inulin/chicory extract, psyllium husk, polydextrose
Gastrointestinal bacteria improvement (improvement of beneficial flora/ suppression of harmful flora)	Guar gum/guar gum hydrolyte
Blood triglyceride	Digestion-resistant maltodextrin

Regulations of Korean Functional Foods 531

21.3.3 Product-Specific Functional Ingredients

When manufacturers or distributors want to launch a product, including new functional ingredients not included in the list of HFF codes, they should register their ingredient as a functional ingredient. The product-specific ingredient registration was based on scientific evidence prepared by industries, so manufacturers or distributors should submit evidence of the standardization, safety, and efficacy of the ingredient to MFDS. Only the industry (business licenser) that has submitted to MFDS has the right to use the ingredient and claim from MFDS. Even if it is the same ingredient, each licenser should go through a registration process.

Product-specific functional ingredients can be converted to generic functional ingredients after the qualification, including the number of products in market and elapsed time.

21.4 Functional Ingredient/Product Approval

21.4.1 Evaluation Process

As a route for new ingredient registration, MFDS has a product-specific ingredients/products registration process. According to the "Regulation on HFF Functional Ingredients/Products Registration," MFDS reviews the standardization, safety, and efficacy of ingredients and products. To register a new ingredient that is not listed in the HFF code, 120 working days will be needed. If manufacturers or distributors want to register the finished product with generic functional ingredients or product-specific ingredients that are already registered, 90 working days will be needed. However, if manufacturers or distributors want to revise the daily intake level and manufacturing standardization of registered functional ingredients, or if they want to add claims on it, 60 working days are required.

In the evaluation process, MFDS can request advice from advisory committees for HFFs. The advisory committees for functional ingredient/product registration comprise 20~30 experts with backgrounds in nutrition, food technology and medicine.

The principle of MFDS review is the balanced satisfaction of standardization, safety, and efficacy. They should be considered together for the evaluation (Figure 21.3).

21.4.2 Standardization

The importance of standardization cannot be overlooked in the process of ingredient/product development. However, if standardization is not achieved and homogeneous ingredients/products cannot be manufactured,

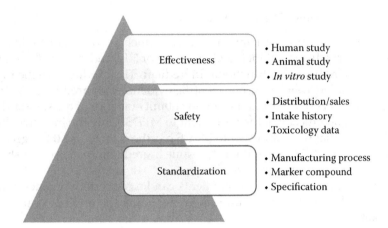

FIGURE 21.3
The principles of MFDS review for functional ingredients.

safety and efficacy cannot be achieved. With this perspective, the basis of evaluation can be standardization.

Standardization documents, including the raw material information (scientific name, part, origin, etc.) and manufacturing process (yield and change in content of functional/marker compounds) are essential details for understanding properties of ingredients/products (Figure 21.4). The production of a preparation should be consistent in terms of chemical composition and effectiveness.

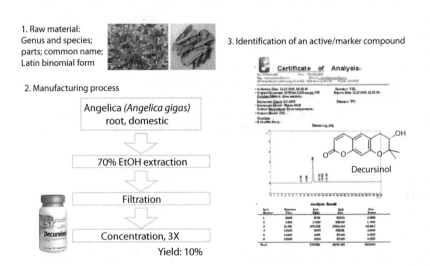

FIGURE 21.4
Examples for standardization.

Regulations of Korean Functional Foods

21.4.3 Safety Evaluation

Safety documents include the history of use, side effects and toxicity of ingredients in the released scientific data, consumption quantity, nutritional impact, bioavailability data, and toxicity tests (Figure 21.5). The decision tree for safety documents has been presented by MFDS. Standards of decision trees are properties of raw material, manufacturing process of ingredients, and exposure assessments. In other words, requirements of safety documents can be different for properties of raw materials, manufacturing process of ingredients, and exposure levels. If the ingredient is nearly a raw material itself, if it is used generally, if the usual exposure level is similar to

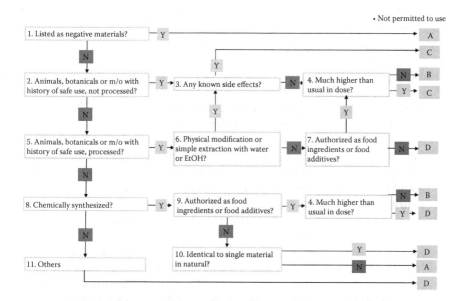

FIGURE 21.5
Decision tree of safety documents.

534

the daily intake suggested by the applicant, required documents are general level to confirm the safety in ordinary use. However, if the ingredient is not used or if the exposure level is lower than the daily intake suggested by the applicant, toxicological data, if necessary even reproductive toxicity data, can be required (MFDS, 2016b).

21.4.4 Efficacy Evaluation

Efficacy evaluation for HFFs is conducted based on scientific evidence. This process is called evidence-based evaluation, and it is used for health claims on foods in global markets, including Korea. Scientific evidence that can support health claims for foods should not rely on a single scientific opinion or experts' experiences in small groups.

To evaluate the efficacy documents for HFFs provided from applicants, MFDS reviews individual studies as well as the totality of work. In other words, the process of efficacy evaluation is as follows:

- Evaluation of individual studies: The first evaluation point is the research type. Human studies are considered competent and reliable scientific evidence to substantiate a health claim for foods. Especially, randomized, double-blind, parallel-group, placebo-controlled intervention studies are considered the gold standard. Other types of research, including animal and *in vitro* studies, can be considered as supporting data to explain the activity or its mechanism that is shown in human studies. Secondary analysis research, including meta-analysis and review articles, would be considered background information. The reason why human studies are required is that consumers can get the information of efficacy and expect efficacy from the health claim on the food. For the same reason, the manner of intake in research should be the same as that required by the actual product. Therefore, research using intravenous injection can be excluded. The second evaluation point for individual studies is the quality of study. Study population, data collection, outcome measures, statistical analysis, and confounding variables can be considered as factors relevant to the scientific quality of individual studies.
- Evaluation of totality: After review and evaluation of individual studies, the totality should be evaluated. In the context of all available information, the result and quality of individual studies should be considered. If there is one low-quality study with a positive result and two high-quality studies with negative results, how should the health claim be handled? Are they enough, or not? To answer the question, totality based on quantity, consistency, and relevance should be evaluated. MFDS has introduced an evidence-based

Regulations of Korean Functional Foods

rating system, which is determined according to the type and quality of individual studies, as well as the quantity, consistency, and relevance of all studies.

In the review and approval of functional ingredients for HFFs, daily dose is one of the important factors. Daily dose for functional ingredients is provided considering both the safety and the efficacy. In other words, the daily dose should be considered in the range of a safe dose. If the range of safe dose is lower than efficacy dose and is supported by human studies, approval is not possible (MFDS, 2008b).

21.4.5 Specification Evaluation

Specifications are important to homogeneous approved ingredients/products with documents for standardization. For the evaluation, the applicant should submit documentation regarding the analytical method for functional/marker compounds, with samples. The analytical method should be validated from the point of selectivity, precision, accuracy, linearity, and range of the method. In addition to functional/marker compounds, the specification of contaminants such as heavy metals, coliforms, and mycotoxins, if necessary, should be suggested by applicants. MFDS reviews whether specifications suggested by applicants are acceptable and have enough scientific evidence or not.

21.5 Health Claims

Claims regarding prevention or cure of specific diseases and misleading consumers about HFFs as drugs are prohibited. Claims for HFFs comprise three types:

- Nutrient function claims: These claims describe the physiological role of the nutrient in the growth, development, and normal functions of the body. Such claims apply to the nutrients, which have their own recommended daily allowance (RDA) and must be based on current, university-level nutrition texts as a source of evidence. For example, "Calcium is necessary for formation of bone and teeth" and "Folic acid is necessary for normal growth of the fetus neural tube" are nutrient function claims.
- Bioactive function claims: These claims concern specific beneficial effects of HFFs on normal functions or biological activities of the body in the context of the total diet. Such claims relate to positive contributions toward health, the specific improvement of a function, or to the modification or preservation of health. For example, "Red

ginseng may help to improve immunity" and "Glucosamine may help the health of joints and cartilage" are bioactive function claims.

- Reduction of disease risk claims: These claims describe the relationship between the consumption of HFFs (in the context of the total diet) and the reduced risk of developing a disease or health-related condition. For example, "Calcium helps to reduce the risk of osteoporosis" is a reduction of disease risk claim.

There were three classes in bioactive function claims according to the level of scientific evidence by 2016. If the strength of scientific evidence is convincing, bioactive function claims, class I, can be applied. If the strength of scientific evidence is not sufficient—for example, in the case that appropriate human clinical studies have not been conducted—bioactive function claims, class III, can be applied. According to the grade, the expression is different. The products of class I can claim that they "can have a beneficial effect on…", but the products of class III should claim that they "may improve…, but the scientific evidence is insufficient." (Table 21.3). After 2013, MFDS recognized that a lot of consumers could not understand the difference between classes. Even if these classes indicated the strength of scientific evidence, consumers were considering classes as grades of product quality or the strength of the health benefit. As a result, MFDS has decided that class information of functional ingredients is not necessary for consumers and industries. The regulations on functional ingredients classes were revised in 2016.

The principle and structure in health claims for HFFs are similar to Codex and US regulations (CCFL, 2004; FDA, 2013). Claims for prevention and cure are prohibited for foods globally; claims for foods and supplements are usually divided into nutrient function claims, reduction of disease risk claims, and bioactive function claims. The bioactive function claim is relevant to other function claims of Codex and structure function claims of the United States. The different point is the management; some countries are managing by industries; others are requiring approvals from government.

In Korea, there is no limitation to getting an approval of claims unless the claim is about sexual behaviors, hallucination, arousal, etc. These prohibited claims are not relevant to public health.

TABLE 21.3

Bioactive Function Claims and Reduction of Disease Risk Claims for HFFs

Type of Claim	Level of Scientific Evidence	Available Statement
Reduction of disease risk	Significant scientific agreement	"…is help to reduce the risk of… (disease)"
Bioactive function	Emerging evidence	"…may improve…" "…may increase (decrease)…"

21.6 Advertisement for HFFs

All labels and advertisements for HFFs should be reviewed in advance by an authorized institution from MFDS. The Korea Health Supplement Association (KHSA) is one of the authorized institutions from MFDS. For prereview, the approval of the advisory committees for HFFs is required. The advisory committees for advertisement prereview comprise about 20 experts in nutrition, food technology, medicine, consumer protection, and advertisement backgrounds.

21.7 Management for Manufacturer

When the regulation of HFFs was legislated, the supplement industry was quite small. Therefore, industries could not follow the regulation even if MFDS wanted to manage the manufacturer with a high-level regulation. However, the supplement industry has grown in the aspects of market size, research funds, trade scale, etc. Therefore, MFDS has decided to change over the GMP requirements to be mandatory.

21.8 Postmarket Surveillance

For HFFs, MFDS has collected all cases estimated as adverse events via various routes, including experts (medical doctors, pharmacists, etc.), consumer agencies, and industries. The difference from other countries is the severity of reported cases. In other countries, severe cases such as operations, hospitalizations, and death are required, whereas all cases should be reported and the analysis of adverse events be conducted in the authorized institution from MFDS. They analyze the relevance between the symptoms of adverse events and ingredients. If the result is significant, MFDS can take actions such as urgent recall, prohibition of sale, and addition of warning labels.

References

CCFL. 2004. Codex guidelines for use of nutritional and health claims.
FDA. 2013. Guidance for industry: A food labeling guide. Washington, DC: Food Drug and Administration.

MFDS. 2008a. The past, the present and the future of health functional foods. Korea: Ministry of Food and Drug Safety.

MFDS. 2008b. The efficacy evaluation on health functional foods. Korea: Ministry of Food and Drug Safety.

MFDS. 2010. Food code. Korea: Ministry of Food and Drug Safety.

MFDS. 2016a. Health/Functional Food Act. Korea: Ministry of Food and Drug Safety.

MFDS. 2016b. Regulations on the premarket approvals of functional ingredients of product-specific health/functional food and food type health food (prenotice), no. 2016-715. Korea: Ministry of Food and Drug Safety.

22

Future of Functional Foods in Korea

Ki Won Lee, Jong Hun Kim, Sanguine Byun, and Jong-Eun Kim

CONTENTS

22.1 Change in Demand for Functional Foods 539
  22.1.1 Growing Demands for Functional Foods Attributed
    to the Aging Population 539
  22.1.2 Growing Interests in Quality of Life due to Increased
    Income 540
  22.1.3 Demands for Functional Foods Catering to Personal Needs... 540
22.2 Limitations on Functional Foods 541
  22.2.1 Regulations on Functional Foods 541
  22.2.2 Public Perception of Health Functional Food 543
22.3 Prospects for the Future of Health Functional Foods 544
  22.3.1 Development of Functional Foods through the Scientific
    Approach 544
  22.3.2 Development of Functional Foods through Scientific
    Convergence 546
  22.3.3 Development of Functional Foods in the Era of the
    Fourth Industrial Revolution 548
  22.3.4 Functional Foods Bracing for Social Changes 548
  22.3.5 The Sixth Industrialization of Functional Food
    under Globalization 549
  22.3.6 Raising Proper Awareness of Functional Food 549
22.4 Conclusion 550
Acknowledgments 551
References 552

22.1 Change in Demand for Functional Foods

22.1.1 Growing Demands for Functional Foods Attributed to the Aging Population

The Republic of Korea (ROK) has been witnessing a change in demographic structure attributed to the low birth rate and the rapidly aging population with life expectancy projections consistently rising. The demand for functional foods has also increased due to the increase in chronic diseases,

539

540   *Korean Functional Foods*

mainly caused by the aging population. Given this changing trend in recent years, it seems logical that people's interests would go beyond simply pursuing longevity—that they would also seek to live a healthy and dignified life. To that end, the concept of disease prevention has been in the limelight and focuses on maintaining a healthy state in order to reduce the possibility of acquiring diseases, instead of seeking medical help after the fact. Thus, functional foods, which target the elderly, are expected to gain momentum along with the rising demand for food markets catering to the needs of the elderly in the future, as illustrated by antiaging food products and the demand for living a long and healthy life.

22.1.2 Growing Interests in Quality of Life due to Increased Income

Income levels are closely related to the quality of one's life. Other factors affecting the quality of life include health, leisure time, and environment, along with the economic factors. Those factors, without exception, are firmly based on the income required for meeting our basic needs of clothes, food, and housing and improving our living standard. Therefore, the enhanced level of income naturally leads people to turn their focus toward increasing their quality of life.

In fact, the Korea Statistical Yearbook from Statistics Korea (2015) suggests that the domestic income level has been steadily rising. Gross national income (GNI) already surpassed $10,000 in 2000 at $11,865, reaching the $20,000 threshold in 2006 at $20,823, and peaked at $27,339 in 2015 (Economic Statistics System of the Bank of Korea, 2016).

As the income level in Korea has improved, thanks in part to its economic success and social development, the general public has become increasingly interested in enhancing the quality of life. While Koreans strive to enhance the level of health and happiness at the individual level, various policies—designed to improve public welfare—have been implemented at the state level. In particular, the growing interests in individual health have played a huge role in spreading a trend toward well-being, which led to a boost in the demand for functional foods (Korea Institute for Health and Social Affairs, 2007).

22.1.3 Demands for Functional Foods Catering to Personal Needs

The area of bioengineering has undergone rapid development in recent years. It was confirmed that various diseases occurred as a result of abnormalities in the function and the structure of genes ever since the genetic functions and structures were unveiled. The Human Genome Project, with the objective of determining the DNA sequence of the entire human genome, was declared completed in 2003 (Hong, 2007). Ever since the sequencing of the human genome, expectations have been growing regarding the possibility of preventing or curing diseases. Especially, there have been increasing attempts

Future of Functional Foods in Korea

to utilize the unique genetic characteristics of individuals to prevent, discover, diagnose, and treat diseases and manage health. The ability to predict the risk of occurrences, prognosis of diseases, and possibility of recurrences, based on individual genetic information, prompted the shift from a treatment-oriented approach to a prevention-centered one (Jeong et al., 2015). In the future, therefore, there will be more foods put on the table that cater to individual needs—food products that provide the benefits of medical treatment, reflect an individual's constitution, and help prevent certain diseases.

However, there is a big difference in how human bodies react to the same food due to variances in individuals' metabolism caused by genetic differences. Despite these distinct differences, people have been pushed toward standardized nutrition and food without considering their individual genetic differences. Therefore, we should develop foods catering to unique individual needs that consider an individual's constitution and help prevent specific diseases, as opposed to merely developing foods for nonspecific populations. The completion of the Human Genome Project made it possible to provide a specific nutrition plan and foods tailored to each individual's needs through genetic testing. In other words, food catering to genetic information can be designed in the future. Individually tailored functional foods can also be developed to deter the occurrence of diseases and ensure their prevention (National Law Information Center, 2017).

22.2 Limitations on Functional Foods

22.2.1 Regulations on Functional Foods

Functional foods in Korea can be divided largely into two categories: the first is general food—often referred to as "healthy food"; the second is the health functional food, which was legally approved by the Ministry of Food and Drug Safety (hereinafter referred to as MFDS). The regulation of health functional food, the purpose of which must be indicated on its label, has been more strictly managed and supervised than for general healthy food. However, not all of the foods categorized as functional foods are officially certified as functional foods. Therefore, it is essential to distinguish general health food from health functional food.

The current Health Functional Food Act (hereinafter referred to as the Act) stipulates that health functional food indicates food manufactured and processed with raw materials and ingredients that provide health benefits to the human body (National Law Information Center, 2017). The Act also decrees that the term "functionality" means controlling nutrients for the structure or functions of the human body or providing beneficial effects for health purposes, such as physiological effects. It is the job of the MFDS to determine and publicly announce the raw materials and ingredients in functional foods.

Only food products whose functionality is certified in accordance with the Act can be labeled as "health functional food" and be eligible for sales with an emphasis on its functionality. The production and distribution history is tracked to record and manage information at every level from manufacturing to sales through a process of "tracking the management of records on functional health foods" as stipulated by the Act. In cases when the safety of functional foods is questioned, the following steps are carried out under such a management system: examining the manufacturing and distribution history of the functional food in question, searching for problems, and taking the necessary steps to resolve any safety issues that were detected.

However, concerns have been growing regarding the need to regulate health functional foods to coincide with increases in the size of the health functional foods market. There are two competing sides on the regulation on health functional foods; one side argues for deregulation for the sake of boosting the health functional food market and the other makes the case for a regulation, claiming that deregulation might confuse consumers. Although this controversy became heated in 2016 during the process of implementing a deregulation policy, the MFDS fully approved 15 proposals and partially approved five proposals out of the 34 regulation revisions recommended by relevant industries, declaring a de facto deregulation on health functional foods. The steps taken by the MFDS have left many wondering whether this lenient decision weakens its legal effectiveness.

A newly implemented regulation that features some differences from the existing one states that an addition of roughly 50 functional raw materials are eligible for MFDS notification, and thus the scope of functional raw materials suitable for MFDS notification has been expanded by a huge margin. The previous deliberation system for labels or advertisements regarding functionality (hereinafter referred to as the prior deliberation process) was abolished and replaced with an autonomous deliberation process. Through such measures, the health functional food market, which used to be sluggish due to unnecessary regulations, is predicted to expand, with economic benefits of as much as 340.9 billion dollars won and the creation of 750 jobs (Korea Rural Economic Institute, www.krei.re.kr/). However, over the past 4 years, as many as 2,697 reports on the side effects of health functional foods have been filed with the MFDS, with the number of reported cases totaling 136 in 2013, 1,744 in 2014, and 502 in 2015. In only the first half of 2016, 326 reports on side effects from health functional foods were filed with the MFDS—65% of the reports filed in 2015 (Ministry of Food and Drug Safety, 2016).

According to the Act, the rights for determining false and exaggerated advertisements under the prior deliberation process are to be comprehensively delegated to a deliberation committee on functionality labels or advertisements (hereinafter referred to as "deliberation committee"). Its members consist of stakeholders from relevant industries, which makes it hard to guarantee fair assessments and objective deliberations. Such concerns have been well evidenced using the following examples: 1,349 cases were reported

Future of Functional Foods in Korea 543

to the MFDS as being false and exaggerated advertisements of businesses in the health functional foods market from 2010 to 2015; the MFDS demanded in 2015 that 4,403 cases out of a total of 5,551 filed for deliberation on labels or advertisements regarding functionality be revisited. Of those cases, 168 were judged ineligible to be labeled or be advertised as functional foods (Ministry of Food and Drug Safety, 2016).

Although responsibility for the safe management of health functional foods lies with the MFDS, safety management is mostly carried out by the manufacturing businesses' own quality control even without proper regulations for periodic examinations. Most of the examinations are conducted via a voluntary report generated by the manufacturing/importing businesses or reports from consumers. Therefore, it is worth considering whether deregulation under nonfunctioning management and supervision can have a positive effect on the health functional food market over the long term.

The cases stated previously are precisely the reason why consumers rarely trust the MFDS's ability to regulate the health functional food industry, which requires an enhanced level of management and supervision of health functional foods along with deregulation in the market.

22.2.2 Public Perception of Health Functional Food

Many consumers find it hard to distinguish the differences between health functional foods and general health foods due to a lack of promotion and education informing them of the differences. Thus, there have been many occurrences where people mistakenly believe that dietary supplements and general health food are equal to health functional food. There have also been many reports of side effects filed for misusing and abusing health functional foods by people fooled by some of the businesses' false, exaggerated, and negative advertisements.

The consumer awareness survey on health functional foods was conducted by the Citizens Consumer Group of the Korea National Council of Consumer Organizations (Consumerskorea, http://consumerskorea.org/), targeting 1,521 consumers aged 20 to over 60 residing in major cities including Seoul and other metropolitan cities. The survey found that 24.9% of consumers responded saying that "the false and exaggerated advertisements for the effectiveness of the products" is the biggest problem, followed by "the safety of food products" at 20.7%, and "the lack of concrete and objective proof confirming its effectiveness" at 19.6%.

Health functional foods cannot be advertised as being effective in treating diseases. In fact, according to Article 17 of the Act, warnings that health functional foods are not medicine for preventing or treating diseases must be indicated on the containers or packaging of health functional foods. Many consumers reported that they saw advertisements giving them the false impression that health functional foods are effective in treating illnesses. Therefore, it would be fair to say that the false, exaggerated, and negative advertisements have prevented consumers from recognizing the effectiveness of health functional foods in a proper way. There are also many accounts of consumers voicing their concerns over exaggerated TV home-shopping ads for health functional foods that have evoked a negative impression toward the health functional food industry.

The survey also found that the majority of consumer opinions were increasingly concentrated on the need to reinforce the health functional food system and its management, which also highlights the large number of consumers urging the government to impose tougher regulations on the system and its management. To elaborate, the most dominant view holds that the certification process for health functional foods should be stricter for proving the effectiveness of food products, followed by arguing for the need to enhance the management of raw materials and quality of foods and to strengthen the government's follow-up management.

In spite of awareness of the existence of side effects, health maintenance was cited as the biggest reason for taking health functional foods, according to the consumer survey. For such reasons, consumers naturally demand accurate information on health functional foods and what they are made of. Related industries—ready for reaping profits driven by commercial gains—are actively engaged in promoting health functional foods targeting health-conscious consumers. In contrast, public institutions and academic communities are thought to be lacking in the area of raising consumer awareness on health functional foods. Therefore, many consumers believe that proper education and thorough promotional activities should be undertaken, thereby shining a light on all kinds of functional foods, including health functional foods.

22.3 Prospects for the Future of Health Functional Foods

22.3.1 Development of Functional Foods through the Scientific Approach

As scientific technology has advanced over time, consumer awareness has also been rising, which has led to qualitative improvements in consumption habits. Various functional foods that are being distributed in the market, but are restricted by existing regulations, fall short of meeting the mounting expectations of the highly educated and informed consumers of our time. Therefore, consumer confidence regarding functional foods currently available in the market remains at a very low level.

The most fundamental reason behind the low level of consumer confidence for functional foods is the poor infrastructure in the domestic functional food industry. Most of the health functional foods in Korea are manufactured by small- and medium-sized companies. Even those sold by large conglomerates

Future of Functional Foods in Korea   545

are mostly manufactured by original equipment manufacturing (OEM) companies, roughly 95% of which are produced and distributed in very poor working conditions (Kim, 2012). Given the nature of the food industry, which requires economies of scale, tangible results can only be expected when massive amounts of capital are invested in the industry. However, the functional food industry often entices investments on a relatively smaller scale, unable to concentrate on developing new products due to a lack of investment assets and thereby manufacturing food products that lack solid scientific evidence.

Additionally, the ambiguous place in which functional food has positioned itself, between science and food, could also give consumers the unfair impression that functional foods lack rock-solid scientific grounds. While the prescriptions of licensed medical experts allow for health management and disease treatment in the fields of medical science and pharmacy, functional foods sit somewhere between medical and pharmaceutical science— unraveling the science of the human body—and the general food industry. Therefore, it seems natural for consumers to have a relatively negative perception of functional foods. Even when there is an abundance of scientific evidence behind a specific functional food available in the market, promoting the food product through a channel that lacks expertise could easily give consumers a misguided impression.

As the boundary between study and technology has become blurry, along with an advancement of scientific technology, various changes are being made not only in the production of products, but also in how people consume them. However, the domestic functional food industry does not seem to be able to keep up with the rapid pace of technological advancement. The functional food market in Korea, therefore, needs to recognize changing trends, produce the products that satisfy the demands of consumers, and develop technology that leads to the creation of new markets and new fields in the industry, moving away from simply focusing on a short-sighted strategy to secure more market share.

To that end, domestic food companies should establish firm scientific grounds for the effectiveness of functional foods by concentrating investments on building their own research and development capacities. Based on such a foundation, they should launch functional foods that have a competitive advantage in the market both at home and abroad and achieve a qualitative and technological advancement in the domestic functional food market. Large conglomerates and leading enterprises in the domestic food industry should make investments for creating new markets, rather than investing further in the already saturated general food market. They should also put forth efforts to increase the size of the market itself by investing in the promising functional food market. Such efforts can help them formulate a strategy to guarantee the permanence of businesses and maximize operating profits. An investment of this kind should be promoted so that research and development on the functional food market can be improved and sufficient scientific grounds regarding functionality can be established, which will enhance

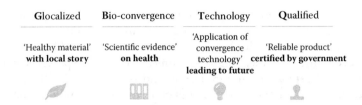

FIGURE 22.1
A model of functional foods developed through the scientific approach.

the level of consumer confidence and help achieve qualitative growth in the domestic food market over the long term (Figure 22.1).

22.3.2 Development of Functional Foods through Scientific Convergence

To overcome the image of the functional food market, which is seen as lacking in professionalism, expertise should be secured at the academic level through continuous basic research into food science, engineering, and nutritional science. At the state level, experts in the food industry should be nurtured so that firm scientific grounds can be well established, not just for general food but also for functional food.

In particular, sustainable development in bioscience technology, which is being mobilized for various fields, is projected to have a positive effect on the functional food markets. Bioscience technology is already being utilized as an essential element for developing each stage of processing, manufacturing, producing, and researching functional food products in the form of technology that refines and modifies active materials according to their physiochemical properties, technology that enables the separation of a specific material from natural materials, and bioconversion technology that enables the mass production of effective components with the use of microorganisms. Those technologies will be more actively utilized in the future when creating new markets as well as staying in line with the rising demand for functional foods, through which scientific evidence for functional foods can be established, consumer confidence can be strengthened, and the functional food market can experience qualitative growth.

Food processing technology to this day has evolved with a focus on the taste and nutrition of food products. The area of functional food, too, has emphasized purifying, separating certain materials, and discovering the functionality and efficacy in the process of developing various food ingredients. However, as the existing research has given birth to advanced scientific technology, expectations are growing high for the prospect of conducting research on functional foods that goes beyond the boundary of existing studies. For example, developments in functional food and its subsequent production will be made possible by strengthened functionality as a result of analysis done on functional materials that were extracted from natural materials, artificial ingredients that can be developed by combining the existing analysis technology—polymer synthesis technology—and various other bioscience technology advances.

There will also be more instances where the enhancement of fermentation efficiency, made possible by an analysis of the metabolic flux of microorganisms, will produce active materials within food products on a massive scale and increase the manufacturing of new ingredients. Further research into dielectric materials of food will also be conducted. Bioengineering technology that enables the mass production of high-value-added food ingredients is emerging as a promising future technology along with existing fermentation engineering using microorganisms. The development of genome sequencing and editing technology enables controlling the metabolic flux of microorganisms, which will lead to an increase in the number of cases where microorganisms function, not just as cells but also as microbial cell factories. In particular, Korea has long developed various fermented foods involving mixed fermentation processes with the use of various microorganisms, which has helped lay the foundation for storing abundant microorganism resources. Such abundant resources will become the subject for microbial metabolic engineering in the future. The characteristics of each microorganism should be analyzed, researched, and evolved into an engineered form, which can serve as tailored microbial cell factories depending on the specific need (Seo, 2008).

Engineering technology has, thus far, been advanced mainly through researchers' intuition. In the future, however, advanced omics technology, protein design technology, and bioengineering technology will control the metabolic pathways of microorganisms, help engineer microorganisms, produce food ingredients, and eventually allow their mass production in the industries of functional food and food ingredients.

Converging nanotechnology (NT) also holds significance for maximizing the effectiveness of functional foods. NT applications in the area of food products are being utilized during the producing and processing stages, rather than on the food itself. NT is also being applied in the production machinery, production method, and packaging technology. Once technological improvements have been made and regulations revised, NT can be directly applied in the components and substances of functional food itself, maximizing the absorption rate of food, controlling its effectiveness, and restricting possible toxic substances in foods.

Judging by the accounts described so far, both large conglomerates and start-up companies should expand the scope of functional foods and work together to develop a system that can help people prevent diseases and manage their health in their daily lives. Their primary concern should not be recording sales and operating profits but improving the general effectiveness of functional foods in society as a whole through health management and an improved quality of life.

22.3.3 Development of Functional Foods in the Era of the Fourth Industrial Revolution

It has become increasingly important for the food industry in its research and development process to look further outside the realm of biotechnology and combine technology from other fields, due to the Fourth Industrial Revolution, the emergence of artificial intelligence (AI), and the sustainable development of information technology (IT). From the perspective of supplying functional foods, a system can be built that enables checking the personal health status of consumers in real time and recommending and selling the functional foods that help prevent or treat various diseases with the use of AI, applications installed on smartphones, and big data technology.

Technology should evolve away from the existing approach of having consumers choose products designed for nonspecific populations to a new approach that guarantees the sustainable development of a system in which suppliers make individually tailored products for specific customer groups. Recently, various channels have been popping up to fulfill the desires of consumers in terms of service, thanks to advancements in IT and the subsequent development of kits or applications that enable self-diagnoses and management of health. Relevant stakeholders should establish a system that allows for recommending and offering consumer-specific products and storing such information in a database, as opposed to dismissing this trend as being irrelevant to their work. An algorithm derived from the analysis of the data collected could present an opportunity to predict future challenges and explore possible resolutions in advance. Furthermore, the food industry as a whole, including the functional food industry, should play a leading role in advancing convergence technology in BT and IT—not just reaping the benefits of IT—so that agile and proper responses to social trends can create high-value-added products, thereby enhancing the living standard of the general public.

22.3.4 Functional Foods Bracing for Social Changes

As with all consumer goods, the rise of the functional food market can also be interpreted and analyzed in the social context. Ever since the mid-2000s, the rapid emergence of the trend for well-being has led the development of functional food products for diet control and, specifically for Korea, the aesthetic industry for beauty management. For example, in 2012, cosmetic products and other products related to weight control, liver health, and boosting immunity were at the forefront of their market growth. In 2015, the market was dominated by products that were known to have antioxidant effects, boosted the immune system, and targeted blood circulation, fatigue, and memory, when evaluated by profits (Kim, 2012; Korea Institute for Food Safety Management Accreditation, 2016). Given the changing dynamics of social trends, the ROK is expected to join the ranks of hyperaging societies

Future of Functional Foods in Korea

with the percentage of the elderly, aged over 65, surpassing 20% of the entire population after 2026 (Statistics Korea, 2015). Products designed to help prevent the effects of aging, such as muscle degeneration, will continue to grow and technology for functional foods that allow the elderly to manage their own health should be developed in response to such social changes. As people's movement in daily life, including housework, becomes reduced thanks to increases in automation in every fabric of society, and changing lifestyles, caused by less manual labor, lead to a lack of exercise, there will be increases in the prevalence of skeletal diseases, the degeneration of muscle mass, weight increases, and obesity in the future.

Therefore, in a bid to address such concerns, there will be continuous development in functional food products—products that have been actively manufactured in recent days, contain low calories but offer high satiety (a sense of fullness), resolve nutritional imbalances, and either help managing weight or minimizing muscle loss for health-conscious customers.

22.3.5 The Sixth Industrialization of Functional Food under Globalization

Unlike other industries, where standardization is strengthened under globalization, diversity including culture, geography, and history is highlighted in the modern food industry. This is because the foreigners who experience local food are also interested in the local culture, geography, and history. The globalization of the food industry has become a chance to reexamine traditional values such as the characteristics of food culture in each country. As a result, "glocalization," which means a strategy to pursue globalization and localization at the same time, is expected to spread more in the future.

A representative approach for glocalization in Korea is the "sixth industrialization," which is linking and combining the cultivation of local agricultural products (first industry), the manufacturing processes of local agricultural products (second industry), and providing services for tourism (third industry). With the rapid growth of the wellness industry in recent years, the development of sixth industrialization in local areas of Korea will continue to accelerate and diversify. Especially for functional and medicinal agricultural products, it will be developed into a manufactured functional food linked with healing tourism such as physical therapy, horticultural therapy, etc.

22.3.6 Raising Proper Awareness of Functional Food

Today, many consumers do not distinguish among general food, functional food, and health functional food. Such terms are often considered confusing to consumers, and the differences are not properly appreciated by those who are not relevant stakeholders and policy researchers.

Creating a thriving market and boosting consumer confidence in any field of society requires consumers' increased interest and an enhanced level of education in that specific area. One of the reasons behind Korea's phenomenal success as an IT powerhouse could be its efforts to maximize the level of research and development through intensive investment and acquired technological capacity to form a competitive edge in leading the world market. This technological advancement has attracted the public's interest at the societal level and thus become very closely connected to every aspect of our lives. Thanks to such improvements, technology subjects make up more of the mandatory educational courses, consumers are given increased opportunities for acquiring technology, and information has become more accessible to the general public. All of this has contributed to building the foundation to keep public awareness at a high level and help nurture experts.

This also applies to the future direction that functional food needs to take. If consumers continue to feel deceived by being provided with information that lacks expertise and purposely omits information on the labels of products, especially when consumer confidence is spiraling downward, the market will regress and people will face a rapidly diminishing living standard. Therefore, the government should initiate more education for raising people's awareness and promote functional foods so that consumers can have more access to them and make proper purchasing decisions. This, in turn, will help to enhance consumer confidence.

At the same time, large conglomerates should invest in research and development to gain a competitive advantage in the world market so that they can make achievements—not in the already saturated industry, but rather in areas that hold the potential to realize the value of wellness going forward. For small-scale businesses it is also important to strive to establish solid and sensible scientific evidence for ideas and make intensive investments for enhancing R&D capacity, rather than merely for marketing. Under these conditions, good products will be given a fair chance to compete in the market and consumers can purchase the products in the market without worries. Additionally, the public can make sound purchasing decisions owing to their raised awareness of the products. Conditions should be established to respond to new trends by pioneering a new market, under which consumers want to catch two birds with one stone: maintain the effectiveness of food as well as maximize health and body maintenance.

22.4 Conclusion

Korean functional foods have been developed based on traditional Korean foods with known health benefits and bioactive compounds found by widely

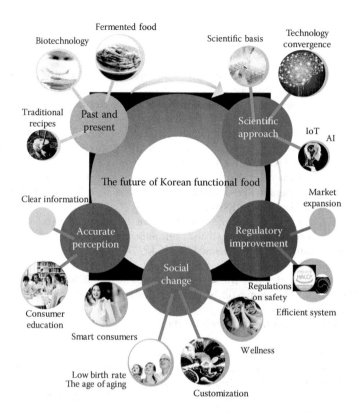

FIGURE 22.2
Prospects for the future of health functional food in Korea.

used scientific approaches. In the future, Korean functional foods should aim to adopt new technologies including the Internet of Things (IoT), artificial intelligence (AI), and new biotechnologies. The complex regulatory system is another barrier that must be overcome. It is also necessary to prepare countermeasures against rapidly changing social environments such as the aging population and the rise in income levels (Figure 22.2).

Acknowledgments

This work was supported by the Korea Institute of Planning and Evaluation for Technology in Food, Agriculture, Forestry and Fisheries (IPET) through the Agri-Bio Industry Technology Development Program (514004), funded by the Ministry of Agriculture, Food and Rural Affairs (MAFRA), Republic of Korea.

References

Consumerskorea. 2017. The consumer awareness survey on health functional foods. http://consumerskorea.org

Economic statistics system of the Bank of Korea. 2016. Annual indicators. https://ecos.bok.or.kr

Hong, K. H. 2007. The present and the future of personalized nutrigenomic foods: Applications of nutrigenomics and personal nutrition in food development. *Food Industry and Nutrition*. 12(2):37–43.

Jeong, K. C., S. K. Kim, S. H. Kim., and M. H. Lee. 2015. Status and challenges of genome -based personalized medicine. www.stepi.re.kr/module/publishDownFile.jsp?categCd=A0501&ntNo=181

Kim, J. Y. 2012. Current status and prospects for the domestic and international health functional food industries. Foundation of agri. tech. commercialization and transfer. http://yesme.kiom.re.kr/Trend/articles/view/tableid/tech/page/6/id/576/view_type/webzine

Korea Institute for Food Safety Management Accreditation. 2016. Analysis on trends of the size of the domestic health functional food market in 2015. http://www.haccpkorea.or.kr

Korea Institute for Health and Social Affairs. 2007. Study on quality of life for Koreans.

Korea Rural Economic Institute. www.krei.re.kr/

Ministry of Food and Drug Safety. 2016. Food and drug statistical yearbook, no.18. www.mfds.go.kr/index.do?mid=1571&pageNo=1&seq=24878&cmd=v

National Law Information Center. 2017. Functional Health Foods Act. www.law.go.kr/LSW/lsInfoP.do?lsiSeq=103971

Seo, J. H. 2008. Trends on technology of producing food ingredients with the use of microbial metabolic engineering. www.bioin.or.kr/board.do?bid=report&cmd=view&num=163696

Statistics Korea. 2015. Statistics for the elderly in 2015. http://kostat.go.kr/portal/eng/index.action

Index

A

Acetic acid bacteria, 221–222
Acetylcholinesterase (AChE), 489
Acid-hydrolyzed soy sauce (AHSS), 129
Activator protein-1 (AP-1), 273
AD, *see* Alzheimer's disease (AD)
Adenosine diphosphate (ADP), 197
Adenosine monophosphate (AMP), 197
Adenosine triphosphate (ATP), 184, 197
Aging population, 539–540
AHSS, *see* Acid-hydrolyzed soy sauce (AHSS)
AIDS, effects of Korean ginseng on, 252
Alcohol dehydrogenase (ADH), 221
Alcoholic beverages, *see* Korean alcoholic beverages (makgeolli/yakju)
Aldehyde dehydrogenase (ALDH), 221
Alginic acid, 368–369
Allergic hypersensitivity, perilla seeds and, 311–312
Allergic rhinitis (AR), 334
Allergy, jukyeom and, 333
Alzheimer's disease (AD), 487
AMPK, 487
Angiotensin-converting enzyme (ACE), 206, 453
Antioxidant effects
    of doenjang, 113–115
    of edible Korean seaweed, 372–374
    of garlic, 276
    of ginger, 271–272
    of jukyeom, 323–324
    of kanjang, 126–129
    of kimchi, 58–60
    of Korean ginseng, 240
    of namul, 404
    of red pepper, 263–264
    of sesame seed, 302
    of yakju, 454–455
Antioxidant response element (ARE), 271

Antiradical efficiency (AE), 128
Artificial intelligence (AI), 551

B

Bamboo salt, *see* Jukyeom (bamboo salt), health benefit effects of
Bapsang, 30–34
Bibimbap (balanced one-dish meal), 421–439
    background, 423–428
    community cuisine, 425
    convenience, 425
    geographical locations, varieties based on, 430
    health benefits, 430–433
    industrialization, 435
    metabolic diseases and, 494
    modernization and globalization, strategy for, 433–435
    mutual generation sequence, 426
    origin, 424–425
    philosophical background, 426–428
    provincial background, 428
    royal court food, 425
    sauces or condiments (jang), varieties based on, 430
    science of yin–yang and five elements theory, 430–431
    toppings, varieties based on, 429–430
    transitions in bibimbap's name, 428
    varieties and characteristics, 429–430
Bioengineering technology, 547
Bioflavonoid (quercetin), 404
Black pepper, 278
Blood flow, effects of makgeolli on, 452–453
Blood pressure, effect of namul on, 410
Blood vessel occlusion test, 478
Body mass index (BMI), 66
Brain health, perilla seeds and, 311

553

C

Cancer
- doenjang and, 115–120
- edible Korean seaweed and, 374–375
- garlic and, 277–278
- ginger and, 272–273
- jukyeom and, 325–327
- kanjang and, 129–132
- kimchi and, 60–65
- Korean ginseng and, 252
- makgeolli and, 450–452
- namul and, 406
- perilla seeds and, 312
- red pepper and, 266–268
- sesame seed and, 302
- yakju and, 455

Capsaicin, 173
- desensitization, 264
- receptor, 38, 263

Cardiovascular disease (CVD), 25
- doenjang and, 123–125
- namul and, 409

Carotenoids, 370–371, 396, 407

Carrageenans, 369

Caspases, 375

Chemical soy sauce, 128

Cheongkukjang, 145–164
- bioactive compounds, 154
- changes in soybean composition, 148–150
- clinical trials of, 495–496
- food composition, 148
- food processing, 147–148
- health benefits, 153, 160
- history, 145–147
- human research, 158–159
- isoflavone glucosides and aglycones, 155–156
- metabolite profiling, 151–153
- modernized, 147
- peptides and proteins, 156–157
- poly-γ-glutamic acid, 154–155
- polysaccharides and lipopeptides, 157
- vitamins K and B_{12}, 157–158
- whole food, cheongkukjang as, 158

Cheonilyeom (solar sea salt), beneficial effects of, 341–357

- effects on fermented foods, 349–353
- fermented seafood (jeotgal), 353
- fermented soybeans, 352
- fermented vegetables, 350–352
- health effects, 346–349
- immune system, activation of, 342–343
- mineral composition, 345–346
- mineral-rich salt, 342, 345
- new physiological roles, salt in, 342–343
- obesity control, 343
- oxidative stress, effect of heat-treated mineral-rich salt on, 347–348
- purified salt, 345
- reactive oxygen species formation, 348
- recent debate on salt restriction, 343–344
- recrystallized salt, 345
- rock salt, 344
- solar sea salt, 345
- types of salt, 344–345

Chito-oligosaccharide, 516

Chlorophyll, 407

Cholesterol
- garlic and, 275
- kimchi and, 92–93
- makgeolli and, 452

Cisplatin ototoxicity, prevention of, 334–335

Citrate lyase inhibitor, 515

Clinical trials, 463–504
- basics in functional foods, 465–466
- bibimbap and kimbap and metabolic diseases, 494
- blood vessel occlusion test, 478
- cases, 480–498
- challenge of customized nutrition, 470
- cheonggukjang, 495–496
- clinical study, 467–470
- Clinical Trial Center for Functional Foods, 479–480
- *Cordyceps sinensis*, 490–491
- crossover design, 470
- *Curcuma longa* (fermented), 483–484
- detection bias, 468
- doenjang, 496

Index 555

gochujang, 497–498
good clinical practice, 471
heart rate variability, 477–478
high-fat diet, 477
information bias, 468
intake of Korean foods and
generative function, 492
intervention study, 469
investigational new drug application,
476
Muju Gastrodiae rhizome, 487–490
NCD dietetic treatments, Korean
foods and, 492–494
noncommunicable diseases, 464
parallel design, 469–470
persimmon leaf extract, 485–486
pomegranate, 480–483
preclinical study, 466–467
preclinical study, pilot clinical study
for increasing success rate of,
478–479
randomization, 469
rice-oriented meals (mixed grains), 494
safety data, 475
selection bias, 468
strategy for developing healthy
functional foods, 474–476
stress loading methods, 476–478
study types, 466–470
successful development strategy,
476–479
traditional soy bean fermented
products, 495–498
understanding clinical study of
foods and procedures, 470–473
verification of clinical excellence in
Korean foods, 492–494
yuja, 485
Cognitive performance, effects of
Korean ginseng on, 251
Colon health, kimchi and, 55–58
Colony-forming units (CFUs), 350
Community cuisine, 425
Conjugated linoleic acid (CLA), 207
Coronary heart disease, perilla seeds
and, 310–311
CVD, *see* Cardiovascular disease (CVD)
Cytidine monophosphate (CMP), 197
Cytidine triphosphate (CTP), 197

D

Detection bias, 468
Diabetes
doenjang and, 126
edible Korean seaweed and,
377–378
garlic and, 275
Korean ginseng and, 250
namul and, 404–405
Dietary approaches to stop
hypertension (DASH) diet,
410
Dietary fiber, 397
Diethylnitrosamine (DEN), 271
Docosahexaenoic acid (DHA), 197, 207
Doenjang (soybean paste) and kanjang
(soybean sauce), health benefits
of, 101–144
anticancer effects of doenjang,
115–120
anticancer properties of kanjang,
129–132
antihypertension functions of
kanjang, 134
anti-inflammation functions of
kanjang, 133
antiobesity effects of doenjang,
120–123
antioxidative effects of doenjang,
113–115
antioxidative effects of kanjang,
126–129
chemical soy sauce, 128
diabetes, 126
doenjang, health benefit effects of,
113–126
history, 103–104
immune function, promotion of, 125
immunomodulation, 132–133
kanjang, functionality of, 126–134
kanjang polysaccharides, 132
miso, 103
modified commercial doenjang,
108–109
modified commercial kanjang,
109–110
nutritional and functional
components, 110–113

Index

prevention of cardiovascular
diseases, 123–125
probiotic function of *Bac. subtilis*,
125–126
processing methods and
microorganisms used in
fermentation, 104–110
traditional doenjang and kanjang,
105–108
Doxorubicin (DOX), 273

E

Eastern medicine, 14–16
Eicosapentaenoic acid (EPA), 197, 207
Endoplasmic reticulum (ER) stress, 349
Evidence-based evaluation, 534

F

Fasting blood glucose (FBG), 71
Fatty acid synthase (FAS), 175, 332
Fermented fish, *see* Jeotgal (fermented
fish) (secret of Korean
seasonings)
Fermented sesame sauce (FseS), 129
Fermented soy sauce (FSS), 129
Five elements theory, 430–431
Five Phases theory, 11–12
Folic acid, 408
Fourth Industrial Revolution,
development of functional
foods in the era of, 548
French paradox, 25
Fructo-oligosaccharide, 512
Fucoidans, 367–368
Functional food industry (processing
and sanitation), 505–521
background and history, 505–506
chito-oligosaccharide, 516
fructo-oligosaccharide, 512
functional food processing, 511–519
function assessment, 509–511
function claims, 510
health claims, 510
hen comb, extract of, 514
nutrition claims, 509
pathogen elimination, 519
raw materials, 506–508

safety assessment, 508–509
sanitation, 518–519
standardization of ingredients, 508
Future of functional foods in Korea,
539–552
aging population, 539–540
change in demand for functional
foods, 539–541
Fourth Industrial Revolution,
development of functional
foods in the era of, 548
globalization, sixth industrialization
of functional food under, 549
limitations on functional foods,
541–544
nanotechnology, 547
personal needs, functional foods
catering to, 540–541
public perception of health
functional food, 543–544
quality of life due to increased
income, 540
raising proper awareness of
functional food, 549–550
regulations on functional foods,
541–543
scientific approach, development
of functional foods through,
544–546
scientific convergence, development
of functional foods through,
546–547
social changes, functional foods
bracing for, 548–549

G

Garlic, 273–278
antidiabetic effect, 275
antihypertensive and cholesterol-
lowering effects, 275
antioxidant effects, 276
cancer preventive and anticancer
effects, 277–278
cardioprotective effect, 274
immune boosting effects, 276
xenobiotic toxicity, protective effects
against, 277
Gas chromatography (GC), 351

Index

Gastric adenocarcinoma cells (AGS), 352
Ginger, 269–273
    analgesic effects, 271
    antiemetic effects, 270
    antioxidant effects, 271–272
    chemopreventive and
        anticarcinogenic effects, 272–273
Ginseng, *see* Korean ginseng
        (composition, processing, and
        health benefits)
Globalization, sixth industrialization of
        functional food under, 549
Glucose tolerance test (GTT), 485
Glucose transporter type 4 (GLUT4), 349
Glutathione (GSH), 448
Glutathione peroxidase (GSH-Px), 129
Glutathione S-transferase (GST), 448
GMP, *see* Guanosine monophosphate
        (GMP)
Gochujang, clinical trials of, 497–498
Good clinical practice (GCP), 471, 510
Good laboratory practice (GLP), 509
Good manufacturing practice (GMP),
        519
Gross national income (GNI), 540
GTT, *see* Glucose tolerance test (GTT)
Guanosine monophosphate (GMP), 112

H

Hangover reduction, effects of Korean
        ginseng on, 252
Hazard analysis and critical control
        points (HACCP) management,
        519
Health/Functional Food Act (HFFA),
        524
Health/functional foods (HFFs), 524
    advertisement for, 537
    generic functional ingredients,
        529–530
    ingredients for, 526–531
    nutrients, 527–528
    product-specific functional
        ingredients, 531
    public perception of, 543–544
Heart rate variability (HRV), 477–478
Hen comb, extract of, 514
Hepatic damage, prevention of, 336

High-density lipoprotein (HDL), 66
High-density lipoprotein cholesterol
        (HDL-C), 481
High-fat diet (HFD), 377, 477
History, culture, and characteristics of
        Korean foods, 1–21
    dietary changes during the last
        century, 9–10
    Eastern medicine and Sasang
        typology, 14–16
    future of Korean functional food,
        16–19
    health concept of Korean functional
        food, 10–16
    historic age, 8–9
    history of Korean dietary culture,
        1–10
    Neolithic age and the era of myth,
        5–8
    Paleolithic age, 2–3
    Primitive Pottery Age, 4
    Taoism, 10–11
    traditional Chinese medicine, 13–14
    yin and yang and Five Phases theory,
        11–12
Human immunodeficiency virus (HIV),
        252
Human mast cell line (HMC), 207
Hwaju, 443
Hydroxy citric acid (HCA), 515
Hyperlipidemia, effects of Korean
        ginseng on, 250
Hypertension
    garlic and, 275
    jukyeom and, 334
    kanjang and, 134
Hypoxanthine (Hx), 184, 197

I

IFG, *see* Impaired fasting glucose (IFG)
Immune function
    doenjang and, 125
    garlic and, 276
    high salt intake and, 342–343
    jukyeom and, 332–333
    Korean ginseng and, 247–248
    namul and, 405–406
    sesame seed and, 302

558   *Index*

IMP, *see* Inosine monophosphate (IMP)
Impaired fasting glucose (IFG), 485
Information bias, 468
Inosine monophosphate (IMP), 112, 197
Institutional Review Board (IRB), 471, 475
Internet of Things (IoT), 551
Investigational new drug (IND) application, 476

J

Jang, 184
Jeotgal (fermented fish) (secret of Korean seasonings), 183–215
   amino acids, 196–197
   classification by main ingredients, 188–189
   classification by seasoning, 189–191
   composition, 195–205
   fatty acids, 197–199
   fermentation, microbial community during, 200–204
   flavor compounds, 199
   health benefits, 205–208
   history, 185–187
   jang, 184
   microbial ecology, 199–205
   microflora, 199–200
   microorganisms, 204–205
   nucleotides, 197
   regional jeotgals, 192–194
   volatile basic nitrogen, 204
Jinchae, 386
Jukyeom (bamboo salt), health benefit effects of, 319–340
   allergic rhinitis, 334
   allergy, 333
   anticancer activity, 325–327
   antimicrobial activity, 336
   antioxidative activity, 323–324
   atopy, 334
   cisplatin ototoxicity, prevention of, 334–335
   composition, 322–323
   enamel remineralization by dentifrice, 336
   functionality, 323–336

   hepatic damage, prevention of, 336
   history, 319–320
   hypertension, 334
   immunity, 332–333
   inflammation, 336
   obesity, 329–332
   processing, 320

K

Kanjang (soybean sauce), *see* Doenjang (soybean paste) and kanjang (soybean sauce), health benefits of
Kanjang polysaccharides, 132
K-diet, *see* Korean diets and their tastes
Kimbap, metabolic diseases and, 494
Kimchi, lactic acid bacteria in, 79–100
   allergic alleviatory effects, 91–92
   antifungal activities, 80–83
   anti-*Helicobacter pylori* effects, 85
   anti-inflammatory effects, 91
   antimicrobial activities, 80–85
   antimutagenic and anticancer effects, 85–88
   antiobesity and cholesterol- and lipid-lowering effects, 92–93
   bacteriocin production, 83–84
   degradation of NO_2 and insecticide, 93–94
   immunomodulatory effects, 88–90
   miscellaneous physiological functions, 94–95
Kimchi and its health benefits, 43–77
   antiobesity effect, 66–69
   antioxidative and antiaging effects, 58–60
   cancer preventive effects, 60–65
   classification, 47–48
   colon health, improvement of, 55–58
   fermentation and LAB, 51–54
   functionalities, 54–72
   history, 44–47
   hypolipidemic effect and control of metabolic syndrome, 69–72
   lactic acid bacteria, 43
   processing and recipes, 49–51
   raw ingredients, 49

Index

Kochujang (red pepper paste), biological functions and traditional therapeutic uses of, 165–181
  biological functions, 172–178
  functionality of kochujang, 174–178
  functionality of red pepper and capsaicin, 173–174
  history and tradition, 166–169
  medicinal effects written in literature, 172
  nutritional and functional components, 173
  nutritional and functional effects, 172–178
  production methods, 169–172
Korea Citation Index (KCI), 475
Korea Health Supplement Association (KHSA), 537
Korean alcoholic beverages (makgeolli/yakju), 441–461
  anticancer effects, 450–452, 455
  anticarcinogenic effects, 455
  antioxidant effect, 454–455
  bioactive compounds 2,6-dimethoxy-1,4-benzoquinone, 449
  characteristics and categories, 443
  cholesterol and activities of hepatic oxygen free radical metabolizing enzymes, 446–449
  cholesterol-lowering effect, 452
  cytotoxic and anti-inflammatory activity, 446
  fermentation agent (nuruk), 444
  fibrinolytic activity, 455–456
  history, 442–443
  improved blood flow effect, 452–453
  improvement of liver function, 452
  inhibiting hypertension (ACE-inhibiting effect), 453
  lactic acid bacteria, 450
  liver protection, 457
  Maillard reaction, 454
  makgeolli, composition of, 449–450
  makgeolli, functionality of, 450–453
  manufacturing method, 443–444
  nuruk, composition of, 445–446
  nuruk, functionality of, 446–449

  removing reactive oxygen species (antioxidant effect), 453
  yakju, composition of, 454
  yakju, functionality of, 454–457
Korean diets and their tastes, 23–42
  characteristics, 27–30
  definition, 26–27
  French paradox, 25
  healthy diet, K-diet as, 25
  Korean diet (K-diet), 23–24
  origin of siwonhada, 36–37
  siwonhan-mat (determining factors of), 39
  siwonhan-mat (third taste of Korean foods), 34–36
  siwonhan-mat (understanding from linguistic and literary approaches, 36–39
  siwonhan-mat (understanding from scientific approach), 37–39
  structure of bapsang and representative k-diet, 30–34
  third taste, 36
Korean ginseng (composition, processing, and health benefits), 233–256
  antiaging effect, 248
  anticarcinogenic and cancer-preventive effects, 252
  antidiabetic effect, 250
  antifatigue and antistress effects, 248
  antiobesity and antihyperlipidemia effects, 250
  antioxidant components, 240
  antioxidative stress effect, 248
  antiviral and anti-AIDS effects, 252
  Arg-Fru-Glc, 240
  blood circulation improvement and lowered blood pressure, effects of, 250–251
  category, 234–235
  cognitive performance, enhancement of, 251
  comparison of ginsenosides of Korean ginseng and foreign ginsengs, 240–241
  cultivation history, 235–236
  cultivation technology and shape, 236–237

excellence of Korean ginseng, 243–244

functional effects proved by modern science, 247–252

functional ingredients, 237–243

ginsenosides, 237–239

hangover reduction effect, 252

history, 234–235

immune function, enhancement of, 247–248

maltol, 240

manufacturing method, ginsenosides, and functionality of Korean black ginseng, 243

naming, 235

polyacetylenes, 239

polysaccharides, 239

processed products, 246–247

production and ginsenosides of Korean red ginseng, 241–242

sexual performance, enhancement of, 251

traditional herbal prescriptions, Korean ginseng in, 244–246

Korean paradox, 25

Korean seaweed (edible), 359–384

alginic acid, 368–369

anticancer properties, 374–375

antidiabetic and antiobese properties, 377–378

anti-inflammation properties, 375–377

antioxidant properties, 372–374

bioactive compounds, 367–372

carotenoids, 370–371

carrageenans, 369

caspases, 375

description of seaweed, 361–363

edible brown seaweed, 365–366

edible green seaweed, 364–365

edible red seaweed, 365

fucoidans, 367–368

laminarin, 368

polyphenols, 370

polysaccharides, 367–370

potential bioactive properties as functional ingredients, 372–378

sterols, 372

traditional Korean foods from seaweed, 363–366

ulvan, 370

L

Lactic acid bacteria (LAB), 43, 350, 450, *see also* Kimchi, lactic acid bacteria in

Laminarin, 368

Lipid metabolism, effects of sesame seed on, 301

Lipopolysaccharides (LPS), 376

Liquid chromatography (LC), 351

Liver function, effects of makgeolli on, 452

Low density lipoprotein (LDL), 66, 302

Low-density lipoprotein cholesterol (LDL-C), 175, 481, 495

LPS, *see* Lipopolysaccharides (LPS)

Lutein, 404

M

Maillard reaction, 454

Makgeolli, *see also* Korean alcoholic beverages (makgeolli/yakju)

anticancer effects, 450–452

cholesterol-lowering effect, 452

composition of, 449–450

functionality of, 450–453

improved blood flow effect, 452–453

improvement of liver function, 452

inhibiting hypertension (ACE-inhibiting effect), 453

lactic acid bacteria, 450

removing reactive oxygen species (antioxidant effect), 453

Maltol, 240

MAPK, *see* Mitogen-activated protein kinases (MAPK)

Mass spectrometry (MS), 351

Memory improvement, rice-oriented meals and, 494

Metabolic syndrome, kimchi and, 69–72

Microsomal triglyceride transfer protein (MTP), 332

Mineral-rich salt (MRS), 342, 345

Ministry of Food and Drug Safety (MFDS), 465, 474, 524, 541
Miso, 103
Mitochondrial dysfunction (MD), 349
Mitogen-activated protein kinases (MAPK), 376
MRS, *see* Mineral-rich salt (MRS)
Muju Gastrodiae rhizome, clinical trials of, 487–490
Mustard, 278–279
Myulchikinase (MK), 207

N

Namul (Korean vegetable dish), 386–419
    anticancer effects, 406
    antidiabetic effects, 404–405
    antioxidative effects, 404
    bioflavonoid (quercetin), 404
    blood pressure, 410
    cardiovascular disease, 409
    carotenoids, 396, 407
    chlorophyll, 407
    classification of edible vegetables, 391
    dietary fiber, 397, 408–409
    folic acid, 408
    food composition, 394–397
    health benefits, 397–410
    history, 387–388
    immunoenhancing effects, 405–406
    lutein and zeaxanthin, 404
    meaning of namul, 389
    minerals, 396
    preparation, 389–394
    preparation of namul dishes, 391–394
    sulforaphane, 408
    total antioxidant capacity, 396
    vitamin K, 396
    water-soluble vitamins, 395–396
Nanotechnology (NT), 547
Natural killer (NK) cells, 408
Nausea and vomiting in early pregnancy (NVEP), 270
NCD dietetic treatments, Korean foods and, 492–494
Nicotinamide adenine dinucleotide (NAD), 221
Noncommunicable diseases (NCD), 464
NT, *see* Nanotechnology (NT)

Nuclear magnetic resonance (NMR), 351
Nuruk, *see* Korean alcoholic beverages (makgeolli/yakju)
Nutrient reference value (NRV), 527

O

Obesity
    capsaicin and, 173
    doenjang and, 120–123
    edible Korean seaweed and, 377–378
    high salt intake and, 343
    jukyeom and, 329–332
    kimchi and, 66–69, 92–93
    kochujang and, 175
    Korean ginseng and, 250
    red pepper and, 265
One-dish meal, *see* Bibimbap (balanced one-dish meal)
Optimal Macronutrient Intake Trial for Heart Health (OmniHeart), 410
Oral glucose tolerance test (OGTT), 485
Osteoarthritis (OA), 271
Oxidative fermentation, 221
Oxidative stresses, excessive, 477

P

Painful diabetic neuropathy (PDN), 264
Pain relief
    ginger and, 271
    red pepper and, 264–265
Perilla seeds and perilla seed oil, 303–312
    adverse effects, 312
    anticarcinogenic activity, 312
    fatty acid composition, 305–306
    health-promoting minor components, 306–308
    health-related functionality, 310–312
    improvement of brain health, 311
    leaves, seed, and seed oil in cuisine, 303–305
    nutty flavors of roasted oil, 309
    oxidative stability, 309–310
    reduction of allergic hypersensitivity, 311–312
    reduction of risk for coronary heart disease, 310–311

562   *Index*

Peroxisome proliferator-activated
receptor gamma (PPARγ), 175
Persimmon leaf extract, clinical trials of,
485–486
Personal needs, functional foods
catering to, 540–541
Phosphorylated AMPK (PAMPK), 273
Polyphenols, 370
Polysaccharides, 367–370
alginic acid, 368–369
carrageenans, 369
fucoidans, 367–368
laminarin, 368
ulvan, 370
Polyunsaturated fatty acid (PUFA), 197,
207, 302
Pomegranate, clinical trials of, 480–483
Postprandial plasma glucose (PPG), 485
Prostaglandins, 302
Protopanaxadiol (PPD), 238
Protopanaxatriol (PPT), 238
Purified salt, 345

Q

Quality of life, 264, 271, 540
Quercetin, 404

R

Reactive oxygen species (ROS), 94, 348,
453
Ready to eat (RTE) functional food, 518
Recommended daily allowance (RDA),
535
Recrystallized salt, 345
Red ginseng acidic polysaccharide
(RGAP), 239
Red pepper, 263–269
anti-inflammatory and antiallergic
effects, 264
antiobesity effects, 265
antioxidant effects, 263–264
cancer chemopreventive and
therapeutic effects, 266–268
cardioprotective effects, 268–269
gastroprotective effects, 266
neuroprotective effects, 266
pain-relieving effects, 264–265

paste, *see* Kochujang (red pepper
paste), biological functions
and traditional therapeutic
uses of
powder (RPP), 46
Regulations of Korean functional foods,
523–538, 541–543
advertisement for HFFs, 537
bioactive function claims, 535–536
efficacy evaluation, 534–535
evaluation process, 531
functional ingredient/product
approval, 531–535
health claims, 535–536
Health/Functional Food Act and
its subordinate regulation,
524–526
ingredients for HFFs, 526–531
management for manufacturer, 537
nutrient function claims, 535
postmarket surveillance, 537
reduction of disease risk claims, 536
safety evaluation, 533–534
specification evaluation, 535
standardization, 531–532
Rock salt, 344
ROS, *see* Reactive oxygen species (ROS)
Royal court food, 425
RPP, *see* Red pepper powder (RPP)

S

Salt, *see* Cheonilyeom (solar sea salt),
beneficial effects of
Sasang typology, 14–16
Science Citation Index (SCI), 475, 518
Scientific approach, development of
functional foods through,
544–546
Scientific convergence, development
of functional foods through,
546–547
Seasonings, *see* Jeotgal (fermented fish)
(secret of Korean seasonings)
Seaweed, *see* Korean seaweed (edible)
Seed oil, *see* Perilla seeds and perilla
seed oil; Sesame seed and
sesame seed oil
Selection bias, 468

Index

Sesame seed and sesame seed oil, 292–302
    antihypertensive, anticancer effects, and blood sugar regulation, 302
    antioxidant properties and immunomodulating effects, 302
    chemical composition, 297
    cultivation, 296
    effects on lipid metabolism, 301
    history as food ingredients, 293–294
    history of harvesting, 292–293
    importance, 292–296
    processing, 297–301
    recipes, 294
Sexual performance, effects of Korean ginseng on, 251
Sikcho (Korean vinegar), 217–232
    acetic acid bacteria, 221–222
    history of vinegar fermentation, 217–219
    major constituents, 224–226
    oxidative fermentation, 221
    physiological functions, 226–228
    production, 219–220
    varieties, 222–224
Single nucleotide polymorphisms (SNPs), 17
Siwonhan-mat
    determining factors of, 39
    third taste of Korean foods, 34–36
    understanding from linguistic and literary approaches, 36–39
    understanding from scientific approach, 37–39
SNPs, *see* Single nucleotide polymorphisms (SNPs)
Social changes, functional foods bracing for, 548–549
Solar sea salt, *see* Cheonilyeom (solar sea salt), beneficial effects of
Sonodynamic therapy, 273
Soybean sauce, *see* Doenjang (soybean paste) and kanjang (soybean sauce), health benefits of
Spices, *see* Yangnyeom (spices) and health benefits
Sterol-regulatory element-binding protein 1c (SREBP-1c), 175
Sterols, 372
Sulforaphane, 408

T

TEWL, *see* Transepidermal water loss (TEWL)
TG, *see* Triglyceride (TG)
Thiobarbituric acid-reactive substances (TBARS), 159
Third taste, 36
Total antioxidant capacity (TAC), 396
Total antioxidant status (TAS), 71
Total cholesterol (TC), 66, 481, 495
Total dietary fiber (TDF), 397
Traditional Chinese medicine (TCM), 13–14
Traditional kanjang-derived polysaccharides (TKP), 132
Transepidermal water loss (TEWL), 482
Transient receptor potential cation channel subfamily V member 1 (TRPV1), 173, 263
Tricarboxylic acid (TCA), 221
Triglyceride (TG), 66, 483, 495
Tumor necrosis factor alpha (TNF-α), 376, 490

U

Ulvan, 370
Uncoupling protein 2 (UCP2), 174

V

Vanilloid receptor 1, 263
Vascular occlusion, 478
Vinegar, *see* Sikcho (Korean vinegar)
Vitamin K, 396
Volatile basic nitrogen (VBN), 204

W

Waist–hip ratio (WHR), 70, 176
Water-soluble vitamins, 395–396
Whole food, cheongkukjang as, 158

Y

Yakju, *see also* Korean alcoholic beverages (makgeolli/yakju)
    anticancer effects, 455
    anticarcinogenic effects, 455

antioxidant effect, 454–455
composition of, 454
fibrinolytic activity, 455–456
functionality of, 454–457
liver protection, 457
Yangnyeom (spices) and health benefits, 257–290
active substances, 260
black pepper, 278
disease prevention and other beneficial health effects, 263–278
garlic, 273–278
ginger, 269–273
history, 258
mustard, 278–279
nutritional composition, 258
red pepper, 263–269
sesame seed and oil, 279–280
sonodynamic therapy, 273
Yin–yang, 11–12, 430–431
Yuja, clinical trials of, 485

Z

Zeaxanthin, 404
Zidovudine (ZDV), 252